# Biomaterial Engineering

**Series Editor**

Youqing Shen, Zhejiang Key Laboratory of Smart BioMaterials and Center for Bionanoengineering, and Key Laboratory of Biomass Chemical Engineering of the Ministry of Education, College of Chemical and Biological Engineering, Zhejiang University, Hangzhou, China

The aim of this work is as a complete reference for researchers, engineers and graduate students who are engaged in R&D of biomaterials. The book facilitates the newcomers to grasp the most updated status in all the related topics in biomaterial's fields with a comprehensive, self-contained, and authoritative knowledge. The unique feature of the book will be the combination of a collection of standard/ advanced experimental protocols in preparing and fabricating biomaterials and related bioassays. This book is a step-by-step guide for new comers, who may not be equipped with appropriate hands-on laboratory skills and experiences, to follow and repeat those important works in the field. This style is particularly important in this interdisciplinary field. This reference work comprises 10 volumes and covers the most popular topics of biomaterials from drug delivery to gene and protein delivery, from biomedical biodetection to diagnosis, from cardiovascular diseases to tissue engineering. The content is created by the leading scientists in the each field and will evolve constantly, thus it presents both high -quality and up-to-date scientific and technical information.

More information about this series at https://link.springer.com/bookseries/13484

Huayu Tian • Xuesi Chen
Editors

# Gene Delivery

With 233 Figures and 9 Tables

Springer

*Editors*
Huayu Tian
Changchun Institute of Applied Chemistry
Chinese Academy of Sciences
Changchun, China

Xuesi Chen
Changchun Institute of Applied Chemistry
Chinese Academy of Sciences
Changchun, China

ISSN 2523-8809 ISSN 2523-8817 (electronic)
ISBN 978-981-16-5418-3 ISBN 978-981-16-5419-0 (eBook)
ISBN 978-981-16-5420-6 (print and electronic bundle)
https://doi.org/10.1007/978-981-16-5419-0



This Springer imprint is published by the registered company Springer Nature Singapore Pte Ltd.
The registered company address is: 152 Beach Road, #21-01/04 Gateway East, Singapore 189721, Singapore

# Series Preface

The use of human body compatible materials for medical diagnosis, treatment, and surgery is always critical in enhancing life-saving therapies and quality of life of patients. With the massive research efforts in this field in both universities and industries, there is a continuous growth in our knowledge/technique in design and use of such biomaterials to effectively deliver specific therapeutics, including DNA, protein, and contrast reagents, to the targeted cells and organs for treatment or diagnosis; to repair or replace tissues; or even to construct artificial organs like cartilages, bones, and skins to regain the body functions. The inherent interdisciplinary nature of biomaterials makes researchers often use methods to prepare a wide range of materials and various bioassays to evaluate their diverse bio-related properties. However, it is generally very difficult to find and tell reliable sources and detailed know-how for the needed methods and protocols, which are buried in the vast literature and only described in general lack of details. One still has to find the best by trial and error.

The aim of this series is to provide a complete reference for researchers, engineers, and graduate students who are engaged in R&D of biomaterials. It provides newcomers the fundamental concepts and overall status of the areas they work on and provides researchers comprehensive, in-depth, and authoritative information including preparation/fabrication protocols of most biomaterials and bioassay protocols as well as a wide variety of advanced experimental methods used in practice, numerous examples, and practical applications.

This reference work, tentatively composed of 10 volumes, covers the most popular topics of biomaterials, from drug delivery to gene and protein delivery, from biomedical biodetection to diagnosis, from cardiovascular diseases to tissue engineering. The content is created by leading scientists in each field and will evolve constantly, thus it presents both high-quality and up-to-date scientific and technical information.

June, 2021 Youqing Shen

# Volume Preface

Gene therapy has been regarded as a great potential for specific treatment of gene-related human diseases, such as cancer, and genetic and epidemic diseases. Gene therapy refers to the biomedical technology that inserts normal or therapeutic exogenous genes into target cells to repair or replace defective genes in target cells, so as to achieve the purpose of treating diseases. With the rapid development of biotechnology, the design of therapeutic genes and their expression regulation technology have made rapid progress, such as CAR-T therapy, gene silencing, mRNA vaccine, and gene editing technology. However, naked genes are difficult to be endocytosed by target cells to achieve their therapeutic effects due to nuclease degradation and elimination by immune systems. Therefore, efficient gene delivery systems have the crucial role of successful implementation of gene therapy.

This book mainly describes the protocols for fabrication of non-viral delivery systems, including inorganic, cationic lipid, polyethylenimine, and polypeptide-based carriers. It unearths the detailed preparation methods of various gene delivery systems or newly synthesized materials. Furthermore, the construction and characterization of several gene and drug co-delivery systems are summarized in detail. Overall, this book provides a platform for young scholars and students to systematically understand the preparation and characterization of the existing gene delivery systems, as well as providing a technology platform for clinical gene therapy.

However, gene therapy is still in the stage of exploration, and there are still many obstacles and challenges, including safety risks, ethical issues, lack of clinical data, immune rejection of the body, expensive treatment costs, and so on. We anticipate that gene therapy will be a routine treatment for major human diseases in the near future.

We would like to express our sincere gratitude to all the authors of each chapter for their contributions to the book and for the effort and time they put into the writing process. Thanks to the reviewers for their efforts to improve the scientificity and rationality for this book. In addition, we wish to thank Professor Youqing Shen, Dr. Jie Chen, Dr. Jacob Arun Raj. Z, Dr. Mengchu Huang, and Dr. Haiqin Dong, for their help in organizing this book.

# Contents

# About the Series Editor

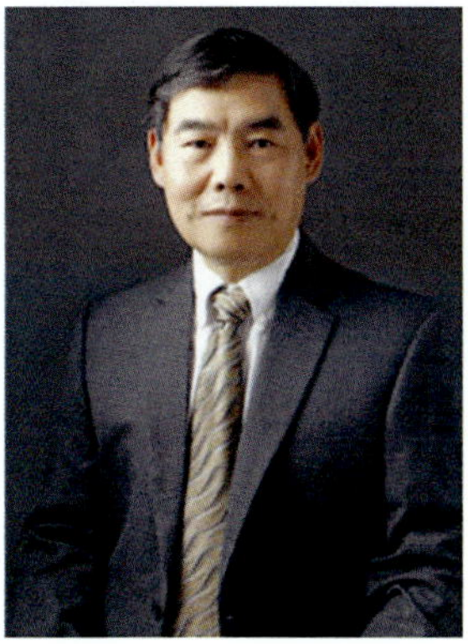

**Youqing Shen**
College of Chemical and Biological Engineering
Zhejiang University
Hangzhou, China

Prof. Youqing Shen is a national Changjiang scholar chair professor in the College of Chemical and Biological Engineering and Deputy Dean of the Faculty of Engineering at Zhejiang University, China, and a fellow of the American Institute of Medical and Biological Engineering (AIMBE). He received his B.Sc. and Dr. Sc. degrees from Zhejiang University and Ph.D. Eng. degree from McMaster University in 2002. After working shortly at Akzo Nobel Canada, he joined the Department of Chemical Engineering at the University of Wyoming, Laramie, Wyoming, USA, as an assistant professor in 2002 and then was early promoted to tenured associate professor in 2007. In 2008, he moved back to Zhejiang University as a Qiushi chair professor and director of the Center for Bionanoengineering. His research, funded by the US and Chinese funding agencies, focuses on designing and synthesizing stimulusresponsive polymers as functional excipients for drug and gene nanomedicines. He has (co-)authored over 300 peer-reviewed articles and edited two books published by RSC and Wiley. Elsevier Scopus has listed him as a "Most Cited Chinese Scholar" in material science since 2014. He has received a number of awards, including the Distinguished Young Investigator Award from China National Natural Science Foundation and the Leading Young Innovator award from the Chinese Ministry of Science and Technology. He serves as editor-in-chief of Biomaterials Engineering, a Springer Nature book series, an associate editor for the American Chemical Society journal *Industrial Engineering Chemistry Research*, and an executive editor for Elsevier journal Advanced *Drug Delivery Review*. He is also vice chair of the nanomedicine committee in the Chinese Pharmaceutical Association and China Medicinal Biotechnology Association.

# About the Volume Editors

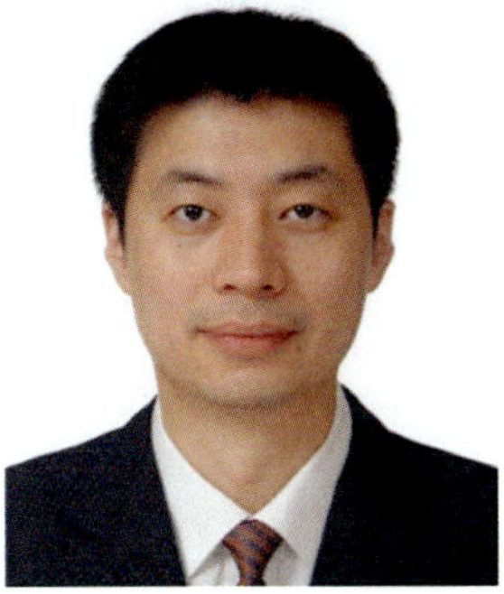

**Huayu Tian** Prof. Tian is currently a professor at Changchun Institute of Applied Chemistry, Chinese Academy of Sciences, Jilin, China.

Prof. Tian was born in 1977 in Nanyang, China. He obtained his bachelor's (1998) and master's (2000) degrees from Harbin Institute of Technology, and PhD degree from Changchun Institute of Applied Chemistry (CIAC), Chinese Academy of Sciences (CAS), in 2006 (supervised by Prof. Xuesi Chen). From 2006 to 2012, he worked at Changchun Institute of Applied Chemistry as an assistant professor and associate professor. He was a visiting scholar at the University of Utah from 2009 to 2010. Prof. Tian was appointed as a full professor at Changchun Institute of Applied Chemistry in 2012.

In 2014, he was supported by the National Program for Support of Top-Notch Young Professionals. In 2019, he was supported by the National Science Fund for Distinguished Young Scholars of China.

Prof. Tian's research interests include design and synthesis of biomedical polymer materials, polymeric gene/drug intelligent delivery systems, polymeric nanocarriers for nucleic acid diagnosis and therapy, polymeric nanocarriers for tumor immunotherapy, and development of materials for bio-manufacturing. He has published more than 160 peer-reviewed scientific articles and holds more than 50 China invention patents. Currently, he is the deputy general secretary of the Biomedical Polymer Materials Branch of the Chinese Society of Biomaterials and chairman of the Jilin Provincial Testing Society.

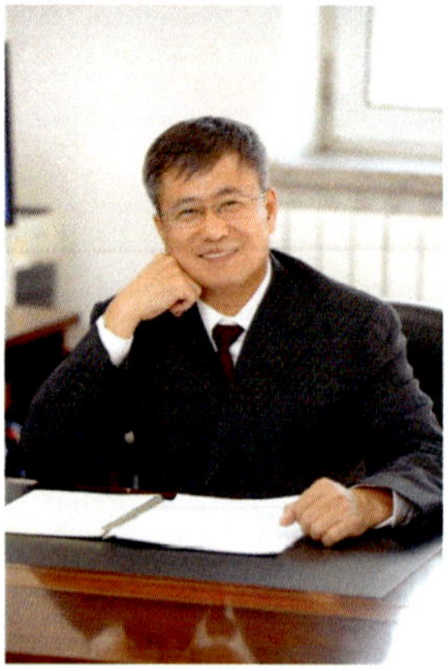

**Xuesi Chen** Prof. Chen is currently a professor at Changchun Institute of Applied Chemistry, CAS, Jilin, China.

Prof. Chen was born in 1959 in Changchun, China. He obtained his bachelor's degree from the Department of Chemistry at Jilin University in 1982; master's degree from Changchun Institute of Applied Chemistry (CIAC), Chinese Academy of Sciences (CAS), in 1988; and doctoral degree from Waseda University in 1997 (supervised by Hiroyuki Nishide). After postdoctoral study at the University of Pennsylvania, he joined the faculty at CIAC as a professor in 1999.

In 2009, he was made the vice director of the academic committee of Key Laboratory of Polymer Ecomaterials, CAS. In 2004, he was supported by the National Science Fund for Distinguished Young Scholars of China. In 2012, he was made the vice director of the academic committee of CIAC, CAS. In 2013, he was the recipient of the "Ten-thousand Talents Program" and the Science and Technology Innovation and Entrepreneurship Talents. In 2016, he was elected to be the Fellow of Biomaterials Science and Engineering. In 2019, he was elected to be the academician of the Chinese Academy of Sciences.

Prof. Chen's research interests include synthesis of Schiff base catalysts for ring-opening polymerization of lactides, preparation of biodegradable polymers for biomedical applications such as bone fracture repair, drug and gene carriers, hydrogels, and industrialization of polylactide (PLA) as green plastics. He has authored or co-authored more than 800 papers with an H-index of 99 (total citations more than 37,000 times). He is also the holder or coholder of more than 310 Chinese invention patents and 1 US-authorized patent. Currently, Prof. Chen is board member of *Advanced Healthcare Materials*, the *Journal of the Controlled Release*, *Biomacromolecules*, and *Acta Biomaterialia*, among others.

# Contributors

**Lintao Cai** Guangdong Key Laboratory of Nanomedicine, CAS-HK Joint Lab for Biomaterials, Shenzhen Engineering Laboratory of Nanomedicine and Nanoformulations, Shenzhen Institute of Advanced Technology (SIAT), Chinese Academy of Sciences, Shenzhen, China

**Xiaobing Chen** National Engineering Research Center for Biomaterials, College of Biomedical Engineering, Sichuan University, Qingyang, Chengdu, Sichuan, P.R. China

**Siqin Chen** Zhejiang Key Laboratory of Smart BioMaterials and Center for Bionanoengineering, and Key Laboratory of Biomass Chemical Engineering of the Ministry of Education, College of Chemical and Biological Engineering, Zhejiang University, Hangzhou, China

**Xuesi Chen** Key Laboratory of Polymer Ecomaterials, Changchun Institute of Applied Chemistry, Chinese Academy of Sciences, Changchun, China

**Du Cheng** School of Materials Science and Engineering, Sun Yat-sen University, Guangzhou, China

**Liang Cheng** Biomedical Polymers Laboratory, College of Chemistry, Chemical Engineering and Materials Science, and State Key Laboratory of Radiation Medicine and Protection, Soochow University, Suzhou, People's Republic of China

**Yilong Cheng** School of Chemistry, Xi'an Jiaotong University, Xi'an, Shaanxi, China

**Anjie Dong** Department of Polymer Science and Technology, School of Chemical Engineering and Technology, Key Laboratory of Systems Bioengineering of the Ministry of Education, Tianjin University, Tianjin, China

**Huapan Fang** Institute of Functional Nano and Soft Materials (FUNSOM), Jiangsu Key Laboratory for Carbon-Based Functional Materials & Devices, Soochow University, Suzhou, Jiangsu, China

**Jun Feng** Key Laboratory of Biomedical Polymers of Ministry of Education, Department of Chemistry, Wuhan University, Wuhan, P. R. China

**Chenglong Ge** Jiangsu Key Laboratory for Carbon-Based Functional Materials and Devices, Institute of Functional Nano & Soft Materials (FUNSOM), Collaborative Innovation Center of Suzhou Nano Science & Technology, Soochow University, Suzhou, China

**Zhongwei Gu** Research Institute for Biomaterials, Tech Institute for Advanced Materials, College of Materials Science and Engineering, Suqian Advanced Materials Industry Technology Innovation Center, Jiangsu Collaborative Innovation Center for Advanced Inorganic Function Composites, Nanjing Tech University, Nanjing, People's Republic of China

Huaxi MR Research Center (HMRRC), Department of Radiology, Functional and Molecular Imaging Key Laboratory of Sichuan Province, West China Hospital, Sichuan University, Chengdu, People's Republic of China

**Xiuwen Guan** College of Pharmacy, Weifang Medical University, Weifang, China

**Tianying Guo** College of Chemistry, Nankai University, Tianjin, China

**Yiyan He** Research Institute for Biomaterials, Tech Institute for Advanced Materials, College of Materials Science and Engineering, Suqian Advanced Materials Industry Technology Innovation Center, Jiangsu Collaborative Innovation Center for Advanced Inorganic Function Composites, Nanjing Tech University, Nanjing, People's Republic of China

**Jinlin He** College of Chemistry, Chemical Engineering and Materials Science, State and Local Joint Engineering Laboratory for Novel Functional Polymeric Materials, Jiangsu Key Laboratory of Advanced Functional Polymer Design and Application, Suzhou Key Laboratory of Macromolecular Design and Precision Synthesis, Soochow University, Suzhou, P. R. China

**Yuanyu Huang** School of Life Science, Advanced Research Institute of Multidisciplinary Science, and Institute of Engineering Medicine, Key Laboratory of Molecular Medicine and Biotherapy, Beijing Institute of Technology, Beijing, China

**Jinsheng Huang** School of Materials Science and Engineering, Sun Yat-sen University, Guangzhou, China

Department of Urology, The Seventh Affiliated Hospital of Sun Yat-sen University, Shenzhen, China

**Shuaidong Huo** Fujian Provincial Key Laboratory of Innovative Drug Target Research, School of Pharmaceutical Sciences, Xiamen University, Xiamen, Fujian, China

**M. Zubair Iqbal** Institute of Smart Biomedical Materials, School of Materials Science and Engineering, Zhejiang Sci-Tech University, Hangzhou, China

Zhejiang-Mauritius Joint Research Center for Biomaterials and Tissue Engineering, Hangzhou, China

**T. Jiang** Henan-Macquarie University Joint Centre for Biomedical Innovation, School of Life Sciences, Henan University, Kaifeng, China

Henan Key Laboratory of Brain Targeted Bio-nanomedicine, School of Life Sciences & School of Pharmacy, Henan University, Kaifeng, China

**Rongrong Jin** National Engineering Research Center for Biomaterials, College of Biomedical Engineering, Sichuan University, Qingyang, Chengdu, Sichuan, P.R. China

**Lingjie Ke** Fujian Provincial Key Laboratory of Innovative Drug Target Research and State Key Laboratory of Cellular Stress Biology, School of Pharmaceutical Sciences, Xiamen University, Xiamen, China

**Xiangdong Kong** Institute of Smart Biomedical Materials, School of Materials Science and Engineering, Zhejiang Sci-Tech University, Hangzhou, China

Zhejiang-Mauritius Joint Research Center for Biomaterials and Tissue Engineering, Hangzhou, China

**Chunhui Li** School of Life Science, Advanced Research Institute of Multidisciplinary Science, and Institute of Engineering Medicine, Key Laboratory of Molecular Medicine and Biotherapy, Beijing Institute of Technology, Beijing, China

**Yachao Li** Department of Pharmacy, College of Biology, Hunan University, Changsha, Hunan, China

**Xing-Jie Liang** Chinese Academy of Sciences (CAS) Key Laboratory for Biomedical Effects of Nanomaterials and Nanosafety, CAS Center for Excellence in Nanoscience, National Center for Nanoscience and Technology of China, Beijing, China

**Zhihuan Liao** Fujian Provincial Key Laboratory of Innovative Drug Target Research, School of Pharmaceutical Sciences, Xiamen University, Xiamen, Fujian, China

**Jie Liu** College of Chemistry, Chemical Engineering and Materials Science, State and Local Joint Engineering Laboratory for Novel Functional Polymeric Materials, Jiangsu Key Laboratory of Advanced Functional Polymer Design and Application, Suzhou Key Laboratory of Macromolecular Design and Precision Synthesis, Soochow University, Suzhou, P. R. China

**Lanlan Liu** Guangdong Key Laboratory of Nanomedicine, CAS-HK Joint Lab for Biomaterials, Shenzhen Engineering Laboratory of Nanomedicine and Nanoformulations, Shenzhen Institute of Advanced Technology (SIAT), Chinese Academy of Sciences, Shenzhen, China

**Q. Liu** Key Laboratory of Functional Polymer Materials of Ministry of Education, State Key Laboratory of Medicinal Chemical Biology, College of Chemistry, National Demonstration Center for Experimental Chemistry Education, Nankai University, Tianjin, China

**Shuai Liu** College of Chemistry, Nankai University, Tianjin, China

**Xun Liu** Jiangsu Key Laboratory for Carbon-Based Functional Materials and Devices, Institute of Functional Nano & Soft Materials (FUNSOM), Collaborative Innovation Center of Suzhou Nano Science & Technology, Soochow University, Suzhou, China

**Yang Liu** Key Laboratory of Functional Polymer Materials of Ministry of Education, State Key Laboratory of Medicinal Chemical Biology, College of Chemistry, National Demonstration Center for Experimental Chemistry Education, Nankai University, Tianjin, China

**Asim Mushtaq** Institute of Smart Biomedical Materials, School of Materials Science and Engineering, Zhejiang Sci-Tech University, Hangzhou, China

Zhejiang-Mauritius Joint Research Center for Biomaterials and Tissue Engineering, Hangzhou, China

**Peihong Ni** College of Chemistry, Chemical Engineering and Materials Science, State and Local Joint Engineering Laboratory for Novel Functional Polymeric Materials, Jiangsu Key Laboratory of Advanced Functional Polymer Design and Application, Suzhou Key Laboratory of Macromolecular Design and Precision Synthesis, Soochow University, Suzhou, P. R. China

**Yu Nie** National Engineering Research Center for Biomaterials, College of Biomedical Engineering, Sichuan University, Qingyang, Chengdu, Sichuan, P.R. China

College of Biomedical Engineering, Sichuan University, Chengdu, Sichuan, China

**Hong Pan** Guangdong Key Laboratory of Nanomedicine, CAS-HK Joint Lab for Biomaterials, Shenzhen Engineering Laboratory of Nanomedicine and Nanoformulations, Shenzhen Institute of Advanced Technology (SIAT), Chinese Academy of Sciences, Shenzhen, China

**Zhiyong Qian** State Key Laboratory of Biotherapy and Cancer Center, West China Hospital, West China Medical School, Sichuan University, Chengdu, People's Republic of China

**Youqing Shen** Zhejiang Key Laboratory of Smart BioMaterials and Center for Bionanoengineering, and Key Laboratory of Biomass Chemical Engineering of the Ministry of Education, College of Chemical and Biological Engineering, Zhejiang University, Hangzhou, China

**Bingyang Shi** Henan-Macquarie University Joint Centre for Biomedical Innovation, School of Life Sciences, Henan University, Kaifeng, China

Henan Key Laboratory of Brain Targeted Bio-nanomedicine, School of Life Sciences & School of Pharmacy, Henan University, Kaifeng, China

Department of Biomedical Sciences, Faculty of Medicine & Health Sciences, Macquarie University, Sydney, NSW, Australia

**Jun Shi** Biomedical Polymers Laboratory, College of Chemistry, Chemical Engineering and Materials Science, and State Key Laboratory of Radiation Medicine and Protection, Soochow University, Suzhou, People's Republic of China

**Shuai Shi** Institute of Biomedical Engineering, School of Ophthalmology & Optometry and Eye Hospital, Wenzhou Medical University, Wenzhou, China

**Xun Sun** Key Laboratory of Drug Targeting and Drug Delivery Systems, Ministry of Education, West China School of Pharmacy, Sichuan University, Chengdu, China

**Huayu Tian** Key Laboratory of Polymer Ecomaterials, Changchun Institute of Applied Chemistry, Chinese Academy of Sciences, Changchun, China

**Guowei Wang** Zhejiang Key Laboratory of Smart BioMaterials and Center for Bionanoengineering, and Key Laboratory of Biomass Chemical Engineering of the Ministry of Education, College of Chemical and Biological Engineering, Zhejiang University, Hangzhou, China

**Long-Hai Wang** CAS Key Laboratory of Soft Matter Chemistry, Department of Polymer Science and Engineering, University of Science and Technology of China, Hefei, Anhui, China

**Qin Wang** Key Laboratory of Drug Targeting and Drug Delivery Systems, Ministry of Education, West China School of Pharmacy, Sichuan University, Chengdu, China

Key Laboratory of Advanced Technologies of Materials, Ministry of Education and School of Materials Science and Engineering, Southwest Jiaotong University, Chengdu, China

**Yuhua Weng** School of Life Science, Advanced Research Institute of Multidisciplinary Science, and Institute of Engineering Medicine, Key Laboratory of Molecular Medicine and Biotherapy, Beijing Institute of Technology, Beijing, China

**Yun-Long Wu** Fujian Provincial Key Laboratory of Innovative Drug Target Research and State Key Laboratory of Cellular Stress Biology, School of Pharmaceutical Sciences, Xiamen University, Xiamen, China

**Caina Xu** Key Laboratory of Polymer Ecomaterials, Changchun Institute of Applied Chemistry, Chinese Academy of Sciences, Changchun, China

**Fu-jian Xu** Key Laboratory of Biomedical Materials of Natural Macromolecules, Beijing Laboratory of Biomedical Materials, Beijing University of Chemical Technology, Ministry of Education, Beijing, China

College of Materials Science and Engineering, Beijing University of Chemical Technology, Beijing, China

**Xianghui Xu** Department of Pharmacy, College of Biology, Hunan University, Changsha, Hunan, China

**Xianzhu Yang** School of Biomedical Sciences and Engineering, South China University of Technology, Guangzhou, China

**Yi Yang** State Key Laboratory of Biotherapy and Cancer Center, West China Hospital, West China Medical School, Sichuan University, Chengdu, People's Republic of China

Precision Medicine Institute, The Second Affiliated Hospital of Xi'an Jiaotong University, Xi'an, Shaanxi Province, China

**Lichen Yin** Jiangsu Key Laboratory for Carbon-Based Functional Materials and Devices, Institute of Functional Nano & Soft Materials (FUNSOM), Collaborative Innovation Center of Suzhou Nano Science & Technology, Soochow University, Suzhou, China

**Ye-Zi You** CAS Key Laboratory of Soft Matter Chemistry, Department of Polymer Science and Engineering, University of Science and Technology of China, Hefei, Anhui, China

**Kai Zhang** Key Laboratory of Biomedical Materials of Natural Macromolecules, Beijing Laboratory of Biomedical Materials, Beijing University of Chemical Technology, Ministry of Education, Beijing, China

College of Materials Science and Engineering, Beijing University of Chemical Technology, Beijing, China

**Mingzu Zhang** College of Chemistry, Chemical Engineering and Materials Science, State and Local Joint Engineering Laboratory for Novel Functional Polymeric Materials, Jiangsu Key Laboratory of Advanced Functional Polymer Design and Application, Suzhou Key Laboratory of Macromolecular Design and Precision Synthesis, Soochow University, Suzhou, P. R. China

**Xian-Zheng Zhang** Key Laboratory of Biomedical Polymers of Ministry of Education, Department of Chemistry, Wuhan University, Wuhan, P. R. China

Key Laboratory of Biomaterials of Guangdong Higher Education Institutes, Department of Biomedical Engineering, Jinan University, Guangzhou, P. R. China

**Liang Zhao** School of Biomedical Sciences and Engineering, South China University of Technology, Guangzhou, China

**Nana Zhao** Key Laboratory of Biomedical Materials of Natural Macromolecules, Beijing Laboratory of Biomedical Materials, Beijing University of Chemical Technology, Ministry of Education, Beijing, China

College of Materials Science and Engineering, Beijing University of Chemical Technology, Beijing, China

**M. Zheng** Henan-Macquarie University Joint Centre for Biomedical Innovation, School of Life Sciences, Henan University, Kaifeng, China

Henan Key Laboratory of Brain Targeted Bio-nanomedicine, School of Life Sciences & School of Pharmacy, Henan University, Kaifeng, China

**Zhiyuan Zhong** Biomedical Polymers Laboratory, College of Chemistry, Chemical Engineering and Materials Science, and State Key Laboratory of Radiation Medicine and Protection, Soochow University, Suzhou, People's Republic of China

**Jing-Yi Zhu** Key Laboratory of Biomedical Polymers of Ministry of Education, Department of Chemistry, Wuhan University, Wuhan, P. R. China

Key Laboratory of Biomaterials of Guangdong Higher Education Institutes, Department of Biomedical Engineering, Jinan University, Guangzhou, P. R. China

# Molecular Strings Modified Gene Delivery System

**1**

Huapan Fang, Huayu Tian, and Xuesi Chen

## Contents



H. Fang (✉)
Institute of Functional Nano and Soft Materials (FUNSOM), Jiangsu Key Laboratory for Carbon-Based Functional Materials & Devices, Soochow University, Suzhou, Jiangsu, China
e-mail: hpfang@suda.edu.cn

H. Tian · X. Chen
Key Laboratory of Polymer Ecomaterials, Changchun Institute of Applied Chemistry, Chinese Academy of Sciences, Changchun, China
e-mail: thy@ciac.ac.cn; xschen@ciac.ac.cn



H. Tian and X. Chen (eds.), *Gene Delivery*, Biomaterial Engineering,
https://doi.org/10.1007/978-981-16-5419-0_12

**Abstract**

Gene therapy as a novel therapeutic tool has shown great potential for curing cancer thoroughly. However, gene carriers are necessary for gene therapy. Polycationic gene carriers have attracted increasing attention due to non-immunogenicity, easy manufacture, and flexible properties. However, high transfection efficiency and low cytotoxicity is a dilemma in the design of polycationic gene carriers. In this chapter, a simple and versatile strategy is described by introducing "molecular string" RT (i.e., p-toluylsulfonyl arginine) onto polylysine (PLL) and the resulting polycationic gene carrier is named PLL-RT. Introducing RT string contributes to the formation of multiple interactions (electrostatic, hydrogen bonding, and hydrophobic interactions) between gene carriers and cell membrane or DNA, as well as adopting α-helix conformation, all of which would be beneficial to enhance gene transfection. Additionally, other polycations such as hyperbranched polyethylenimine (PEI) and dendrimer polyamidoamine (PAMAM) modified with RT string can also acquire improved transfection efficiency and lower cytotoxicity. Moreover, PLL-RT mediated therapeutic gene showed a significant antitumor effect in vivo. This work provides an effective method for developing polycationic gene carriers with efficient transfection and excellent biocompatibility.

**Keywords**

Gene therapy · Polycationic gene carrier · Molecular string · Transfection efficiency · Cytotoxicity · Multiple interactions · α-Helix conformation

## 1 Overview

Cancers are malignant diseases, which threaten human life severely. The traditional treatments including chemotherapy, radiotherapy, and surgery cannot efficiently cure cancer. Gene therapy as a novel therapeutic tool presents great potential for curing cancer (Gutierrez et al. 1992; Weichselbaum and Kufe 1997; Verma and Somia 1997; Cross and Burmester 2006). Generally speaking, gene carriers are necessary for the success of gene therapy. Among them, polycationic gene carriers have drawn great attention because of nonimmunogenicity, easy manufacture, and flexible properties (Kim et al. 2007; Liu et al. 2010). Although some traditional polycations such as polyethylenimine (PEI) (Akinc et al. 2005; Kim et al. 2013), polylysine (PLL) (Choi et al. 1998), and polyamidoamine (PAMAM) (Kukowska et al. 1996; Tang et al. 1996) have already been used for gene transfection, these gene carriers were urgently needed to improve transfection performance and reduce cytotoxicity for clinical application.

## 2 Protocol and Discussion

It is well known to that the electrostatic interactions between gene carriers and cell membrane or DNA will influence transfection capability of polycations (Guo and Huang 2012; Sun et al. 2015; Liu et al. 2016). In general, proper electrostatic interactions will contribute to DNA loading, condensation, and endocytosis, which are beneficial to gene transfection. However, too large charge density will cause deadly cytotoxicity, hindering transfection performance. Therefore, introducing other types of interactions or characteristics can be regarded as one alternative strategy for acquiring efficient transfection and low cytotoxicity.

Cheng's group modified PAMAM with hydrophobic perfluorinated alkyl hydrocarbon, which remarkably improved transfection efficiency (Wang et al. 2014, 2015). Schmuck and his collaborators utilized hydrogen bonding interactions between oligopeptide and cell membrane or DNA to acquire efficient gene transfection (Li et al. 2015). Additionally, Cheng et al. synthesized a series of cationic polypeptides adopting α-helix conformation with excellent transfection performance (Gabrielson et al. 2012; Yin et al. 2013). Nevertheless, there were few reports on designing highly efficient gene carrier by simultaneously introducing multiple interactions or characteristics to one polycation. Combining multiple interactions or characteristics into one polymer molecule can hardly be accomplished unless various molecules are involved in the construction of polycation. The reason is that multistep reactions are needed, which is tedious and difficult to repeat. Moreover, introduction of various molecules tends to consume amino groups of polycation, resulting in poor transfection efficiency.

The protocol provided a comprehensive "all in one" strategy to develop a highly efficient polycationic gene carrier by introducing multiple interactions (electrostatic interaction, hydrogen bonding interaction, and hydrophobic interaction) or characteristics (α-helix conformation) into one polycation. A "molecular string," arginine protected by tosyl group (abbreviated as RT string, R refers to arginine, T refers to tosyl) is grafted onto PLL to promote the transfection performance (Fig. 1). This method possesses the following advantages: (1) Not only the conformation of polycationic gene carrier is transformed from a random coil to a α-helix conformation after introducing "RT string" but also multiple interactions (i.e., electrostatic interaction, hydrogen bonding interaction and hydrophobic interaction) are formed simultaneously between gene carrier and cell membrane or DNA. The multiple interactions and α-helix conformation can synergistically improve the transfection efficiency. (2) The number of amino groups of polycationic gene carrier will remain unchanged. One amino group is consumed, in the meantime, another amino group will be supplemented. (3) "RT string" modified PLL (the resulting polycation is defined as PLL-RT) not only significantly promotes DNA transfection but also exhibits excellent serum resistance and RNA silencing efficiency. (4) Introducing "RT string" onto polycations can be used as a universal strategy of enhancing transfection for polycations, such as PEI25k and PAMAM. (5) PLL-RT can accomplish excellent in vivo antitumor efficacy by combining therapeutic genes. The molecular structure of PLL-RT and control polycations are characterized in detail, and the influence of "RT string" on transfection behaviors of polycations are systematically investigated. "RT string" provides an enlightened strategy for developing polycationic gene carriers with high transfection efficiency and low cytotoxicity.

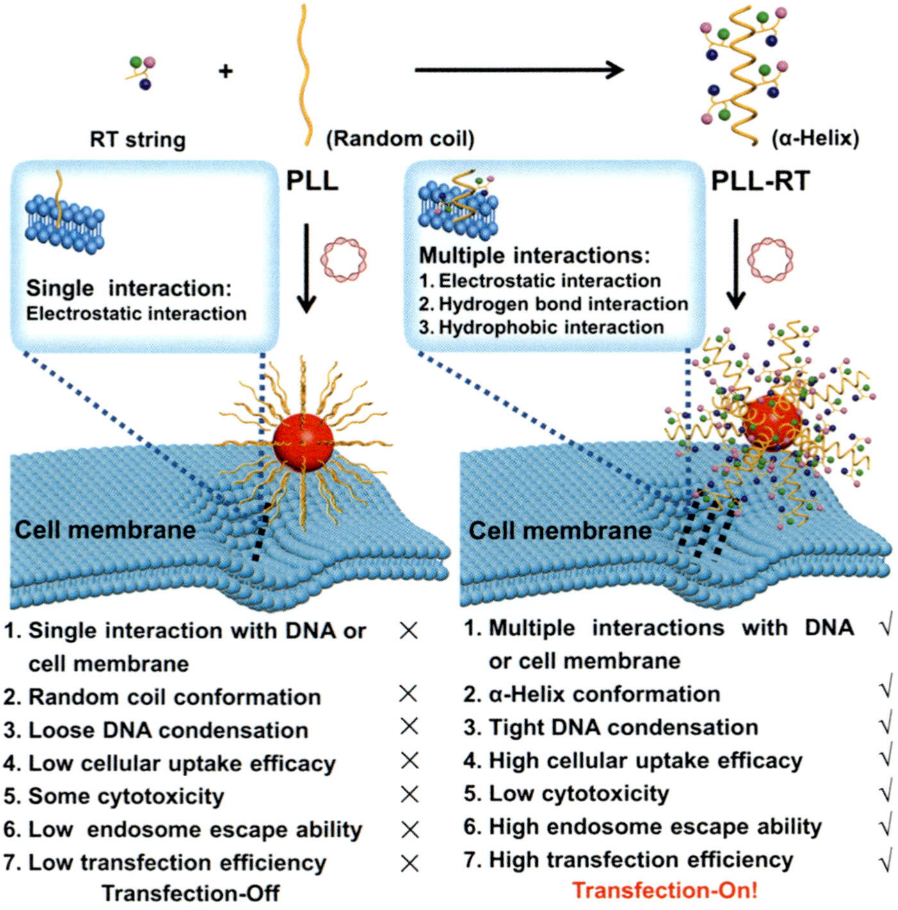


**Fig. 1** Construction of highly efficient gene carriers by introducing multiple interactions and α-helix characteristic into polycations. (Adapted from Fang et al. 2018, with permission)

# 3 Materials

## 3.1 Synthesis of Lys(Z)-NCA

1. H-Lys(Z)-OH (GL Biochem Ltd., Shanghai, China)
2. Triphosgene (Xiya Reagent Co., Ltd. (Linyi, Shandong, China))
3. Tetrahydrofuran (THF)
4. Hexane
5. Ethyl acetate
6. $CDCl_3$
7. Bruker AV 400 M NMR spectrometer (Bruker, Ettlingen, Germany)

### 3.2 Synthesis of PLL

1. N, N-dimethyl formamide (DMF)
2. n-Hexylamine
3. Trifluoroacetic acid (TFA)
4. Hydrobromic acid in 33% acetic acid (ACROS)
5. Anhydrous ether
6. Dialysis bag: Cut off 3500 Dalton (Yuanye Biological Technology Co., Ltd., Shanghai, China)
7. DMSO-$d_6$
8. $D_2O$
9. Bruker AV 400 M NMR spectrometer (Bruker, Ettlingen, Germany)

### 3.3 Synthesis of PLL-RT4

1. Boc-Arg(Tos)-OH
2. PLL
3. EDCI
4. HOBT
5. DIPEA
6. DMSO-$d_6$
7. $D_2O$
8. Bruker AV 400 M NMR spectrometer (Bruker, Ettlingen, Germany)

### 3.4 Synthesis of PLL-MS

1. Methylsufonyl chloride
2. PLL
3. DIPEA
4. THF
5. Dialysis bag: Cut off 3500 Dalton (Yuanye Biological Technology Co., Ltd., Shanghai, China)
6. DMSO-$d_6$
7. $D_2O$
8. Bruker AV 400 M NMR spectrometer (Bruker, Ettlingen, Germany)

### 3.5 Synthesis of PLL-Too

1. PLL
2. p-Toluoyl chloride
3. THF
4. DIPEA

5. Dialysis bag: Cut off 3500 Dalton (Yuanye Biological Technology Co., Ltd., Shanghai, China)
6. DMSO-$d_6$
7. $D_2O$
8. Bruker AV 400 M NMR spectrometer (Bruker, Ettlingen, Germany)

### 3.6 Synthesis of PLL-Tos

1. PLL
2. p-Toluene sulfonyl chloride
3. THF
4. DIPEA
5. Dialysis bag: Cut off 3500 Dalton (Yuanye Biological Technology Co., Ltd., Shanghai, China)
6. DMSO-$d_6$
7. $D_2O$
8. Bruker AV 400 M NMR spectrometer (Bruker, Ettlingen, Germany)

### 3.7 Synthesis of PLL-Orn

1. PLL
2. Boc-Orn(Boc)-OH
3. EDCI
4. HOBT
5. DMF
6. DIPEA
7. TFA
8. Dialysis bag: Cut off 3500 Dalton (Yuanye Biological Technology Co., Ltd., Shanghai, China)
9. DMSO-$d_6$
10. $D_2O$
11. Bruker AV 400 M NMR spectrometer (Bruker, Ettlingen, Germany)

### 3.8 Synthesis of PLL-Arg

1. PLL
2. Boc-Arg(Pbf)-OH
3. EDCI
4. HOBT
5. DMF
6. DIPEA
7. TFA

8. Dialysis bag: Cut off 3500 Dalton (Yuanye Biological Technology Co., Ltd., Shanghai, China)
9. DMSO-$d_6$
10. $D_2O$
11. Bruker AV 400 M NMR spectrometer (Bruker, Ettlingen, Germany)

### 3.9 Synthesis of PLL-Orn(Tos)

1. PLL
2. Boc-Orn(Tos)-OH
3. EDCI
4. NHS
5. DMF
6. TFA
7. Dialysis bag: Cut off 3500 Dalton (Yuanye Biological Technology Co., Ltd., Shanghai, China)
8. DMSO-$d_6$
9. $D_2O$
10. Bruker AV 400 M NMR spectrometer (Bruker, Ettlingen, Germany)

### 3.10 Synthesis of PLL-Arg($NO_2$)

1. PLL
2. Boc-Arg($NO_2$)-OH
3. EDCI
4. NHS
5. DMF
6. TFA
7. Dialysis bag: Cut off 3500 Dalton (Yuanye Biological Technology Co., Ltd., Shanghai, China)
8. DMSO-$d_6$
9. $D_2O$
10. Bruker AV 400 M NMR spectrometer (Bruker, Ettlingen, Germany)

### 3.11 Synthesis of PEI25k-RT2

1. PEI25k
2. Boc-Arg(Tos)-OH
3. EDCI
4. HOBT
5. DIPEA

6. TFA
7. Dialysis bag: Cut off 3500 Dalton (Yuanye Biological Technology Co., Ltd., Shanghai, China)
8. $CD_3CN$
9. $D_2O$
10. Bruker AV 400 M NMR spectrometer (Bruker, Ettlingen, Germany)

## 3.12 Synthesis of G4-RT2

1. G4 PAMAM
2. Boc-Arg(Tos)-OH
3. EDCI
4. HOBT
5. DIPEA
6. TFA
7. Dialysis bag: Cut off 3500 Dalton (Yuanye Biological Technology Co., Ltd., Shanghai, China)
8. $CD_3CN$
9. $D_2O$
10. Bruker AV 400 M NMR spectrometer (Bruker, Ettlingen, Germany)

## 3.13 Preparation of Carrier/DNA Nanoparticles

1. Calf thymus DNA (Sigma, St. Louis, MO, USA)
2. PLL/DNA, PLL-RT4/DNA and control carriers/DNA
3. Vortex finder
4. pH Meter

## 3.14 Measurements of Zeta Potential and Particle Size

1. PLL/DNA, PLL-RT4/DNA and control carriers/DNA
2. Zeta potential/BI-90Plus particle size analyzer (Brookhaven, USA)
3. XL-30ESEM-FEG SEM system (SEI, USA)

## 3.15 Determination of Molecular Weight and Molecular Weight Distribution

1. PLL
2. Gel permeation chromatography (GPC) with 515 GPC (Waters, USA)
3. 0.5 mol/L $CH_3COONa/CH_3COOH$
4. mPEG2k (JenKem Technology Co., Ltd. Beijing, China)

## 3.16 In Situ Surface-Enhanced Infrared Absorption Spectroscopy (SEIRAS)

1. 0.1 mol/L $H_2SO_4$
2. Au film
3. FTIR spectrometer
4. Liquid nitrogen-cooled MCT detector
5. Cardiolipin
6. $N_2$
7. 1-Dodecanethiol (Sigma-Aldrich, USA)
8. Ethanol
9. HCl
10. NaOH
11. pH Meter
12. PLL
13. PLL-RT4

## 3.17 Isothermal Titration Calorimetry (ITC) Measurement

1. ITC200 (MicroCal)
2. Cardiolipin
3. Sodium cacodylate
4. Lys4
5. Lys4-RT2
6. Calf thymus DNA (Sigma, St. Louis, MO, USA)

## 3.18 Measurement of Circular Dichroism (CD) Spectra

1. J-815 CD spectrometer (JACS, Easton, MD, USA)
2. pH Meter (Oakton Instruments, Vernon Hills, IL, USA)
3. PLL
4. PLL-RT4 and control polycations
5. HCl
6. NaOH

## 3.19 Cell Culture

1. MCF-7 cells, HeLa cells, CT26 cells, and B16F10 cells (Shanghai Cell Bank of the Chinese Academy of Sciences, China)
2. Dulbecco's modified Eagle's medium (DMEM) culture medium (Gibco, Grand Island, USA)
3. RPMI 1640 culture medium (FBS, Gibco, Grand Island, USA)

4. Fetal bovine serum (FBS, Gibco, Grand Island, USA)
5. Cell incubator

### 3.20 In Vitro DNA Transfection

1. MCF-7 cells, HeLa cells, CT26 cells and B16F10 cells (Shanghai Cell Bank of the Chinese Academy of Sciences, China)
2. Dulbecco's modified Eagle's medium (DMEM) culture medium (Gibco, Grand Island, USA)
3. RPMI 1640 culture medium (FBS, Gibco, Grand Island, USA)
4. Fetal bovine serum (FBS, Gibco, Grand Island, USA)
5. Luciferase plasmid DNA (pGL3, Promega, Mannheim, Germany)
6. 96-Well plates
7. PLL/pGL3 at various mass ratios
8. PLL-RT4/pGL3 and control polycations/pGL3 at various mass ratios
9. Luciferase reporter gene assay kit (Promega, Mannheim, Germany)
10. Luminometer (Turner Biosystems & Promega)
11. BCA protein assay

### 3.21 Flow Cytometry Assay

1. MCF-7 cells, HeLa cells, CT26 cells, and B16F10 cells (Shanghai Cell Bank of the Chinese Academy of Sciences, China)
2. Dulbecco's modified Eagle's medium (DMEM) culture medium (Gibco, Grand Island, USA)
3. RPMI 1640 culture medium (FBS, Gibco, Grand Island, USA)
4. Fetal bovine serum (FBS, Gibco, Grand Island, USA)
5. 12-Well plates
6. Cyanine 5 labeled DNA (Cy5-DNA, RiboBio, Guangzhou, China)
7. PLL/Cy5-DNA
8. PLL-RT4/Cy5-DNA and control polycations/Cy5-DNA
9. pH Meter (Oakton Instruments, Vernon Hills, IL, USA)
10. HCl
11. NaOH
12. Guava EasyCyte flow cytometer (Guava Technologies)

### 3.22 Confocal Laser Scanning Microscopy (CLSM) to Observe the Cellular Uptake

1. MCF-7 cells, HeLa cells, CT26 cells, and B16F10 cells (Shanghai Cell Bank of the Chinese Academy of Sciences, China)

2. Dulbecco's modified Eagle's medium (DMEM) culture medium (Gibco, Grand Island, USA)
3. RPMI 1640 culture medium (FBS, Gibco, Grand Island, USA)
4. Fetal bovine serum (FBS, Gibco, Grand Island, USA)
5. 6-Well plates
6. Cyanine 5 labeled DNA (Cy5-DNA, RiboBio, Guangzhou, China)
7. PLL/Cy5-DNA
8. PLL-RT4/Cy5-DNA and control polycations/Cy5-DNA
9. DAPI
10. Alexa Fluor 488 phalloidin
11. Glass slides
12. Glycerol
13. CLSM (ZEISS LSM780, Germany)

## 3.23 CLSM to Observe Endosomal Escape

1. MCF-7 cells, HeLa cells, CT26 cells, and B16F10 cells (Shanghai Cell Bank of the Chinese Academy of Sciences, China)
2. Dulbecco's modified Eagle's medium (DMEM) culture medium (Gibco, Grand Island, USA)
3. RPMI 1640 culture medium (FBS, Gibco, Grand Island, USA)
4. Fetal bovine serum (FBS, Gibco, Grand Island, USA)
5. 6-Well plates
6. Cyanine 5 labeled DNA (Cy5-DNA, RiboBio, Guangzhou, China)
7. PLL/Cy5-DNA
8. PLL-RT4/Cy5-DNA and control polycations/Cy5-DNA
9. DAPI
10. Lysotracker Green
11. Glass slides
12. Glycerol
13. CLSM (ZEISS LSM780, Germany)

## 3.24 Cytotoxicity Assay

1. MCF-7 cells, HeLa cells, CT26 cells, and B16F10 cells (Shanghai Cell Bank of the Chinese Academy of Sciences, China)
2. Dulbecco's modified Eagle's medium (DMEM) culture medium (Gibco, Grand Island, USA)
3. RPMI 1640 culture medium (FBS, Gibco, Grand Island, USA)
4. Fetal bovine serum (FBS, Gibco, Grand Island, USA)
5. 96-Well plates
6. pGL3 DNA
7. PLL/pGL3 DNA

8. PLL-RT4/pGL3 DNA and control polycations/pGL3 DNA
9. MTT
10. Bio-Rad 680 microplate reader

### 3.25 Antiserum Transfection

1. MCF-7 cells, HeLa cells, CT26 cells, and B16F10 cells (Shanghai Cell Bank of the Chinese Academy of Sciences, China)
2. Dulbecco's modified Eagle's medium (DMEM) culture medium (Gibco, Grand Island, USA)
3. RPMI 1640 culture medium (FBS, Gibco, Grand Island, USA)
4. Fetal bovine serum (FBS, Gibco, Grand Island, USA)
5. pGL3
6. 96-Well plates
7. PLL/pGL3 at various mass ratios
8. PLL-RT4/pGL3 and control polycations/pGL3 at various mass ratios
9. Luciferase reporter gene assay kit (Promega, Mannheim, Germany)
10. Luminometer (Turner Biosystems & Promega)
11. BCA protein assay

### 3.26 In Vitro Gene Silencing

1. Huh-7 Luc cells
2. Dulbecco's modified Eagle's medium (DMEM) culture medium (Gibco, Grand Island, USA)
3. siRNA (GL3 luciferase-siRNA double strands (sense: 5'-CUUACGCUGAGU-ACUUC GAdTdT-3′ and antisense: 5'-UCGAAGUACUCAGCGUAAGdTdT-3′, FASMAC, Japan)
4. 96-Well plates
5. PLL/siRNA
6. PLL-RT4/siRNA and control polycations/siRNA
7. Luciferase reporter gene assay kit (Promega, Mannheim, Germany)
8. Luminometer (Turner Biosystems & Promega)
9. BCA protein assay

### 3.27 Construction of Tumor Model

1. Five to six-week-old female BALB/c mice (Vital River Company, Beijing)
2. CT26 cells
3. RPMI 1640 culture medium (FBS, Gibco, Grand Island, USA)
4. Fetal bovine serum (FBS, Gibco, Grand Island, USA)
5. PBS

## 3.28 Antitumor Treatment

1. CT26 tumor bearing BALB/c mice
2. pDNA expressed shRNA VEGF (shVEGF, Sangon, Shanghai, China)
3. PBS
4. PLL/shVEGF
5. PLL-RT4/shVEGF
6. Vernier caliper
7. Electronic balance

## 3.29 Hematoxylin-Eosin (H&E) Staining

1. Major organs (heart, liver, spleen, lung and kidney) of mice after treatment
2. Tumors of mice after treatment
3. Hematoxylin-eosin (H&E)
4. Paraffin
5. Dimethylbenzene
6. Ethanol
7. Glass slides
8. Glycerol

## 3.30 Immunofluorescent Staining for Tumor Vessels

1. Anti-CD31 antibody
2. FITC-labeled secondary antibody
3. Paraffin
4. Dimethylbenzene
5. Ethanol
6. Glass slides
7. Glycerol
8. CLSM (ZEISS LSM780, Germany)

## 3.31 qRT-PCR Assay

1. Tumors of mice after treatment
2. Trizol (Invitrogen, Carlsbad, CA, USA)
3. Centrifuge
4. Prime Script® RT reagent kit with gDNA Eraser (Perfect Real Time) (TaKaRa, Dalian, China)
5. SYBR® Premix Ex Taq™ II (Tli RNaseH Plus) (TaKaRa, Dalian, China)
6. VEGF primers: Forward, 5‘-GGT GAG AGG TCT AGT TCC CGA-3’; Reverse, 5‘-CCA TGA ACT TTC TGC TCT TC-3’

7. GAPDH primers: Forward, 5‘-GTT CCA GTA TGA CTC TAC CC-3’; Reverse, 5‘-AGT CTT CTG AGG CAG TGA TG-3’
8. Mx3005P instrument (Stratagene, USA)

### 3.32 Enzyme Linked Immunosorbent Assay (ELISA)

1. Tumors of mice after treatment
2. Centrifuge
3. Homogenizer
4. Mouse VEGF ELISA kit (R&D Systems, MA, USA)
5. Tecan infinite M200 Microplate Readers (Tecan, Austria)

## 4 Methods

### 4.1 Synthesis of Lys(Z)-NCA

1. H-Lys(Z)-OH and triphosgene were added into dry three-mouth flask, and THF was added inside and reacted for 1.5 h at 50 °C until the mixture solution was clear.
2. Mixture solution was cooled to room temperature naturally, and 2 L of cold hexane was added inside for precipitation, filtered, and the white power was dissolved ethyl acetate.
3. Cold deionized water was added into above solution, the organic layer was extracted and dried with anhydrous magnesium sulfate, put in fridge at −20 °C overnight. Next filtered, the filtrate was dried under vacuum and recrystallized with THF and hexane, and white solid powder was obtained.
4. The product was characterized by $^1$H NMR spectra, the measurement was conducted at room temperature and $CDCl_3$ was used as solvent (Fig. 2).

### 4.2 Synthesis of PLL

1. Lys(Z)-NCA and n-hexylamine was dissolved dry DMF and stirred for 72 h at room temperature.
2. The reaction mixture was dialyzed for 72 h and freeze-dried to get white power.
3. The white powder was dissolved in TFA, and hydrobromic acid in 33% acetic acid was added to react for 4 h at room temperature. After that, anhydrous ether was used for precipitation, then filtered, dried under vacuum, and dialyzed for 72 h, freeze-dried, and white solid was obtained.
4. The product was characterized by $^1$H NMR spectra, the measurement was conducted at room temperature and $D_2O/DMSO\text{-}d_6 = 1/1$ (v/v) was used as solvent (Fig. 3).

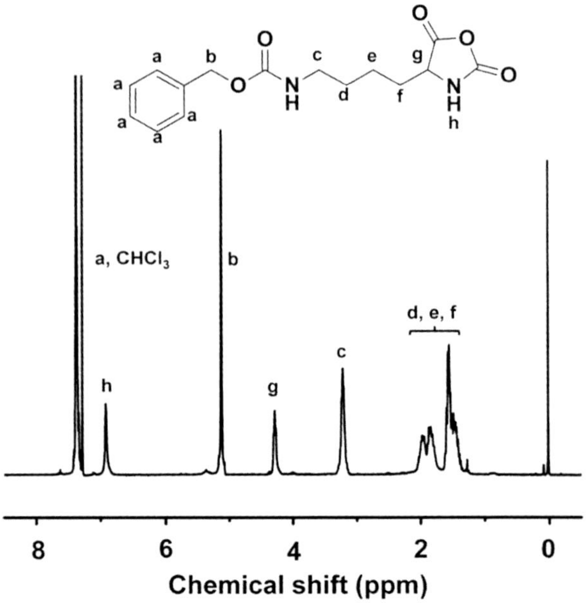


**Fig. 2** $^1$H NMR spectrum of Lys(Z)-NCA (400 MHz, $CDCl_3$). (Adapted from Fang et al. 2018, with permission)

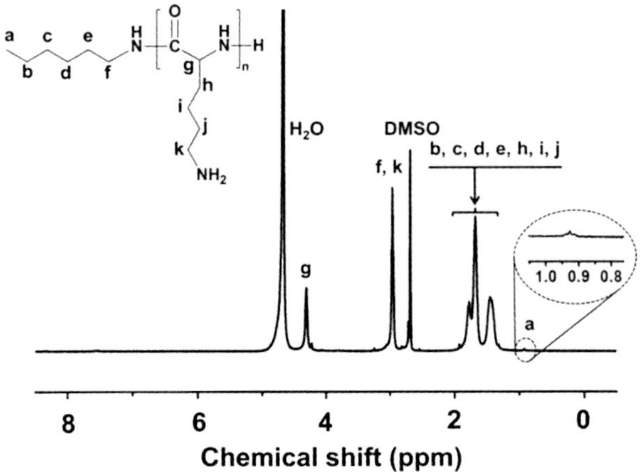


**Fig. 3** $^1$H NMR spectrum of PLL (400 MHz, DMSO-$d_6$/$D_2O$ (v/v = 1/1)). (Adapted from Fang et al. 2018, with permission)

## 4.3 Synthesis of PLL-RT4

1. The mixture of Boc-Arg(Tos)-OH, EDCI, and HOBT were dissolved DMF and stirred for 30 min at room temperature.
2. PLL was dissolved in deionized water. Then PLL solution and DIPEA were added into above mixture solution, stirred for 72 h at room temperature, then dialyzed for 72 h, freeze-dried, and white solid was obtained.

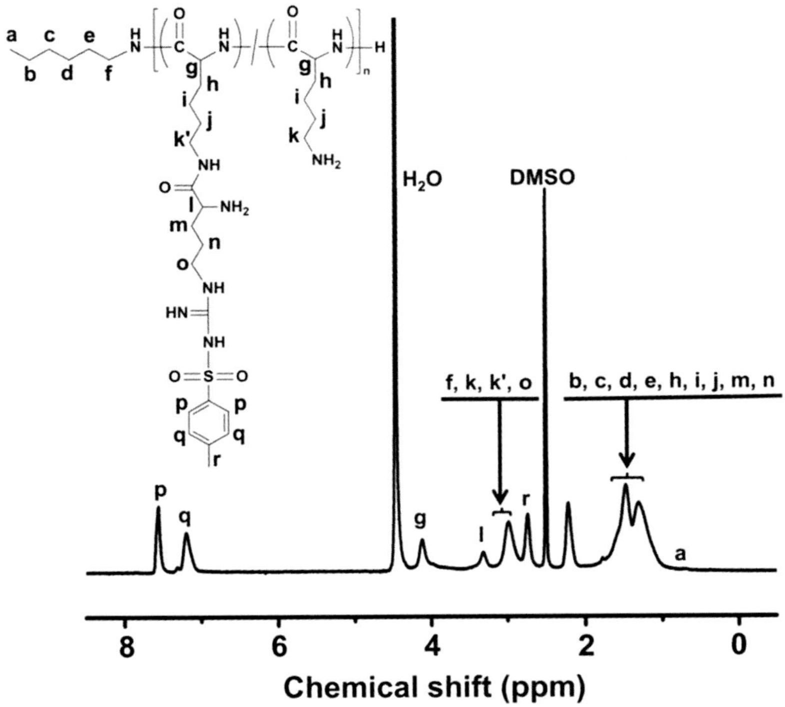


**Fig. 4** [1]H NMR spectrum of PLL-RT4 (400 MHz, DMSO-$d_6$/$D_2O$ (v/v = 1/1)). (Adapted from Fang et al. 2018, with permission)

3. The white solid was added into TFA and stirred for 4 h at room temperature, precipitated with anhydrous ether, filtered and dried under vacuum, dialyzed for 72 h and freeze-dried, and the white floc solid was obtained.
4. The product was characterized by $^1$H NMR spectra, the measurement was conducted at room temperature and $D_2O$/DMSO-$d_6$ = 1/1 (v/v) was used as solvent (Fig. 4).

## 4.4 Synthesis of PLL-MS

1. Methylsufonyl chloride was dissolved in THF, and PLL was dissolved in deionized water.
2. Methylsufonyl chloride solution was dropwise added into PLL solution in an ice bath, and DIPEA was added and stirred for 12 h in ice bath.
3. The mixture was dialyzed for 72 h, freeze-dried, white solid product was obtained.
4. The product was characterized by $^1$H NMR spectra, the measurement was conducted at room temperature and $D_2O$/DMSO-$d_6$ = 1/1 (v/v) was used as solvent (Fig. 5).

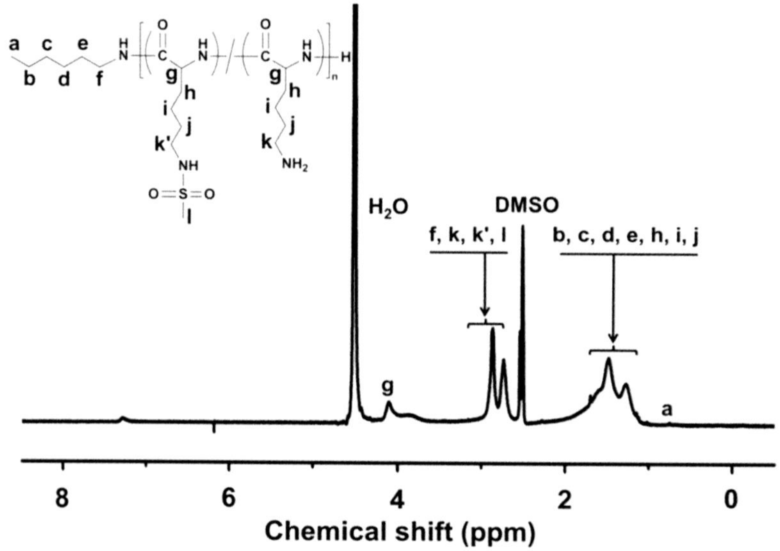


**Fig. 5** $^{1}$H NMR spectrum of PLL-MS (400 MHz, DMSO-$d_6$/$D_2O$ (v/v = 1/1)). (Adapted from Fang et al. 2018, with permission)

## 4.5 Synthesis of PLL-Too

1. P-toluoyl chloride was dissolved in THF, and PLL was dissolved in deionized water.
2. P-toluoyl chloride solution was dropwise added into PLL solution in an ice bath, and DIPEA was added and stirred for 12 h in an ice bath.
3. The mixture was dialyzed for 72 h, freeze-dried, white solid product was obtained.
4. The product was characterized by $^{1}$H NMR spectra, the measurement was conducted at room temperature and $D_2O$/DMSO-$d_6$ = 1/1 (v/v) was used as solvent (Fig. 6).

## 4.6 Synthesis of PLL-Tos

1. P-toluene sulfonyl chloride was dissolved in THF, and PLL was dissolved in deionized water.
2. P-toluene sulfonyl chloride solution was dropwise added into PLL solution in an ice bath, and DIPEA was added and stirred for 12 h in an ice bath.
3. The mixture was dialyzed for 72 h, freeze-dried, white solid product was obtained.
4. The product was characterized by $^{1}$H NMR spectra, the measurement was conducted at room temperature and $D_2O$/DMSO-$d_6$ = 1/1 (v/v) was used as solvent (Fig. 7).

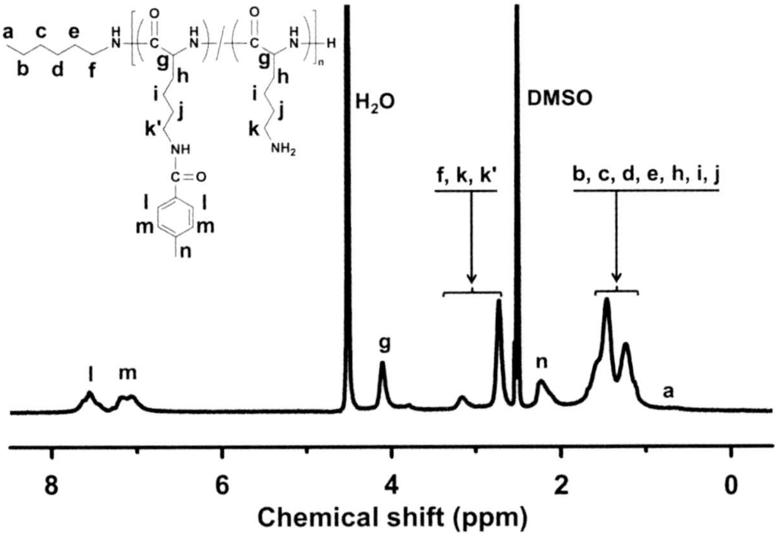


**Fig. 6** $^1$H NMR spectrum of PLL-Too (400 MHz, DMSO-$d_6$/$D_2O$ (v/v = 1/1)). (Adapted from Fang et al. 2018, with permission)

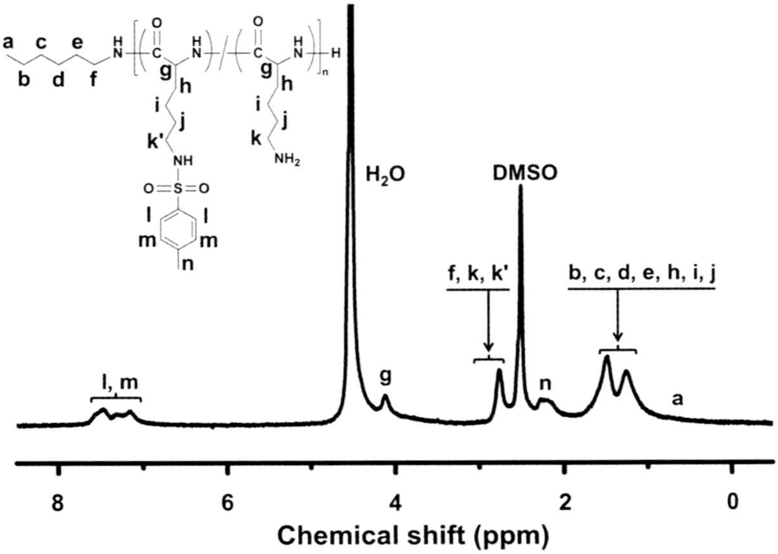


**Fig. 7** $^1$H NMR spectrum of PLL-Tos (400 MHz, DMSO-$d_6$/$D_2O$ (v/v = 1/1)). (Adapted from Fang et al. 2018, with permission)

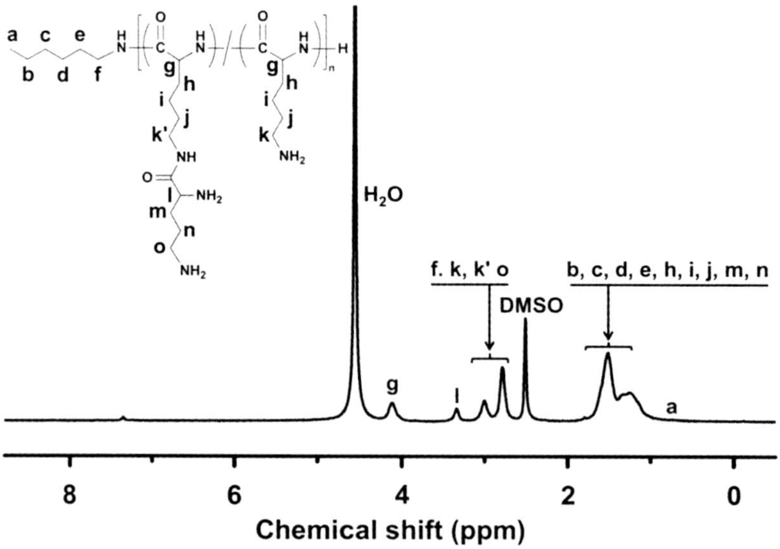


**Fig. 8** $^1$H NMR spectrum of PLL-Orn (400 MHz, DMSO-$d_6$/$D_2O$ (v/v = 1/1)). (Adapted from Fang et al. 2018, with permission)

## 4.7 Synthesis of PLL-Orn

1. The mixture of Boc-Orn(Boc)-OH, EDCI, and HOBT was dissolved in DMF and stirred for 1 h at room temperature.
2. PLL was dissolved in deionized water. PLL solution and DIPEA was added into the above solution and stirred for 72 h at room temperature.
3. The above mixture was dialyzed, freeze-dried, white solid powder was obtained.
4. The white solid powder was dissolved in TFA and stirred for 4 h at room temperature. After that, the mixture solution was precipitated with anhydrous ether, filtered, dried under vacuum, dialyzed, and freeze-dried, the white power was obtained.
5. The product was characterized by $^1$H NMR spectra, the measurement was conducted at room temperature and $D_2O$/DMSO-$d_6$ = 1/1 (v/v) was used as solvent (Fig. 8).

## 4.8 Synthesis of PLL-Arg

1. The mixture of Boc-Arg(Pbf), EDCI, and HOBT was dissolved in DMF and stirred for 1 h at room temperature.
2. PLL was dissolved in deionized water. PLL solution and DIPEA was added into the above solution and stirred for 72 h at room temperature.
3. The above mixture was dialyzed, freeze-dried, white solid powder was obtained.

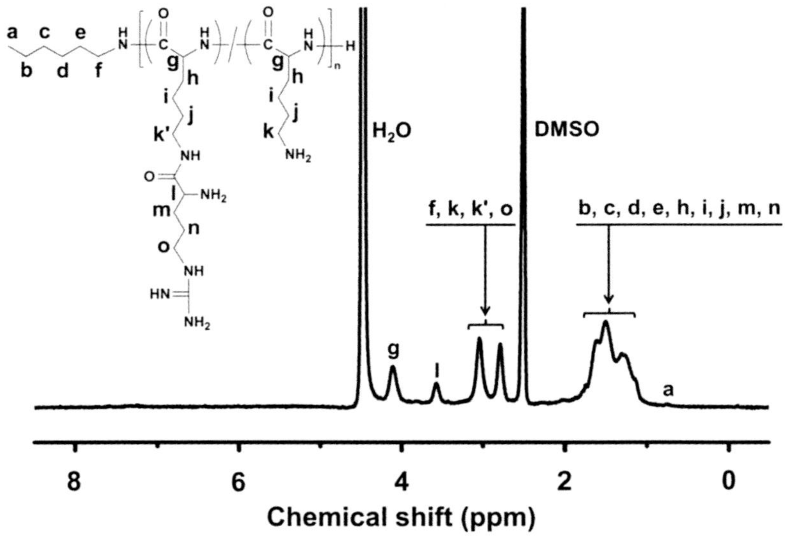


**Fig. 9** $^1$H NMR spectrum of PLL-Arg (400 MHz, DMSO-d$_6$/D$_2$O (v/v = 1/1)). (Adapted from Fang et al. 2018, with permission)

4. The white solid powder was dissolved in TFA and stirred for 4 h at room temperature. After that, the mixture solution was precipitated with anhydrous ether, filtered, dried under vacuum, dialyzed, and freeze-dried, the white power was obtained.
5. The product was characterized by $^1$H NMR spectra, the measurement was conducted at room temperature and D$_2$O/DMSO-d$_6$ = 1/1 (v/v) was used as solvent (Fig. 9).

## 4.9 Synthesis of PLL-Orn(Tos)

1. The mixture of Boc-Orn(Tos)-OH, EDCI, and NHS was dissolved in methanol and stirred for 1 h at room temperature.
2. PLL was dissolved in deionized water. PLL solution was added into the above solution and stirred for 72 h at room temperature.
3. The above mixture was dialyzed, freeze-dried, white solid powder was obtained.
4. The white solid powder was dissolved in TFA and stirred for 4 h at room temperature. After that, the mixture solution was precipitated with anhydrous ether, filtered, dried under vacuum, dialyzed, and freeze-dried, the white power was obtained.
5. The product was characterized by $^1$H NMR spectra, the measurement was conducted at room temperature and D$_2$O/DMSO-d$_6$ = 1/1 (v/v) was used as solvent (Fig. 10).

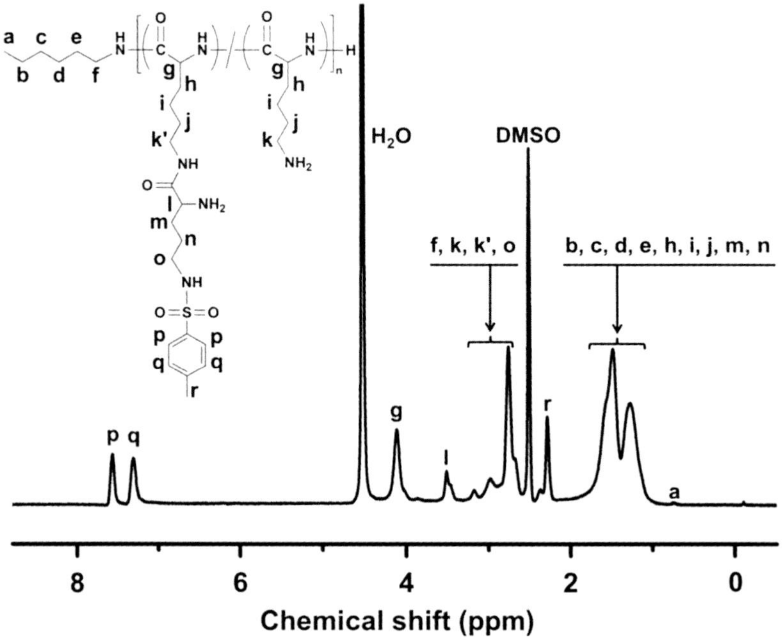


**Fig. 10** $^{1}H$ NMR spectrum of PLL-Orn(Tos) (400 MHz, DMSO-$d_6$/$D_2O$ (v/v = 1/1)). (Adapted from Fang et al. 2018, with permission)

## 4.10 Synthesis of PLL-Arg($NO_2$)

1. The mixture of Boc-Orn(Tos)-OH, EDCI, and NHS was dissolved in DMSO and stirred for 1 h at room temperature.
2. PLL was dissolved in deionized water. PLL solution was added into the above solution and stirred for 72 h at room temperature.
3. The above mixture was dialyzed, freeze-dried, white solid powder was obtained.
4. The white solid powder was dissolved in TFA and stirred for 4 h at room temperature. After that, the mixture solution was precipitated with anhydrous ether, filtered, dried under vacuum, dialyzed, and freeze-dried, the white power was obtained.
5. The product was characterized by $^{1}H$ NMR spectra, the measurement was conducted at room temperature and $D_2O$/DMSO-$d_6$ = 1/1 (v/v) was used as solvent (Fig. 11).

## 4.11 Synthesis of PEI25k-RT2

1. The mixture of Boc-Arg(Tos)-OH, EDCI, and HOBT was dissolved in DMF and stirred for 1 h at room temperature.
2. PEI25k was dissolved in DMF, then PEI25k solution and DIPEA were added and stirred for 5 days at room temperature.

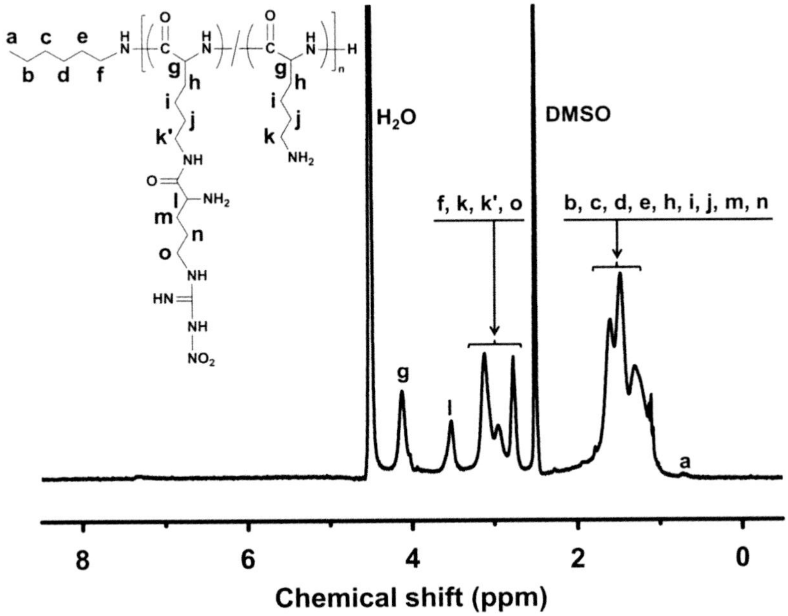


**Fig. 11** $^1$H NMR spectrum of PLL-Arg($NO_2$) (400 MHz, DMSO-$d_6$/$D_2O$ (v/v = 1/1)). (Adapted from Fang et al. 2018, with permission)

3. The mixture solution was dialyzed, freeze-dried, the white solid was obtained. Next, the white solid was dissolved in TFA and stirred for 4 h at room temperature. Then precipitated with anhydrous ether, filtered and dried under vacuum, dialyzed for 72 h and freeze-dried, the white solid was obtained.
4. The product was characterized by $^1$H NMR spectra, the measurement was conducted at room temperature and $D_2O/CD_3CN$ = 1/1 (v/v) was used as solvent (Fig. 12).

## 4.12 Synthesis of G4-RT2

1. The mixture of Boc-Arg(Tos)-OH, EDCI, and HOBT was dissolved in methanol and stirred for 2 h at room temperature.
2. G4 PAMAM was dissolved in methanol, then G4 PAMAM solution and DIPEA were added and stirred for 7 days at room temperature.
3. The mixture solution was dialyzed, freeze-dried, the white solid was obtained. Next, the white solid was dissolved in TFA and stirred for 4 h at room temperature. Then precipitated with anhydrous ether, filtered and dried under vacuum, dialyzed for 72 h and freeze-dried, the white solid was obtained.
4. The product was characterized by $^1$H NMR spectra, the measurement was conducted at room temperature and $D_2O$ was used as solvent (Fig. 13).

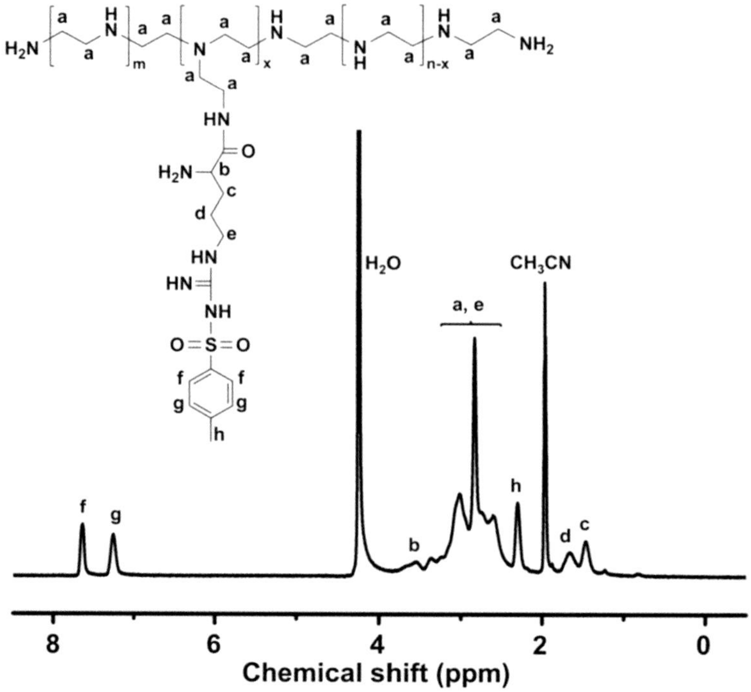


**Fig. 12** [1]H NMR spectrum of PEI25k-RT (400 MHz, $CD_3CN/D_2O$ (v/v = 1/1)). (Adapted from Fang et al. 2018, with permission)

## 4.13 Preparation of Polymer/DNA Nanoparticles

1. PLL-RT4/DNA complexes were prepared by mixing 0.1 mg/mL of DNA aqueous solution with 0.25 mg/mL of PLL-RT4 aqueous solution in equal volume. After 20 s vortex and 20 min incubation at room temperature, PLL-RT4/DNA complexes at mass ratio of 2.5/1 was obtained. Other polycations/DNA complexes were prepared in the similar way.
2. The preparation of PLL-RT4/DNA complexes at different pH values (pH 7.4, 6.8, and 6.0) was similar to the above method, the difference only lies in the pH values of aqueous solution.

## 4.14 Measurements of Zeta Potential and Particle Size

1. Zeta potential and particle size of PLL-RT4/DNA and other carrier/DNA complexes were measured at room temperature by zeta potential/BI-90Plus particle size analyzer (Brookhaven, USA).
2. Morphological characterization of PLL-RT4/DNA and PLL/DNA complexes were observed by scanning electron microscopy (SEM) containing XL-30ESEM-FEG SEM system (SEI, USA) (Figs. 14 and 15).

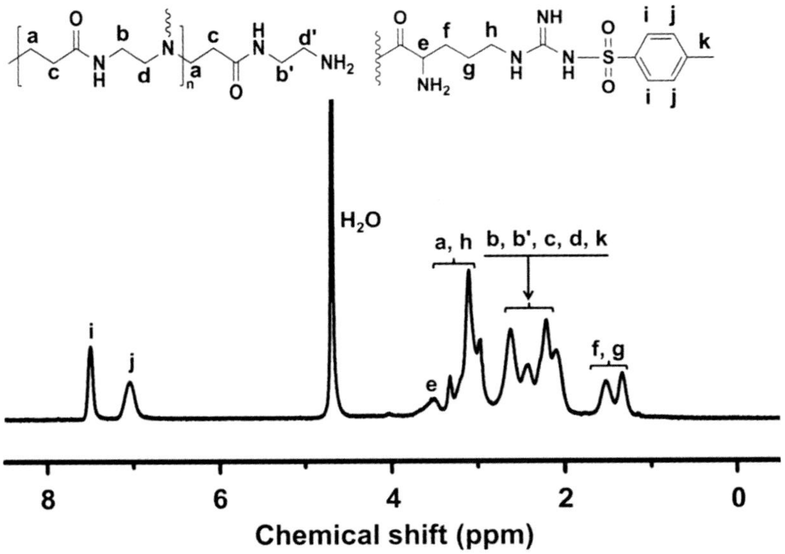


**Fig. 13** [1]H NMR spectrum of G4 PAMAM-RT (400 MHz, $D_2O$). (Adapted from Fang et al. 2018, with permission)

## 4.15 Determination of Molecular Weight and Molecular Weight Distribution

1. Gel permeation chromatography (GPC) was used to measure the molecule weight (Mn) and molecular weight distribution (PDI) of PLL and 0.5 mol/L of $CH_3COONa/CH_3COOH$ as the eluent.
2. The molecular weight of PLL was calibrated with mPEG2k (Fig. 16).

## 4.16 In Situ Surface-Enhanced Infrared Absorption Spectroscopy (SEIRAS)

1. A thin gold film was deposited on the surface of a triangular silicon prism by chemical deposition.
2. The gold-coated prism was put into a polytrifluorochloroethylene cell.
3. All spectra were recorded in a spectral range from 4000 to 800 $cm^{-1}$ and a resolution of 4 $cm^{-1}$ using an FTIR spectrometer by a liquid nitrogen-cooled MCT detector.
4. Cardiolipin was dissolved with chloroform, the solvent was removed under a $N_2$ stream to form a thin lipid layer on the glass vial. The film was dried under vacuum and hydrated and re-suspended in vial containing deionized water to yield a final concentration at 1 mg/mL by vortex, then the solution was sonicated until it was clear. Then the solution was centrifuged for 20 min at 12000 rpm to remove the metal particles, then stored at 4 °C.

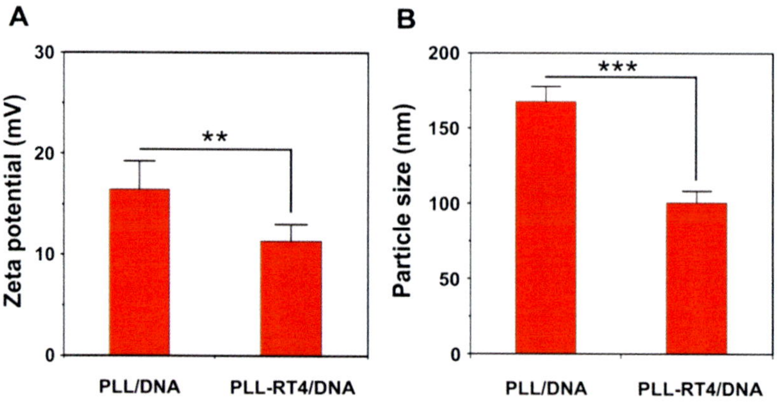


**Fig. 14** (**a**) Zeta potential and (B) particle size of PLL/DNA and PLL-RT4/DNA. (Adapted from Fang et al. 2018, with permission)

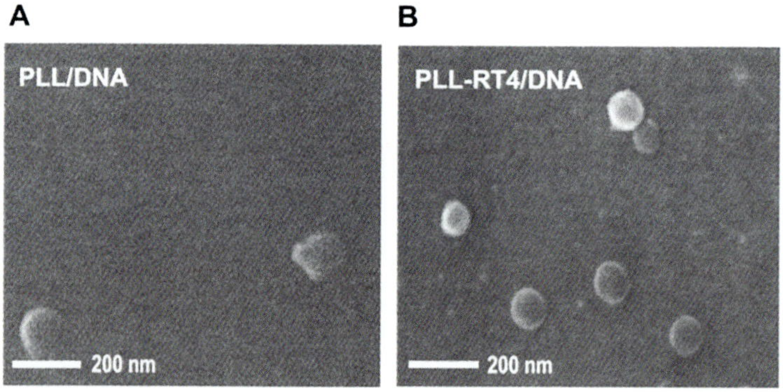


**Fig. 15** SEM images of (**a**) PLL/DNA and (B) PLL-RT4/DNA.. (Adapted from Fang et al. 2018, with permission)

5. A prepared gold film was immersed into 1 mmol/L 1-dodecanethiol (ethanol as solvent) overnight, then rinsed with ethanol and dried with $N_2$ stream, vesicle solution was added and the final concentration was 0.5 mg/mL to enable formation of planar membrane on the surface by vesicle spreading and fusion. Next, the surface was rinsed with water.
6. A reference spectrum of background solution was recorded before sample spectra were obtained.
7. With the addition of PLL-RT or PLL solution, a series of spectra with interval of 1 min have been recorded. The pH value of the solution used throughout the experiment was adjusted to 7.4 (Figs. 17 and 18).

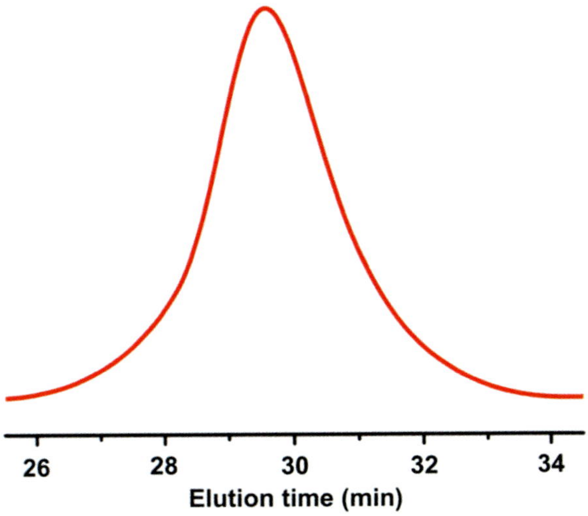


**Fig. 16** GPC trace of PLL (PDI = 1.23). (Adapted from Fang et al. 2018, with permission)

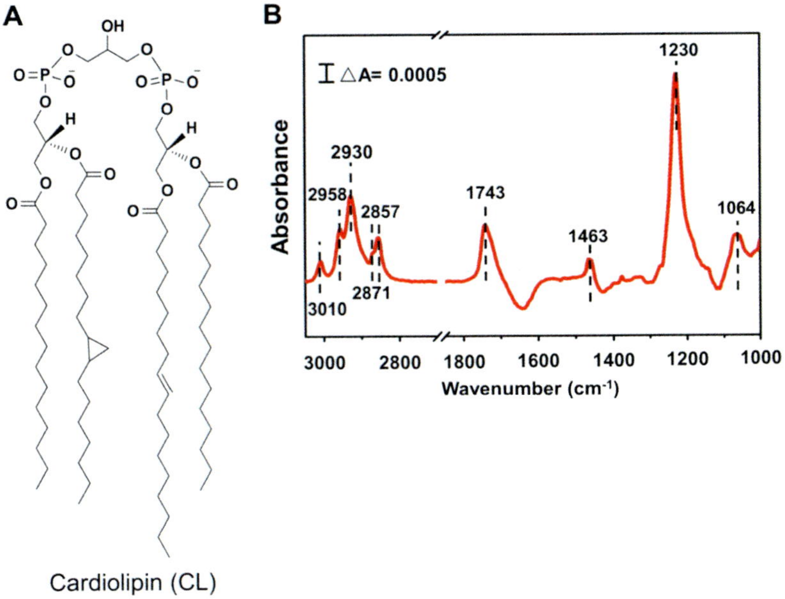


**Fig. 17** (**a**) Molecular structure of cardiolipin and (**b**) cardiolipin induced SEIRA spectra in the aqueous solution. (Adapted from Fang et al. 2018, with permission)

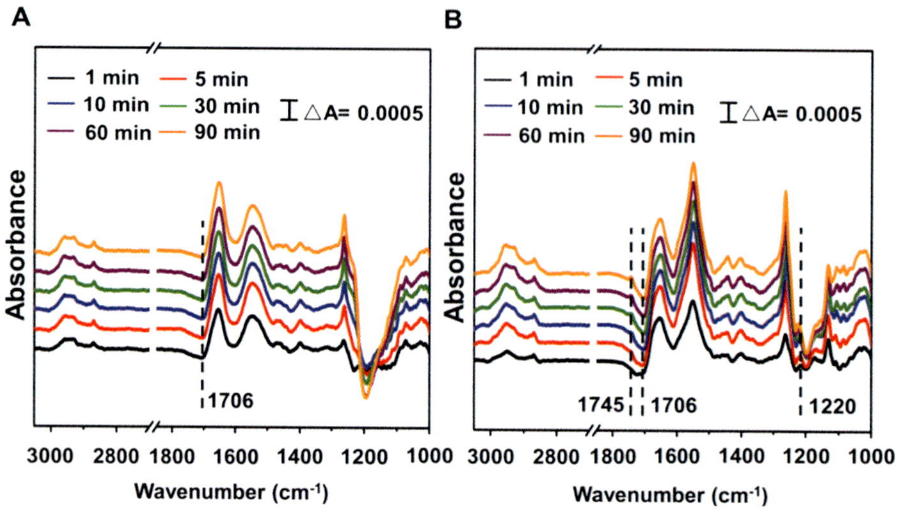


**Fig. 18** (a) PLL or (B) PLL-RT4 induced SEIRA difference spectra of lipid membrane at selected time point in aqueous solution. (Adapted from Fang et al. 2018, with permission)

## 4.17 Isothermal Titration Calorimetry (ITC) Measurement

1. ITC200 (MicroCal) was used to determinate the binding interactions between model molecules (Lys4 and Ly4-RT2) and cardiolipin.
2. Sodium cacodylate solution (0.01 M) was used as buffer. Cardiolipin solution was added into sample cell ($V_{cell}$ = 204.9 μL). Model molecule (Lys4 and Ly4-RT2) solution in a syringe was injected into cardiolipin buffer solution (1 injection of 0.4 μL and 29 more injections of 2 μL each).
3. The duration of each injection was 4 s, and the interval between each injection was 120 s. The injector stirred the buffer solution at rate of 1000 rpm.
4. Calorimetric data was analyzed by Origin 7.0 software (MicroCal) and the temperature was 25 °C.
5. ITC titration was conducted as follows: (1) titration of Lys4 or Lys4-RT2 with cardioplin buffer solution, (2) titration of Lys4 or Lys4-RT2 with buffer solution (blank). The titration procedure of Lys4 or Lys4-RT2 titrating into DNA was similar to the procedure of Lys4 or Lys4-RT2 titrating into cardiolipin (Figs. 19 and 20).

## 4.18 Measurement of Circular Dichroism (CD) Spectra

1. The CD spectra of PLL, PLL-RT4, and control polycations were detected with J-815 CD spectrometer (JACS, Easton, MD, USA) (Fig. 21).

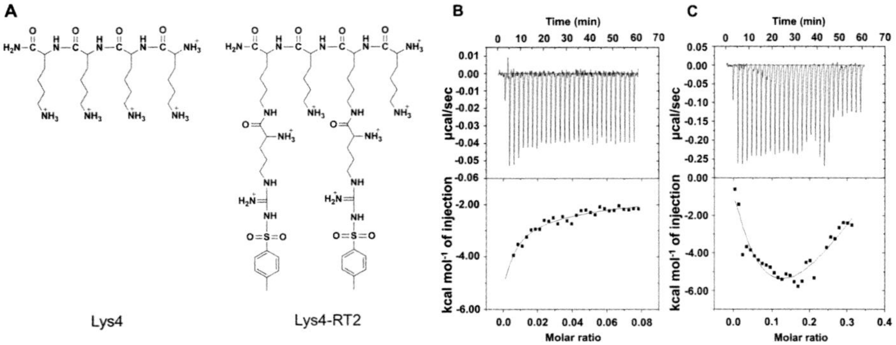

**Fig. 19** **(a)** Molecular structure of model molecules. ITC curves obtained by titrating **(b)** Lys4 or **(c)** Lys4-RT2 into DNA in sodium cacodylate buffer (0.01 M) at pH 7.4 and 25 °C. (Adapted from Fang et al. 2018, with permission)

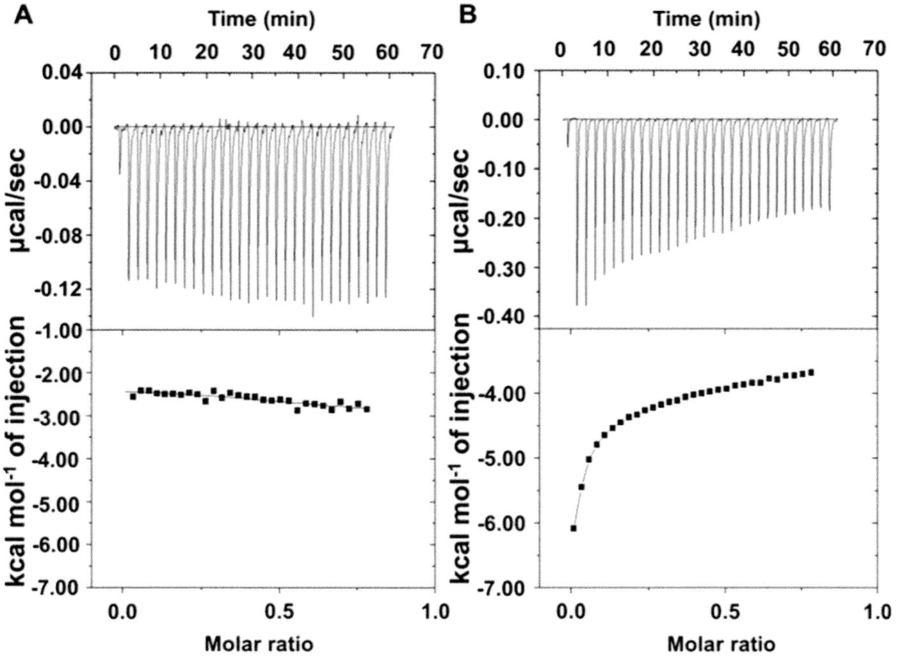

**Fig. 20** ITC curves obtained by titrating **(a)** Lys4 or **(b)** Lys4-RT2 into cardiolipin in sodium cacodylate buffer (0.01 M) at pH 7.4 and 25 °C. (Adapted from Fang et al. 2018, with permission)

2. The concentration of all the samples solution were 0.1 mg/mL, and solution was adjusted to the specific pH value (pH 7.4, 6.8, or 6.0).
3. The mean residue molar ellipticity of polymers was calculated based on the following

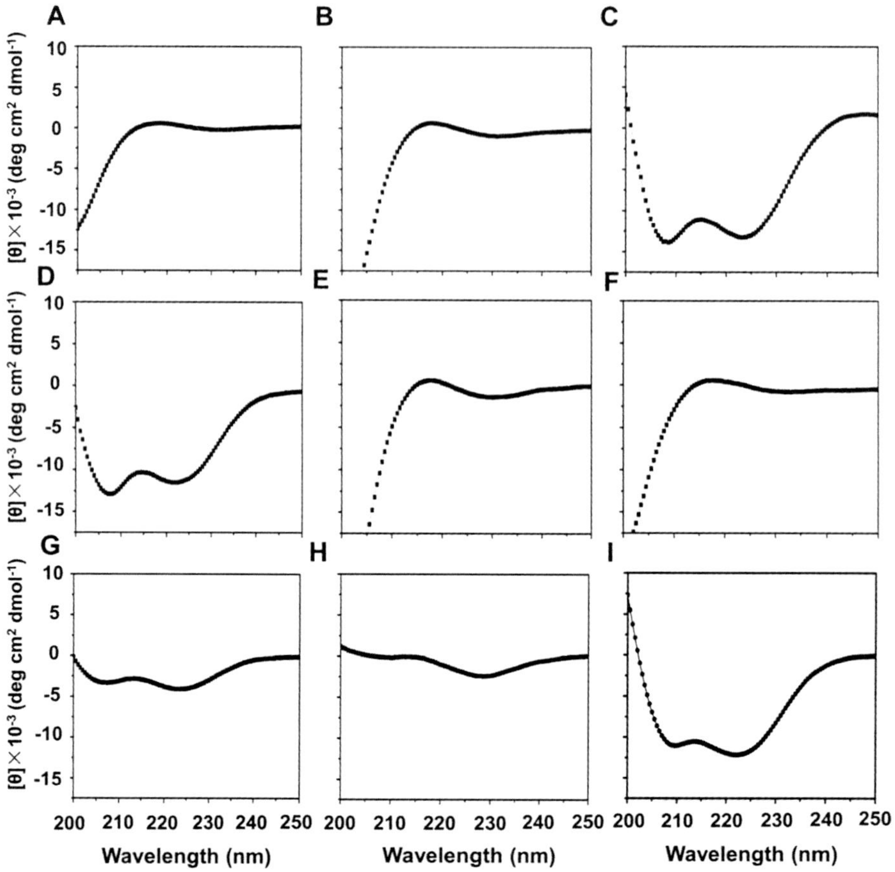


**Fig. 21** The CD spectra of polymers containing different "molecular strings" in aqueous solution. **(a)** PLL, **(b)** PLL-MS, **(c)** PLL-Too, (D) PLL-Tos, (E) PLL-Orn, (F)PLL-Arg, (G) PLL-Orn(Tos), (H) PLL-Arg ($NO_2$), and (I) PLL-RT4. (Adapted from Fang et al. 2018, with permission)

$$\text{formulas : Ellipticity } \left([\theta] \text{ in deg.cm}^2/\text{dmol}\right) = (\text{millidegrees} \times \text{mean residue weight})/(\text{path length in millimeters} \times \text{concentrations of polypeptide in mg/mL}).$$

## 4.19 Cell Culture

1. MCF-7 cells, HeLa cells, and B16F10 cells were cultured with DMEM medium containing 10% (v/v) FBS at 37 °C in 5% (v/v) carbon dioxide ($CO_2$) (Thermo Forma, USA).
2. CT26 cells cultured with RPMI 1640 medium containing 10% (v/v) FBS at 37 °C in 5% (v/v) carbon dioxide ($CO_2$) (Thermo Forma, USA).

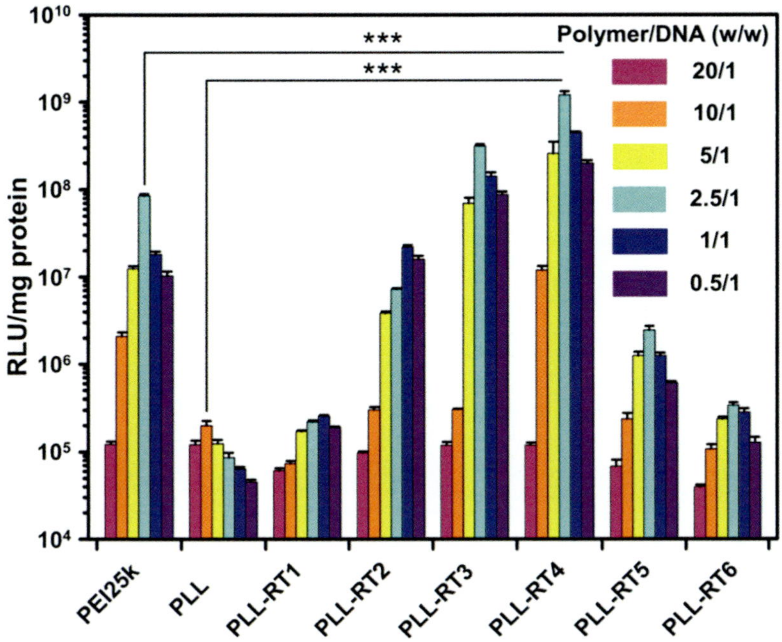


**Fig. 22** Transfection efficiency of PLL-RTs in MCF-7 cells, PEI25k, and PLL were included as control. (Adapted from Fang et al. 2018, with permission)

## 4.20 In Vitro DNA Transfection

1. Luciferase plasmid DNA (pGL3) was used as reporter gene. MCF-7 cells (or other kinds of cell lines) were seeded in 96-well plate at a density of $10^4$ cells per well and cultured at 37 °C in 5% $CO_2$ overnight.
2. Carrier/pGL3 complexes with various mass ratios (20:1, 10:1, 5:1, 2.5:1, 1:1) were added into 96-well plate and incubated for 48 h. Afterwards, the cells were lysed with cell lysate and frozen at −80 °C for 30 min. After melting, the luciferase substrate was added.
3. The relative light units (RLU) were measured by luminometer and normalized to total protein content (BCA protein assay kit, Sigma). Luciferase activity was expressed as RLU/mg protein) (Figs. 22 and 23).

## 4.21 Flow Cytometry Assay

1. Cellular uptake efficiency of carrier/DNA complexes was determined by flow cytometry assay. Cells were seeded in 12-well plates at a density of $10^5$ cells per well and cultured at 37 °C in 5% $CO_2$ overnight.

2. Carrier/Cy5-DNA complexes were added into 12-well plates and incubated for 3 h, then cells were digested, centrifuged, and washed three times with PBS. The cells were tested with Guava EasyCyte low cytometer.
3. For the cellular uptake of carrier/Cy5-DNA complexes at different pH values, the difference only lay in the culture medium at different pH values before the addition of carrier/Cy5-DNA complexes.

## 4.22 CLSM to Observe the Cellular Uptake

1. Cells were seeded in 6-well plates containing coverslip at a density of $10^5$ cells per well and cultured at 37 °C in 5% $CO_2$ overnight.
2. PLL-RT4/Cy5-DNA complexes (or PLL/Cy5-DNA complexes) were added into 6-well plates and incubated for 3 h. Then cells were washed three times with PBS and fixed with 4% paraformaldehyde for 10 min at room temperature. Cell nucleus was stained with DAPI for 10 min at room temperature. Cell membrane was stained with Alexa Fluor 488 phalloidin at 37 °C for 30 min.
3. Finally, coverslips were taken out carefully and put on the glass slides, enclosed with glycerol, and observed by CLSM.

## 4.23 CLSM to Observe Endosomal Escape

1. Cells were seeded in 6-well plates containing coverslip at a density of $10^5$ cells per well and cultured at 37 °C in 5% $CO_2$ overnight.
2. PLL-RT4/Cy5-DNA complexes (or PLL/Cy5-DNA complexes) were added into 6-well plates and incubated for 1, 3, and 6 h.
3. Then cells were washed three times with PBS and fixed with 4% paraformaldehyde for 10 min at room temperature. Nucleus was stained with DAPI for 10 min, and endosome was stained with Lysotracker Green.
4. Coverslips were taken out carefully and put on the glass slides, enclosed with glycerol, and observed by CLSM, the correlation coefficient R values were obtained from CLSM images (ZEN software).

## 4.24 Cytotoxicity Assay

1. Cells were seeded in 96-well plates at a density of $10^4$ cells per well and cultured at 37 °C in 5% $CO_2$ overnight.
2. Carrier/pGL3 complexes at various mass ratios (20:1, 10:1, 5:1, 2.5:1, 1:1) were added into 96-well plates and incubated for 48 h. Then MTT was added and incubated for 4 h.

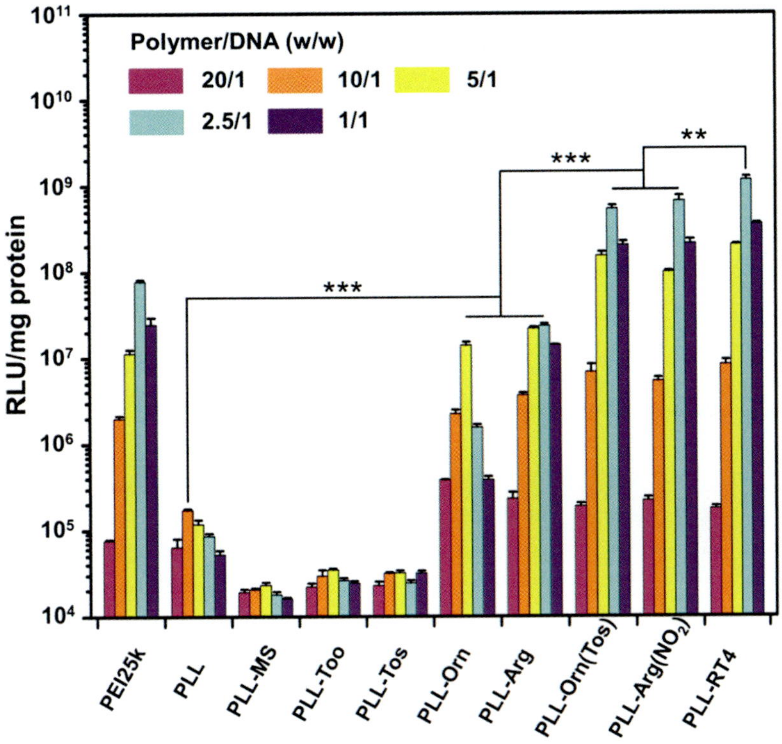


**Fig. 23** DNA transfection of PLL grafted with different types of "molecular strings" in MCF-7 cells. (Adapted from Fang et al. 2018, with permission)

3. After that, the solution was removed and DMSO was added to dissolve the formazan crystals. The samples were determined with a Bio-Rad 680 microplate reader at 492 nm.
4. Cell viability (%) was calculated by this equation: cell viability (%) = ($A_{sample}$/$A_{control}$) × 100, where $A_{sample}$ was the absorbance of sample well and $A_{control}$ was the absorbance of control well.

## 4.25 Antiserum Transfection

1. The antiserum ability was studied by evaluating the transfection efficiency in serum containing media.
2. The antiserum transfection assay was similar to in vitro DNA transfection. The only difference was that the culture medium was replaced with culture medium containing different percentages of FBS (10%, 30%, 50%, 70%, and 90%) before the addition of carrier/pDNA complexes.

## 4.26 In Vitro Gene Silencing

1. Huh-7 Luc cells were seeded in 96-well plates at a density of $10^4$ cells/well and incubated for 24 h.
2. Carrier/siRNA complexes were added into 96-well plates and incubated for 48 h, then cells were lysed with cell lysate and frozen at −80 °C for 30 min. After melting, the luciferase substrate was added.
3. The relative light units (RLU) were measured by luminometer and normalized to total protein content (BCA protein assay kit, Sigma). (Luciferase activity was expressed as RLU/mg protein).

## 4.27 Construction of Tumor Model

1. CT26 cells were large-scale expanded in culture medium and collected in PBS. Cell suspensions were injected into the left armpit of BABL/c mice.
2. Tumor growth was monitored and tumor bearing mice (average tumor volume, 100 mm3) were randomly divided into four groups: PBS, shVEGF, PLL/shVEGF, PLL-RT4/shVEGF.

## 4.28 Antitumor Treatment

1. PLL-RT4/shVEGF complexes and control groups were intratumorally injected every other day into tumor-bearing mice for six times (Fig. 24).
2. Body weight and tumor size were measured every other day, and the tumor growth was observed for 2 weeks.

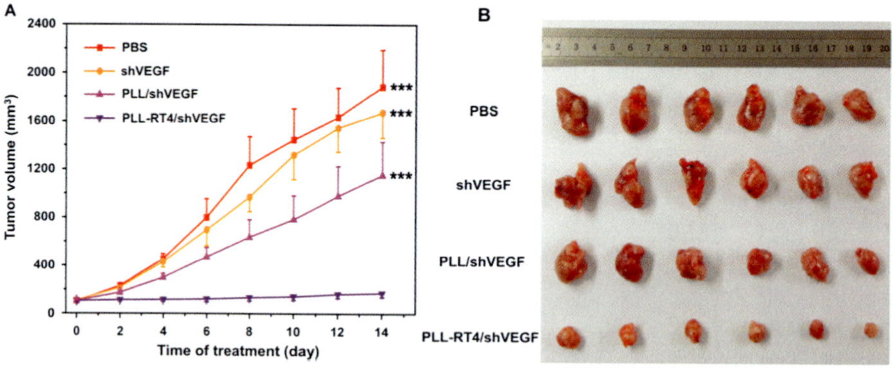


**Fig. 24** **(a)** Changes of tumor volume of BABL/c mice administered with PBS, shVEGF, PLL/shVEGF, and PLL-RT4/shVEGF. **(b)** Images of excised tumors at the end of treatment. (Adapted from Fang et al. 2018, with permission)

3. After treatment, the animals were euthanized, and the major organs (heart, liver, spleen, lung, and kidney) and tumor were collected for the further analysis.

## 4.29 Histological Analyses

1. The major organs (heart, liver, spleen, lung, and kidney) and tumors were collected and the sections were stained by H&E for pathological analysis.
2. The samples were observed with optical microscope.

## 4.30 Immunofluorescent Staining for Tumor Vessels

1. The tumor tissues were embedded in paraffin and bound with anti-CD31 antibody and FITC-labeled secondary antibody for immunofluorescence analysis of tumor vessels.
2. The samples were observed with CLSM.

## 4.31 qRT-PCR Assay

1. Tumor tissue (100 mg) of each group was ground up with mortar under liquid nitrogen and RNA was extracted with 1 mL of Trizol.
2. The RNA was reversely transcribed to cDNA by Prime Script® RT reagent kit with gDNA Eraser (Perfect Real Time) according to the specification.
3. Real-time PCR experiment was carried out by SYBR® Premix Ex Taq™ II (Tli RNaseH Plus) according to the specification.
4. The primers for VEGF: Forward, 5‘-GGT GAG AGG TCT AGT TCC CGA-3’; Reverse, 5‘-CCA TGA ACT TTC TGC TCT TC-3’. The primers for GAPDH: Forward, 5‘-GTT CCA GTA TGA CTC TAC CC-3’; Reverse, 5‘-AGT CTT CTG AGG CAG TGA TG-3’.
5. The amplification condition was as follows: pre-denaturated at 95 °C for 30 s. conducted 40 cycles of denaturation at 95 °C for 5 s, annealed at 58 °C for 34 s, and amplificated at 72 °C for 30 s with Mx3005P instrument.

## 4.32 Elisa

1. The tumor tissues were homogenized. The supernatants of tumor tissues were added into the plate together with anti-VEGF antibody and streptomycin-HRP and incubated for 60 min at 37 °C.
2. After washing for five times with washing buffer, chromogenic reaction was carried out and then stop buffer was added.
3. The OD value was obtained under 450 nm by a Tecan infinite M200 Microplate Readers.

4. According to the protocol, the standard sample was diluted into different concentrations of gradients and a calibration curve was obtained for calculating the concentrations of the samples, and the OD value of blank sample was subtracted.

### 4.33 Statistical Analysis

1. All measurements were carried out in triplicate and presented as mean ± standard deviation.
2. Student's t-test was conducted to compare the statistical significance. Statistical significance was set at $*p < 0.05$, $**p < 0.01$, and $***p < 0.001$ were deemed extremely significant.

## 5 Conclusion

This chapter describes an efficient strategy of introducing "molecular string" RT to traditional gene carriers, which can significantly improve the transfection efficiency and reduce the cytotoxicity. "RT string" grafted onto PLL introduces multiple interactions (i.e., electrostatic interaction, hydrogen bonding interaction, and hydrophobic interaction) between polycation and cell membrane or DNA. Additionally, PLL grafted with "RT string" adopts α-helix conformation, which is also helpful for gene transfection by improving the cellular uptake. "RT string" introduced into PEI25k and PAMAM can also improve the transfection efficiency and lower the cytotoxicity. Finally, in vivo experiment shows that PLL-RT4/shVEGF has an excellent antitumor effect and negligible pathological abnormalities. This work provides an ideal strategy for constructing polycationic gene carriers with high transfection efficiency and low cytotoxicity. More polycations modified by introducing RT string will be developed for researching high-performance gene carriers in the future.

## References

Akinc A, Thomas M, Klibanov AM, Langer RJ (2005) Genet Med 7:657–663
Choi YH, Liu F, Kim JS, Choi YK, Park JS, Kim SWJ (1998) Controlled Release 54:39–48
Cross D, Burmester JK (2006) Clin Med Res 4:218–227
Fang H, Guo Z, Lin L, Chen J, Sun P, Wu J, Xu C, Tian H, Chen X (2018) J Am Chem Soc 140:11992–12000
Gabrielson NP, Lu H, Yin L, Li D, Wang F, Cheng J (2012) Angew Chem Int Ed 51:1143–1147
Guo X, Huang L (2012) Acc Chem Res 45:971–979
Gutierrez AA, Lemoine NR, Sikora K (1992) Lancet 339:715–721
Kim TI, Baek JU, Bai CZ, Park JS (2007) Biomaterials 28:2061–2067
Kim J, Park J, Kim H, Singha K, Kim WJ (2013) Biomaterials 34:7168–7180
Kukowska Latallo JF, Bielinska AU, Johnson J, Spindler R, Tomalia DA, Baker JR (1996) Proc Natl Acad Sci U S A 93:4897–4902
Li M, Schlesiger S, Knauer SK, Schmuck C (2015) Angew Chem Int Ed 54:2941–2944

Liu X, Xiang J, Zhu D, Jiang L, Zhou Z, Tang J, Liu X, Huang Y, Shen Y (2016) Adv Mater 28:1743–1752
Liu Z, Zhang Z, Zhou C, Jiao Y (2010) Prog Polym Sci 35:1144–1162
Sun CY, Shen S, Xu CF, Li HJ, Liu Y, Cao ZT, Yang XZ, Xia JX, Wang J(2015) J Am Chem Soc 137:15217–15224
Tang MX, Redemann CT, Szoka FC (1996) Bioconjug Chem 7:703–714
Verma IM, Somia N (1997) Nature 389:239–242
Wang M, Liu H, Li L, Cheng Y (2014) Nat Commun 5:3053–3060
Wang H, Wang Y, Wang Y, Hu J, Li T, Liu H, Zhang Q, Cheng Y (2015) Angew Chem Int Ed 54:11647–11651
Weichselbaum RR, Kufe D (1997) Lancet 349:S10–S12
Yin L, Tang H, Kim KH, Zheng N, Song Z, Gabrielson NP, Lu H, Cheng J (2013) Angew Chem Int Ed 52:9182–9186

# Charge/Size Dual-Rebound Gene Delivery System

**2**

Xiuwen Guan, Huayu Tian, and Xuesi Chen

## Contents



X. Guan
College of Pharmacy, Weifang Medical University, Weifang, China
e-mail: gxw2603@wfmc.edu.cn

H. Tian (✉) · X. Chen
Key Laboratory of Polymer Ecomaterials, Changchun Institute of Applied Chemistry, Chinese Academy of Sciences, Changchun, China
e-mail: thy@ciac.ac.cn; xschen@ciac.ac.cn



H. Tian and X. Chen (eds.), *Gene Delivery*, Biomaterial Engineering,
https://doi.org/10.1007/978-981-16-5419-0_11

**Abstract**

This chapter presents a facile strategy for constructing an ultrasensitive pH-triggered charge/size dual-rebound gene delivery system for cancer therapy. Therapeutic gene was condensed by polycation polyethylenimine (PEI) and polyanion poly-L-glutamate (PLG), further in situ tightened by aldehyde-modified polyethylene glycol (PEG) via Schiff-base reaction. The Schiff-base bonds were stable in neutral physiological pH but cleavable in acidic tumor extracellular pH. The gene delivery system possessed the following highlights: (1) this tunable gene delivery system was prepared by a chemical bench-free "green" and fast process which would be favored by the majority of users, (2) PEG shielded the positive surface charges and tightened the gene-loaded complex particles, leading to decreased systemic cytotoxicity, improved stability, and prolonged in vivo circulation, (3) PEG shielding was rapidly peeled off by acidic pH as soon as stepping into tumor area, and (4) the higher positive surface potential and bigger size after the ultrasensitive charge/size dual-rebounding was contributing to realize highly enhanced tumor cellular uptake. Superior antitumor efficacy was achieved when an anti-angiogenesis gene–targeted vascular endothelial growth factor (VEGF) was loaded in the charge/size dual-rebound gene delivery system as a model therapeutic gene for treating CT26 colonic tumors in mice. The charge/size dual-rebound gene delivery system displayed great potential for cancer therapy.

**Keywords**

Gene delivery system · Cancer therapy · Ultrasensitive pH response · Charge/size dual-rebound · PEG shielding · Aldehyde modification · Schiff base · Polyethylenimine · VEGF

## 1 Overview

Gene therapy has been one of the most prospective approaches for cancer treatment (Hatakeyama et al. 2007; Cring and Sheffield 2020). The past few decades have witnessed the rapid development of various polycationic gene delivery systems with good safety and multifunctionality (Merdan et al. 2002; Morille et al. 2008; Tian et al. 2012; Chen et al. 2018). As a negatively charged biomacromolecule, gene can be condensed by positively charged polycations via electrostatic interactions and formed complex nanoparticles (NPs) (Liu et al. 2015). The NPs have to overcome many biological barriers to perform gene transfection in the targeted cells (Kircheis et al. 2001; Lima et al. 2001). The complicated in vitro and in vivo delivery process demands the NPs possessing different adaptative properties in coping with different delivery phases. However, these requirements are usually ineluctably contradictory (Sun et al. 2014). For example, the NPs with low positive charges or negative charges have advantages for maintaining stability and decreasing nonspecific adsorptions in circulation, but these NPs are not favorable for tumor cell attaching and cellular uptake (Pearce et al. 2012; Xu et al. 2011; Jin et al. 2013). On the other hand, the size of the NPs is also under different preference. Smaller size will be conducive to long circulation, and appropriately bigger size is proven to be helpful for cellular uptake (Liang et al. 2015; Tasciotti et al. 2008). In another case, PEGylation can improve the in vivo circulation time of NPs, but it also compromises tumor cell uptake (Dufort et al. 2012; Mishra et al. 2004; Hatakeyama et al. 2011). Meanwhile, the NPs are awaited to exhibit lower cell uptake in normal cells but higher uptake in tumor cells. These intractable dilemmas have put forward more difficult requirements to the design of practical and efficient gene delivery systems.

To coordinate the above dilemmas, many strategies have been developed (Shetty et al. 2020; Deng et al. 2012; Guo and Huang 2011; Du et al. 2010a). A pH-responsive charge-conversional nanogel was proposed in Wang's work. The nanogel was negatively charged at physiological pH, but it became positively charged in acidic tumor extracellular pH. This charge conversion could facilitate cell uptake and drug release, which realized prominent tumor suppression (Du et al. 2010b). In Gu's study, a dendritic lipopeptide-based gene delivery system with charge-tunable shielding was developed (Zhang et al. 2015). The system presented negatively charged surface in normal pH during circulation, and further transformed into positively charged in tumor extracellular pH. In another study, Zhou's group reported a novel size-changeable nanocarrier (Guo et al. 2015). The micelles were small in normal physiological conditions. At acidic tumor area, the micelles had increased size and further readily internalized by tumor cells. Furthermore, the micelles could be changed much smaller after endosomes escape under the elevated glutathione (GSH) concentration in the cytoplasm. The smaller-sized NPs easily entered into cell nuclei and released the cargos. In the research of Wang's work (Sun et al. 2016), tumor-pH-labile polymeric NPs were developed. The PEGylated NPs shown long circulation and lowered cell uptake in normal cells. When at acidic tumor tissue, PEG was detached from the NPs leading to the exposure of the amino groups with positive zeta potential, which would facilitate tumor cellular uptake and improved the in vivo tumor inhibition rate. There were many similar studies; however, these strategies only focused on one or two dilemmas, while most of them inevitably involved complicated and tedious synthesis and preparations. Therefore, it will be really encouraging to design a comprehensive solution covering all the dilemmas by a simple and convenient method. A gene delivery system which is adaptive for different phases in the delivery process is highly desirable.

This protocol provides a facile coping strategy for the different requirements during transportation process by an ultrasensitive pH-triggered charge/size dual-rebound gene delivery system (Guan et al. 2016). Therapeutic gene was condensed by PEI and PLG via electrostatic interaction. The generated gene-loaded complex NPs were further tightened by aldehyde-modified PEG through the in situ Schiff-base reaction between the aldehyde groups on both terminal of PEG and the amino groups of PEI. The Schiff-base reaction could rapidly progress in neutral or alkaline aqueous solution with high efficiency. The Schiff-base bonds between PEG and PEI were stable in physiological pH 7.4, but labile and cleavable in the slightly acidic tumor extracellular pH (Fig. 1).

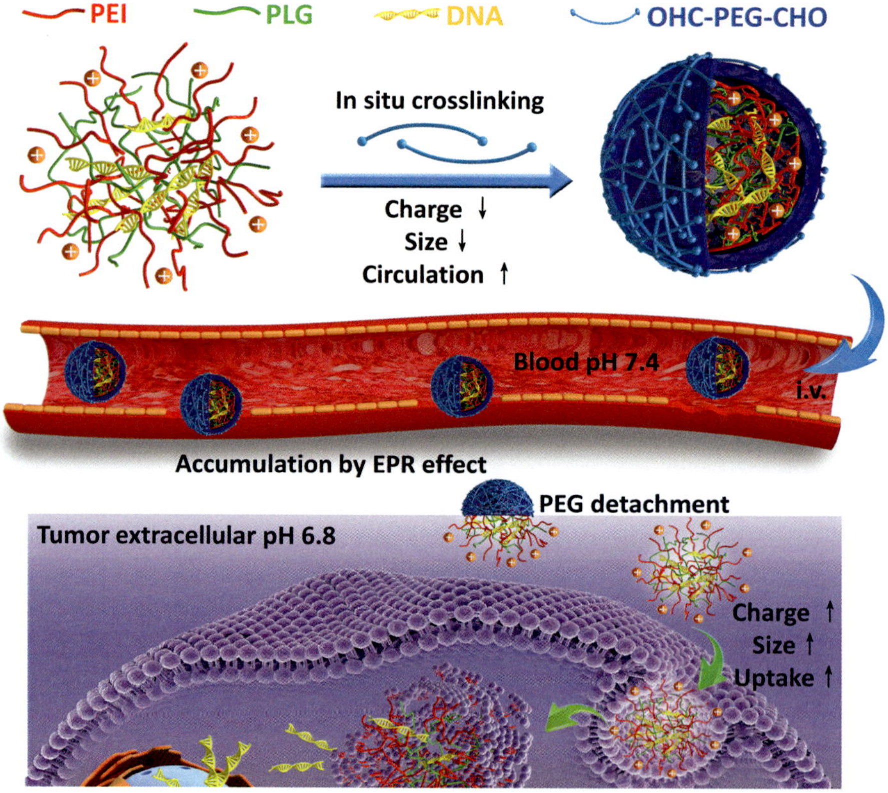


**Fig. 1** The schematic of the ultrasensitive pH-triggered charge/size dual-rebound gene delivery system. (Adapted from Guan et al. 2016, with permission)

Moreover, the acidic stimuli response of this ultra-pH-sensitive Schiff-base bonds was much faster than that of the most reported acidic cleavable chemical bonds (Ko et al. 2007; Liu et al. 2014; Prabaharan et al. 2009; Bae et al. 2003), which would facilitate the rapid detachment of PEG shielding. The ultrasensitive pH-triggered charge/size dual-rebound gene delivery system was proved to possess the following favorable properties: (1) Fast and efficient Schiff-base reaction was recruited to in situ strengthen the gene complex NPs in organic solvent-free system, constructing a facile gene delivery system with tunable PEG density and crosslinking degree. (2) PEG shielded the positive surface charges and tighten the complex NPs, leading to decreased systemic cytotoxicity, improved stability, and prolonged circulation. (3) PEG deshielding was rapidly triggered by acidic tumor extracellular pH, accelerating further tumor cellular uptake. (4) Charge/size dual-rebounding to higher positive potential and bigger size enhanced tumor uptake efficiency. In the following protocol, the material synthesis, gene delivery system preparation, and characterization were mentioned in detail. A plasmid DNA (*p*DNA) expressed small hairpin RNA (shRNA) targeting vascular endothelial growth factor (VEGF) that was loaded in the system to verify the antitumor therapeutic efficacy in vivo. This ultrasensitive pH-triggered charge/size dual-rebound gene delivery system has presented excellent therapeutic efficacy and great potential for cancer therapy.

## 2 Materials

### 2.1 Synthesis and Characterization of Poly-L-Glutamate (PLG)

1. N-Hexylamine
2. N-Carboxyanhydride of γ-benzyl-L-glutamate (BLG-NCA, GL Biochem Ltd., Shanghai, China)
3. Chloroform ($CHCl_3$)
4. Diethyl ether
5. Hydrobromic acid (HBr)
6. Dichloroacetic acid
7. Bruker AV-400 NMR spectrometer (Bruker, Ettlingen, Germany)
8. Trifluoroacetic acid-d ($CF_3COOD$)

### 2.2 Synthesis of Aldehyde Group Modified PEG (OHC-PEG-CHO) and Characterization

1. PEG (Mw = 2,000 Da, Aldrich)
2. 4-Carboxybenzaldehyde (Aladdin, Shanghai, China)
3. EDC·HCl
4. DMAP
5. Dichloromethane (DCM)
6. Rotary evaporator
7. NaCl

8. Anhydrous magnesium sulfate
9. Diethyl ether
10. Bruker AV-300 NMR spectrometer (Bruker, Ettlingen, Germany)
11. Chloroform-d ($CDCl_3$)
12. $D_2O$

## 2.3 Preparation of NPs

1. Deionized water
2. PEI (Mw = 25,000 Da, Aldrich)
3. Calf thymus DNA (Sigma, St. Louis, MO, USA)
4. Vortex finder
5. PLG
6. OHC-PEG-CHO

## 2.4 Zeta Potential, Particle Size, and Morphology

1. PEI/DNA (PD) NPs
2. PLG/(PEI/DNA) (G(PD)) NPs
3. (PLG/PEI)/DNA ((GP)D) NPs
4. PEG[(PLG/PEI)/DNA] (P[(GP)D]) NPs
5. $H_2O$
6. HCl
7. NaOH
8. Zeta potential/BI-90Plus particle size analyzer (Brookhaven, USA)
9. JEM-1200EX TEM system (NEC, Tokyo, Japan)
10. 200-mesh carbon-coated copper grid

## 2.5 In Vitro DNA Transfection

1. Mouse colon carcinoma (CT26) cell line
2. Dulbecco's modified Eagle's medium (DMEM) culture medium (Gibco, Grand Island, USA)
3. Fetal bovine serum (FBS, Gibco, Grand Island, USA)
4. Cell incubator
5. Luciferase plasmid DNA (*p*GL3-control, Promega, Mannheim, Germany)
6. 96-well plates
7. (GP)D NPs at various mass ratios
8. P[(GP)D] NPs at various mass ratios
9. Luciferase reporter gene assay kit (Promega, Mannheim, Germany)
10. Luminometer (Turner Biosystems & Promega)
11. BCA protein assay

## 2.6 Cytotoxicity Assay

1. CT26 cells
2. 96-well plates
3. PD NPs
4. G(PD) NPs
5. (GP)D NPs
6. P[(GP)D] NPs
7. DMEM culture medium
8. Cell incubator
9. Methyl thiazolyl tetrazolium (MTT, Amresco, Solon, Ohio, USA)
10. Dimethyl sulfoxide (DMSO)
11. Bio-Rad 680 microplate reader

## 2.7 Cell Uptake

1. CT26 cells
2. Six-well plates
3. Cyanine 5 labeled DNA (Cy5-DNA, RiboBio, Guangzhou, China)
4. PD NPs
5. G(PD) NPs
6. (GP)D NPs
7. P[(GP)D] NPs
8. DMEM culture medium
9. Cell incubator
10. Guava EasyCyte flow cytometer (Guava Technologies)

## 2.8 Confocal Laser Scanning Microscopy (CLSM)

1. CT26 cells
2. Coverslips
3. Six-well plates
4. Cy5-DNA
5. PD NPs
6. G(PD) NPs
7. (GP)D NPs
8. P[(GP)D] NPs
9. DMEM culture medium
10. Cell incubator
11. Paraformaldehyde
12. 4′-6-Diamidino-2-phenylindole (DAPI)
13. Alexa Fluor 488 phalloidin
14. Glass slides

15. Glycerol
16. CLSM (ZEISS LSM780, Germany)
17. Cy5 monosuccinimidyl ester (AAT Bioquest, Inc., Sunnyvale, CA, USA)
18. DMSO
19. PEI
20. Cy5-PEI
21. Lyophilizer

## 2.9 Tumor Accumulation

1. CT26 cells
2. BALB/C nude mice (4–5 weeks, female, Vital River Company, Beijing, China)
3. Cy5-DNA
4. Cy5-PEI
5. Phosphate buffered saline (PBS)
6. PD NPs
7. G(PD) NPs
8. (GP)D NPs
9. P[(GP)D] NPs
10. Syringe
11. Pentobarbital sodium
12. Maestro In Vivo Imaging System (Cambridge Research & Instrumentation, Inc., USA)

## 2.10 In Vivo Antitumor Therapeutic Efficacy

1. BALB/C mice (4–5 weeks, female, Vital River Company, Beijing, China)
2. CT26 cells
3. *p*DNA expressed shRNA-VEGF (shVEGF, Sangon, Shanghai, China)
4. PBS
5. PD NPs
6. G(PD) NPs
7. (GP)D NPs
8. P[(GP)D] NPs
9. Syringe
10. Vernier caliper
11. Chemical balance

## 2.11 Histology and Immunofluorescence Analyses

1. Major organs (heart, liver, spleen, lung, and kidney) of mice after therapy
2. Tumors of mice after therapy
3. Hematoxylin-eosin (H&E)

4. Paraffin
5. Ethanol
6. Anti-CD31 antibody
7. FITC-labeled secondary antibody
8. DAPI
9. Glass slides
10. Glycerol
11. CLSM (ZEISS LSM780, Germany)

## 2.12 Photoacoustic Imaging

1. BALB/C nude mice (4–5 weeks, female, Vital River Company, Beijing, China)
2. CT26 cells
3. *p*DNA expressed shRNA-VEGF (shVEGF, Sangon, Shanghai, China)
4. PBS
5. PD NPs
6. G(PD) NPs
7. (GP)D NPs
8. P[(GP)D] NPs
9. Syringe
10. Isoflurane
11. MSOT scanner equipped with 128 ultrasound transducer elements (MSOT inVision 128, iThera Medical GmbH, Munich, Germany)

## 2.13 VEGF Gene Expression

1. Tumor tissues
2. Trizol (Invitrogen, Carlsbad, CA, USA)
3. Centrifuge
4. Prime Script® RT reagent kit with gDNA Eraser (Perfect Real Time) (TaKaRa, Dalian, China)
5. SYBR® Premix Ex Taq™ II (Tli RNaseH Plus) (TaKaRa, Dalian, China)
6. VEGF primers: Forward, 5′-GGT GAG AGG TCT AGT TCC CGA-3′; Reverse, 5′-CCA TGA ACT TTC TGC TCT TC-3′
7. GAPDH primers: Forward, 5′-GTT CCA GTA TGA CTC TAC CC-3′; Reverse, 5′-AGT CTT CTG AGG CAG TGA TG-3′
8. Mx3005P instrument (Stratagene, USA)

## 2.14 Enzyme-Linked Immunosorbent Assay (ELISA)

1. Tumor tissues
2. Centrifuge
3. Homogenizer

4. Mouse VEGF ELISA kit (R&D Systems, Minneapolis, MA, USA)
5. Tecan infinite M200 Microplate Readers (Tecan, Austria)

### 2.15 Western Blot

1. Tumor tissues
2. Cell lysis buffer for Western and IP (KeyGEN, Jiangsu, China)
3. BCA protein assay kit (Thermo Scientific, Rockford, USA)
4. Loading buffer
5. Marker
6. SDS-PAGE equipment
7. PVDF film
8. Bovine serum albumin (BSA)
9. VEGF antibody (Santa Cruz Biotechnology, Santa Cruz, CA, USA)
10. Tubulin antibody (Santa Cruz Biotechnology, Santa Cruz, CA, USA)
11. HRP-labeled second antibody
12. ECL kit (GE, London, UK)

## 3 Methods

### 3.1 Synthesis and Characterization of PLG (Note 1)

1. N-Hexylamine and BLG-NCA were dissolved in 100 mL dried chloroform.
2. The mixture was stirred for 72 h at 30 °C, then deposited with excess diethyl ether and obtained the poly (benzyl-L-glutamate) (PBLG).
3. The final product PLG was obtained by removing the protecting benzyl groups on the PBLG with HBr.
4. The polymer was characterized by $^{1}$H NMR spectra, the measurement was carried out at room temperature, and CF3COOD was used as the solvent.

### 3.2 Synthesis of OHC-PEG-CHO and Characterization (Note 2)

1. PEG (10 g, 5 mmol), 4-carboxybenzaldehyde (2.25 g, 15 mmol), EDC·HCl (9.585 g, 50 mmol), and DMAP (0.244 g, 2 mmol) were dissolved in 150 mL DCM and stirred for 48 h at 25 °C.
2. After the reaction was completed, the solution was concentrated by rotary evaporator, and then the mixture was washed for five times with saturated NaCl solution and another three times with 5% NaCl solution, respectively.
3. The organic layer was collected and 50 ~ 100 g anhydrous magnesium sulfate as dehydration agent was added and stood for about 12 h.

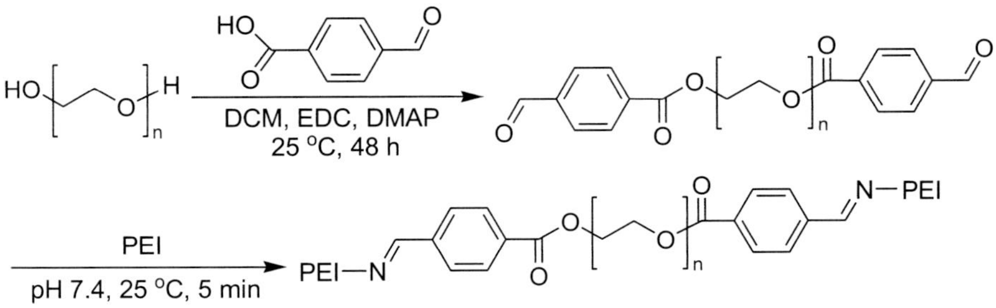


**Fig. 2** The synthesis procedure of OHC-PEG-CHO and the further reaction between OHC-PEG-CHO and PEI

4. After filtration, the filtrate was concentrated and deposited twice with excess diethyl ether.
5. The final product was dried under vacuum at room temperature overnight.
6. The product was characterized by $^1$H NMR spectra in $CDCl_3$.
7. To verify the pH-sensitivity of the reaction between OHC-PEG-CHO and PEI, OHC-PEG-CHO and PEI were dissolved in $D_2O$ (the pH of the solution should be adjusted to 7.4) and reacted for 20 min. Then the pH of the solution was adjusted to different pH values; the $^1$H NMR spectra were detected and analyzed (Fig. 2).

### 3.3 Preparation of NPs (Note 3)

1. **P**EI/**D**NA (PD) complexes were prepared by mixing 0.1 mg/mL DNA aqueous solution with 0.25 mg/mL PEI aqueous solution in equal volume. After 15 s vortex and 20 min incubation at room temperature, the PD complexes with mass ratio of 2.5:1 for PEI/DNA were obtained.
2. PL**G**/(**P**EI/**D**NA) (G(PD)) complexes were prepared by adding 0.125 mg/mL PLG aqueous solution into the preprepared PD solution, also for 15 s vortex and 20 min incubation. G(PD) complexes with mass ratio of 1.25:2.5:1 for PLG/(PEI/DNA) were obtained.
3. (PL**G**/**P**EI)/**D**NA ((GP)D) complexes were prepared by mixing different concentration of PLG aqueous solution with 0.25 mg/mL PEI aqueous solution in equal volume first and incubated at room temperature for 20 min, then 0.1 mg/mL DNA aqueous solution was added. After 15 s vortex and 20 min incubation at room temperature, (GP)D complexes with mass ratio of (0.625 ~ 5):2.5:1 for (PLG/PEI)/DNA were obtained.
4. The PEG crosslinked NPs were further prepared by adding different concentration of OHC-PEG-CHO aqueous solution into the above-prepared (GP)D in pH 7.4 and incubated at room temperature for 5 min. **P**EG[(PL**G**/**P**EI)/**D**NA] (P[(GP)D]) with mass ratio of (2.5 ~ 20):1.25:2.5:1 for PEG[(PLG/PEI)/DNA] was obtained.

### 3.4 Zeta Potential, Particle Size, and Morphology (Note 4)

1. Prepared the PD, G(PD), (GP)D, and P[(GP)D] NPs freshly, and incubated at different pH values (pH 7.4 and 6.8).
2. The zeta potential and particle size of PD, G(PD), (GP)D, and P[(GP)D] NPs were immediately measured at room temperature by zeta potential/BI-90Plus particle size analyzer. Data were shown as mean ± standard deviation (SD) based on triplicate independent experiments.
3. The morphological characteristic of the NPs was observed by transmission electron microscope (TEM), which was operated at 50 kV. A drop of NPs aqueous solution was deposited onto a 200-mesh carbon-coated copper grid, standing at room temperature until the samples completely dried.

### 3.5 In Vitro DNA Transfection (Note 5)

1. CT26 cells were seeded in 96-well plates at a density of 8000 cells/well and then cultured at 37 °C in a 5% $CO_2$ atmosphere for 24 h.
2. The (GP)D NPs at various mass ratios were prepared and added into the plates; the cells were then incubated for 48 h.
3. The P[(GP)D] NPs (with various PEG mass ratios) were prepared. The culture medium (DMEM) in the plates was replaced with 180 μL/well fresh DMEM with different pH values (7.4 and 6.8). After the NPs were added to each well, the plates were returned to the incubator for 2 h. Then culture medium was replaced with 200 μL/well fresh DMEM, and the plates were returned to the incubator for another 46 h.
4. After incubation, 50 μL cell lysate was added to each well and the plates were frozen in −80 °C for 0.5 ~ 1 h.
5. After thawing, the supernatant of the cell lysate (20 μL) was mixed with 100 μL luciferase substrate.
6. The relative light units (RLU) were measured by luminometer and normalized to total protein content measured by BCA protein assay.
7. Luciferase activity was expressed as RLU/mg protein.

### 3.6 Cytotoxicity Assay

1. CT26 cells were seeded in 96-well plates at 8000 cells/well and cultured at 37 °C in a 5% $CO_2$ atmosphere for 24 h.
2. PD, G(PD), (GP)D, and P[(GP)D] NPs were prepared.
3. The plates were taken out and 180 μL/well fresh DMEM in different pH values (7.4 and 6.8) was added. After the NPs were added to each well, the plates were returned to the incubator for 2 h.

4. Then culture medium was replaced with 200 μL/well fresh DMEM, and the plates were returned to the incubator for another 46 h.
5. MTT (20 μL, 5 mg/mL) was then added to each well.
6. After 4 h of incubation, the medium was removed carefully and 200 μL DMSO was added to each well for dissolving the formazan crystals.
7. The samples were measured by using a Bio-Rad 680 microplate reader at 492 nm.
8. The cell viability (%) was calculated as: cell viability (%) = $(A_{sample}/A_{control}) \times 100\%$, where $A_{sample}$ was the absorbency of the sample well and $A_{control}$ was the absorbency of the control well.

### 3.7 Cell Uptake

1. CT26 cells were seeded in six-well plates at a density of $2.0 \times 10^5$ cells/well and cultured at 37 °C in a 5% $CO_2$ atmosphere for 24 h.
2. Then PD, G(PD), (GP)D, and P[(GP)D] NPs were prepared (Cy5-DNA was used for NPs preparation).
3. The growth medium was replaced by fresh medium of pH 7.4 and 6.8.
4. PD, G(PD), (GP)D, and P[(GP)D] NPs were added into each well, the cells were incubated for another 2 h.
5. After incubation, the cells were digested with pancreatin and collected after washed twice with cold PBS.
6. The cells were tested with a Guava EasyCyte flow cytometer.

### 3.8 CLSM

1. CT26 cells were seeded on coverslips in six-well plates at a density of $1.0 \times 10^5$ cells/well and grown for 24 h.
2. The naked DNA (D), PD, G(PD), (GP)D, and P[(GP)D] NPs (Cy5-DNA) were used for NPs preparation and intracellular tracking.
3. Before the NPs were added, the growth medium was replaced with fresh DMEM of pH 7.4 or 6.8.
4. D, PD, G(PD), (GP)D, and P[(GP)D] NPs were added to each well for 2 h incubation.
5. The cells were washed with PBS and fixed with 3.7% paraformaldehyde for 15 min at room temperature.
6. The cell nuclei were stained by DAPI (1 mg/mL, 1 μL/well) for 15 min.
7. The cell membranes were stained with 5 μL Alexa Fluor 488 phalloidin for 20 min at 37 °C.
8. The coverslips were carefully taken out and placed on the slides, enclosed with glycerol.
9. The samples were observed by CLSM.

### 3.9 Tumor Accumulation (Note 6)

1. Subcutaneous tumor model was generated by injecting CT26 cells ($1 \times 10^6$ cells/100 μL) into the left flank of nude mice.
2. After implantation, it needed about 1–2 weeks to develop into tumors which were about 0.5 cm in diameter.
3. Then the mice were injected with 0.2 mL solutions of D, PD, G(PD), (GP)D, and P[(GP)D] (1 mg/kg body weight on DNA basis) via tail vein (Cy5-DNA and Cy5-PEI were both used for tracking the tumor accumulation of the NPs).
4. After 24 h, the mice were anesthetized and sacrificed, the tumors were excised and imaged by a Maestro In Vivo Imaging System (excited by a yellow excitation filter, the fluorescence was detected through 645 nm emission filter, and the exposure time was 2000 ms).

### 3.10 In Vivo Antitumor Therapeutic Efficacy (Note 7)

1. Subcutaneous tumor model was generated by injecting CT26 cells ($1 \times 10^6$ cells/100 μL) into the left flank of BALB/C mice (4–5 week, female).
2. The CT26 tumor-bearing mice were randomly divided into six groups and respectively injected with PBS, D, PD, G(PD), (GP)D, and P[(GP)D] via tail vein (*p*DNA expressed shVEGF was loaded as the therapeutic gene).
3. The tumor volume and body weight were monitored every other day.
4. After treatment, the animals were sacrificed and the tumors and major organs were collected for further analysis.

### 3.11 Histology and Immunofluorescence Analyses

1. The major organs (heart, liver, spleen, lung, and kidney) and tumors were collected and the sections were stained by H&E for pathological analysis.
2. The tumor tissues were embedded in paraffin and the sections were examined for immunofluorescence by using anti-CD31 antibody and FITC-labeled secondary antibody to assess the suppression of tumor angiogenesis.

### 3.12 Photoacoustic Imaging (Note 8)

1. BALB/C nude mice bearing CT26 tumors were injected with PBS, D, PD, G (PD), (GP)D, and P[(GP)D] via tail vein every other day for a total of four times, the dosage was 1 mg/kg body weight on DNA basis.
2. The mice were anesthetized with 2% isoflurane and placed into the MSOT system. Multispectral process scanning (MSP) was performed at 680, 730, 760, 800, 850, and 900 nm.

3. The results were reconstructed in a linear model, and linear regression was used for the multispectral processing.

### 3.13 VEGF Gene Expression

1. The tumor tissues were grinded in mortar with liquid nitrogen and the RNA was extracted by Trizol.
2. The RNA was reversely transcribed to cDNA with Prime Script® RT reagent kit with gDNA Eraser (Perfect Real Time) according to the instructions.
3. Real-time PCR experiment was performed using SYBR® Premix Ex Taq™ II (Tli RNaseH Plus) according to the instructions.
4. The primers for VEGF were as follows: forward, 5′-GGT GAG AGG TCT AGT TCC CGA-3′; reverse, 5'-CCA TGA ACT TTC TGC TCT TC-3′. For GAPDH: forward, 5′-GTT CCA GTA TGA CTC TAC CC-3′; reverse, 5′-AGT CTT CTG AGG CAG TGA TG-3′.
5. Amplification condition was as follows: predenaturation at 95 °C for 30 s, 40 cycles of denaturation at 95 °C for 5 s, annealing at 58 °C for 34 s, and extension at 72 °C for 30 s with Mx3005P instrument.

### 3.14 Elisa

1. The tumor tissues were homogenized. The supernatants were collected and added into the well of the plate together with anti-VEGF antibody and streptavidin-HRP, and incubated in 37 °C for 60 min.
2. After washing and chromogenic reaction, the stop buffer was added.
3. The OD value of each well was measured under 450 nm by a Tecan infinite M200 Microplate Readers.
4. According to the manufacturer's protocol, the standard sample was diluted into different concentrations and used to construct a calibration curve to calculate the concentrations of the samples, and the OD value of the blank sample was subtracted.

### 3.15 Western Blot

1. Tumor tissues were lysed and the supernatants were collected after centrifuging at 10,000 g for 10 min to obtain the proteins.
2. Protein quantification was performed with BCA protein assay kit.
3. SDS-PAGE was used for protein isolation.
4. Transferred the proteins to PVDF film.
5. Blocked the nonspecific binding site by 5% BSA for 1 h.

6. Incubated with homologous first antibody overnight at 4 °C and HRP labeled second antibody at room temperature for 1 h.
7. The result was finally obtained after the exposure and development of the film using the ECL kit.

### 3.16 Statistical Analysis

1. All measurements were conducted in triplicate and expressed as mean ± standard deviation.
2. Student's t-test was performed to compare the statistical significance. $*p < 0.05$ was considered statistically significant. $**p < 0.01$ and $***p < 0.001$ were considered extremely significant.

## 4 Notes

1. PLG was synthesized according to the previously reported method (Xia et al. 2010). PBLG was obtained by ring opening polymerization of BLG-NCA with N-hexylamine as the initiator. The protecting benzyl groups on PBLG were removed by HBr. The final product PLG was obtained after dialysis and lyophilization.
2. The synthesis of aldehyde-modified PEG was according to the reported method with slight modification (Gu et al. 2007). 4-carboxybenzaldehyde was conjugated on both terminal of PEG with the help of EDC·HCl and DMAP. The aldehyde groups of OHC-PEG-CHO could react with the amino groups of PEI via Schiff-base reaction in neutral or alkaline aqueous solution. Hence, PEG shielding could be realized in situ on the surface of PEI-based NPs through this "click" reaction. And the generated Schiff-base bonds were labile and cleavable in slightly acidic tumor extracellular pH, which was precisely convenient for PEG detaching. The pH sensitivity of the formation and cleavage of the Schiff-base bonds was verified by $^{1}$H NMR. The different pH values were obtained by adjusting $D_2O$ with $CF_3COOD$. The peak of aldehyde groups ($^{1}$H NMR spectrum, at 10 ppm) had completely disappeared in pH 7.4, demonstrating that all the aldehyde groups had reacted with PEI to form Schiff-base bonds. In slightly acidic pH 6.8, the signal of aldehyde groups reappeared due to the rapidly dynamic cleavage of the Schiff-base bonds.
3. PD, G(PD), and (GP)D were prepared by electrostatic interaction through mixing DNA, PEI, and PLG aqueous solutions in different orders under equal volume. And the PEG shielded NPs were prepared by simply adding different amount of OHC-PEG-CHO aqueous solution into the (GP)D complexes to obtain the P[(GP)D] NPs. Significantly, for this step, the pH of the solution should be adjusted to 7.4 for ensuring the formation of the Schiff-base bonds.
4. The zeta potential and particle size should be measured right after the PD, G(PD), (GP)D, and P[(GP)D]. NPs were freshly prepared. PEG had effectively shielded

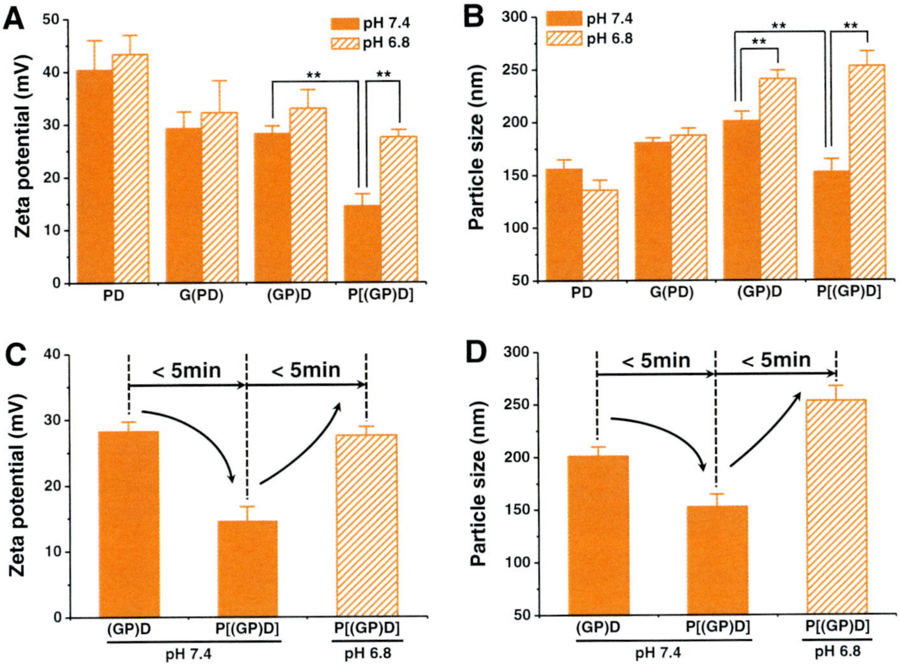


**Fig. 3** (**a**) Zeta potential and (**b**) particle size of the NPs. (**c**, **d**) Charge/size dual-rebound property of the gene delivery system.. (Adapted from Guan et al. 2016, with permission)

the positive potential of the NPs. Furthermore, the potential of P[(GP)D] NPs was much higher in pH 6.8 than 7.4 (Fig. 3a). The crosslinking of PEG on (GP)D surface could tighten particle size in pH 7.4. And in pH 6.8, the size was restored due to the PEG detachment from P[(GP)D] (Fig. 3b). The speed of PEG shielding and charge/size rebound along with pH variations were monitored, these mentioned processes were proven to be happened within 5 min (Fig. 3c and d).

5. DNA transfection was carried out in CT26 cells by utilizing the luciferase *p*DNA (*p*GL3-control) as the reporter gene. The gene transfection of (GP)D was detected first for screening the optimal mass ratio (PLG:PEI:DNA = 1.25:2.5:1). The transfection efficiencies of P[(GP)D] NPs (various PEG mass ratios) in different pH were analyzed, and all the tested ratios have shown significant transfection efficiency difference between pH 7.4 and 6.8, confirming that the practicability of the pH-responsive PEG shielding. The NPs with PEG:PLG:PEI:DNA mass ratio of 5:1.25:2.5:1 presented the highest transfection efficiency and biggest difference between pH 6.8 and 7.4 (Fig. 4).
6. The tumor accumulation of the different NPs was evaluated by ex vivo imaging on subcutaneous tumor model. The tumor-bearing mice were injected with the NPs via tail vein. The Cy5-DNA and Cy5-PEI were respectively used for NPs preparation and tracking. For P[(GP)D], both Cy5-DNA and Cy5-PEI exhibited the most effective accumulation in tumors among all the groups. The result also

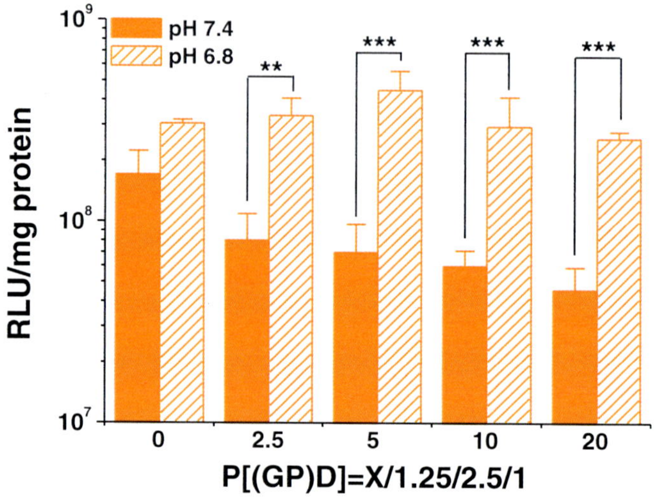


**Fig. 4** Transfection efficiency of P[(GP)D] (with various PEG mass ratios) at different pH values (7.4 and 6.8) in CT26 cells. (Adapted from Guan et al. 2016, with permission)

revealed that DNA and PEI in P[(GP)D] could be synchronously delivered to the tumors, and the DNA could be stably complexed with PEI during systemic delivery process.

7. BALB/C mice (4–5 weeks, female) were obtained from Vital River Company in Beijing. All experimental procedures were in accordance with the guidelines for laboratory animals established by the Animal Care and Use Committee of Northeast Normal University. The CT26 subcutaneous tumor-bearing mice were randomly divided into six groups and respectively injected with PBS, D, PD, G(PD), (GP)D, and P[(GP)D] via tail vein. *p*DNA expressed shVEGF was loaded as the therapeutic gene, and the shVEGF could downregulate the expression of VEGF. VEGF was known to be crucial in tumor growth, infiltration, and metastasis. It could stimulate the proliferation of endothelial cells and promote tumor angiogenesis. Thus, inhibition of VEGF expression was beneficial for the treatment of tumor (Liu et al. 2011; Inai et al. 2004). The therapeutic gene injection dosage was 1 mg/kg body weight on *p*DNA basis by every other day for a total of six times. Tumor volume was calculated by the formula: $L \times S^2/2$, where L refers to the longer diameter and S refers to the shorter diameter.
8. The Hb and $HbO_2$ in the blood could be detected by photoacoustic imaging, and utilized to reflect the location of blood vessels inside the tumors (Mallidi et al. 2011). Therefore, photoacoustic imaging could help to estimate the anti-angiogenesis effect (Song et al. 2015; Jose et al. 2009). P[(GP)D] NPs displayed lower intensity of Hb and $HbO_2$, indicating that less blood vessels were in the tumor tissue, and the P[(GP)D] NPs could effectively silence the VEGF expression and suppress the tumor angiogenesis.

## 5 Conclusion

This protocol presents an ultrasensitive pH-triggered charge/size dual-rebound gene delivery system developed by facile strategy for efficient cancer treatment. This system possesses the following favorable properties: (1) the gene delivery system is constructed by a chemical bench-free "green" and fast process which will be favored by wide audience, (2) powerful PEG shielding decreases charges and sizes of the complex NPs, leading to good biocompatibility, stability, and long circulation, (3) "stealthy coating" can be rapidly peeled off as soon as NPs arriving tumors, and (4) ultrasensitive charge/size dual-rebounding synergistically elaborate an excellent gene delivery efficiency. In the chapter, the material synthesis and the gene delivery system preparation characterizations, in vitro and in vivo, have been introduced in detail for systematically demonstrating the gene delivery system. The superior properties had been well proved by sufficient biological evidences. This ultrasensitive pH-triggered charge/size dual-rebound gene delivery system has great potentials for cancer therapy in the future.

## References

Bae Y, Fukushima S, Harada A, Kataoka K (2003) Design of environment-sensitive supramolecular assemblies for intracellular drug delivery: polymeric micelles that are responsive to intracellular pH change. Angew Chem Int Edit 115(38):4788–4791

Chen J, Wang K, Wu J, Tian H, Chen X (2018) Polycations for gene delivery: dilemmas and solutions. Bioconjug Chem 30(2):338–349

Cring MR, Sheffield VC (2020) Gene therapy and gene correction: targets, progress, and challenges for treating human diseases. Gene Ther 1–10. https://doi.org/10.1038/s41434-020-00197-8

Deng C, Jiang Y, Cheng R, Meng F, Zhong Z (2012) Biodegradable polymeric micelles for targeted and controlled anticancer drug delivery: promises progress and prospects. Nano Today 7(5): 467–480

Du JZ, Sun TM, Song WJ, Wu J, Wang J (2010a) A tumor-acidity-activated charge-conversional nanogel as an intelligent vehicle for promoted tumoral-cell uptake and drug delivery. Angew Chem Int Edit 122(21):3703–3708

Du FS, Wang Y, Zhang R, Li ZC (2010b) Intelligent nucleic acid delivery systems based on stimuli-responsive polymers. Soft Matter 6(5):835–848

Dufort S, Sancey L, Coll JL (2012) Physico-chemical parameters that govern nanoparticles fate also dictate rules for their molecular evolution. Adv Drug Deliv Rev 64(2):179–189

Gu J, Cheng WP, Liu J, Lo SY, Smith D, Qu X, Yang Z (2007) pH-triggered reversible "stealth" polycationic micelles. Biomacromolecules 9(1):255–262

Guan X, Guo Z, Lin L, Chen J, Tian H, Chen X (2016) Ultrasensitive pH triggered charge/size dual-rebound gene delivery system. Nano Lett 16(11):6823–6831

Guo S, Huang L (2011) Nanoparticles escaping RES and endosome: challenges for siRNA delivery for cancer therapy. J Nanomater 2011:1–12. Article ID 742895

Guo X, Wei X, Jing Y, Zhou S (2015) Size changeable nanocarriers with nuclear targeting for effectively overcoming multidrug resistance in cancer therapy. Adv Mater 27(41):6450–6456

Hatakeyama H, Akita H, Kogure K, Oishi M, Nagasaki Y, Kihira Y, Ueno M, Kobayashi H, Kikuchi H, Harashima H (2007) Development of a novel systemic gene delivery system for cancer therapy with a tumor-specific cleavable PEG-lipid. Gene Ther 14(1):68–77

Hatakeyama H, Akita H, Harashima HA (2011) Multifunctional envelope type nano device (MEND) for gene delivery to tumours based on the EPR effect: a strategy for overcoming the PEG dilemma. Adv Drug Deliv Rev 63(3):152–160

Inai T, Mancuso M, Hashizume H, Baffert F, Haskell A, Baluk P, Hu-Lowe DD, Shalinsky DR, Thurston G, Yancopoulos GD (2004) Inhibition of vascular endothelial growth factor (VEGF) signaling in cancer causes loss of endothelial fenestrations, regression of tumor vessels, and appearance of basement membrane ghosts. Am J Pathol 165(1):35–52

Jin E, Zhang B, Sun X, Zhou Z, Ma X, Sun Q, Tang J, Shen Y, Van Kirk E, Murdoch WJ (2013) Acid-active cell-penetrating peptides for in vivo tumor-targeted drug delivery. J Am Chem Soc 135(2):933–940

Jose J, Manohar S, Kolkman RG, Steenbergen W, van Leeuwen TG (2009) Imaging of tumor vasculature using twente photoacoustic systems. J Biophotonics 2(12):701–717

Kircheis R, Wightman L, Wagner E (2001) Design and gene delivery activity of modified polyethylenimines. Adv Drug Deliv Rev 53(3):341–358

Ko J, Park K, Kim YS, Kim MS, Han JK, Kim K, Park RW, Kim IS, Song HK, Lee DS (2007) Tumoral acidic extracellular pH targeting of pH-responsive mPEG-poly (β-amino ester) block copolymer micelles for cancer therapy. J Control Release 123(2):109–115

Liang S, Yang XZ, Du XJ, Wang HX, Li HJ, Liu WW, Yao YD, Zhu YH, Ma YC, Wang J (2015) Optimizing the size of micellar nanoparticles for efficient siRNA delivery. Adv Funct Mater 25(30):4778–4787

Lima MCP, Simoes S, Pires P, Faneca H, Düzgüneş N (2001) Cationic lipid-DNA complexes in gene delivery: from biophysics to biological applications. Adv Drug Deliv Rev 47(2–3):277–294

Liu T, Ye L, He Y, Chen X, Peng J, Zhang X, Yi H, Peng F, Leng A (2011) Combination gene therapy using VEGF-shRNA and fusion suicide gene yCDglyTK inhibits gastric carcinoma growth. Exp Mol Pathol 91(3):745–752

Liu J, Huang Y, Kumar A, Tan A, Jin S, Mozhi A, Liang XJ (2014) pH-sensitive nano-systems for drug delivery in cancer therapy. Biotechnol Adv 32(4):693–710

Liu X, Xiang J, Zhu D, Jiang L, Zhou Z, Tang J, Liu X, Huang Y, Shen Y (2015) Fusogenic reactive oxygen species triggered charge-reversal vector for effective gene delivery. Adv Mater 28(9): 1743–1752

Mallidi S, Luke GP, Emelianov S (2011) Photoacoustic imaging in cancer detection, diagnosis, and treatment guidance. Trends Biotechnol 29(5):213–221

Merdan T, Kopeček J, Kissel T (2002) Prospects for cationic polymers in gene and oligonucleotide therapy against cancer. Adv Drug Deliv Rev 54(5):715–758

Mishra S, Webster P, Davis ME (2004) PEGylation significantly affects cellular uptake and intracellular trafficking of non-viral gene delivery particles. Eur J Cell Biol 83(3):97–111

Morille M, Passirani C, Vonarbourg A, Clavreul A, Benoit JP (2008) Progress in developing cationic vectors for non-viral systemic gene therapy against cancer. Biomaterials 29(24–25):3477–3496

Pearce TR, Shroff K, Kokkoli E (2012) Peptide targeted lipid nanoparticles for anticancer drug delivery. Adv Mater 24(28):3803–3822

Prabaharan M, Grailer JJ, Pilla S, Steeber DA, Gong S (2009) Amphiphilic multi-arm-block copolymer conjugated with doxorubicin via pH-sensitive hydrazone bond for tumor-targeted drug delivery. Biomaterials 30(29):5757–5766

Shetty C, Noronha A, Pontarelli A, Wilds CJ, Oh JK (2020) Dual-location dual-acid/glutathione-degradable cationic micelleplexes through hydrophobic modification for enhanced gene silencing. Mol Pharm 17(10):3979–3989

Song W, Tang Z, Zhang D, Yu H, Chen X (2015) Coadministration of vascular disrupting agents and nanomedicines to eradicate tumors from peripheral and central regions. Small 11(31): 3755–3761

Sun Q, Sun X, Ma X, Zhou Z, Jin E, Zhang B, Shen Y, Van Kirk EA, Murdoch WJ, Lott JR (2014) Integration of nanoassembly functions for an effective delivery cascade for cancer drugs. Adv Mater 26(45):7615–7621

Sun C, Liu Y, Du J, Cao Z, Xu C, Wang J (2016) Facile generation of tumor-pH-labile linkage-bridged block copolymers for chemotherapeutic delivery. Angew Chem Int Ed 128(3):1022–1026

Tasciotti E, Liu X, Bhavane R, Plant K, Leonard AD, Price BK, Cheng MC, Decuzzi P, Tour JM, Robertson F (2008) Mesoporous silicon particles as a multistage delivery system for imaging and therapeutic applications. Nat Nanotechnol 3(3):151–157

Tian H, Tang Z, Zhuang X, Chen X, Jing X (2012) Biodegradable synthetic polymers: preparation, functionalization and biomedical application. Prog Polym Sci 37(2):237–280

Xia J, Chen J, Tian H, Chen X (2010) Synthesis and characterization of a pH-sensitive shielding system for polycation gene carriers. Sci China Chem 53(3):502–507

Xu CH, Sui MH, Tang JB (2011) What can we learn from virus in designing nonviral gene vectors. Chin J Polym Sci 29(3):274–287

Zhang Z, Zhang X, Xu X, Li Y, Li Y, Zhong D, He Y, Gu Z (2015) Virus-inspired mimics based on dendritic lipopeptides for efficient tumor-specific infection and systemic drug delivery. Adv Funct Mater 25(33):5250–5260

# Pulmonary Co-delivery of DOX and siRNA 3

Caina Xu, Huayu Tian, and Xuesi Chen

## Contents



**Abstract**

Pulmonary delivery is a noninvasive route, which can deliver drugs and therapeutic genes to pulmonary epithelia. Developing co-delivery system for delivering doxorubicin (DOX) and siRNAs by the pulmonary delivery provides a promising local treatment strategy for lung cancer. DOX was conjugated onto polyethyleneimine (PEI) by using cis-aconitic anhydride (CA), and PEI-CA-DOX conjugate was prepared. And then PEI-CA-DOX/siRNA complex nanoparticles were formed through electrostatic interaction. The prepared complex nanoparticles were tested in B16F10 cells, and the results showed that the co-delivery system exhibited higher cytotoxicity than that of DOX or siRNA alone. The antitumor efficiency of pulmonary administered PEI-CA-DOX/siRNA complex nanoparticles was assessed through the treatment of metastatic lung cancer on C57BL/6 mice. Tumors in B16F10-implanted mice treated with PEI-CA-DOX/siRNA complex nanoparticles were obviously smaller and fewer in numbers than mice treated with DOX or siRNA alone, which could be due to

C. Xu · H. Tian (✉) · X. Chen
Key Laboratory of Polymer Ecomaterials, Changchun Institute of Applied Chemistry, Chinese Academy of Sciences, Changchun, China
e-mail: thy@ciac.ac.cn; xschen@ciac.ac.cn



H. Tian and X. Chen (eds.), *Gene Delivery*, Biomaterial Engineering,
https://doi.org/10.1007/978-981-16-5419-0_10

the synergistic antitumor effects of DOX and siRNA. Furthermore, most DOX and siRNA were found in the tumor of lungs after pulmonary administration, but rarely restrained in the normal lung tissue. All the results proved that pulmonary co-delivery of DOX and siRNA was an effective way to treat metastatic lung cancer. This noninvasive route of pulmonary administration was very potential for delivering drugs and genes.

**Keywords**

Pulmonary delivery · Co-delivery · Antitumor effect · DOX · siRNA · Metastatic lung cancer

## 1 Overview

Cancer has become one of the biggest problems that threaten human health; cancer treatment has attracted many attentions of the researchers (Guo and Huang 2020; Martin et al. 2020). Lung cancer is also known as primary bronchial carcinoma, one of the common malignant tumors (Haddad et al. 2020; Siegel et al. 2019). In recent years, the incidence of lung cancer in various countries has risen sharply. About 80–85% is non-small cell lung cancer (NSCLC) based on cell origin (Herbst et al. 2018; Yuan et al. 2019). According to reports, the average 5-year survival rate of lung cancer is below 20%, and the survival time of most lung cancer patients is about 2 years (Siegel et al. 2019, 2020). At present, traditional methods for treating lung cancer are surgery, chemotherapy, and radiotherapy (Miller et al. 2019). However, a large side effect occurred after chemotherapy or radiotherapy, such as high recurrence rate and multidrug resistance. In addition, it is difficult to achieve good therapeutic effect for a single gene or drug due to the heterogeneity of tumors (Zappa and Mousa 2016). Therefore, it is required to develop new treatment methods by combining drugs and genes for cancer therapy.

Pulmonary drug delivery system (PDDS) refers to a drug delivery system, which can deliver drugs to the lungs, producing local or systemic therapeutic effects. Pulmonary administration has been used in clinic to treat disease of respiratory system (Otterson et al. 2007, 2010). Compared with traditional intravenous administration, pulmonary delivery system has many advantages (Shen and Minko 2020): (1) the drugs can be delivered to the lung directly, thereby reducing the amount of drug dosage and the side effect (Bivas-Benita et al. 2005; Roa et al. 2011); (2) the lung has a huge surface area, which benefits the efficient delivery of the protein and polypeptide drugs with large molecular weight; (3) the pulmonary administration can avoid the first-pass metabolism, thereby improving the bioavailability of drugs (Yu and Chien 1997). Therefore, the lung administration is great potential in the treatment of pneumonia (Iwabuchi et al. 2020), lung cancer (Lee et al. 2018), asthma (Campa et al. 2018), pulmonary fibrosis (Garbuzenko et al. 2017), chronic obstructive pulmonary disease (Tashkin and Strange 2018), and pulmonary hypertension (Gupta et al. 2011).

Combining drug and gene treatment can improve the therapeutic effect with reducing the resistance and side effects (Chen et al. 2009; Creixell and Peppas 2012; He et al. 2016; Khan et al. 2012; Wang et al. 2006). However, efficient delivery of drug and gene to tumor tissue will impact the therapeutic effect. Some delivery carriers were developed for co-delivery drugs and genes, such as lipid-based nanoparticles (Saad et al. 2008; Zununi Vahed et al. 2017), silica nanoparticles (Paris and Vallet-Regí 2020), and polymeric nanoparticles (Elmowafy et al. 2017). However, the construction of co-delivery carriers was rarely reported on the use of drugs and genes to cancer treatment via pulmonary administration. Among them, Tamara Minko' group successfully constructed the cationic liposome carrier system, which could deliver drug and gene to lung with a good accumulation in the lung tissue. And the results showed that the combination of drug and gene had significant antitumor effects (Garbuzenko et al. 2009, 2010; Taratula et al. 2013). In addition, Tamara Minko' group developed porous silicon nanoparticles for pulmonary co-delivery drug and gene, which had achieved expected results (Taratula et al. 2011). Moreover, some polymers were used for delivery therapeutic genes or drugs to the lungs (Na et al. 2019). Therefore, it is still necessary to exploit the efficient carriers for pulmonary co-delivery drugs and genes with good biocompatibility and degradability properties.

In this chapter, chemotherapy drug (DOX) was modified on polyethyleneimine (PEI) by an acid-sensitive bond, and then PEI-CA-DOX/siRNA complex particles were prepared via electrostatic interaction (Xu et al. 2015). The as-prepared complex particles were sprayed directly into the lungs through the mice of trachea using a liquid aerosol device. The DOX was released in a relative low pH in tumor tissue and entered into nucleus to damage tumor cells. In addition, siRNA was released from the PEI-CA-DOX/siRNA complex particles, and participated in the subsequent transfection process for gene silencing, thereby causing apoptosis of tumor cells and ultimately inhibiting lung cancer. The synthesis of PEI-CA-DOX conjugate was verified by $^{1}$H NMR, and CA-DOX/siRNA complex particles were studied by a series of in vitro characteristics and cell experiments, and the in vivo antitumor effects were studied. Finally, the distribution of DOX and gene was analyzed on B16F10 tumor bearing mice. The main purpose of this chapter is to prepare polymer drug and gene co-delivery carriers with low cytotoxicity and high transfection efficiency, which is suitable for spray administration trachea and lungs in vivo, and provides a new treatment for lung metastasis treatment, as well as applications in the clinical studies (Fig. 1).

## 2 Protocol

### 2.1 Materials

#### 2.1.1 Synthesis of PEI-CA-DOX

1. Polyethyleneimine (PEI, molecular weight of 25,000 Da)
2. Doxorubicin hydrochloride (DOX·HCl)
3. Cis-aconitic anhydride (CA)

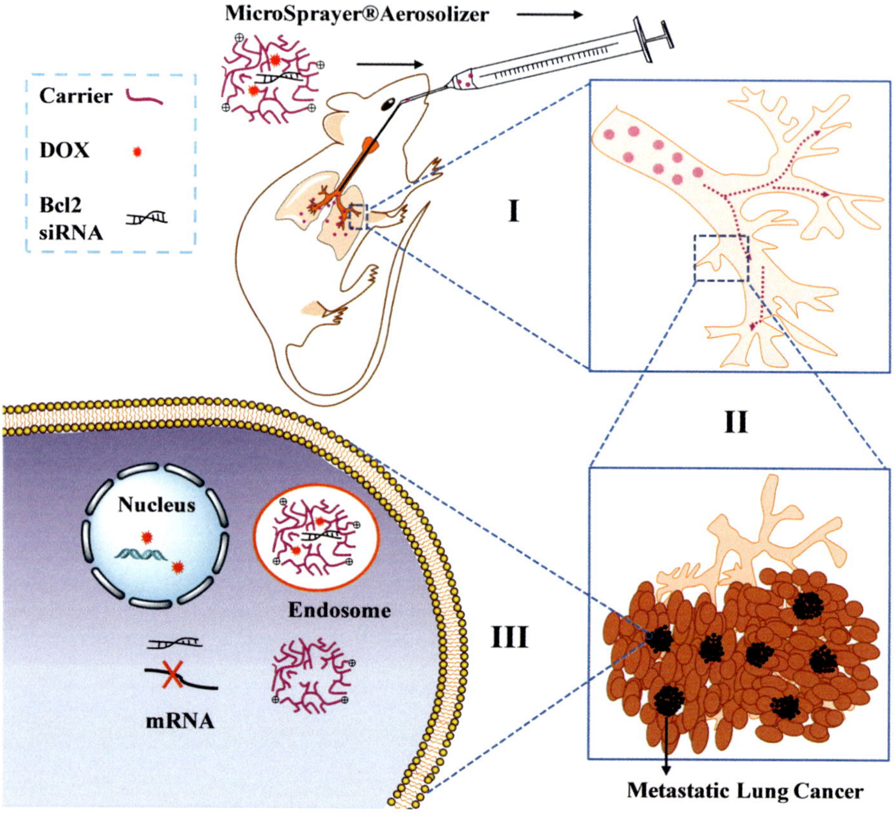


**Fig. 1** Schematic illustration of pulmonary co-delivery DOX and siRNA to the lung. (Adapted from XU et al. 2015, with permission, Copyright Wiley VCH)

4. Dimethylformamide (DMF)
5. Dimethyl sulfoxide (DMSO)
6. Triethanolamine (TEA)
7. N-Hydroxysuccinimide (NHS)
8. 1-ethyl-3-[3-dimethylaminopropyl]carbodiimide hydrochloride (EDC)

### 2.1.2 Characterization

1. $^{1}H$ NMR at 400 MHz (Bruker, Ettlingen, Germany)
2. Deuterated water ($D_2O$)

### 2.1.3 Preparation of PEI/siRNA and PEI-CA-DOX/siRNA

1. Deionized water
2. Bcl2 siRNA
3. Negative control siRNA (Nc siRNA)

#### 2.1.4 Drug Release Experiment

1. Phosphate buffered saline (PBS, pH = 5.0, 6.8 and 7.4)
2. Dialysis bag (MWCO 7,000 Da)
3. Deionized water
4. Fluorescence spectrophotometer

#### 2.1.5 Particle Sizes and Zeta Potential Analysis

1. Zeta potential/BI-90Plus particle size analyzer (Brookhaven, USA)
2. Deionized water

#### 2.1.6 Cell Uptake Study

1. Confocal laser scanning microscopy (CLSM, ZEISS LSM 780, Germany)
2. Fluorescent dye Cy5
3. B16F10 cells
4. Bcl2 siRNA
5. Negative control siRNA (Nc siRNA)
6. Phosphate buffered saline (PBS)
7. 4% paraformaldehyde
8. 4′,6-diamidino-2-phenylindole (DAPI)
9. 6-well plates
10. Dulbecco's Modified Eagle Medium (DMEM)
11. Trypsin-EDTA
12. Fetal bovine serum (FBS)
13. Glycerol
14. $CO_2$ incubator
15. Penicillin
16. Streptomycin
17. Optical microscope

#### 2.1.7 Quantification of Bcl2 Gene Expression by qRT-PCR

1. B16F10 cells
2. Phosphate buffered solution (PBS)
3. Nc siRNA, Bcl2 siRNA, or PEI/Bcl2 siRNA
4. Reverse transcription kit from Takara Biotechnology Co., Ltd. (Dalian, China)
5. PrimeScript™ RT Master Mix and SYBR® Premix Ex Taq™
6. Mxpro 3005P Real-Time PCR Detection system (Stratagene, USA)
7. Trizol reagent (Invitrogen)
8. Takara Biotechnology Co., Ltd. (Dalian, China)

#### 2.1.8 Cytotoxicity Assay

1. B16F10 cells
2. Phosphate buffered solution (PBS)
3. 3-(4,5-dimethylthiazol-2-yl)-2,5-diphenyltetrazolium bromide (MTT)
4. 96-well plates
5. $CO_2$ incubator

6. Dimethyl sulfoxide (DMSO)
7. Bio-Rad 680 Microplate Reader

#### 2.1.9 In Vivo Antitumor Therapy

1. Male C57BL/6 mice
2. B16F10 cells
3. Doxorubicin hydrochloride (DOX·HCl)
4. Liquid aerosol device (MicroSprayer® Aerosolizer, Penn-Century, Philadelphia, PA)
5. Phosphate buffered solution (PBS)
6. Bcl2 siRNA
7. Negative control siRNA (Nc siRNA)
8. PEI-CA-DOX/siRNA complex nanoparticles

#### 2.1.10 Biodistribution

1. Cy5-Nc siRNA
2. Liquid aerosol device (MicroSprayer® Aerosolizer, Penn-Century, Philadelphia, PA)
3. PEI-CA-DOX/Cy5-Nc siRNA complex nanoparticles
4. Male C57BL/6 mice
5. B16F10 cells
6. Doxorubicin hydrochloride (DOX·HCl)
7. Phosphate buffered solution (PBS)
8. Maestro in vivo Imaging System (Cambridge Research & Instrumentation, Inc., USA)

#### 2.1.11 Intracellular Uptake of DOX and siRNA In Vivo

1. Cy5-Nc siRNA
2. Liquid aerosol device (MicroSprayer® Aerosolizer, Penn-Century, Philadelphia, PA)
3. Male C57BL/6 mice
4. B16F10 cells
5. PEI-CA-DOX/Cy5-Nc siRNA complex nanoparticles
6. Phosphate buffered solution (PBS)
7. 4′,6-diamidino-2-phenylindole (DAPI)
8. Confocal laser scanning microscopy (CLSM, ZEISS LSM 780, Germany)

## 2.2 Methods

#### 2.2.1 Synthesis of PEI-CA-DOX and Characterization (Note 1)

1. DOX (50 mg) and CA were dissolved in DMF (10 mL) according to the molar ratio of 1:1.1, and then TEA was added (TEA and DOX molar ratio of 1:1). Under room temperature, the reaction was carried out for 24 h in the dark.

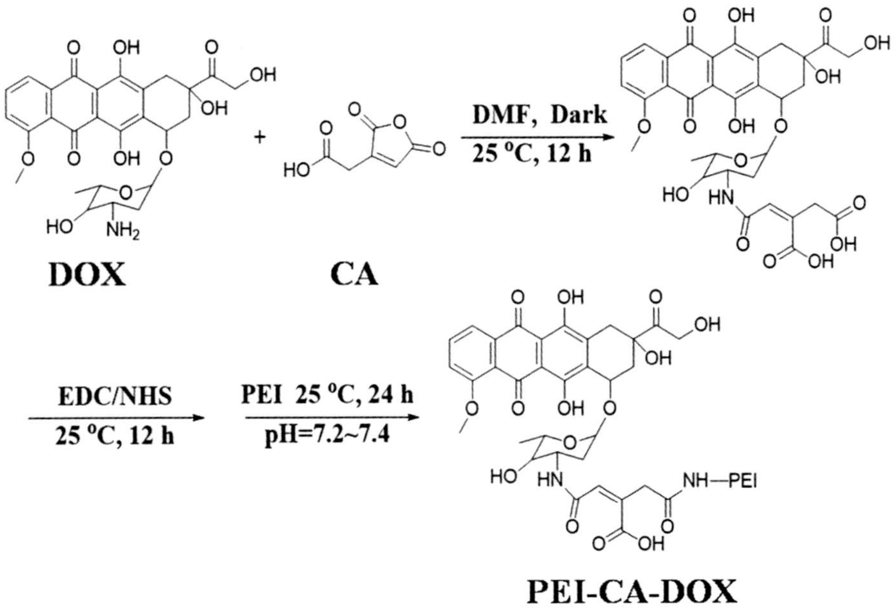


**Fig. 2** Synthesis route of PEI-CA-DOX. (Adapted from XU et al. 2015, with permission, Copyright Wiley VCH)

2. The reaction solution was poured into excess ethyl acetate, and then washed 7–8 times using saturated sodium chloride. The organic phase was collected and was added to anhydrous sodium sulfate for 4–6 h in dark. The organic phase was filtered and dried. The product of CA-DOX was obtained.
3. The CA-DOX (144.7 mg) was dissolved in DMSO (6–8 mL), EDC (47.6 mg), and NHS (28.6 mg) were added in the above solution for 12 h in the dark.
4. The pH of PEI was adjusted to 7.2–7.4 in deionized water (3 mL), and the CA-DOX solution was mixed with PEI solution for 24 h at room temperature in the dark.
5. The reaction solution was dialyzed for 3 days (MWCO 7,000 Da), and the final product was obtained following lyophilization (Fig. 2).

### 2.2.2 Characterization of PEI-CA-DOX (Note 2)

1. The PEI-CA-DOX was characterized by $^1$H NMR spectra. NMR was used to detect the NMR hydrogen spectra of CA-DOX and PEI-CA-DOX, respectively.
2. The $^1$H NMR spectra was measured at room temperature, and the $D_2O$ was used as the solvent (Fig. 3).

### 2.2.3 Preparation of PEI/siRNA and PEI-CA-DOX/siRNA (Note 3)

1. PEI/siRNA and PEI-CA-DOX/siRNA were prepared by mixing siRNA (0.1 mg/mL) with PEI (0.5 mg/mL) or PEI-CA-DOX (0.5 mg/mL).

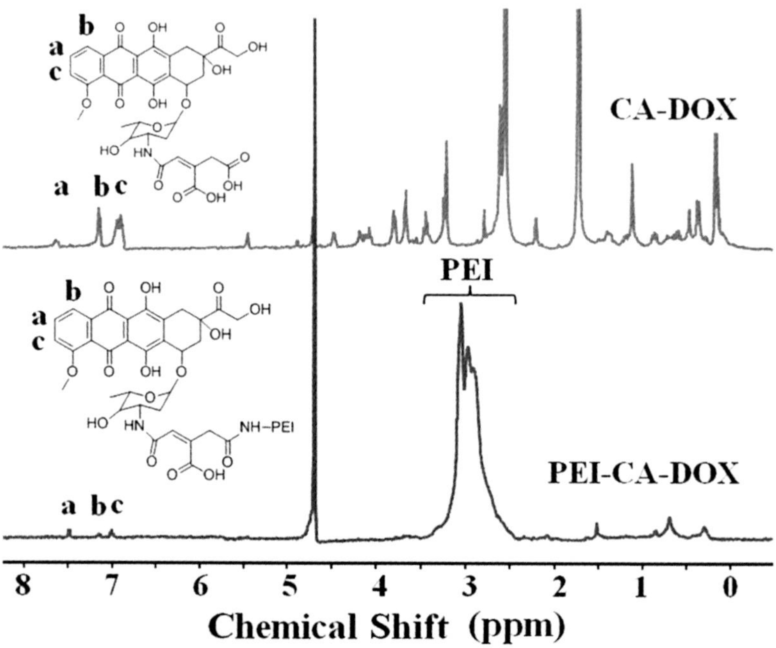


**Fig. 3** [1]H NMR spectra of CA-DOX and PEI-CA-DOX in $D_2O$. (Adapted from XU et al. 2015, with permission, Copyright Wiley VCH)

2. After gently vortexing and 30 min incubation at room temperature, PEI/siRNA and PEI-CA-DOX/siRNA complex nanoparticles at a 5/1 (wt/wt) ratio were obtained.

### 2.2.4 Drug Release Experiment (Note 4)

1. The PEI-CA-DOX or PEI-CA-DOX/DNA was diluted into PBS (2 mL, pH = 5.0, 6.8, and 7.4, respectively) with a concentration equivalent to 50 μg/mL free DOX.
2. The solution was dialyzed at 37 °C in a dialysis bag (MWCO 7,000 Da) for 72 h at 58 mL of PBS container with continuous shaking.
3. At predetermined intervals, 2 mL PBS from container was collected for test, and then 2 mL fresh PBS was added to the container.
4. The fluorescence of released DOX was detected at the excitation and emission wavelength of 480 nm and 590 nm, respectively.

### 2.2.5 Zeta Potential and Particle Size Analysis (Note 5)

1. The PEI/siRNA or PEI-CA-DOX/siRNA complex nanoparticles (0.1 mg/mL) were prepared in deionized water.
2. The particle size and zeta potential of the PEI/siRNA or PEI-CA-DOX/siRNA complex nanoparticles were measured by a zeta potential/BI-90Plus particle size analyzer (Brookhaven, USA).

### 2.2.6 Cell Uptake Study

1. B16F10 cells were seeded into 6-well plates at a density of $1 \times 10^5$ cells/well and incubated for 24 h. The siRNA was labeled with fluorescent dye Cy5.
2. The cells were treated with PEI-CA-DOX/siRNA complex nanoparticles (5/1, wt/wt) at the concentration 2 μg of siRNA/well for 3 h and 24 h.
3. The cells were washed with PBS five times and fixed with 4% paraformaldehyde for 15 min at room temperature.
4. The cell nuclei were stained with 4′,6-diamidino-2-phenylindole (DAPI, 1 mg/mL) for 2 min.
5. The coverslips were placed on slides and enclosed in glycerol.
6. The samples were investigated using confocal laser scanning microscopy (CLSM, ZEISS LSM 780, Germany).

### 2.2.7 Quantification of Bcl2 Gene Expression by qRT-PCR (Note 6)

1. The cells were seeded into 6-well plates at a density of $1 \times 10^5$ cells/well and then incubated overnight at 37 °C in a 5% $CO_2$ atmosphere.
2. The cells were treated with Nc siRNA, Bcl2 siRNA, or PEI/Bcl2 siRNA (5/1, wt/wt, 2.0 μg of siRNA/well) for 48 h.
3. The Trizol reagent (Invitrogen) was used to extract the total mRNA.
4. The cDNA was synthesized using reverse transcription kit from Takara Biotechnology Co., Ltd. (Dalian, China).
5. Quantitative real-time PCR was performed by Mxpro 3005P real-time PCR detection system using SYBR® Premix Ex Taq™ and PrimeScript™ RT Master Mix.

### 2.2.8 Cytotoxicity Assay

1. The cells were seeded into 96-well plates at a density of $1 \times 10^4$ cells/well and then incubated overnight at 37 °C in a 5% $CO_2$ atmosphere.
2. PEI/Bcl2 siRNA (5/1, wt/wt, 0.2 μg of siRNA/well), free DOX (0.5 μg/mL), PEI-CA-DOX/Nc siRNA (5/1, wt/wt, 0.2 μg of siRNA/well), and PEI-CA-DOX/Bcl2 siRNA (5/1, wt/wt, 0.2 μg of siRNA/well) were prepared and added into cells for 48 h.
3. 20 μL of MTT (5 mg/mL) was added into each well.
4. After incubation for extra 4 h, the medium was removed and 160 μL of DMSO was added to each well.
5. The plate was determined using a Bio-Rad 680 microplate reader at 492 nm.
6. Cell viability (%) was calculated with the following equation: Cell viability (%) = $(A_{sample}/A_{control}) \times 100\%$; where $A_{sample}$ represented the absorbencies of the sample wells, and $A_{control}$ represented the absorbencies of control wells.

### 2.2.9 In Vivo Antitumor Therapy (Note 7)

1. The antitumor efficacy of pulmonary co-delivery of DOX and siRNA was evaluated using male C57BL/6 mice (18–20 g).

2. B16F10 cells (1 × $10^4$ cells per mouse) were injected to C57BL/6 mice by intravenous injection to obtain an animal model of metastatic lung cancer.
3. The mice bearing tumors were randomly divided into six groups ($n = 6$ for each group): control, PBS, PEI/Bcl2 siRNA nanoparticles, free DOX, PEI-CA-DOX/Nc siRNA nanoparticles, and PEI-CA-DOX/Bcl2 siRNA nanoparticles, respectively.
4. The complex nanoparticles (DOX 10 μg, siRNA 20 μg) were delivered directly to the lungs for three times at 3, 10, and 17 days after B16F10 cells implantation through the mouse of trachea using a liquid aerosol device (MicroSprayer® Aerosolizer, Penn-Century, Philadelphia, PA).
5. The body weight was monitored every 3 days.
6. After 24 days, the mice were sacrificed and the lungs and major organs were collected for further analysis.

### 2.2.10 Biodistribution

1. The mice were treated with PEI-CA-DOX/Cy5 siRNA (DOX 10 μg, siRNA 20 μg), free DOX (DOX 10 μg), and free Cy5 siRNA (siRNA 20 μg) by pulmonary administration or intravenous injection.
2. After the injection, major organs (heart, liver, spleen, lung, and kidney) of mice were excised and washed with saline at 0.5 h, 3 h, 6 h, 12 h, 1 d, 2 d, 3 d, 5 d, and 7 d, respectively.
3. At excitation and emission wavelengths, respectively, of 523 and 560 nm for DOX and of 650 and 670 nm for Cy5 siRNA, the fluorescence distribution was observed by a Maestro in vivo Imaging System (Cambridge Research & Instrumentation, Inc., USA).

### 2.2.11 Intracellular Uptake of DOX and siRNA In Vivo (Note 8)

1. The mice were treated with PEI-CA-DOX/Cy5 siRNA complex nanoparticles (DOX 10 μg, siRNA 20 μg) by pulmonary administration or intravenous injection.
2. After 24 h, all the lungs of mice were collected and frozen at −80 °C overnight.
3. The iced lungs were sectioned into 5 μm/slice and stained nuclei using DAPI for 5 min.
4. The lung sections were observed with ZEISS LSM 780 CLSM.

## 3 Discussion

Here are some notes which can be used to solve possible problems.

1. Acidic and neutral saturated sodium chloride were prepared, respectively, and then were placed in the –20 °C refrigerator overnight. The target product was first washed twice with an acidic saturated sodium chloride, and then washed five times with neutral saturated sodium chloride, and finally dried over anhydrous sodium sulfate.
2. The peaks in the $^1$H NMR spectra of PEI-CA-DOX at 2.5–3.5 ppm were attributed to PEI and the peaks at 7.0–8.0 ppm were belonged to DOX (Hu et al. 2009; Tang et al. 2006).

3. PEI/siRNA and PEI-CA-DOX/siRNA were prepared by electrostatic interaction through mixing PEI or PEI-CA-DOX and siRNA.
4. The substitute for siRNA was calf thymus DNA to save costs. The DOX release from PEI-CA-DOX and PEI-CA-DOX/DNA exhibited both in a time- and pH-dependent manner, and were higher in acidic conditions than that in physiological condition (pH 7.4). This phenomenon might attribute to that the cis-aconityl linkage of PEI-CA-DOX could easily cleave in acidic conditions (Guan et al. 2013).
5. The zeta potential of the PEI/siRNA and PEI-CA-DOX/siRNA (5/1, wt/wt) were positive charged. Based on the electrostatic interactions between the positively charged complex nanoparticles and negatively charged cell surface, the positive charged complex nanoparticles might enhance the cellular uptake (Mintzer and Simanek 2009). The particle size of PEI-CA-DOX/siRNA was about 76 nm, which would be beneficial for tumor accumulation (Dufort et al. 2012).
6. The real-time PCR program was carried out with the following procedure: the initial heating at 95 °C for 10 min, 40 cycles of 95 °C for 30 s, 56 °C for 1 min, 72 °C for 1 min.
7. All the animals were cared for in compliance with the guidelines of the Animal Care and Use Committee of Northeast Normal University. The healthy mice were control group without B16F10 cells injection.
8. The mice treated by pulmonary administration of PEI-CA-DOX/siRNA complex nanoparticles showed higher fluorescent intensity of DOX and Cy5 in the tumor tissues than that treated with systemic administration, which indicated that the pulmonary delivery DOX and siRNA to the lung tumor tissues was better than that systemic administration.

## 4 Conclusion

This chapter presented the PEI-CA-DOX/siRNA complex nanoparticles for pulmonary co-delivery DOX and Bcl2 siRNA. At first, the chemotherapy drugs (DOX) could bond to PEI to obtain acid-sensitive drug conjugate (PEI-CA-DOX), and then PEI-CA-DOX could combine with Bcl2 siRNA to prepare PEI-CA-DOX/siRNA complex particles through the electrostatic interaction. The results showed that DOX from PEI-CA-DOX conjugate could be released largely under acidic conditions compared with physiological environment. MTT results showed that the cell survival rate in the co-delivery of DOX and siRNA was significantly lower than that in the DOX or siRNA alone, which indicated the co-delivery system of DOX and siRNA has good antitumor effects. The anti-tumor experiments in vivo showed that the pulmonary co-delivery of DOX and siRNA could significantly inhibit tumor growth compared with the single-delivery system, which might due to the higher accumulation of DOX and Bcl2 siRNA in the tumor tissues in lungs. The distribution results in vivo showed that pulmonary administration could improve the accumulation DOX and siRNA in the lungs compared with intravenous administration. The intracellular uptake of DOX and siRNA showed that the DOX and siRNA accumulated more at the tumor site than that in the normal tissue after pulmonary administration, which suggested that the DOX and siRNA could exhibit good antitumor effects at the tumor site with low side effects to normal tissues. The pulmonary co-delivery DOX and siRNA system has the great potentials for the metastatic lung cancer treatment.

## References


Bivas-Benita M, Zwier R, Junginger HE, Borchard G (2005) Non-invasive pulmonary aerosol delivery in mice by the endotracheal route. Eur J Pharm Biopharm 61(3):214–218

Campa CC, Silva RL, Margaria JP, Pirali T (2018) Inhalation of the prodrug PI3K inhibitor CL27c improves lung function in asthma and fibrosis. Nat Commun 9(1):5232

Chen AM, Zhang M, Wei D, Stueber D, Taratula O, Minko T, He H (2009) Co-delivery of doxorubicin and Bcl-2 siRNA by mesoporous silica nanoparticles enhances the efficacy of chemotherapy in multidrug-resistant cancer cells. Small 5(23):2673–2677

Creixell M, Peppas NA (2012) Co-delivery of siRNA and therapeutic agents using nanocarriers to overcome cancer resistance. Nano Today 7(4):367–379

Dufort S, Sancey L, Coll J-L (2012) Physico-chemical parameters that govern nanoparticles fate also dictate rules for their molecular evolution. Adv Drug Deliv Rev 64(2):179–189

Elmowafy E, Osman R, Ishak RA (2017) Polymer-based novel lung targeted delivery systems. Curr Pharm Des 23(3):373–392

Garbuzenko OB, Saad M, Betigeri S, Zhang M, Vetcher AA, Soldatenkov VA, Reimer DC, Pozharov VP, Minko T (2009) Intratracheal versus intravenous liposomal delivery of siRNA, antisense oligonucleotides and anticancer drug. Pharm Res 26(2):382–394

Garbuzenko OB, Saad M, Pozharov VP, Reuhl KR, Mainelis G, Minko T (2010) Inhibition of lung tumor growth by complex pulmonary delivery of drugs with oligonucleotides as suppressors of cellular resistance. Proc Natl Acad Sci U S A 107(23):10737–10742

Garbuzenko OB, Ivanova V, Kholodovych V, Reimer DC, Reuhl KR, Yurkow E, Adler D, Minko T (2017) Combinatorial treatment of idiopathic pulmonary fibrosis using nanoparticles with prostaglandin E and siRNA(s). Nanomedicine 13(6):1983–1992

Guan X, Li Y, Jiao Z, Chen J, Guo Z, Tian H, Chen X (2013) A pH-sensitive charge-conversion system for doxorubicin delivery. Acta Biomater 9(8):7672–7678

Guo J, Huang L (2020) Membrane-core nanoparticles for cancer nanomedicine. Adv Drug Deliv Rev 156:23–39

Gupta V, Davis M, Hope-Weeks LJ, Ahsan F (2011) PLGA microparticles encapsulating prostaglandin E1-hydroxypropyl-β-cyclodextrin (PGE1-HPβCD) complex for the treatment of pulmonary arterial hypertension (PAH). Pharm Res 28(7):1733–1749

Haddad DN, Sandler KL, Henderson LM, Rivera MP, Aldrich MC (2020) Disparities in lung cancer screening: a review. Ann Am Thorac Soc 17(4):399–405

He C, Tang Z, Tian H, Chen X (2016) Co-delivery of chemotherapeutics and proteins for synergistic therapy. Adv Drug Deliv Rev 98:64–76

Herbst RS, Morgensztern D, Boshoff C (2018) The biology and management of non-small cell lung cancer. Nature 553(7689):446–454

Hu F-Q, Liu L-N, Yong-Zhong D, Yuan H (2009) Synthesis and antitumor activity of doxorubicin conjugated stearic acid-g-chitosan oligosaccharide polymeric micelles. Biomaterials 30(36): 6955–6963

Iwabuchi K, Yoshie K, Kurakami Y, Takahashi K, Kato Y, Morishima T (2020) Therapeutic potential of ciclesonide inhalation for COVID-19 pneumonia: report of three cases. J Infect Chemother 26(6):625–632

Khan M, Ong ZY, Wiradharma N, Attia AB, Yang YY (2012) Advanced materials for co-delivery of drugs and genes in cancer therapy. Adv Healthc Mater 1(4):373–392

Lee WH, Loo CY, Ghadiri M, Leong CR, Young PM, Traini D (2018) The potential to treat lung cancer via inhalation of repurposed drugs. Adv Drug Deliv Rev 133:107–130

Martin JD, Cabral H, Stylianopoulos T, Jain RK (2020) Improving cancer immunotherapy using nanomedicines: progress, opportunities and challenges. Nat Rev Clin Oncol 17(4):251–266

Miller KD, Nogueira L, Mariotto AB, Rowland JH, Robin Yabroff K, Alfano CM, Jemal A, Kramer JL, Siegel RL (2019) Cancer treatment and survivorship statistics, 2019. CA Cancer J Clin 69(5):363–385

Mintzer MA, Simanek EE (2009) Nonviral vectors for gene delivery. Chem Rev 109(2):259–302

Na DH, Emami F, Yazdi SJM (2019) Poly(lactic acid)/poly(lactic-co-glycolic acid) particulate carriers for pulmonary drug delivery. J Pharm Investig 49(4):427–442

Otterson GA, Villalona-Calero MA, Sharma S, Kris MG, Imondi A, Gerber M, White DA, Ratain MJ, Schiller JH, Sandler A, Kraut M, Mani S, Murren JR (2007) Phase I study of inhaled doxorubicin for patients with metastatic tumors to the lungs. Clin Cancer Res 13(4):1246–1252

Otterson GA, Villalona-Calero MA, Hicks W, Pan X, Ellerton JA, Gettinger SN, Murren JR (2010) Phase I/II study of inhaled doxorubicin combined with platinum-based therapy for advanced non-small cell lung cancer. Clin Cancer Res 16(8):2466–2473

Paris JL, Vallet-Regí M (2020) Mesoporous silica nanoparticles for co-delivery of drugs and nucleic acids in oncology: a review. Pharmaceutics 12(6):526

Roa WH, Azarmi S, Al-Hallak MH, Finlay WH, Magliocco AM, Löbenberg R (2011) Inhalable nanoparticles, a non-invasive approach to treat lung cancer in a mouse model. J Control Release 150(1):49–55

Saad M, Garbuzenko OB, Minko T (2008) Co-delivery of siRNA and an anticancer drug for treatment of multidrug-resistant cancer. Nanomedicine (Lond) 3(6):761–776

Shen AM, Minko T (2020) Pharmacokinetics of inhaled nanotherapeutics for pulmonary delivery. J Control Release 326:222–244

Siegel RL, Miller KD, Jemal A (2019) 2019 Cancer statistics. CA Cancer J Clin 69(1):7–34

Siegel RL, Miller KD, Jemal A (2020) 2020 Cancer statistics. CA Cancer J Clin 70(1):7–30

Tang GP, Guo HY, Alexis F, Wang X, Zeng S, Lim TM, Ding J, Yang YY, Wang S (2006) Low molecular weight polyethylenimines linked by beta-cyclodextrin for gene transfer into the nervous system. J Gene Med 8(6):736–744

Taratula O, Garbuzenko OB, Chen AM, Minko T (2011) Innovative strategy for treatment of lung cancer: targeted nanotechnology-based inhalation co-delivery of anticancer drugs and siRNA. J Drug Target 19(10):900–914

Taratula O, Kuzmov A, Shah M, Garbuzenko OB, Minko T (2013) Nanostructured lipid carriers as multifunctional nanomedicine platform for pulmonary co-delivery of anticancer drugs and siRNA. J Control Release 171(3):349–357

Tashkin DP, Strange C (2018) Inhaled corticosteroids for chronic obstructive pulmonary disease: what is their role in therapy? Int J Chron Obstruct Pulmon Dis 13:2587–2601

Wang Y, Gao S, Ye WH, Yoon HS, Yang YY (2006) Co-delivery of drugs and DNA from cationic core-shell nanoparticles self-assembled from a biodegradable copolymer. Nat Mater 5(10): 791–796

Xu C, Wang P, Zhang J, Tian H, Park K, Chen X (2015) Pulmonary codelivery of doxorubicin and siRNA by pH-sensitive nanoparticles for therapy of metastatic lung cancer. Small 11(34): 4321–4333

Yu J, Chien YW (1997) Pulmonary drug delivery: physiologic and mechanistic aspects. Crit Rev Ther Drug Carrier Syst 14(4):395–453

Yuan M, Huang LL, Chen JH, Wu J, Xu Q (2019) The emerging treatment landscape of targeted therapy in non-small-cell lung cancer. Signal Transduct Target Ther 4:61

Zappa C, Mousa SA (2016) Non-small cell lung cancer: current treatment and future advances. Transl Lung Cancer Res 5(3):288–300

Zununi Vahed S, Salehi R, Davaran S, Sharifi S (2017) Liposome-based drug co-delivery systems in cancer cells. Mater Sci Eng C Mater Biol Appl 71:1327–1341

# Fluorinated α-Helical Polypeptides Toward Pulmonary siRNA Delivery

4

Chenglong Ge, Xun Liu, and Lichen Yin

## Contents



**Abstract**

The mucus layer and cell membrane are two major barriers against pulmonary siRNA delivery. Commonly used polycationic gene carriers can hardly penetrate the mucus layer due to the adsorption of mucin glycoproteins that trap and destabilize the polyplexes. In this study, a series of fluorinated cationic polypeptides were constructed based on ring-opening polymerization and click chemistry, aiming to synchronize mucus permeation and cell penetration to realize efficient pulmonary siRNA delivery against acute lung injury (ALI). Studies have shown that the introduction of an appropriate amount of fluorine chains can not only improve the cellular uptake and gene silencing efficiency but also greatly promote the stability of the polypeptide/siRNA polyplexes, which further enhance the permeation in the mucus layer based on hydrophobic and lipophobic properties of fluorine chains. Moreover, the in vivo anti-inflammatory results indicated that the P3F16/siTNF-α and P7F7/siTNF-α polyplexes can significantly

C. Ge · X. Liu · L. Yin (✉)
Jiangsu Key Laboratory for Carbon-Based Functional Materials and Devices, Institute of Functional Nano & Soft Materials (FUNSOM), Collaborative Innovation Center of Suzhou Nano Science & Technology, Soochow University, Suzhou, China
e-mail: lcyin@suda.edu.cn



H. Tian and X. Chen (eds.), *Gene Delivery*, Biomaterial Engineering,
https://doi.org/10.1007/978-981-16-5419-0_9

reduce the expression of pro-inflammatory factors, such as TNF-α and IL-6. It thus renders promising potentials toward the treatment of pulmonary diseases via noninvasive, localized delivery.

**Keywords**

Helical polypeptide · Fluorination · Pulmonary siRNA delivery · Mucus permeation · Cell penetration · Anti-inflammation

## 1 Overview

Pneumonia has become one of the most common infectious diseases in the world, and severe pneumonia may cause acute lung injury (ALI) or acute respiratory distress syndrome (ARDS) (Matthay et al. 2018). In this process, the imbalance of the anti-inflammatory factors and pro-inflammatory factors often causes a lung cytokine storm, which in turn induces a systemic cytokine storm and leads to multiple organ dysfunction (Mehta et al. 2020). Acute lung injury (ALI) is a serious form of diffuse lung inflammation, characterized by the increased permeability of the alveolar-capillary barrier and lung edema with protein-rich fluid that result in the impairment of arterial oxygenation (Levy and Serhan et al. 2014). Studies have shown that the macrophages can release inflammatory factors induced lipopolysaccharide (LPS), such as tumor necrosis factor-α (TNF-α), interleukin-1 (IL-1), and interleukin-6 (IL-6) (Shen et al. 2018; Bhattacharya and Matthay 2013; Peng et al. 2019; Zhang et al. 2018). Thus, small interfering RNA (siRNA)-mediated gene silencing that can specifically and efficiently inhibit the expression of pro-inflammatory cytokines at the mRNA level has become a promising paradigm for the treatment of ALI (Khan et al. 2014; Li et al. 2017).

Naked siRNA is prone to hydrolysis by nucleases in the body, and it is thus difficult to penetrate the cell membrane alone to effectively treat ALI. As a common gene delivery carrier, cationic polymers can effectively condense nucleic acids through electrostatic interactions to promote the intracellular delivery (Guan et al. 2016; Duro-Castano et al. 2017; Cheng et al. 2016; Kim et al. 2018). However, cationic polyplexes are often easily captured by endosomes/lysosomes, which greatly reduces gene transfection ability (Fang et al. 2018; Kim et al. 2019; He et al. 2016; Song et al. 2017; Wei et al. 2013). Recently, cationic α-helical polypeptides have been widely used in gene and drug delivery systems. They can efficiently deliver nucleic acids into cells through a "punch" mechanism, thereby avoiding endosome capture and significantly improving gene transfection efficiency (Ge et al. 2020a, b; Liu and Yin 2021).

However, during the pulmonary siRNA delivery, the positively charged polyplexes are often easily entrapped by mucin glycoproteins. The mucus layer covering the pulmonary epithelia contains densely glycosylated and negatively charged regions, which greatly reduce the gene transfection efficiency of polyplexes. Simultaneously, the frequent turn-over of the mucin layer further leads to fast mucociliary clearance of polyplexes (Shan et al. 2015; Vllasaliu et al. 2011; Chen et al. 2020; Ding et al. 2021; Yang et al. 2021). To address such a critical issue, Hanes and coworkers reported pioneering work to densely decorate the polyplexes surface with poly(ethylene glycol) (PEG), which facilitated trans-mucus penetration as a result of diminished adhesive interaction with mucus (Yang et al. 2011; Ensign et al. 2012). Nevertheless, the dense PEG decoration may compromise the interaction between polyplexes and cell membranes, which hurdles effective cellular internalization and gene transfection.

Fluoropolymers have been widely used in gene and protein delivery due to their unique fluorine effect in recent years. In 2014, Cheng reported for the first time that fluorinated dendrimers possess excellent serum stability and gene transfection efficiency. The excellent serum stability of fluorinated polymers originated from the lipophobic as well as hydrophobic feature of fluorocarbon compounds, which improves the physiological stability of polyplexes against serum by resisting adsorption of serum proteins onto polyplexes surfaces as well as preventing nonspecific exchanges with serum proteins (Wang et al. 2014). Inspired by these understandings, we hypothesized that fluorination modification can also enhance the stability and permeability of cationic polyplexes in the mucus layer via steric hindrance against the adsorption of mucin glycoproteins, which further resolves the contradiction between polyplexes-mediated mucus transport and cell membrane penetration. To verify this hypothesis, we herein developed a series of guanidinated and fluorinated bifunctional polypeptides with stable α-helical conformation for the pulmonary delivery of siRNA against tumor necrosis factor-α (siTNF-α). In this system, the positive charge and rod-like helix of the polypeptide can render strong cell membrane penetration, and the introduction of fluorocarbon in the side chain further enables trans-mucus penetration, thus allowing effective siTNF-α delivery into alveolar macrophages to provoke anti-inflammatory effect against ALI (Ge et al. 2020a, b).

## 2 Protocol

### 2.1 Materials

#### 2.1.1 Synthesis of 3F-Cl and 5F-Cl

1. 6-Chlorohexanol.
2. Trifluoroacetic anhydride.
3. Pentafluoropropionic anhydride.
4. Pyridine.
5. 4-Dimethylaminopyridine (DMAP).
6. Dichloromethane.
7. HCl (1 M).
8. Saturated sodium chloride.
9. Anhydrous sodium sulfate.
10. Nuclear magnetic resonance spectroscopy.

### 2.1.2 Synthesis of 7F-Cl

1. 6-Chlorohexanol.
2. Heptafluorobutyric anhydride.
3. Pyridine.
4. 4-Dimethylaminopyridine (DMAP).
5. Dichloromethane.
6. HCl (1 M).
7. Saturated sodium chloride.
8. Distilled water (DI $H_2O$).
9. Saturated sodium bicarbonate.
10. Anhydrous sodium sulfate.
11. Nuclear magnetic resonance spectroscopy.

### 2.1.3 Synthesis of *n*F-$N_3$ ($n = 3, 5$, and 7)

1. *n*F-Cl ($n = 3, 5$, and 7).
2. Sodium azide ($NaN_3$) (see Sect. 3 “1”).
3. Dimethylformamide (DMF).
4. Hexane.
5. Saturated sodium chloride.
6. Anhydrous sodium sulfate.
7. Nuclear magnetic resonance spectroscopy.

### 2.1.4 Synthesis of Polypeptide PPOBLG

1. γ-(4-Propargyloxybenzyl)-L-glutamic acid based *N*-carboxyanhydride (POBLG-NCA) (Zhang et al. 2014) (see Sect. 3 “2”).
2. Dimethylformamide (DMF).
3. *n*-Butylamine/DMF stock solution (0.1 M).
4. Distilled water (DI $H_2O$).
5. Nuclear magnetic resonance spectroscopy.
6. Gel permeation chromatography.

### 2.1.5 Synthesis of P*m*F*x* and PG1

1. PPOBLG (see Sect. 3 “3”).
2. *n*F-$N_3$ ($n = 3, 5$, and 7).
3. 6-Azidohexyl guanidine (Zhang et al. 2014).
4. *N,N,N′,N″,N″*-pentamethyldiethylenetriamine (PMDETA).
5. Copper(I) bromide (CuBr) (see Sect. 3 “4”).
6. Dimethylformamide (DMF).
7. HCl (1 M).
8. Distilled water (DI $H_2O$).
9. Dialysis bag (MWCO = 3500 Da).
10. Nuclear magnetic resonance spectroscopy.
11. Circular dichroism.

#### 2.1.6 Preparation of Polypeptide/siRNA Polyplexes

1. P*m*F*x* and PG1.
2. TNF-α siRNA (siTNF-α).
3. Negative control siRNA (siNC).
4. DI $H_2O$ pretreated with diethyl pyrocarbonate (DEPC).
5. Vortex mixer (IKA, VORTEX 2).
6. Dynamic light scattering (DLS).

#### 2.1.7 Gel Electrophoresis

1. Agarose.
2. 50× TAE buffer (40 mM Tris-acetic acid, 1 mM EDTA (pH 8)).
3. Ethidium bromide (EB), store away from light.
4. Polypeptide/siRNA polyplexes at various polypeptide/siRNA weight ratios.
5. Loading buffer (6×).
6. 1.5 mL Micro centrifuge tubes (DNase/RNase free).
7. Gel imaging system.
8. Microplate reader.

#### 2.1.8 Cell Culture

1. RAW 264.7 (mouse monocyte macrophage) cells.
2. Calu-3 (human lung adenocarcinoma) cells.
3. Dulbecco's Modified Eagles Medium (DMEM).
4. Fetal bovine serum (FBS).
5. Phosphate-buffered saline (PBS, 1×, pH 7.4) (see Sect. 3 "5").
6. $CO_2$ incubator.
7. Disposable sterile cell scraper.
8. Cell culture dish (60 × 15 mm).

#### 2.1.9 Cell Uptake

1. RAW 264.7 cells.
2. DMEM and DMEM containing 10% FBS.
3. 96-Well plates.
4. PBS (1×, pH 7.4) and PBS containing heparin (20 U/mL) (see Sect. 3 "5").
5. Cy3-siRNA.
6. Polypeptide/siRNA polyplexes (w/w = 15) were prepared as described in Sect. 2.2.6.
7. RIPA lysis buffer (0.394 g Tris·HCl, 0.438 g NaCl, 0.5 mL nonidet P-40, 0.05 g SDS, and 50 mL DI $H_2O$).
8. BCA kit.
9. Microplate reader.

### 2.1.10 In Vitro TNF-α Knockdown Efficiency

1. RAW 264.7 cells.
2. DMEM and DMEM containing 10% FBS.
3. 96-Well plate and 6-well plate.
4. PBS (1×, pH 7.4) (see Sect. 3 "5").
5. siTNF-α (same as in Table 1) and polypeptide/siTNF-α polyplexes (w/w = 15) were prepared as described in Sect. 2.2.6.
6. Lipopolysaccharide (LPS).
7. $H_2SO_4$ (1 M).
8. ELISA kit.
9. Polyethylenimine (PEI, MW = 25,000).
10. Total RNA isolation agent.
11. Chloroform.
12. Isopropanol.
13. PrimeScript.
14. SYBR Premix Ex Taq kit (Primer sequences are shown in Table 2).
15. Nano drop.
16. Real-time PCR system (Bio-Rad CFX connect).
17. Microplate reader.

### 2.1.11 In Vitro Permeation Across Calu-3 Cell Monolayers (Huang et al. 2017) (See Sect. 3 "6")

1. Calu-3 cells.
2. DMEM and DMEM containing 10% FBS.
3. 24-Well plate.
4. Transwells (0.33 $cm^2$, pore size of 3.0 μm, Corning, NY).
5. Cy3-siRNA.
6. Polypeptide/Cy3-siRNA polyplexes (w/w = 15) were prepared as described in Sect. 2.2.6.

**Table 1** Sequences of siTNF-α and siNC

| Sequence | |
|---|---|
| siTNF-α sense | 5′-GUCUCAGCCUCUUCUCAUUCCUGCT-3′ |
| siTNF-α antisense | 5′-AGCAGGAAmUGmAAmGAGGmCUGAmGACmAmU-3′ |
| siNC sense | 5′-UUCUCCGAACGUGUCACGUTT-3′ |
| siNC antisense | 5′-ACGUGACACGUUCGGAGAATT-3′ |

**Table 2** Primer sequences of TNF-α and GAPDH

| Sequence | |
|---|---|
| TNF-α F | 5′-CCCTCACACTCAGATCATCTTCT-3′ |
| TNF-α R | 5′-GCTACGACGTGGGCATCAG-3′ |
| GAPDH F | 5′-TTCACCACCATGGAGAAGGC-3′ |
| GAPDH R | 5′-GGCATGGACTGTGGTCATGA-3′ |

7. KRB buffer (114.2 mM NaCl, 3 mM KCl, 1.5 mM $K_2HPO_4$, 10 mM HEPES, 4 mM D-glucose, 1.4 mM $CaCl_2$, 2.56 mM $MgCl_2$).
8. Transmembrane resistance analyzer.
9. Microplate reader.

#### 2.1.12 Multiple Particle Tracking (Huang et al. 2017)

1. Cystic fibrosis (CF) mucus (see Sect. 3 "7").
2. Polypeptide/Cy3-siRNA polyplexes (w/w = 15) were prepared as described in Sect. 2.2.6.
3. Confocal laser scanning microscopy (CLSM).

#### 2.1.13 In Vivo Gene Knockdown Efficiency

1. Male Balb/c mice (6–8 weeks).
2. Lipopolysaccharide (LPS).
3. PBS (1×, pH 7.4).
4. siTNF-α (same as in Sect. 2.2.6) and polypeptide/siTNF-α polyplexes (w/w = 15) were prepared as described in Sect. 2.2.6.
5. ELISA kit.
6. Polyethylenimine (PEI, MW = 25,000) (see Sect. 3 "8").
7. Microplate reader.
8. Vertical electrophoresis.
9. 12% SDS-PAGE separation gel.
10. 5% SDS-PAGE concentration gel.
11. 1× Electrophoresis buffer (3.03 g Tris, 18.8 g glycine, 1 g SDS, 1000 mL DI $H_2O$).
12. 1× Transfer buffer (3.03 g Tris, 14.4 g glycine, 200 mL methanol, 800 mL DI $H_2O$).
13. 1× TBST (6.057 g Tris, 9 g NaCl, 3.5 mL HCl, 1 mL Tween20, 1000 mL DI $H_2O$).
14. Primary antibody, secondary antibody.
15. Photographic developer.
16. Gel imaging system.

#### 2.1.14 Lung Function Assessment

1. Male Balb/c mice (6–8 weeks).
2. Lipopolysaccharide (LPS).
3. PBS (1×, pH 7.4).
4. siTNF-α (same as in Sect. 2.2.6) and polypeptide/siTNF-α polyplexes (w/w = 15) were prepared as described in Sect. 2.2.6
5. 10% PFA.
6. Paraffin.
7. Hematoxylin/eosin (HE).
8. Optical microscopy.
9. Blood-gas analyzer.

## 2.2 Methods

### 2.2.1 Synthesis of 3F-Cl and 5F-Cl

1. Add 6-chlorohexanol (1.00 g, 7.32 mmol), trifluoroacetic anhydride (2.00 g, 9.51 mmol), pyridine (1.74 g, 21.96 mmol), and DMAP (60 mg, 0.488 mmol) into a 10-mL vial in an ice-water bath.
2. Transfer the vial in room temperature and stir the system for 84 h (see Sect. 3 "9").
3. Dissolve the mixture in 50 mL of dichloromethane.
4. Wash the mixture with brine (50 mL × 1), 1 M HCl (50 mL × 4), and brine (50 mL × 2) (see Sect. 3 "10").
5. Separate the organic phase and dry with anhydrous sodium sulfate.
6. Remove the solvent under vacuum, and obtain a light yellow liquid.
7. Determine the structure of the resulting 3F-Cl using nuclear magnetic resonance spectroscopy.
8. Use the same method to synthesize 5F-Cl (see Sect. 3 "11").

### 2.2.2 Synthesis of 7F-Cl

1. Add 6-chlorohexanol (1.00 g, 7.32 mmol), heptafluorobutyric anhydride (3.60 g, 8.78 mmol), pyridine (1.74 g, 21.96 mmol), and DMAP (60 mg, 0.488 mmol) into a 10-mL vial in an ice-water bath.
2. Transfer the vial in room temperature and stir the system for 84 h (see Sect. 3 "9").
3. Dissolve the mixture in 50 mL of dichloromethane.
4. Wash the mixture with brine (50 mL × 1), 1 M HCl (50 mL × 4), and brine (50 mL × 2) (see Sect. 3 "10").
5. Remove the solvent to obtain a light yellow oil.
6. Add 20 mL of DI $H_2O$ and stir the mixture at 60 °C for 1 h (see Sect. 3 "12").
7. Dissolve the mixture in 50 mL of dichloromethane.
8. Wash the mixture with saturated $NaHCO_3$ solution (50 mL × 2) and brine (50 mL × 2) (see Sect. 3 "10").
9. Separate the organic phase and dry with anhydrous sodium sulfate.
10. Remove the solvent under vacuum, and obtain a light yellow liquid.
11. Determine the structure of the resulting 7F-Cl using nuclear magnetic resonance spectroscopy.

### 2.2.3 Synthesis of *n*F-$N_3$ (*n* = 3, 5, and 7)

1. Dissolve 3F-Cl (0.8 g, 3.44 mmol) and $NaN_3$ (1.12 g, 17.19 mmol) in 2 mL of DMF into a round-bottom flask.
2. Stir the mixture at 60 °C for 48 h.
3. Dissolve the mixture in 50 mL of hexane and wash with brine (50 mL × 4).
4. Separate the organic phase and dry with anhydrous sodium sulfate.
5. Remove the solvent under vacuum, and obtain a transparent liquid.

6. Determine the structure of the resulting 3F-$N_3$ using nuclear magnetic resonance spectroscopy.
7. Use the same method to synthesize 5F-$N_3$ and 7F-$N_3$.

### 2.2.4 Synthesis of Polypeptide PPOBLG

1. Synthesize POBLG-NCA using literature method (see Sect. 3 "13") (Zhang et al. 2014).
2. Synthesize PPOBLG via ring-opening polymerization (ROP) of POBLG-NCA as initiated by *n*-butylamine. Dissolve POBLG-NCA (0.86 g, 2.71 mmol) in 5 mL of anhydrous DMF in a vial under nitrogen.
3. Add a solution of *n*-butylamine in DMF (0.1 M, 271 μL, 0.027 mmol) with a syringe.
4. Stir the mixture at room temperature for 72 h (see Sect. 3 "14").
5. Add the mixture dropwise into 60 mL of cold DI $H_2O$ and collect the white precipitate by centrifuging.
6. Determine the structure using nuclear magnetic resonance spectroscopy, and determine the molecular weight and polydispersity using gel permeation chromatography (see Sect. 3 "3").

### 2.2.5 Synthesis of P*m*F*x* and PG1

1. Synthesize P*m*F*x* and PG1 via click chemistry. Dissolve PPOBLG, 6-azidohexyl guanidine and *n*F-$N_3$ in 5 mL of DMF in glove box (see Table 3).
2. Add *N*,*N*,*N*′,*N*″,*N*″-pentamethyldiethylenetriamine (PMDETA, 34 μL, 0.125 mmol) and CuBr (18 mg, 0.125 mmol) into the mixture.
3. Stir the mixture at room temperature for 36 h.
4. Quench the reaction by exposure to air and add 3–4 mL of HCl (1 M) until the solution became colorless.
5. Dialyze the resulting mixture against distilled water (MWCO = 3500 Da) for 3 days and lyophilize to afford white solid.

**Table 3** Synthesis of P*m*F*x* and PG1 from PPOBLG

| | PPOBLG (mg) | G-6-$N_3$ (mg) | *n*F-$N_3$ (mg) | 7H-$N_3$ (mg) | Yield (%) |
|---|---|---|---|---|---|
| PG1 | 30 | 22.3 | – | – | 91 |
| P3F7 | 30 | 20.7 | 2.1 | – | 94 |
| P3F16 | 30 | 18.9 | 4.3 | – | 87 |
| P3F31 | 30 | 15.6 | 8.7 | – | 86 |
| P5F6 | 30 | 20.7 | 2.5 | – | 90 |
| P5F16 | 30 | 18.9 | 5.3 | – | 90 |
| P5F34 | 30 | 15.6 | 10.5 | – | 88 |
| P7F7 | 30 | 20.7 | 2.9 | – | 92 |
| P7F18 | 30 | 18.9 | 6.2 | – | 85 |
| P7F34 | 30 | 15.6 | 12.3 | – | 87 |

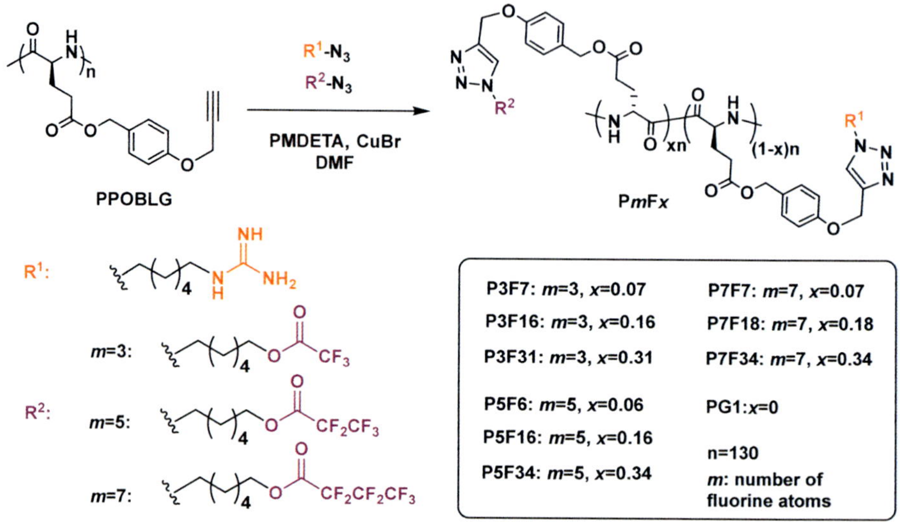


**Fig. 1** Synthetic routes of P*m*F*x* and PG1

6. Determine the structure using nuclear magnetic resonance spectroscopy, and determine the secondary structure using circular dichroism (see Sect. 3 "15") (Fig. 1).

### 2.2.6 Preparation of Polypeptide/siRNA Polyplexes

1. Add polypeptide solution (0.2 mg/mL) into the siRNA solution (0.1 mg/mL) at weight ratios of 2, 5, 10, 15, and 20.
2. Vortex the mixture for 10 s and incubate at 37 °C for 30 min to form polypeptide/siRNA polyplexes.
3. Measure the particle size and zeta potential by Malvern Zetasizer.

### 2.2.7 Gel Electrophoresis

1. Dissolve 3 g of agarose in 150 mL of 1× TAE buffer to prepare 2% agarose solution.
2. Cool down the solution and add 10 μL of EB into the agarose solution.
3. Pour the solution into the acrylic plate and insert a comb to form a gel.
4. Put the gel in the electrophoresis tank, and add 1× TAE buffer to cover the gel.
5. Add 4 μL of 6× loading buffer into the polypeptide/siRNA polyplexes, and then load the mixture into the wells slowly with a pipette (0.1 μg siRNA/well).
6. Cover the tank and subject the loaded samples to electrophoresis for 20 min at 90 V in 1× TAE buffer.
7. Visualize the electrophoretic mobility of the siRNA by gel imaging system (see Sect. 3 "16").

### 2.2.8 Cell Culture

1. Transfer RAW 264.7 (or Calu-3) cells into a cell culture dish (60 × 15 mm) with 4 mL of DMEM containing 10% FBS.
2. Grow the cells to ~80% confluence in the incubator with a 5% $CO_2$ at 37 °C.
3. To subculture the cells, remove the DMEM, wash the cells twice with 2 mL of PBS (pH 7.4), put 3 mL of DMEM containing 10% FBS into the cell culture dish, scrape the cells gently with a disposable sterile cell scraper and disperse the cells evenly in the culture medium, take 1 mL of the mixture into a new cell culture dish, add 3 mL of new DMEM containing 10% FBS, and culture the cells in the incubator (see Sect. 3 "17").

### 2.2.9 Cell Uptake

1. Seed RAW 264.7 cells (~70% confluence) in 96-well plates and culture the cells under 5% $CO_2$ at 37 °C for 24 h.
2. Replace the medium with serum-free DMEM.
3. Add polypeptide/Cy3-siRNA polyplexes (w/w = 15) at 1 μg Cy3-siRNA/mL and incubate for 4 h (see Sect. 3 "18").
4. Wash the cells with cold PBS containing heparin (20 U/mL) for three times and lyse the cells with the RIPA lysis buffer (100 μL/well) for 20 min in the dark.
5. Measure the Cy3-siRNA content in the lysate by spectrofluorimetry ($\lambda_{ex} = 550$ nm, $\lambda_{em} = 565$ nm).
6. Quantify the protein level by using BCA kit, and uptake level was expressed as μg Cy3-siRNA associated with 1 mg of cellular protein (see Sect. 3 "19").
7. Statistical analysis was conducted using the Student's t test, and differences were assessed to be significant at $^*p < 0.05$ and very significant at $^{**}p < 0.01$ and $^{***}p < 0.001$.

### 2.2.10 ELISA Assay

1. Seed RAW 264.7 cells (~70% confluence) in 96-well plates and culture the cells under 5% $CO_2$ at 37 °C for 24 h.
2. Replace the medium with serum-free DMEM.
3. Add polypeptide/siTNF-α polyplexes (w/w = 15) at 1 μg siTNF-α/mL and incubate for 4 h (see Sect. 3 "18").
4. Wash the cells with PBS buffer.
5. Replace the medium with DMEM containing 10% FBS and further incubate for 20 h.
6. Challenge the cells with LPS (7.5 ng/mL) for 5 h.
7. Determine TNF-α level in the medium by ELISA kit, and the knockdown efficiency was denoted as the percentage TNF-α level of control cells that did not receive polyplexes treatment (see Sect. 3 "20").
8. Statistical analysis was conducted using the Student's t test, and differences were assessed to be significant at $^*p < 0.05$ and very significant at $^{**}p < 0.01$ and $^{***}p < 0.001$.

### 2.2.11 PCR Assay

1. Seed RAW 264.7 cells (~70% confluence) in 96-well plates and culture the cells under 5% $CO_2$ at 37 °C for 24 h.
2. Replace the medium with serum-free DMEM.
3. Add polypeptide/siTNF-α polyplexes (w/w = 15) at 1 μg siTNF-α/mL and incubate for 4 h (see Sect. 3 "18").
4. Wash the cells with PBS buffer.
5. Replace the medium with DMEM containing 10% FBS and further incubate for 20 h.
6. Challenge the cells with LPS (7.5 ng/mL) for 5 h.
7. Isolate total RNA from cells using the Trizol reagent and measure the RNA concentration using nano drop.
8. Synthesize cDNA from total RNA using the high-capacity cDNA reverse transcription kit.
9. Mix synthesized cDNA, TNF-α primers, and SYBR Premix Ex Taq and run on the real-time PCR system (Bio-Rad CFX connect).
10. Analyzed the 36B4 expression in parallel in the same run.
11. Calculate the TNF-α mRNA content expressed as percentage TNF-α mRNA level of control cells that were challenged by LPS but not treated with polyplexes (see Sect. 3 "20").
12. Statistical analysis was conducted using the Student's t test, and differences were assessed to be significant at $*p < 0.05$ and very significant at $**p < 0.01$ and $***p < 0.001$.

### 2.2.12 In Vitro Permeation Across Calu-3 Cell Monolayers

1. Construct air-interfaced culture (AIC) model using Calu-3 cells. Seed Calu-3 cells on Transwells (0.33 $cm^2$, pore size of 3.0 μm, Corning, NY) at $5.0 \times 10^5$ cell/$cm^2$ and culture for 14 days (see Sect. 3 "21").
2. Determine the transepithelial electrical resistance (TEER) during days 7–14 until TEER stops increasing.
3. Wash the cells with PBS for three times.
4. Add 500 μL of KRB containing 1% BSA to the basolateral side, and add 200 μL of KRB containing 1% BSA to the apical side.
5. Add polypeptide/Cy3-siRNA polyplexes (w/w = 15) at 2 μg Cy3-siRNA/mL and incubate for 6 h.
6. Harvest the medium in the basolateral side and determine the amount of Cy3-siRNA by microplate reader.
7. Calculate the apparent permeability coefficient ($P_{app}$) using the equation of $P_{app} = Q/Act$, where $Q$ is the amount of permeated Cy3-siRNA (ng), $A$ is the diffusion area of the cell monolayers ($cm^2$), $c$ is the initial concentration of Cy3-siRNA at the apical side (ng/$cm^3$), and $t$ is the transport time (s) (see Sect. 3 "22").

### 2.2.13 Multiple Particle Tracking

1. Prepare 5% CF mucus solution using DI $H_2O$.
2. Add polypeptide/Cy3-siRNA polyplexes (w/w = 15, with 2 μg Cy3-siRNA) into 1 mL of CF mucus solution and transfer to an eight-well chamber slide.
3. Incubate the mixture at 37 °C for 1 h.
4. Acquire 20-s movies at 66.7 ms temporal resolution using an Evolve 512 EMCCD camera (Photometrics, Tucson, AZ) equipped on an inverted epifluorescence microscope (Observer Z1, Zeiss; Thornwood, NY) with a 100× 1.4 NA objective.
5. Analyzed the movies by Imaris software to extract movement orbits and mean square displacement (MSD) for individual polyplexes (see Sect. 3 "23").

### 2.2.14 In Vivo Gene Knockdown Efficiency

1. Divide male Balb/c mice into six groups, and intratracheally inject 50 μL of LPS solution (5 mg/mL in saline) in groups 1–5 to induce ALI.
2. Two hours later, intratracheally inject PBS, PG1/siTNF-α polyplexes (w/w = 15), P3F16/siTNF-α polyplexes (w/w = 15), P7F7/siTNF-α polyplexes (w/w = 15), and PEI/siTNF-α polyplexes (w/w = 5) at 200 μg siRNA/kg in groups 1–5. Mice in group 6 did not receive LPS or polyplexes administration and thus served as the normal control.
3. Sacrifice the mice and collect the lung tissues after another 22 h.
4. Homogenize the tissues with the RBC lysis buffer (see Sect. 3 "24").
5. Evaluate the TNF-α and IL-6 protein levels in lung tissues by ELISA and Western blot (see Sect. 3 "25").
6. Statistical analysis was conducted using the Student's t test, and differences were assessed to be significant at $^{*}p < 0.05$ and very significant at $^{**}p < 0.01$ and $^{***}p < 0.001$.

### 2.2.15 Lung Function Assessment

1. Divide male Balb/c mice into six groups, and intratracheally inject 50 μL of LPS solution (5 mg/mL in saline) in groups 1–5 to induce ALI.
2. Two hours later, intratracheally inject PBS, PG1/siTNF-α polyplexes (w/w = 15), P3F16/siTNF-α polyplexes (w/w = 15), P7F7/siTNF-α polyplexes (w/w = 15), and PEI/siTNF-α polyplexes (w/w = 5) at 200 μg siRNA/kg in groups 1–5. Mice in group 6 did not receive LPS or polyplexes administration and thus served as the normal control.
3. Sacrifice the mice, collect the fresh blood samples and lung tissues after another 22 h.
4. Measure the partial pressure of oxygen ($PaO_2$), partial pressure of carbon dioxide ($PaCO_2$), and pH by using the blood-gas analyzer (see Sect. 3 "26").

5. Collect the lung tissues, fix the lung tissues in 10% PFA, embed in paraffin, sectioned at 8-μm thickness, and stain with hematoxylin/eosin (HE) before histological observation using optical microscopy (see Sect. 3 “27”).
6. Statistical analysis was conducted using the Student’s t test, and differences were assessed to be significant at $*p < 0.05$ and very significant at $**p < 0.01$ and $***p < 0.001$.

## 3 Discussion

1. Avoid shock and high temperature when using $NaN_3$, and it is forbidden to use metal spoons for weighing.
2. NCA monomer is unstable, and it should be used and stored under anhydrous, low-temperature conditions.
3. The degree of polymerization (DP) and the distribution index ($Đ$) were determined to be 130 and 1.10, respectively.
4. CuBr is easily oxidized and should be used and stored under anhydrous and oxygen-free conditions.
5. PBS should be sterilized before using.
6. Air-interfaced culture (AIC) of Calu-3 cells is regarded as a well-established in vitro model of bronchial epithelia with secreted mucus layers, which can be adopted to evaluate the mucus/epithelia penetration capabilities of polyplexes.
7. CF mucus was obtained from CF patients of the Second Affiliated Hospital of Soochow University, and was diluted with DI $H_2O$ for 20-fold before using.
8. PEI is used for control experiments, and the weight ratio of PEI/siRNA is fixed at 5/1.
9. The mixture turned yellow gradually and precipitates appeared during this process.
10. Emulsification may occur in this process. In order to increase the yield, it is necessary to wait until the organic phase and the water phase are completely separated before performing liquid separation.
11. 5F-Cl was prepared from 6-chlorohexanol (1.00 g, 7.32 mmol), pentafluoropropionic anhydride (2.72 g, 8.78 mmol), pyridine (1.74 g, 21.96 mmol), and DMAP (60 mg, 0.488 mmol) using the same procedure as for 3F-Cl.
12. Since heptafluorobutyric acid anhydride possesses a higher boiling point (~111 °C), it can be removed by hydrolyzing it into heptafluorobutyric acid.
13. POBLG-NCA is purified by ethyl acetate/*n*-hexane interface recrystallization. If necessary, it can be further purified by column chromatography using ethyl acetate as the eluent phase after recrystallization.
14. The progress of the ring-opening polymerization can be monitored by Fourier transform infrared spectroscopy (FTIR). The characteristic peaks of NCA at 1835 and 1782 $cm^{-1}$ disappeared after the reaction completed.
15. The resulting polypeptides were named as PG1 and P*m*F*x* ($m = 3, 5$, or 7; $x = 6$, 7, 16, 18, 31, or 34), where *m* represents the number of fluorine atoms on each

fluorocarbon side chain and $x$ (mol%) represents the graft ratio of fluorocarbon side chains. All polypeptides adopted α-helical conformation as evidenced by the double minima at 208 and 222 nm (Fig. 2).

16. The gel retardation assay indicated that all polypeptides can retard siRNA migration after agarose gel electrophoresis at weight ratios $\geq 10$ (Fig. 3).
17. For Calu-3 cells, add 1 mL of trypsin to dissociate the cells instead of using a disposable sterile cell scraper.
18. Considering the unsatisfactory serum stability of the polyplexes, it is necessary to replace the serum-free DMEM before loading the samples.
19. Appropriate levels of fluorination of polyplexes ($\leq 18\%$) can obviously increase the uptake level compared with PG1 polyplexes, while the cellular uptake level decreased when the fluorine content further increased (31–34%), which might be due to the excessive compromise of the cationic guanidine groups. The

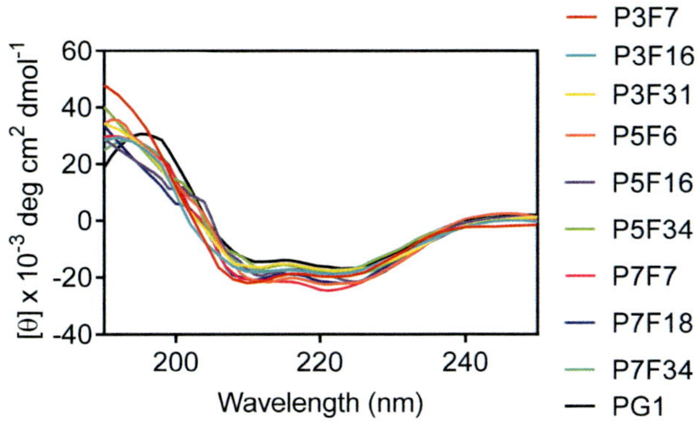


**Fig. 2** CD spectra of P*m*F*x* and PG1 (0.2 mg/mL) in DI water

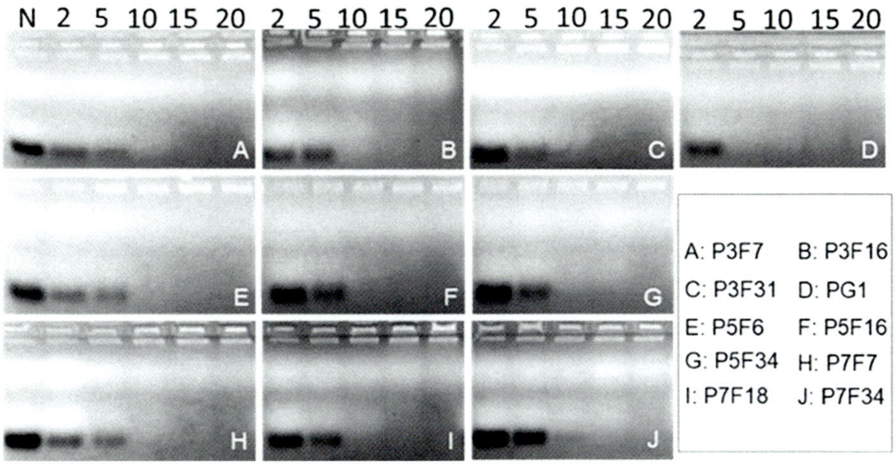


**Fig. 3** siRNA condensation by polypeptides at various polypeptide/siRNA weight ratios as evaluated by the gel retardation assay. N represents naked siRNA

top-performing material, P7F7 (Fig. 4), led to higher cellular uptake level than PG1 by nearly twofold, substantiating the important role of fluorination in potentiating the membrane activity of helical polypeptides.

20. The gene silencing efficiencies of fluorinated polypeptides were higher than PG1 and commercial reagent PEI 25k. Specifically, P3F16 and P7F7 provoked TNF-α silencing by ~70% at either protein or mRNA level (Fig. 5).
21. Within 2 weeks of building the AIC model, the medium in the apical compartment needed to be removed at 4 days post cell seeding while the medium in the basolateral side needed to be replaced every day.
22. All fluorinated polypeptides enabled higher apparent permeability coefficient ($P_{app}$) of Cy3-siRNA across Calu-3 cell monolayers than PG1, indicating the pronounced contribution of fluorination toward mucus penetration. Specifically, P3F16 and P7F7, conferred 22- and 25-fold higher siRNA permeation levels than PG1, respectively (Fig. 6).

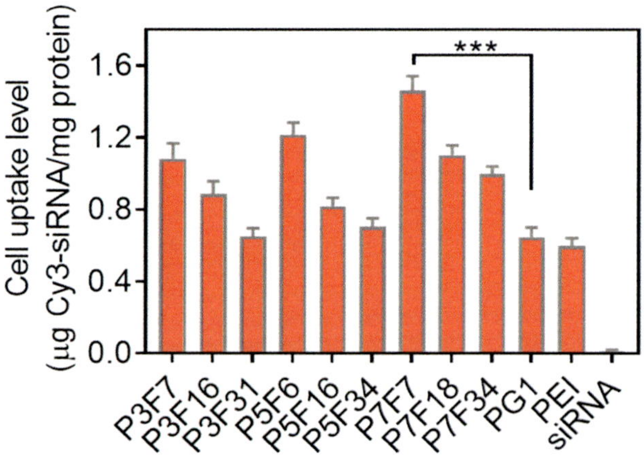


**Fig. 4** Cellular uptake levels of polypeptide/Cy3-siRNA polyplexes following 4-h incubation ($n = 3$). Naked siRNA and PEI/siRNA polyplexes (w/w = 5) served as controls

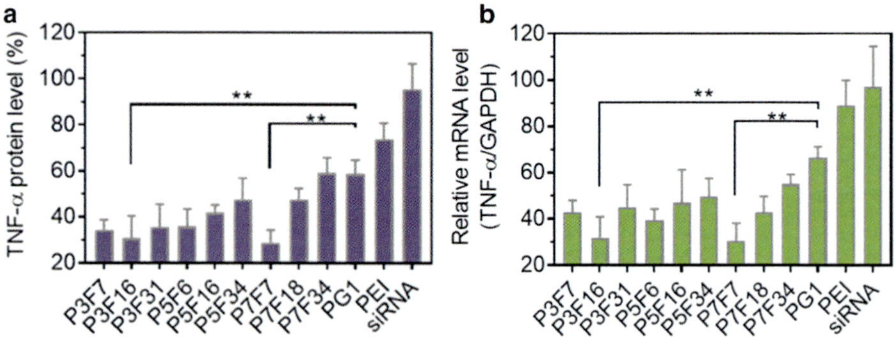


**Fig. 5** TNF-α secretion levels (**a**) and TNF-α mRNA levels (**b**) as determined by ELISA and real-time PCR, respectively ($n = 3$)

**Fig. 6** $P_{app}$ of polypeptide/Cy3-siRNA polyplexes across the AIC model ($n = 3$)

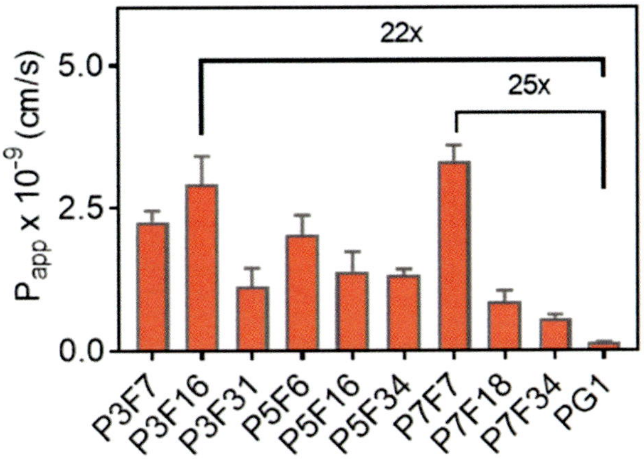


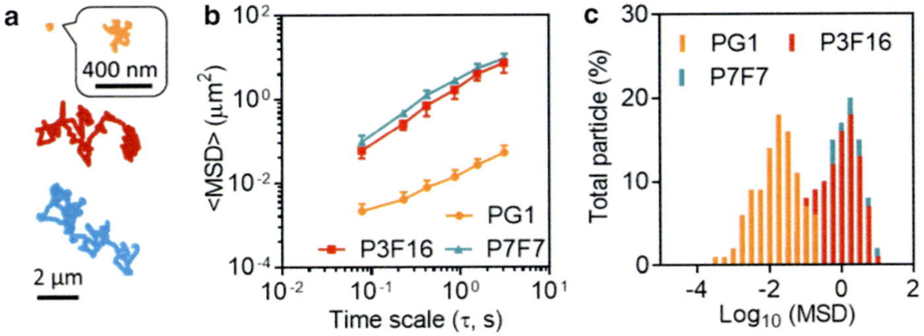


**Fig. 7** (**a**) Representative trajectories of polyplexes in the CF mucus during the 20-s movies. (**b**) <MSD> of polyplexes as a function of the time scale (τ). (**c**) Distribution of the logarithmic MSD of an individual polyplex at $\tau = 1$ s

23. As is shown in Fig. 7, the movement of the PG1/siRNA polyplexes in the mucus was severely impeded. Specifically, the geometric averaged mean square displacement (<MSD>) values of P3F16/siRNA polyplexes and P7F7/siRNA polyplexes were 2.276 and 3.583 $\mu m^2$ at the time scale (τ) of 1 s, which were 152- and 239-fold of the PG1/siRNA polyplexes (0.015 $\mu m^2$), respectively. In addition, P3F16/siRNA polyplexes and P7F7/siRNA polyplexes possessed a uniformly higher individual MSD at $\tau = 1$ s compared with PG1/siRNA polyplexes. These results collectively demonstrated that fluorination of the guanidinated helical polypeptides greatly enhanced the mucus-penetrating capabilities.
24. The mixture is centrifuged and the supernatant is collected for subsequent testing.
25. P3F16 and P7F7 polyplexes provoked remarkably higher TNF-α and IL-6 knockdown efficiencies than PG1 polyplexes (Fig. 8).

**Fig. 8** (**a**) TNF-α and IL-6 expression levels in lung tissues as evaluated by Western blot. TNF-α (**b**) and IL-6 (**c**) expression levels in lung tissues as quantified by ELISA after intratracheal administration ($n = 6$)

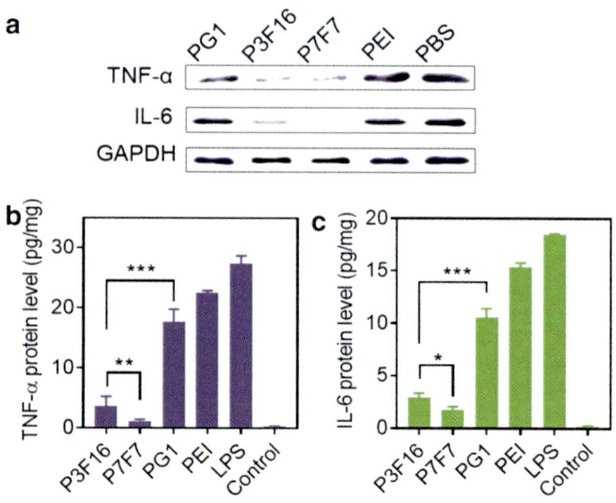


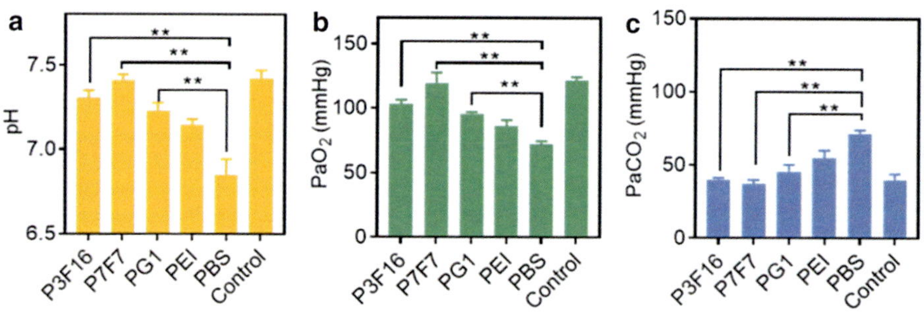


**Fig. 9** Arterial oxygen tension and total thoracic compliance as revealed by pH (**a**), $PaO_2$ (**b**), and $PaCO_2$ (**c**) in the arterial blood after intratracheal administration ($n = 6$)

26. LPS challenge led to significantly decreased partial pressure of oxygen ($PaO_2$) yet increased partial pressure of carbon dioxide ($PaCO_2$) in the arterial blood, and decreased pH of blood, indicating increased permeability of the alveolar-capillary barrier and lung edema with protein-rich fluid that further impaired the arterial oxygenation. In comparison, the blood pH, $PaO_2$, and $PaCO_2$ almost completely recovered to the normal level after administration with P7F7/siTNF-α polyplexes, which substantiated the potent therapeutic outcomes of the fluorinated polyplexes to recover the pulmonary ventilation function (Fig. 9).
27. HE staining demonstrates that the P7F7/siTNF-α polyplexes could notably alleviate LPS-induced tissue damage, including interstitial edema, hemorrhage, and thickening of the alveolar wall (Fig. 10).

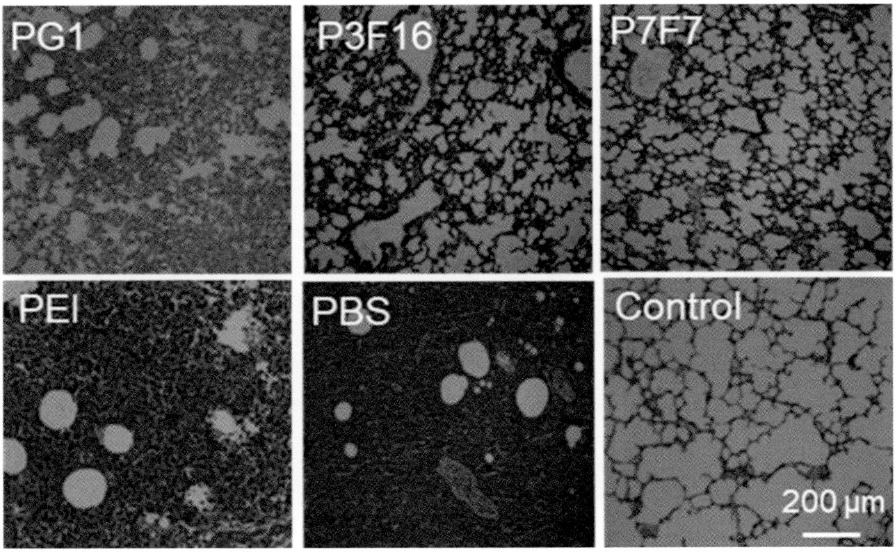


**Fig. 10** HE-stained lung tissue sections after intratracheal administration ($n = 6$)

## 4 Conclusion

In this chapter, a series of guanidinated and fluorinated α-helical polypeptides were synthesized based on ring-opening polymerization and click chemistry for penetrating the mucus layer and macrophage cell membrane to mediate highly effective pulmonary TNF-α silencing against acute lung injury. Studies have shown that the introduction of an appropriate amount of fluoroalkyl chains can not only increase the cell uptake level and gene silencing efficiency in vitro, but also enhance the mucus layer permeability due to reduced interaction between polyplexes and mucin. Moreover, in vivo anti-inflammatory results indicated that P3F16/siTNF-α and P7F7/siTNF-α polyplexes can provoke significant anti-inflammatory effect by reducing the expression of pro-inflammatory factors and inhibiting neutrophil infiltration (Figs. 2, 3, 4, 5, 6, 7, 8, 9, and 10).

## References

Bhattacharya J, Matthay MA (2013) Regulation and repair of the alveolar-capillary barrier in acute lung injury. Annu Rev Physiol 75:593–615

Chen D, Liu J, Wu J, Suk JS (2020) Enhancing nanoparticle penetration through airway mucus to improve drug delivery efficacy in the lung. Expert Opin Drug Deliv 14:1–12

Cheng Y, Yumul RC, Pun SH (2016) Virus-inspired polymer for efficient in vitro and in vivo gene delivery. Angew Chem Int Ed 128:12192–12196

Ding L, Tang S, Wyatt TA, Knoell DL, Oupický D (2021) Pulmonary siRNA delivery for lung disease: review of recent progress and challenges. J Control Release 330:977–991

Duro-Castano A, Nebot VJ, Niño-Pariente A, Armiñán A, Arroyo-Crespo JJ, Paul A, Feiner-Gracia N, Albertazzi L, Vicent MJ (2017) Capturing "extraordinary" soft-assembled charge-like polypeptides as a strategy for nanocarrier design. Adv Mater 29:1702888

Ensign LM, Schneider C, Suk JS, Cone R, Hanes J (2012) Mucus penetrating nanoparticles: biophysical tool and method of drug and gene delivery. Adv Mater 24:3887–3894

Fang H, Guo Z, Lin L, Chen J, Sun P, Wu J, Xu C, Tian H, Chen X (2018) Molecular strings significantly improved the gene transfection efficiency of polycations. J Am Chem Soc 140: 11992–12000

Ge C, Yang J, Duan S, Liu Y, Meng F, Yin L (2020a) Fluorinated α-helical polypeptides synchronize mucus permeation and cell penetration toward highly efficient pulmonary siRNA delivery against acute lung injury. Nano Lett 20:1738–1746

Ge C, Ye H, Wu F, Zhu J, Song Z, Liu Y, Yin L (2020b) Biological applications of water-soluble polypeptides with ordered secondary structures. J Mater Chem B 8:6530–6547

Guan X, Guo Z, Lin L, Chen J, Tian H, Chen X (2016) Ultrasensitive pH triggered charge/size dual-rebound gene delivery system. Nano Lett 16:6823–6831

He H, Zheng N, Song Z, Kim KH, Yao C, Zhang R, Zhang C, Huang Y, Uckun FM, Cheng J, Zhang Y, Yin L (2016) Suppression of hepatic inflammation via systemic siRNA delivery by membrane-disruptive and endosomolytic helical polypeptide hybrid nanoparticles. ACS Nano 10:1859–1870

Huang X, Chisholm J, Zhuang J, Xiao Y, Duncan G, Chen X, Suk JS, Hanes J (2017) Protein nanocages that penetrate airway mucus and tumor tissue. Proc Natl Acad Sci U S A 114:E6595–E6602

Khan OF, Zaia EW, Yin H, Bogorad RL, Pelet JM, Webber MJ, Zhuang I, Dahlman JE, Langer R, Anderson DG (2014) Ionizable amphiphilic dendrimer-based nanomaterials with alkyl-chain-substituted amines for tunable sirna delivery to the liver endothelium in vivo. Angew Chem Int Ed 53:14397–14401

Kim HS, Son YJ, Mao W, Leong KW, Yoo HS (2018) Atom transfer radical polymerization of multishelled cationic corona for the systemic delivery of siRNA. Nano Lett 18:314–325

Kim BS, Chuanoi S, Suma T, Anraku Y, Hayashi K, Naito M, Kim HJ, Kwon IC, Miyata K, Kishimura A, Kataoka K (2019) Self-assembly of siRNA/PEG-*b*-catiomer at integer molar ratio into 100 nm-sized vesicular polyion complexes (siRNAsomes) for RNAi and codelivery of cargo macromolecules. J Am Chem Soc 141:3699–3709

Levy BD, Serhan CN (2014) Resolution of acute inflammation in the lung. Annu Rev Physiol 76: 467–492

Li F, Li Y, Zhou Z, Lv S, Deng Q, Xu X, Yin L (2017) Engineering the aromaticity of cationic helical polypeptides toward "self-activated" DNA/siRNA delivery. ACS Appl Mater Interfaces 9:23586–23601

Liu Y, Yin L (2021) α-Amino acid *N*-carboxyanhydride (NCA)-derived synthetic polypeptides for nucleic acids delivery. Adv Drug Deliv Rev 171:139–163

Matthay MA, Zemans RL, Zimmerman GA, Arabi YM, Beitler JR, Mercat A, Herridge M, Randolph AG, Calfee CS (2018) Acute respiratory distress syndrome. Nat Rev Dis Primers 5: 18–40

Mehta P, McAuley DF, Brown M, Sanchez E, Tattersall RS, Manson JJ (2020) COVID-19: consider cytokine storm syndromes and immunosuppression. Lancet 395:1033–1034

Peng B, Liang H, Li Y, Dong C, Shen J, Mao HQ, Leong KW, Chen Y, Liu L (2019) Tuned cationic dendronized polymer: molecular scavenger for rheumatoid arthritis treatment. Angew Chem Int Ed 58:4254–4258

Shan W, Zhu X, Liu M, Li L, Zhong J, Sun W, Zhang Z, Huang Y (2015) Overcoming the diffusion barrier of mucus and absorption barrier of epithelium by self-assembled nanoparticles for oral delivery of insulin. ACS Nano 9:2345–2356

Shen W, Wang Q, Shen Y, Gao X, Li L, Yan Y, Wang H, Cheng Y (2018) Green tea catechin dramatically promotes RNAi mediated by low-molecular-weight polymers. ACS Cent Sci 4: 1326–1333

Song Z, Han Z, Lv S, Chen C, Chen L, Yin L, Cheng J (2017) Synthetic polypeptides: from polymer design to supramolecular assembly and biomedical application. Chem Soc Rev 46:6570–6599

Vllasaliu D, Fowler R, Garnett M, Eaton M, Stolnik S (2011) Barrier characteristics of epithelial cultures modelling the airway and intestinal mucosa: a comparison. Biochem Biophys Res Commun 415:579–585

Wang M, Liu H, Li L, Cheng Y (2014) A fluorinated dendrimer achieves excellent gene transfection efficacy at extremely low nitrogen to phosphorus ratios. Nat Commun 5:3053

Wei T, Liu J, Ma H, Cheng Q, Huang Y, Zhao J, Huo S, Xue X, Liang Z, Liang XJ (2013) Functionalized nanoscale micelles improve drug delivery for cancer therapy in vitro and in vivo. Nano Lett 13:2528–2534

Yang M, Lai SK, Wang YY, Zhong W, Happe C, Zhang M, Fu J, Hanes J (2011) Biodegradable nanoparticles composed entirely of safe materials that rapidly penetrate human mucus. Angew Chem Int Ed 50:2597–2600

Yang J, Duan S, Ye H, Ge C, Piao C, Chen Y, Lee M, Yin L (2021) Pro-peptide-reinforced, mucus-penetrating pulmonary siRNA delivery mitigates cytokine storm in pneumonia. Adv Funct Mater 31:2008960

Zhang R, Zheng N, Song Z, Yin L, Cheng J (2014) The effect of side-chain functionality and hydrophobicity on the gene delivery capabilities of cationic helical polypeptides. Biomaterials 35:3443–3454

Zhang W, Zhou Y, Li X, Xu X, Chen Y, Zhu R, Yin L (2018) Macrophage-targeting and reactive oxygen species (ROS)-responsive nanopolyplexes mediate anti-inflammatory siRNA delivery against acute liver failure (ALF). Biomater Sci 6:1986–1993

# Preparation and Evaluation of Polymeric Hybrid Micelles to Co-deliver Small Molecule Drug and siRNA for Rheumatoid Arthritis Therapy

# 5

Qin Wang and Xun Sun

## Contents



Q. Wang
Key Laboratory of Drug Targeting and Drug Delivery Systems, Ministry of Education, West China School of Pharmacy, Sichuan University, Chengdu, China

Key Laboratory of Advanced Technologies of Materials, Ministry of Education and School of Materials Science and Engineering, Southwest Jiaotong University, Chengdu, China

X. Sun (✉)
Key Laboratory of Drug Targeting and Drug Delivery Systems, Ministry of Education, West China School of Pharmacy, Sichuan University, Chengdu, China
e-mail: sunxun@scu.edu.cn


H. Tian and X. Chen (eds.), *Gene Delivery*, Biomaterial Engineering,
https://doi.org/10.1007/978-981-16-5419-0_8

**Abstract**

Small interfering RNA (siRNA) has emerged as a potential drug candidate in the treatment of various diseases. However, efficient delivery of siRNA molecules to the cytoplasm of target cells still remains a huge challenge for the application in vivo. Here, this protocol describes a practical approach to prepare a highly flexible polymeric hybrid micelles for the in vivo delivery of siRNA. The micelles consist of cationic polycaprolactone-polyethylenimine (PCL-PEI) and neutral polycaprolactone-polyethylene glycol (PCL-PEG), the ratio of which could be rationally adjusted to obtain various hybrid micelles with different physicochemical properties. The small proportion of PEI segments ensures the sufficient encapsulation of siRNA without causing obvious cytotoxicity. The high proportion of PEG segments renders the hybrid micelles nearly neutral surface charge and prolonged in vivo circulation. In order to efficiently block the key inflammatory signaling NF-κB pathway in rheumatoid arthritis (RA), siRNA targeting p65 (a key subunit of NF-κB family) combined with small molecule drugs dexamethasone (Dex) using the hybrid micelle as a carrier has been developed for the treatment of RA. These hybrid micelles would encapsulate siRNA via the electrostatic interaction between siRNA and PEI and load Dex in the PCL core via the hydrophobic interaction. The dual drugs are expected to be delivered to inflamed sites to synergistically suppress the NF-κB signaling and achieve the improved anti-inflammatory efficacy. Here, the methods for preparation and characterization of the hybrid micelles are described in detail. And the in vitro evaluation including the endosome escape and gene silencing have been systematically indicated. Meanwhile, the in vivo biodistribution and pharmacodynamics of this dual drugs-loaded formulation have been assessed according to the normalized methods. This protocol displays a practical approach for co-delivering genetic drugs and small molecule chemotherapeutics for in vivo application.

**Keywords**

siRNA delivery · Gene silencing · Micelles · Rheumatoid arthritis · NF-κB signaling · Dexamethasone

## 1 Overview

RNA interference (RNAi) is to achieve the sequence-specific knocking down of gene expression via small interfering RNA (siRNA). This technique has gained considerable attention worldwide since the discovery of the mechanism of gene silencing in 1998 (Whitehead et al. 2009). siRNA is a negative, double-strand RNA composed of 21–23 nucleotides, which could be synthetically produced in vitro. Once the siRNA molecule enters the cytoplasm of the target cells, it binds to a protein complex called the RNA-induced silencing complex (RISC). Afterwards, siRNA molecules are unwound by a helicase named argonaute protein 2 (Ago2) and the sense strand of the siRNA is cleaved. The RISC containing the antisense strand of the siRNA binds to the complementary mRNA in the cytoplasm (target mRNA). Subsequently, the mRNA would be cleaved by Ago2 and destroyed quickly, leading to the silence of the specific target genes (Apparailly and Jorgensen 2013). After decades of exploration on siRNA-based treatments, only three kinds of siRNA formulations (patisiran, givosiran, and lumasiran) used for the treatment of genetic diseases have been approved by Food and Drug Administration (FDA) for the application in clinical treatment. In practice, the siRNA can be applied to knock down any gene in living body if the siRNA molecules are properly designed. Any disease that can be ameliorated via the downregulation of a specific protein is expected to be treated by siRNA therapeutics. Therefore, siRNA-based therapeutic strategies also hold great promise for the treatment of rheumatoid arthritis (RA), which is a chronic and refractory autoimmune disease with a high morbidity worldwide. Although various therapeutic strategies have been developed for RA therapy, effective and safe treatment is still in great need (Wang and Sun. 2017).

In RA condition, the nuclear factor-κB (NF-κB) signaling pathway, one of the most intensively investigated pathways in the inflammatory diseases, plays a crucial role in the onset and development of RA (Simmonds and Foxwell 2008; Roman-Blas and Jimenez 2006; Okamoto et al. 2010). Under normal conditions, NF-κB transcription factors are mainly found in the cytoplasm as homodimers or heterodimers, exhibiting an inactive state under the action of the inhibitor of κB (IκB) molecule (Oeckinghaus et al. 2011; Hayden and Ghosh 2008). In the pathogenesis of RA, the stimulus such as inflammatory cytokines would trigger the activation of the NF-κB signaling, leading to the transactivation of a multitude of inflammation-related genes such as TNF-a, IL-6, or IL-1β. And the activation of NF-κB signaling discovered in a variety of inflammation resident cells such as fibroblast-like synoviocytes, macrophages, and lymphocytes would consequently further result in the exacerbation of inflammation and damage of joint tissues (Roman-Blas and Jimenez 2006). The current small molecule inhibitors for NF-κB signaling are often associated with some serious adverse effects due to the lack of specificity (O'Neill 2006; Gaestel et al. 2009). Accordingly, applying siRNA technique to knock down the expression of the key component in NF-κB signaling to effectively suppress the activation of NF-κB signaling would be a practicable approach to achieve the anti-inflammatory therapy (Wang et al. 2017). Here, this protocol offers a method to utilize p65 siRNA to selectively silence the p65 subunit of NF-κB family, which is a principal transcriptional regulator in NF-κB pathway.

Dramatic gene silencing occurs rapidly after intracellular delivery of a suitable and efficient siRNA. However, the direct application of naked siRNAs is unable to produce efficient and predictable therapeutic effects. Within a few minutes after in vivo administration, the majority of the injected siRNA will be cleared from circulation by the reticuloendothelial system (RES) and renal clearance. Only a very small proportion of the administrated siRNA remains available for the target cells or tissues. However, this small percentage of siRNA is easily degraded by nuclease widely distributed in vivo. Moreover, the siRNA alone cannot efficiently penetrate the cellular membrane. Generally speaking, the in vivo application of siRNA therapeutics is hindered by numerous biological barriers in both extracellular matrix and cytoplasm including rapid enzymatic degradation, inability to transport across cell membrane, endosomal destruction, as well as renal elimination (Whitehead et al. 2009; Kim et al. 2016). As a result, developing an effective siRNA delivery vehicle aiming at overcoming these barriers is essential. Although viral vectors such as adenovirus or lentivirus have been demonstrated favorable intracellular delivery efficiency, the strong immunogenicity and potential toxicity limit their further application (Shim and Kwon 2010). As an alternative, the lipid or polymer with positive surface charge have been developed and widely applied for nucleic acid delivery such as cationic 1,2-dioleoyl-3-trimethylammonium-propane (DOTAP), polyethylene imine (PEI), and poly-L-lysine (PLL) (Zhang et al. 2007). Inadequate proportion of cationic segments would not guarantee the sufficient entrapment, protection, and cellular uptake of the siRNA molecules. On the other hand, excess positive charge would probably bring about high risk of cytotoxicity and undesirable in vivo circulation time, as well as the inability of liberating siRNA timely from endosome (van der Aa et al. 2011). In an attempt to address the dilemma existed in the cationic delivery vectors, this protocol introduces a feasible solution by designing a versatile hybrid micelle system consisting of two similar amphiphilic diblock copolymers, neutral PCL-PEI and cationic PCL-PEG. The ratio of the two copolymers can be easily tailored to adjust the physicochemical properties of the hybrid micelles. Based on our previous optimization, Li et al. found that the hybrid micelles composed of 2% (w/w) PCL-PEI and 98% (w/w) PCL-PEG possess the superior in vivo performance (Li et al. 2015). The small proportion of PEI ensured the sufficient encapsulation of siRNA without causing obvious cytotoxicity. On the other hand, the large amount of PEG segments renders the hybrid micelles nearly neutral surface charge and prolonged in vivo circulation.

In view of the complicated and enormous inflammatory network presented in RA, one single siRNA might not be enough to suppress the broadly activated inflammatory signaling. Herein, the combination of p65 siRNA with low-dose anti-inflammatory dexamethasone (Dex) was applied to synergistically suppress the activated NF-κB signaling in RA. Since the Dex could also inhibit the activation of NF-κB signaling by translocating into the nucleus and binding to the specific site of gene sequences (Vandewalle et al. 2018). The combination of Dex (encapsulated in the hydrophobic core of PCL components) and p65 siRNA (complexed with cationic hydrophilic PEI segments) is expected to cooperatively achieve improved therapeutic efficacy by blocking the NF-κB signaling (Fig. 1). In this protocol, we intend to display the detailed instructions for fabricating the p65 siRNA and Dex co-loaded hybrid micelles. More importantly, the characterization of the dual-drugs loaded formulation as well as the in vitro and in vivo evaluation has been comprehensively indicated. Overall, this protocol aims to provide a practical method to prepare and evaluate a co-delivery vehicle (co-delivering nucleic acids and small molecule drugs) to overcome various physiological obstacles appeared in their in vivo application.

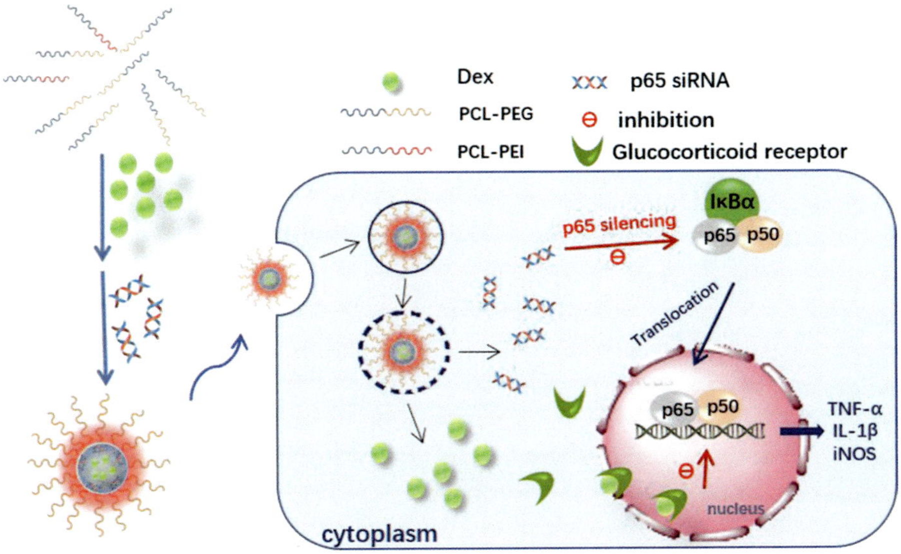


**Fig. 1** Schematic overview illustrating the construction of the dual agents-loaded hybrid micelles and the intracellular fate of these micelles

## 2 Protocol

### 2.1 Materials

#### 2.1.1 Synthesis of PCL-PEG and PCL-PEI Polymers

1. Poly(ε-caprolactone) (PCL-OH) (MWCO = 2000 Da, Sigma-Aldrich, USA)
2. 4-nitrophenyl chloroformate (NPC, Aladdin, China)
3. Ice (obtained from an ice making machine)
4. PEG-$NH_2$(MWCO = 5000 Da, JenKem, China)
5. Polyethyleneimine 2000 (PEI 2 k, Sigma-Aldrich, USA)
6. Anhydrous dichloromethane (analytical purity, Kemiou, China)
7. Pyridine (Kemiou, China)
8. Anhydrous sodium sulfate (Kelong, China)
9. Cold diethyl ether (Kemiou, China)
10. Triethylamine (Kemiou, China)
11. Deionized water (obtained from Milli-Q equipment)
12. Dimethyl sulfoxide (Kemiou, China)
13. Tetrahydrofuran (THF, Kemiou, China)
14. Dialysis bag (MWCO = 8000 ~ 14,000 Da, Biosharp, China)
15. Round-bottom flask (100, 250, and 500 mL, Shuniu, China)
16. Magnetic stirrer bars
17. Buchner funnel

18. Qualitative filter paper (Jiaojie, China)
19. Beakers (100, 500, and 1000 mL, Shuniu, China)

**Equipment**
1. Magnetic stirring apparatus (IKA, Germany)
2. Vacuum drying oven (Jinghong, China)
3. Rotary vacuum evaporator (BUCHI, Switzerland)
4. Circulating water multipurpose vacuum pump (Changcheng, China).
5. Analytical balance (Sartorius, Germany)
6. Milli-Q (Millipore, USA)
7. Lyophilizer (Scientz, China)
8. Freezer (−20 °C) and 4 °C refrigerator (Haier, China)
9. Ice making machine (Xueke, China)

### 2.1.2 Preparation and Characterization of Polymeric Hybrid Micelles

1. Tetrahydrofuran (THF, Kemiou, China)
2. Deionized water
3. Dexamethasone (Meilun, China)
4. p65 siRNA (Riobobio, China, see Table 1 for RNA sequences).
5. RNase-free water (Tiangen, China)
6. Vortex mixer (IKA, Germany)
7. Ultrafiltration tube (MWCO = 30kD, Millipore, USA)
8. Syringe (1 mL)
9. Diethyl pyrocarbonate (DEPC, Beyotime, China)
10. Centrifuge tube (2, 5 and 10 mL, Axygen, USA)
11. Quartz cuvette (Jinghe, China)
12. Acetonitrile (ACN, HPLC grade, Sigma-Aldrich, USA)
13. Methanol (HPLC grade, Sigma-Aldrich, USA)
14. C18 reverse-phase columns (4.6 mm*150 mm*5 um, Shimadzu, Japan)
15. Copper grid (Zhongjing, China)

**Equipment**
1. Centrifuge (Beckman, USA)
2. Micropore filter membrane (0.45 μm, Millipore, USA)
3. Transmission electron microscopy (JEOL, Japan)
4. Dynamic light scattering (DLS) analyzer (Malvern, UK)
5. High performance liquid chromatographic (HPLC) system (Agilent 1260, USA)
6. UV-vis spectrophotometer (Varian, USA)
7. Pipette (50, 200, and 1000 μL, Thermo Fisher, USA)

### 2.1.3 Optimization of N/P Ratio Based on Cellular Internalization

1. Fam-labeled p65 siRNA (Riobobio, China)
2. Phosphate-buffered saline (PBS, 10 mM, pH 7.4, ZSGB, China)
3. Dulbecco's modification of Eagle's medium (DMEM, Hyclone, USA)

**Table 1** The sequences of nucleic acids used in following experiments

| RNA sequence | |
|---|---|
| p65 siRNA | Sense: 5-'GCGACAAGGUGCAGAAAGAdTdT3<br>Antisense: 3-'dTdTCGCUGUUCCACGUCUUUCU5 |
| Scrambled siRNA | Sense: 5-'GAACGAACCGGAGUGAAAG dTdT3<br>Antisense: 3-'dTdTCUUGCUUGGCCUCACUUUC5 |
| DNA primers | |
| Primer for p65 | Forward: 5-'AAAGAAGACATTGAGGTGTA3<br>Reverse: 5-'AGGTACCATGGCTGTGGAAC3 |
| Primer for actin | Forward: 5-'CTACAATGAGCTGCGTGTGG3<br>Reverse: 5-'CAGGTCCAGACGCAGGATGGC3 |
| Primer for TNF-α | Forward: 5-'GCTCCCTCTCATCAGTTCCA3<br>Reverse: 5-'GCTTGGTGGTTTGCTACGAC3 |
| Primer for IL-1β | Forward: 5-'GCCAACAAGTGGTATTCTCCA3<br>Reverse: 5-'TGCCGTCTTTCATCACACAG3 |

4. Fetal bovine serum (FBS, Hyclone, USA)
5. Streptomycin/penicillin (100X, Solarbio, China)
6. Cell culture flask (60 mm, Corning, USA)
7. 12-well culture plate (Corning, USA)
8. 0.25% trypsin containing 0.02%EDTA (Hyclone, USA)
9. Sterile filter (0.45 μm, Millipore, USA)
10. Murine macrophage Raw264.7 (obtained from the American Type Culture Collection, USA), grown in DMEM culture medium supplemented with 1% antibiotics (penicillin and streptomycin), and 10% fetal bovine serum.
11. Sterile saline (Kelun, China)
12. Hypochloric acid (Kelong, China)

**Equipment**
1. Cell incubator (Thermo Fisher, USA)
2. Flow cytometer (Beckman FC500, USA)
3. Benchtop centrifuge (Eppendorf, Germany)

### 2.1.4 RNase Protection Assay of siRNA-Loaded Hybrid Micelles

1. Sodium dodecyl sulfate (SDS, Sigma-Aldrich, USA)
2. RNase (Biosharp, China)
3. GoldView (Biosharp, China)
4. Heparin sodium (Biosharp, China)
5. Tris base (Sigma-Aldrich, USA)
6. EDTA disodium (EDTA-2Na, Sigma-Aldrich, USA)
7. Acetic acid (Kelong, China)
8. Sodium hydroxide (NaOH, Kelong, China)
9. Agarose (Biosharp, China)

**Equipment**

1. Incubator shaker (Minquan, China)
2. Horizontal electrophoresis system (Bio-rad, USA)
3. Gel imaging system (Bio-rad, USA)

### 2.1.5 Measurement of Cell Viability

1. Human umbilical vein endothelial cells (HUVECs) obtained from the American Type Culture Collection, grown in DMEM culture medium supplemented with 1% antibiotics (penicillin and streptomycin), and 10% fetal bovine serum.
2. 96-well plates (Corning, USA)
3. 3-(4,5-dimethylthiazol-2-yl)-2,5-diphenyltetrazolium bromide (MTT) (Biosharp, China). Prepare MTT solution (5 mg/mL) using PBS buffer for subsequent use.
4. Dimethyl sulfoxide (DMSO, Solarbio, China)
5. Sterile filter (0.45 μm, Millipore, USA)

**Equipment**

1. Automated cell counters (Countstar, China)
2. Varioskan Flash microplate reader (Thermo Fisher, USA)

### 2.1.6 Endosome Escape

1. Cell culture flask (sterile, 35 mm, Corning, USA)
2. Lyso tracker Red (Beyotime, China)
3. Lipopolysaccharide (LPS, Biosharp, China)
4. Fam-labeled p65 siRNA (Riobobio, China)

**Equipment**

1. Confocal laser scanning microscopy (Zeiss, Germany)

### 2.1.7 Gene Silencing Study In Vitro

1. HiPerFect transfection reagent (Qiagen, China)
2. Scrambled siRNA (Riobobio, China, see Table 1 for RNA sequences)
3. Primers for p65 (Sangon, China, see Table 1 for DNA sequences; all the sequences of primers are designed by Primer Premier 5.0.)
4. Primers for β-actin (Sangon, China, see Table 1 for DNA sequences)
5. Mercaptoethanol (Kemiou, China)
6. RNAprep pure Cell Kit (Tiangen, China)
7. TIANscript RT Kit (Tiangen, China)
8. EvaGreen® Supermix (Bio-rad, USA)
9. 8-tube Strips (Axygen, China)

**Equipment**

1. iQ-TM 5R real-time PCR detection system (Bio-rad, USA)
2. Clean bench (Sujing, China)
3. Microcentrifuge (IKA, Germany)

### 2.1.8 Ability of Dual Drugs-Loaded Micelles to Inhibit the Production of Inflammatory Cytokines

1. DMEM culture medium
2. DMEM culture medium supplemented with 10% FBS (v/v) and 1% antibiotics
3. Lipopolysaccharide
4. Dexamethasone
5. p65 siRNA stock solution
6. Primers for TNF-α (Sangon, China, see Table 1 for DNA sequences)
7. Primers for IL-1β (Sangon, China, see Table 1 for DNA sequences)

**Equipment**

1. iQ-TM 5R real-time PCR system (Bio-rad, USA)
2. Clean bench (Sujing, China)

### 2.1.9 Immunofluorescent Staining of Nuclear Translocation of p65 Subunit

1. Culture dish (35 mm, Corning, USA)
2. 4% paraformaldehyde (Meilun, China)
3. Triton X-100 (Solarbio, China)
4. Bovine serum albumin (BSA, Solarbio, China)
5. Rabbit anti-p65 antibody (Primary antibody, Cell Signaling Technology, USA)
6. Alexa Fluor 488-labeled secondary antibody (Cell Signaling Technology, USA)
7. 2-(4-Amidinophenyl)-6-indolecarbamidine dihydrochloride (DAPI, Beyotime, China)

**Equipment**

1. Confocal laser scanning microscopy (Zeiss, Germany)

### 2.1.10 Western Blotting

1. Nuclear and Cytoplasmic Protein Extraction Kit (Beyotime, China)
2. BCA assay kit (Thermo Fisher, USA)
3. SDS-PAGE Gel SuperQuick Preparation Kit (Beyotime, China)
4. PVDF membrane (Beyotime, China)
5. Rabbit anti-p65 antibody (Primary antibody, Cell Signaling Technology, USA)
6. Rabbit anti-histone antibody (Proteintech, USA).
7. Peroxidase-conjugated goat anti-rabbit IgG (ZSGB, China)
8. ECL chemiluminescence kit (Millipore, USA)

**Equipment**

1. Varioskan flash microplate reader (Thermo Fisher, USA)
2. Mini-PROTEAN Tetra system (Bio-Rad, USA)
3. Gel imaging system (Bio-rad, USA)

#### 2.1.11 Establishment of Collagen-Induced Arthritis Model

1. Male DBA/1 J mice (weighing 18–20 g, Vitalriver, China)
2. Bovine CII collagen (2 mg/mL, Chondrex, USA)
3. Complete Freund's adjuvant (containing heat-killed *M. tuberculosis* at the concentration of 5 mg/mL, Chondrex, USA)
4. Incomplete Freund's adjuvant (Chondrex, USA)
5. Sterile syringe (1 mL, Kelun, China)
6. Ice bath

**Equipment**

1. Avanti mini-extruder (Avanti, USA)

#### 2.1.12 Accumulation of Hybrid Micelles in Arthritic Joints

1. 1,1′-dioctadecyl-3,3,3′,3′-tetramethylindodicarbocyanine (DiD, Sigma-Aldrich, USA)
2. Propylene glycol (Kemiou, China)
3. Pentasorbital sodium (Biosharp, China)
4. Surgical scissors and tweezers
5. Saline (Kelun, China)

**Equipment**

1. IVIS® Spectrum system

#### 2.1.13 Therapeutic Efficacy of Micelles Co-Loaded with Dex and siRNA In Vivo

1. Healthy male DBA/1 J mice
2. Male DBA/1 J mice with established arthritis
3. Sterile PBS buffer
4. Dexamethasone
5. p65 siRNA stock solution
6. Vernier caliper (Deli, China)
7. TNF-a and IL-1β ELISA kit (Ebioscience, USA)
8. 4% paraformaldehyde (Meilun, China)
9. EDTA-2Na (Kelong, China)

## 3 Methods

### 3.1 Synthesis of PCL-PEG and PCL-PEI Polymers (Fig. 2)

1. Dissolve 1 g PCL-OH and 0.5 g NPC in 5 mL anhydrous dichloromethane in 100 mL round-bottom flask. Add 150 μL pyridine into the mixture under constant stirring at ice bath. Stir the mixture overnight at room temperature under the protection of nitrogen.

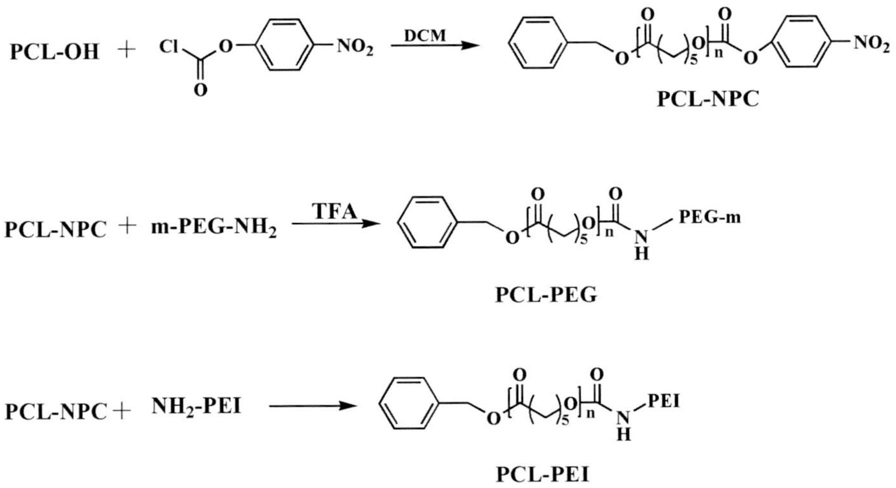


**Fig. 2** The synthesis scheme of PCL-PEG and PCL-PEI copolymers

2. Remove the solvent using a rotary evaporator under vacuum at 30 °C. Redissolve the yellowish and viscous products in 50 mL anhydrous dichloromethane. Dry the organic solution with 10 g anhydrous sodium sulfate and shake the mixture vigorously to fully remove the residual water. Concentrate the volume of solution to approximately 5 mL using a rotary evaporator. Add the solution (5 mL) to the cold diethyl ether (500 mL) to precipitate the PCL-NPC.
3. Use the circulating water vacuum pump to remove the diethyl ether and harvest the PCL-NPC in the Buchner funnel with the filter paper. Dry the obtained products in vacuum drying oven at room temperature (RT) for 12 h.
4. Dissolve 0.4 g PCL-NPC and 1 g PEG-$NH_2$ in anhydrous dichloromethane. Add 150 μL triethylamine into the mixture and allow the reaction proceed under constant stirring at RT for 24 h. Evaporate the solvent and redissolve the mixture in deionized water. Dialyze the suspension against deionized water for 48 h to remove the unreacted PEG-$NH_2$ and excess triethylamine. Lyophilize the suspensions to obtain PCL-PEG.
5. Dissolve 2 g PEI in 10 mL dimethyl sulfoxide. Dissolve 0.5 g PCL-NPC in 5 mL tetrahydrofuran. Inject the PCL-NPC solution into the PEI solution slowly using a constant-speed pump under stirring at RT for 12 h. Dialyze the suspensions against deionized water for 48 h to remove the unreacted PEI and lyophilize the suspensions to obtain PCL-PEI. Store the lyophilized PCL-PEG and PCL-PEI at −20 °C until further use.
6. Confirm the chemical structure of PCL-PEG and PCL-PEI by $H^1$NMR spectrometer and determine the molecular weight of the two copolymers by gel permeation chromatography (GPC).

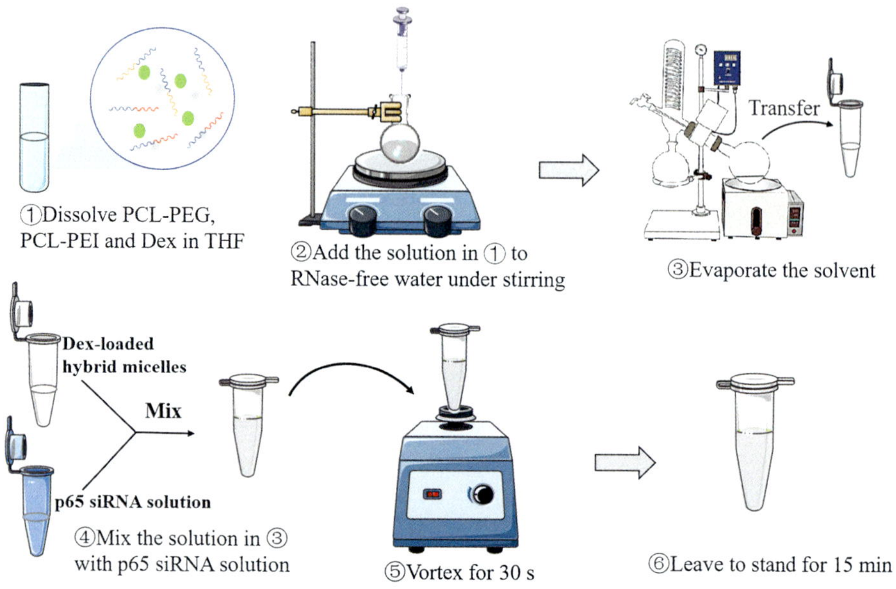


**Fig. 3** Preparation process of polymeric hybrid micelles co-loading Dex and p65 siRNA

## 3.2 Preparation of Polymeric Hybrid Micelles Co-Loading with Dex and siRNA (Fig. 3)

1. Dissolved 0.25 mg PCL-PEI, 11.75 mg PCL-PEG, and 0.25 mg Dex in 1 mL THF. Add the solution to 10 mL RNase-free water drop by drop using a syringe (1 mL) under vigorous stirring. Evaporate the mixture solution subsequently at RT to remove the THF. After the evaporation of THF, turn the temperature of water bath up to 45 °C to evaporate the excess water and concentrate the solution to 500 μL.
2. Take the vial containing the p65 siRNA powder out of the refrigerator (−20 °C) and centrifuge for 1 min at the speed of 200 g. Prepare a siRNA stock solution at the concentration of 20 μM using RNase-free water and store them in aliquots (50 μL) at −80 °C. Avoid repeated freezing and thawing of siRNA stock solution.
3. Mix the obtained Dex-loaded hybrid micelles solution with an equal volume (500 μL) of p65 siRNA in RNase-free water. Vortex for 30 s and leave to stand for a further 15 min to allow the formation of Dex/siRNA-loaded hybrid micelles (M-Dex/siRNA).

## 3.3 Characterization of Polymeric Hybrid Micelles Co-Loading Dex and p65 siRNA

1. Determine the particle size and zeta potential of the M-Dex/siRNA obtained in Sect. 3.2 using dynamic light scattering (DLS, ZetasizerNano ZS90, Malvern, UK).

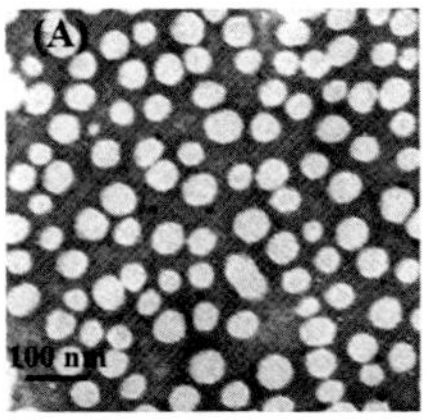


(B)

| Size (nm) | PDI | Zeta Potential (mV) | Encapsulation efficiency | | Drug loading yield | |
|---|---|---|---|---|---|---|
| 98.4±1.0 | 0.167± 0.021 | 4.22±1.34 | Dex | 96.2±3.6% | Dex | 2.0±0.14% |
| | | | siRNA | 97.0±1.1% | siRNA | 0.20±0.01% |

**Fig. 4** (**a**) The morphology of M-Dex/siRNA micelles observed by transmission electron microscopy (TEM). Scale bar, 100 nm. (**b**) M-Dex/siRNA micelles were characterized in terms of hydrodynamic size, polydispersity index (PDI), and zeta potential using dynamic light scattering, as well as in terms of encapsulation efficiency (EE) and drug loading yield (DL). Results are shown as mean ± SD (n = 3)

2. Apply one drop (5 μL) of the micellar solution to the copper grid and wait for 10 min for the absorption and dry in the air. Stain the sample with phosphotungstic acid (1%, w/v) for 10 s. Observe the morphology of the obtained M-Dex/siRNA by TEM at 120 kV (Fig. 4a).
3. Separate the unencapsulated drugs and drug-loaded formulations using an ultrafiltration tube (30 kDa, Millipore, USA) at 5000 rpm for 30 min. Analyze the concentration of unencapsulated Dex and siRNA in the bottom of the ultrafiltration tube using HPLC and UV-vis spectrum, respectively. For quantitative determination of Dex using HPLC, the mobile phase is as follow: 40% ACN (buffer A) and 60% water (buffer B) both containing 0.1% formic acid; flow rate: 1 mL/min; wavelength of detection: 254 nm. For quantitative determination of siRNA using UV-vis spectrophotometer, determine the absorbance of samples at the wavelength of 260 nm.
4. Calculate the encapsulation efficiency (EE) of Dex and siRNA using the following formula (Fig. 4b): EE% = (Weight of drug in micelles/Weight of total feeding drug) *100%. Calculate the drug loading yield (DL) with the following formula: DL (%) = (Weight of drug in micelles/Weight of total formulation) *100%.

## 3.4 Optimization of N/P Ratio Based on Cellular Internalization

1. Inoculate Raw264.7 cells into 12-well plates at the density of $5 \times 10^5$ cells in 1 mL culture medium per well and culture overnight using DMEM culture medium containing 10% FBS at 37 °C, 5% $CO_2$.
2. Prepare Fam-siRNA loaded hybrid micelles at different mass ratios (1:1, 4:1, 6:1, 8:1, 10:1, and 15:1) of polycation nitrogen to RNA phosphate (N/P) as described in Sect. 3.2.
3. Dilute the Fam-siRNA loaded hybrid micelles at different N/P to acquire the final concentration of siRNA at 100 nM using the DMEM culture medium without FBS or antibiotics.
4. Incubate these Fam-siRNA loaded formulations at the same siRNA concentration (100 nM) with Raw264.7 in 12-well plates for 1 h using the DMEM culture medium without FBS or antibiotics.

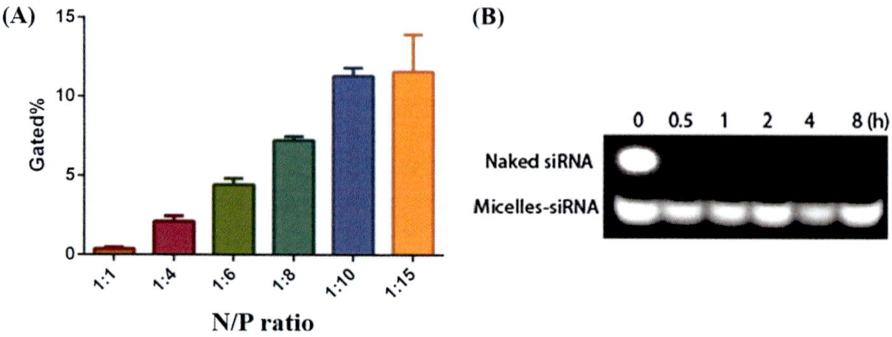


**Fig. 5** (**a**) Efficiency of cellular uptake of Fam-siRNA loaded hybrid micelles prepared at N/P ratios ranging from 1:1 to 1:15 in Raw264.7 cell culture. Results are shown as mean ± SD (n = 4). (**b**) Protection of encapsulated siRNA from RNase at different timepoints

5. Remove the culture medium containing Fam-siRNA loaded hybrid micelles and wash twice with PBS. Add 200 μL 0.25% trypsin containing 0.02% EDTA-2Na to each well and incubate for 1 min. Tap the plate and detach Raw264.7 from the bottom of the 12-well plate by gently pipetting the cells. Immediately add 200 μL of fresh complete DMEM culture medium to each well to neutralize the action of trypsin.
6. Harvest cells by centrifuging at 300 g for 3 min and wash twice with PBS. Resuspend the cell pellets in 500 μL PBS and determine the proportion of Fam-positive cells by flow cytometer in all groups (Fig. 5a).

## 3.5 RNase Protection Assay of siRNA Loaded into Hybrid Micelles

1. Incubate M-Dex/siRNA (at the final siRNA concentration of 500 nM) solution (500 μL) with RNase (at the final concentration of 1 mU) at 37 °C. Take an aliquot (50 μL) at the indicated time point (0.5, 1, 2, 4, 8 h). Add sodium dodecyl sulfate (SDS, final concentration 10%, w/v) and heparin sodium (final concentration 1%, w/v) into the aliquots. Vortex and incubate the mixtures for 15 min at 37 °C to free the siRNA from the hybrid micelles.
2. Prepare TAE buffer (containing 4.88 g tris base, 0.4 g EDTA-2Na, 1 mL acetic acid in 1 L RNase-free water) and use NaOH solution (1 M) to adjust the pH of TAE buffer to 8.3.
3. Dissolve 0.4 g agarose in 50 mL TAE buffer and heat the solution to boiling. When it cools to about 60 °C, add 1 μL GoldView dye into the gel solution. After mixing together, pour the gel solution into an electrophoresis chamber.
4. Insert the comb between the glass plates and avoid air bubbles between the comb and the gel. Let the solution cool to form a gel. Load the siRNA samples obtained in Step 1 in the sample lanes in agarose gel and run the electrophoresis at 90 V for

25 min by connecting to a power supply. Analyze the result using a gel imaging system (Fig. 5b).

## 3.6 Cell Viability

1. Inoculate Raw264.7 and HUVEC in a 96-well plate at the density of $1 \times 10^4$ cells (100 μL) per well respectively and allow them to attach overnight. Avoid using the wells placed at the edges of the plate.
2. Prepare hybrid micelles as described in Sect. 3.2 without drug loading (blank hybrid micelles) at the copolymer concentration of 5 mg/mL. Dilute the blank hybrid micelles solution with FBS-free and antibiotics-free incomplete DMEM culture medium to obtain the final concentration of 2, 5, 10, 20, 50, and 100 μg/mL copolymer.
3. Add the blank hybrid micelles solution with different concentration of copolymer to each well.
4. After incubating blank hybrid micelles with cells for 4 h, remove the culture medium containing blank hybrid micelles. Replenish the fresh complete DMEM culture medium to each well and incubate for 12 h.
5. Add MTT solution (5 mg/mL) to each well at the final MTT concentration of 0.5 mg/mL and incubate with cells for 4 h.
6. Remove the culture medium containing MTT carefully and do not pipette the generated formazan crystals. Add DMSO to each well and incubate for 15 min in a shaker to completely resolve the formazan crystals (150 μL per well).
7. Measure the absorbance of the each well at 490 nm using a microplate reader. Relative cell viability was calculated using the following equation:

$$\text{Cell viability} = \left(A_{\text{Sample}} - A_{\text{Blank}}\right) / \left(A_{\text{Control}} - A_{\text{Blank}}\right) \times 100\%$$

Control group: cells without any treatment of hybrid micelles; Blank group: wells with only culture medium.

## 3.7 Endosome Escape

1. Inoculate Raw264.7 cells into 35 mm culture flask at the density of $2 \times 10^5$ cells (500 μL) per well and incubate overnight.
2. Prepare Fam-siRNA loaded hybrid micelles at the siRNA concentration of 1 μM. Apply the Fam-siRNA loaded hybrid micelles into cell flask at the final Fam-siRNA concentration of 200 nM.
3. After incubating with Raw264.7 for 2 h using the DMEM culture medium without the addition of FBS or antibiotics, replace with fresh complete culture medium and further incubate for 2 h and 6 h, respectively.
4. Discard the culture medium and carefully wash the cells with PBS in culture flask for three times. Add Lyso tracker Red (at the final concentration of 1 mM) to each

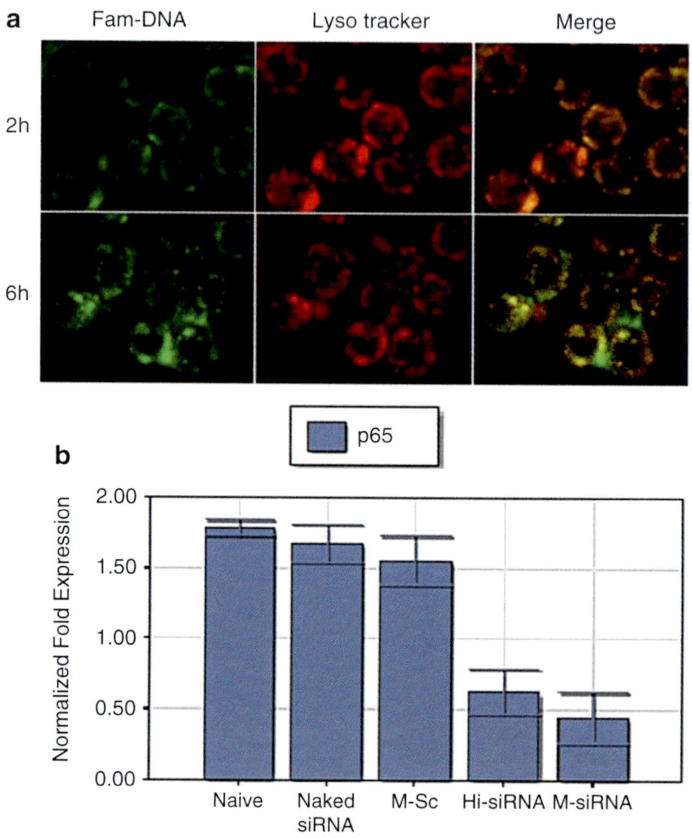


**Fig. 6** (**a**) Escape of internalized micelles loaded with Fam-DNA (green) from the endosomes (red) of macrophages. (**b**) Downregulation of p65 expression in murine macrophages by siRNA encapsulated in micelles. Levels of p65 mRNA were normalized to those of β-actin. M-Sc, micelles containing scrambled siRNA; Hi-siRNA, p65 siRNA encapsulated in HiPerFect transfection reagent; Results are shown as mean ± SD (n = 4)

flask and incubate for 1 h to stain the lysosome within the cytoplasm. Afterwards, gently wash the cell culture three times with cold PBS.

5. Observe the distribution of fluorescence within cells using a confocal laser scanning microscopy (as shown in Fig. 6a).

### 3.8 In Vitro Gene Silencing Study

1. Count the Raw264.7 using an automated cell counters and inoculate Raw264.7 cells into 12-well plate at the density of $1 \times 10^5$ cells per well. Add LPS at final concentration of 1 μg/mL into the cell culture to stimulate the upregulation of p65 level. The transfection experiment can be started when the cell confluence reaches about 40%.

2. Prepare free p65 siRNA solution, micelles encapsulating p65 siRNA (M-siRNA), p65 siRNA complexed with commercially available transfection reagent HiPerFect (Hi-siRNA), and micelles containing scrambled siRNA (M-Sc) in RNase-free water at the equal siRNA concentration of 1 μM. Dilute all these siRNA formulations to the final concentration at 100 nM using DMEM culture medium without FBS or antibiotics and then proceed immediately to the gene silencing experiments.
3. Add free p65 siRNA, M-siRNA, Hi-siRNA, and M-Sc solution diluted in step 2 (1 mL) to each corresponding well respectively at final siRNA concentration of 100 nM and incubate with cells for 4 h.
4. Replace the culture medium with fresh complete medium and further incubate for 24 h.
5. Remove the culture medium from the cell plates and wash cells twice with PBS.
6. Extract total RNA from each well using an RNA isolation kit (RNAprep pure Cell Kit, Tiangen) according to the manufacturer's instruction. Apply TIANscript RT kit to obtain cDNA from the isolated RNA by the reverse transcription process. Start a quantitative real-time PCR by mixing the cDNA sample (3 μL), forward primers of p65 (1.5 μL), reverse primers of p65 (1.5 μL), and EvaGreen® Supermix (6.75 μL) together. Add 7.25 μL RNase-free water to supplement the final volume to 20 μL.
7. Analyze the p65 mRNA level normalized to the control gene of β-actin using quantitative real-time PCR (As shown in Fig. 6b).

### 3.9 Ability of Drugs-Loaded Hybrid Micelles to Inhibit the Production of Inflammatory Cytokines

1. Seed the Raw264.7 cell in 12-well plates at the density of $1 \times 10^5$ cells per well. Add LPS solution at final concentration of 1 μg/mL into the cell cultures and incubate for 12 h to activate the Raw264.7 to an inflammatory state.
2. Prepare free p65 siRNA solution using RNase-free water, free Dex solution using 25% propylene glycol (v/v), micelles encapsulating p65 siRNA (M-siRNA) solution, micelles encapsulating Dex (M-Dex) solution, and micelles co-encapsulating p65 siRNA and Dex (M-Dex/siRNA) solution. Dilute all these formulations to the Dex concentration of 10 μM and p65 siRNA concentration of 100 nM using DMEM culture medium without FBS or antibiotics.
3. Add the abovementioned formulations to each corresponding well respectively and incubate with cells for 4 h.
4. Replace the culture medium with fresh complete medium and further incubate for 24 h.
5. Remove the culture medium from the cell plates. And wash cells twice with PBS.

6. Measure the levels of mRNAs encoding the inflammatory cytokines TNF-a and IL-1β using RT-PCR method. Extract total RNA from each well using an RNA isolation kit (RNAprep pure Cell Kit, Tiangen) according to the manufacturer's instruction. Apply TIANscript RT kit to obtain cDNA from the isolated RNA by reverse transcription process. Start a quantitative real-time PCR by mixing the cDNA sample (3 μL), forward primers (1.5 μL), reverse primers (1.5 μL), and EvaGreen® Supermix (6.75 μL) together. Add 7.25 μL RNase-free water to supplement the final volume to 20 μL.
7. Analyze the mRNA level of TNF-α and IL-1β normalized to the control gene of β-actin using quantitative real-time PCR.

### 3.10 Immunofluorescent Staining of Nuclear Translocation of p65 Subunit

1. Seed Raw264.7 in the culture dishes (35 mm) at the density of $2 \times 10^5$ cells and add LPS solution at final concentration of 1 μg/mL into the cell cultures. Incubate for 12 h to activate the Raw264.7 to an inflammatory state.
2. Prepare free p65 siRNA solution using RNase-free water, free Dex solution using 25% propylene glycol (v/v), micelles encapsulating p65 siRNA (M-siRNA) solution, micelles encapsulating Dex (M-Dex) solution, and micelles co-encapsulating p65 siRNA and Dex (M-Dex/siRNA) solution. Dilute all these formulation to the Dex concentration of 10 μM and p65 siRNA concentration of 100 nM using DMEM culture medium without FBS or antibiotics.
3. Add the abovementioned formulations to each corresponding well respectively and incubate for 4 h. Replace the culture medium with fresh complete medium and further incubate for 24 h.
4. Remove the culture medium from the cell dishes. Wash cells twice with cold PBS and fix the cells with 4% paraformaldehyde for 10 min at RT. Discard the paraformaldehyde solution and wash cells twice with cold PBS. Permeabilize cells for 15 min with 0.2% (w/w) Triton X-100 at RT.
5. Prepare 2% (w/w) BSA buffer (blocking buffer) and incubate cells with blocking buffer for 1 h at 37 °C. Dilute the primary antibody (rabbit anti-p65 antibody) with blocking buffer at the dilute ratio of 1:5000. Incubate cells with diluted primary antibody (1 mL) overnight at 4 °C. Remove the primary antibody solution and wash cells gently in a shaker using cold PBS for three times.
6. Dilute the Alexa Fluor 488-labeled secondary antibody with blocking buffer at the dilute ratio of 1:1000. Incubate cells with diluted secondary antibody (1 mL) for 1 h at RT in a shaker. Remove the secondary antibody solution and wash cells gently in a shaker using PBS for three times.
7. Stain the cell nuclei using DAPI for 5 min at RT and wash cells using PBS for three times. Observe the distribution of fluorescence signal of cells via a confocal laser scanning microscopy.

### 3.11 Western Blotting

1. Seed Raw264.7 in the 6-well plates at the density of $1 \times 10^6$ cells. Add LPS solution at final concentration of 1 μg/mL into the cell culture and incubate for 12 h to activate the Raw264.7 to an inflammatory state.
2. Incubate various drug formulations (prepared as Sect. 3.9 described) with Raw264.7 cultures and incubate for 4 h (The dose of Dex and p65 siRNA in this section is the same with the Sect. 3.9). Replace the culture medium with fresh complete medium and further incubate for 24 h. Remove the culture medium from the cell dishes and wash cells twice with PBS. Harvest cells by a cell scraper and resuspend cells in cold PBS.
3. Extract the nuclear proteins using a Nuclear and Cytoplasmic Protein Extraction Kit following the manufacturer's instructions. Boil the protein samples in boiling water for 3 min to fully denature the proteins. Quantify the total nuclear protein using the BCA assay kit.
4. Separate the proteins by sodium dodecyl sulfate polyacrylamide gel electrophoresis (SDS-PAGE) using the SDS-PAGE Gel SuperQuick Preparation Kit following the manufacturer's instructions. After the process of electrophoresis, transfer proteins to a PVDF membrane using the Mini-PROTEAN Tetra system (Bio-Rad, USA).
5. Block the membrane in 5% (w/w) BSA solution for 2 h at 37 °C. Incubate the PVDF membrane with rabbit anti-p65 antibody and rabbit anti-histone antibody at 4 °C overnight.
6. Wash the membrane for three times and incubate with peroxidase-conjugated goat anti-rabbit IgG (ZSGB, China) for 1 h. Develop the blot using the ECL chemiluminescence kit (Millipore, CA, USA).

### 3.12 Establishment of the Collagen-Induced Arthritis Model (CIA)

1. Vortex the CFA suspension vigorously to ensure the *M. tuberculosis* homogeneously dispersed. Mix the bovine CII collagen (2 mg/mL) with equal volume of CFA using an Avanti mini-extruder. Extrude 10 times on ice bath to obtain uniform emulsion. Ensure that the emulsion is thoroughly mixed and display the appearance and viscosity of dense whipped cream. The obtained emulsion must be prepared for immediate use.
2. Slowly inject 100 μL emulsion obtained in **Step 1** at the base of the tail of DBA/1 mice intradermally on day 0. A booster immunization using the same concentration of CII emulsified in IFA is injected at the base of the tail of DBA/1 mice on day 21 after the primary immunization.
3. Monitor the arthritis progression in DBA/1 mice. Evaluate each paw of mice and score for the joint swelling individually on a scale of 0–4, with 4 indicating the

most severe joint swelling. The basis for scoring the joint swelling is according to the previously reported protocol (Brand et al. 2007).

### 3.13 Biodistribution of the Hybrid Micelles in CIA Mice

1. Select mice with similar degree of established arthritis for the biodistribution study.
2. Prepare DiD-loaded hybrid micelles (at the final DiD concentration of 2 μg/mL) and inject intravenously to the arthritic mice (0.5 μg DiD per mouse) via tail vein. Dissolve free DiD in 25% propylene glycol solution (propylene glycol is used as a solubilizer to facilitate the dissolution of the hydrophobic DiD molecules).
3. Preheat the tail of mice with warm water (45 °C) to make the vein in tail more obvious. Inject DiD-loaded hybrid micelles or free DiD solution intravenously to arthritic mice at the same dose ($n = 3$).
4. Anesthetize the mice by intraperitoneally injecting 2% pentasorbital sodium at the dose of 60 mg/kg at indicated time point (2, 6, 24 h) and visualize the distribution of fluorescent signal in mice using the IVIS® spectrum system.

### 3.14 Therapeutic Efficacy of Hybrid Micelles Co-Loading with Dex and p65 siRNA In Vivo

1. Prepare the following formulations: PBS solution, free Dex dissolved in 25% propylene glycol, naked siRNA solution, Dex encapsulated in micelles (M-Dex), p65 siRNA encapsulated in micelles (M-siRNA), or micelles co-loading with Dex and p65 siRNA (M-Dex/siRNA). All formulations should be passed through a sterile filter (0.45 μm) before administration in vivo.
2. Randomly divide mice with similar degree of arthritis into six groups ($n = 8$). On day 36, 38, 40, and 42 after the arthritis induction, intravenously inject 200 μL one of the following formulations: PBS, naked siRNA, free Dex, M-Dex, M-siRNA, or M-Dex/siRNA to the corresponding group. The dose of Dex is 0.5 mg/kg, and the dose of siRNA is 0.4 mg/kg. In parallel, apply eight healthy mice without bearing arthritis serving as a normal control.
3. Monitor the joint score and body weight of each mouse during the period of treatment (As shown in Fig. 7).
4. On day 44 after first immunization, collect blood samples via orbital venous using a 0.3 mm capillary tube. Sacrifice the mice and dissect the joint tissues from mice in each group. Determine the level of TNF-a and IL-1β in serum and homogenate of joint tissues by ELISA kit according to the manufacturer's instructions. Fix the ankle joints obtained from mice in each group in 4% paraformaldehyde for 48 h. Decalcify the ankle joints by immersing them in 15% neutral EDTA-2Na solution for 3 weeks at 25 °C in a shaker. Embed decalcified tissues in paraffin and cut into thin sections (5 mm). Stain these tissue sections with hematoxylin-eosin.

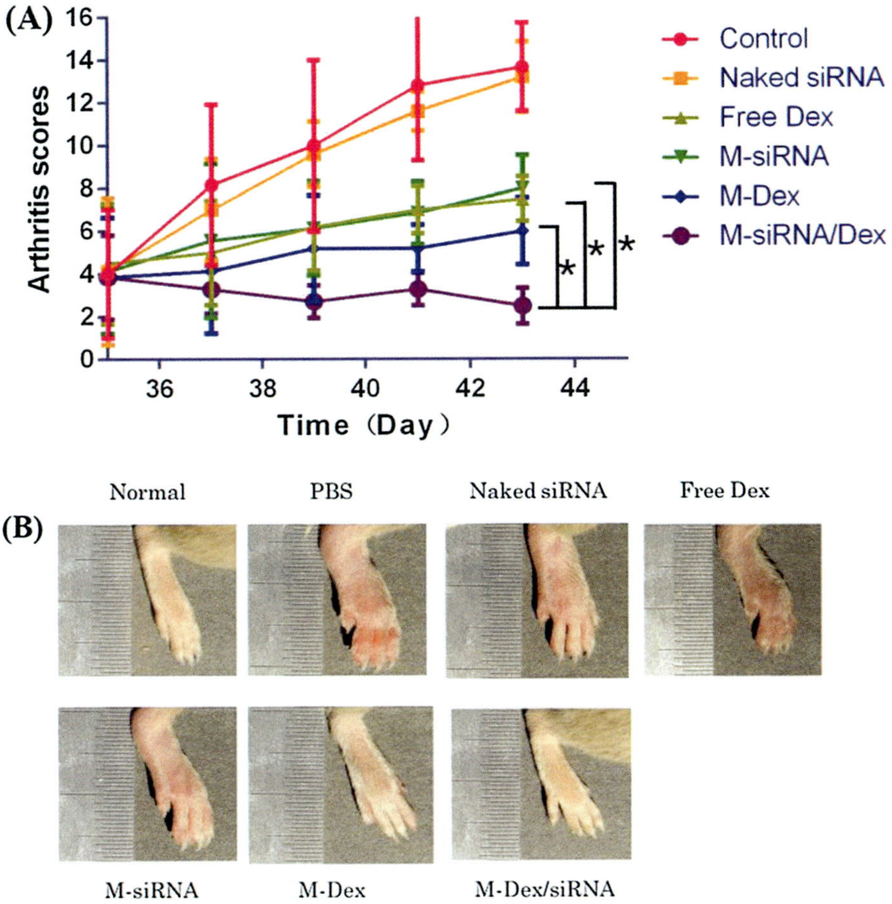


**Fig. 7** (**a**) Arthritic scores of mice treated with various drug formulations. Results are shown as mean ± SD ($n = 8$). *$p < 0.05$. (**b**) Photographs of representative hind legs from mice treated with various drug formulations. M-Dex, micelles containing Dex; M-siRNA, micelles containing siRNA; M-Dex/siRNA, micelles containing both Dex and siRNA

### 3.15 Statistical Analysis

1. Use Graphpad Prism 7.0 (GraphPad Software, USA) to plot the data.
2. Display data as the mean ± standard deviation (SD).
3. Differences and correlations between two groups were evaluated for significance using Student's 2-tailed test. Differences among three or more groups were assessed for significance using one-way analysis of variance. Bonferroni's correction for multiple comparisons is used.
4. Consider a value of $P < 0.05$ to be significant for all analyses.

# 4 Discussion (Table 2)

**Table 2** Common mistake and troubleshooting

| Mistake | Possible reason | Solution |
|---|---|---|
| Too large molecular weight of the synthetic PCL-PEI polymer | 1. Improper feeding speed<br>2. Improper ratio of PCL-NPC and PEI | PEI might easily react with several PCL molecules at the same time due to the multiple amino groups of the PEI. This can be avoided by properly increasing the proportion of PEI and slowing down the feeding speed of PCL-NPC |
| Low encapsulation rate of siRNA | 1. Inadequate time for the complexation of siRNA and delivery systems<br>2. Inappropriate ratio of N/P | Extend the time for the complexation of siRNA and delivery systems (15–30 min is appropriate)<br>Increase the ratio of N/P moderately |
| RNA degradation | 1. Contamination of exogenous RNase<br>2. Inappropriate storage | Process all these tips, tubes, and containers used in this experiment using 0.1% (v/v) DEPC solution<br>Store the RNA samples in −80 °C and avoid repeated freezing and thawing |
| Low efficiency of transfection | 1. Improper density of inoculated cells<br>2. Improper concentration of siRNA<br>3. Inappropriate ratio of N/P and incubation time for the formation of the complexes<br>4. Inappropriate Incubation time of exposure of these complexes to cells | Optimize the cell confluence before transfection study<br>Generally speaking, the siRNA concentration at 100 nM is mostly used in cell transfection assay. However, there might be differences in the optimal siRNA concentration depending on the type of cell and siRNA. Thus, the optimal concentration of siRNA should be investigated in this experiment<br>Similarly, the N/P and the incubation time should be optimized in the target cell |
| Cell contamination when incubating with drug-loaded formulations | Insufficient sterilization before adding formulations to cell cultures | Pass all these formulations through a sterile filter (0.45 μm) before adding to the cell cultures |
| Weak signal in Western blotting | 1. Low expression of the target protein<br>2. Insufficient time for signal development | Increase the loading volume or concentration of the protein samples<br>Extend the time for developing the blot |

## 5 Notes

1. The obtained PCL-PEG and PCL-PEI copolymers should be kept in cool and dry condition to prevent the moisture absorption.
2. As siRNA molecules are highly susceptible to RNase, which would be easily introduced to the siRNA-loaded formulations in preparation process. Therefore, RNase-free reagents, pipette tips and tubes as well as DEPC-treated container such as flasks and beakers should be used. Moreover, all experiments involving siRNA should be handled with gloved hands to avoid the contact with RNase on the surface of skins.
3. The Lyso tracker Red is suitable for fluorescence labeling of lysosome in the living cells, but not for lysosomes in the fixed cells. Therefore, the endosome escape study should be investigated without the procedure of cell fixing.
4. In electrophoresis assay, the addition of SDS is to break down the self-assembly of the hybrid micelles. And the negatively charged heparin sodium is served as a replacement of siRNA to bind to PCL-PEI, liberating the siRNA from the formulations.
5. The low N/P ratio is not sufficient to encapsulate siRNA molecules. While the high N/P is accompanied with too much PEG density on the surface, which would further hinder the cellular uptake. Therefore, the optimization of the N/P ratio is necessary for determine the superior complex ratio between siRNA and cationic polymers.
6. In the section of establishing CIA mice model, make sure the mixture of bovine CII collagen and Freund's adjuvant is fully emulsified. Add a drop of the prepared emulsion on the surface of the water. If it does not spread out, it would be a qualified emulsion.
7. Be careful to choose an appropriate injection site to avoid the vessels nearby when immunization and booster injection for the arthritis induction.
8. The drug-loaded hybrid micelles should be passed through a sterile filter (0.45 μm) to get rid of the bacteria before being incubated with cell cultures or administrated to mice.
9. The p65 siRNA could silence the expression of key subunit p65 in NF-κB family. While Dex is able to suppress the transcription activity of NF-κB signaling. The combination of the two different mechanisms aiming at inhibiting one signaling pathway would ultimately expedite the synergistic therapeutic efficacy. Furthermore, due to the co-delivery strategy and the selective targeting capacity of the hybrid micelles, the Dex dose (0.5 mg/kg) in this study is much lower than the previously reported, which might decrease the risk of side effects associated with Dex treatments.
10. Use the siRNA-loaded hybrid micelles immediately after preparation. This will reduce the risk of siRNA degradation and the contamination of microorganism.
11. The DEPC, GoldView, and paraformaldehyde are harmful to human body. Do not allow exposure to the human skin and mucosal tissues.

## 6 Conclusion

This protocol offers a facile and feasible approach to construct a polymeric hybrid micelle to co-deliver Dex and p65 siRNA to the inflamed joints for the treatment of RA. The method described here mainly focus on the preparation and evaluation of the dual-drugs loaded hybrid micelles, especially highlighting on the siRNA-based delivery both in vitro and in vivo.

## References

van der Aa LJ, Vader P, Storm G et al (2011) Optimization of poly(amido amine)s as vectors for siRNA delivery. J Control Release 150:177–186

Apparailly F, Jorgensen C (2013) siRNA-based therapeutic approaches for rheumatic diseases. Nat Rev Rheumatol 9:56–62

Brand DD, Latham KA, Rosloniec EF (2007) Collagen-induced arthritis. Nat Protoc 2:1269–1275

Gaestel M, Kotlyarov A, Kracht M (2009) Targeting innate immunity protein kinase signalling in inflammation. Nat Rev Drug Discov 8:480–499

Hayden MS, Ghosh S (2008) Shared principles in NF-κB signaling. Cell 132:344–362

Kim HJ, Kim A, Miyata K, Kataoka K (2016) Recent progress in development of siRNA delivery vehicles for cancer therapy. Adv Drug Deliv Rev 104:61–77

Li H, Fu Y, Zhang T et al (2015) Rational design of polymeric hybrid micelles with highly tunable properties to co-deliver MicroRNA-34a and Vismodegib for melanoma therapy. Adv Funct Mater 25:7457–7469

O'Neill LAJ (2006) Targeting signal transduction as a strategy to treat inflammatory diseases. Nat Rev Drug Discov 5:549–563

Oeckinghaus A, Hayden MS, Ghosh S (2011) Crosstalk in NF-κB signaling pathways. Nat Immunol 12:695–708

Okamoto H, Yoshio T, Kaneko H, Yamanaka H (2010) Inhibition of NF-κB signaling by fasudil as a potential therapeutic strategy for rheumatoid arthritis. Arthritis Rheum 62:82–92

Roman-Blas JA, Jimenez SA (2006) NF-κB as a potential therapeutic target in osteoarthritis and rheumatoid arthritis. Osteoarthr Cartil 14:839–848

Shim MS, Kwon YJ (2010) Efficient and targeted delivery of siRNA in vivo. FEBS J 277: 4814–4827

Simmonds RE, Foxwell BM (2008) Signalling, inflammation and arthritis: NF-κB and its relevance to arthritis and inflammation. Rheumatology 47:584–590

Vandewalle J, Luypaert A, De Bosscher K, Libert C (2018) Therapeutic mechanisms of glucocorticoids. Trends Endocrinol Metabol 29:42–54

Wang Q, Sun X (2017) Recent advances in nanomedicines for the treatment of rheumatoid arthritis. Biomater Sci 5:1407–1420

Wang Q, Jiang H, Li Y et al (2017) Targeting NF-kB signaling with polymeric hybrid micelles that co-deliver siRNA and dexamethasone for arthritis therapy. Biomaterials 1:10–22

Whitehead KA, Langer R, Anderson DG (2009) Knocking down barriers: advances in siRNA delivery. Nat Rev Drug Discov 8:129–138

Zhang S, Zhao B, Jiang H et al (2007) Cationic lipids and polymers mediated vectors for delivery of siRNA. J Control Release 123:1–10

# Preparation and Application of MPEG-PCL-g-PEI Cationic Micelles in Cancer Therapy

**6**

Yi Yang, Shuai Shi, and Zhiyong Qian

## Contents



Y. Yang
State Key Laboratory of Biotherapy and Cancer Center, West China Hospital, West China Medical School, Sichuan University, Chengdu, People's Republic of China

Precision Medicine Institute, The Second Affiliated Hospital of Xi'an Jiaotong University, Xi'an, Shaanxi Province, China

S. Shi
Institute of Biomedical Engineering, School of Ophthalmology & Optometry and Eye Hospital, Wenzhou Medical University, Wenzhou, China

Z. Qian (✉)
State Key Laboratory of Biotherapy and Cancer Center, West China Hospital, West China Medical School, Sichuan University, Chengdu, People's Republic of China
e-mail: zhiyongqian@scu.edu.cn


H. Tian and X. Chen (eds.), *Gene Delivery*, Biomaterial Engineering,
https://doi.org/10.1007/978-981-16-5419-0_7

**Abstract**

Gene therapy, as a novel treatment for cancers, needs gene carriers with high transfection efficiency in order to achieve excellent therapeutic efficacy. In recent years, the development of nonviral gene carriers has received great interest worldwide. However, the limitations of safety and low therapeutic efficacy make few nonviral gene vectors be used in clinical therapy of cancer. Therefore, co-delivery of functional genes and chemotherapeutic drugs is a promising method to improve therapeutic efficacy of cancer. Gene and drug delivery vector prepared with copolymers has attracted attention due to the flexibility, safety, and diverse chemical composition, and it is so easy to modify the polymer with an applicable structure in order to get requirements for co-delivery of gene and drug. Self-assembled micelles are usually modified to have multifarious advantages, such as prolonging circulation time, targeting to tumor tissue via enhanced permeability and retention effect. In this regard, this protocol focuses on the functional gene and chemotherapeutic drug co-delivery cationic micelles used in cancer therapy. Here, the preparation and characterization of gene and drug co-delivery micelles are described. Doxorubicin and Msurvivin T34A are used as model drug and gene, respectively. The present data show that the prepared cationic micelles exhibit effective co-delivery of functional gene and chemotherapeutic drug in cancer therapy.

**Keywords**

Block copolymer · Gene delivery · Drug carrier · Cancer therapy

## 1 Overview

A large number of nanomedicines based on copolymers have attracted great attention because of their diverse and flexible chemical composition. Improving the physical and chemical properties through changing the chemical composition of copolymers is very easy (Venkataraman et al. 2011). Meanwhile, due to incorporation of targeted ligand, the drug-loaded nanoparticles based on copolymers deliver drugs to the desired site (Dobson 2009). Many researchers point out that the adsorption properties of nanoparticles is related with lipophilic of nanoparticle's surface, so they modify hydrophilic groups on the nanoparticle's surface for prolonging circulation time of nanoparticles in vivo (Wang et al. 2008). There are many methods to obtain drug-loaded nanoparticles, and block copolymer micelle is one of them with hydrophobic core and hydrophilic shell. Block copolymer micelle is usually prepared by self-assembly of amphiphilic copolymers in aqueous medium. The micelles prepared with block copolymers have many advantages, such as increasing solubility and stability of hydrophobic drug, enhancing drug utilization, and decreasing toxicity by prolonging cycle time of drugs (Rösler et al. 2012).

Poly(ethylene glycol) (short for PEG), as hydrophilic agent, generally links with hydrophobic groups in order to enhance its bioavailability and biocompatibility. Therefore, PEG-PCL copolymers has been a good candidate for advanced drug delivery systems for its amphiphilicity, biodegradability, and biocompatibility. Firstly, to investigate cellular uptake and in vivo enrichment of block copolymer MPEG-PCL, $-C{=}C$ is introduced to increase chemical reaction site (Duan et al. 2012; Xue et al. 2012; Gong et al. 2012). Polyethylenimine (PEI), as nonviral gene vector, can efficiently deliver therapeutic genes into cancer cells. Branched polyethyleneimine (25kD) is an effective and commercial PEI, but high cytotoxicity limits its clinical use (Shi et al. 2010; Shi et al. 2012). In our present work, we link PEI ($MW = 25kD$) to monomethoxy poly(ethylene glycol) (MPEG)-PCL copolymer through chemical reaction, but the physical and chemical properties of the obtained copolymer are changed. Then we adjust the molecular weight of amphiphilic polymer MPEG-PCL and PEI, we gained triblock copolymers $MPEG_{5000}$-$PCL_{2000}$-g-$PEI_{2000}$, and their remarkable properties make us be conscious of their potential use as vectors for chemical drug and gene delivery (Shi et al. 2012).

Doxorubicin, as an anthracycline antibiotics, has become part of stand treatment regiments for multifarious tumor, such as sarcoma, breast cancer, hematological malignancies, and lung cancer (Cai et al. 2010). Doxorubicin can inhibit the growth of cancers by restraining the synthesis of DNA and RNA in subcellular level. However, thrombocytopenia, neutropenia, and cardiac toxicity of doxorubicin limit its clinical use (Takemura and Fujiwara 2007). Survivin is part of apoptosis gene family inhibitor and has relationship with proliferation and differentiation of cancer cells. Furthermore, survivin can only inhibit the growth of tumor and embryonic tissue, and many studies have been made to counteract survivin in cancer cell including anti-sense, RNAi-mediated, and dominant negative mutants (McKay et al. 2003; Aspe and Wall 2010; Grossman et al. 2001). Thus, as a negative mutant, Msurvivin T34A can reduce growth activity of cancer cells and lead to caspase-mediated apoptosis.

In this protocol, we chose doxorubicin and Msurvivin T34A as model drug and plasmid, respectively, to investigate the potential application of MPEG-PCL-g-PEI cationic micelles in delivering chemotherapy drug and gene prodrug in cancer therapy.

## 2 Materials

### 2.1 Preparation of MPEG-PCL-g-PEI Micelles

1. Monomethoxy poly(ethylene glycol) (short for MPEG, Mn = 5000, 2000)
2. ε-caprolactone (short for ε-CL, Mw = 114)
3. Polyethyleneimine (short for PEI, Mw = 2000)
4. Stannous octoate (short for Sn(Oct)2)
5. 97% glycidyl methacrylate (short for GMA)
6. Ethanol
7. Methanol
8. Petroleum ether
9. Micropore filter membrane (0.2 μm)
10. N,N-dimethylaminopyridine (DMAP)
11. 3-Aminobenzoic acid ethyl ester methanesulfonate (MS222)
12. Methylene chloride
13. 100 ml pear-shaped flask
14. Gas partition chromatography (GPC)

### 2.2 Preparation of Doxorubicin and Msurvivin T34A Loaded MPEG-PCL-g-PEI Micelles

1. Ethanol
2. Phosphate-buffered saline (short for PBS)
3. Distilled water
4. Hydrochloric acid
5. Bath-type sonicator
6. 100 ml pear-shaped flask
7. Circulating water multipurpose vacuum pump
8. Magnetic stirrer
9. Doxorubicin chloride (Doxorubicin, short for DOX)
10. Msurvivin T34A plasmid
11. 0.2 μm micropore filter membrane

### 2.3 Evaluation of MPEG-PCL-g-PEI Micelles Morphology

1. Transmission electron microscopy
2. Distilled water
3. 0.2 μm micropore filter membrane
4. Copper grids coated with carbon films
5. 1% uranyl acetate solution
6. Malvern Nano-ZAS 90 laser particle size analyzer
7. Silicon slice

### 2.4 Determination of Doxorubicin and Msurvivin T34A Loaded Micelles In Vitro and In Vivo

1. B16F10 murine melanoma cell line
2. MCF-7 human breast cell line
3. CT26 colon carcinoma cell line
4. C57 female mice (6–8 weeks)
5. BALB/c female mice (6–8 weeks)
6. Dulbecco's modification of Eagle's medium (short for DMEM)
7. Heat-inactivated fetal bovine serum (FBS)
8. Trypsin EDTA
9. CO2 incubator
10. Optical microscope
11. Penicillin
12. Streptomycin
13. l-Glutamine
14. Nile red

## 3 Protocol

### 3.1 Preparation and Characterization of MPEG-PCL-g-PEI Copolymer

The synthesis method of MPEG-PCL-PEI copolymer used in this protocol is according to the previous report (Shi et al. 2012).

#### 3.1.1 Preparation and Characterization of MPEG-PCL Copolymer

1. Add MPEG into 100 ml flask at 90 °C for 30 min.
2. Add ε-caprolactone and Sn(Oct)2 into the flask, then stir at 130 °C for 6 h.
3. Add methylene chloride into the flask when at room temperature and precipitate with precooled petroleum ether repeatedly.
4. Volatilize the solvent in chemical hood, and dry it in vacuum drying oven.
5. Confirm the structure of the product with $^1$H NMR and GPC.

#### 3.1.2 Preparation and Characterization of MPEG-PCL-GMA Copolymer

1. Dissolve MPEG-PCL powder and GMA in 100 mL methylene chloride, respectively.
2. Add MPEG-PCL solution and DMAP into 500 mL flask.
3. Add GMA solution into the flask drop by drop.
4. Stir at room temperature for 48 h.
5. Precipitate with precooled petroleum ether.
6. Purify the product with precooled petroleum ether and methylene chloride, dry it in vacuum drying oven.
7. Confirm the structure of the product with $^1$H NMR and GPC.

### 3.1.3 Preparation and Characterization of MPEG-PCL-g-PEI Copolymer

1. Dissolve MPEG-PCL-GMA powder and PEI in 100 mL methylene chloride, respectively.
2. Add MPEG-PCL-GMA solution into 500 mL flask.
3. Add PEI solution into the flask drop by drop.
4. Stir at 45 °C for 48 h.
5. Precipitate with precooled petroleum ether.
6. Purify the product with precooled petroleum ether and methylene chloride, dry it in vacuum drying oven.
7. Purify through dialysis and lyophilization.
8. Confirm the structure of the product with $^{1}$H NMR and GPC.

## 3.2 Preparation and Characterization of Blank MPEG-PCL-g-PEI Micelles

### 3.2.1 Preparation of Blank MPEG-PCL-g-PEI Micelles

1. Add MPEG–PCL-g–PEI copolymers to deionized water.
2. MPEG–PCL-g–PEI copolymer self-assemble into nanoscale micelles in deionized water when increasing temperature to 55 °C, and the schematic illustration for this process is shown in Fig. 1a.

### 3.2.2 Morphology of Blank MPEG-PCL-g-PEI Micelles

**Determination of Morphology by Malvern Nano-ZAS 90 Laser Particle Size Analyzer**

1. Dissolve MPEG-PCL-PEI copolymer in deionized water.
2. Filter through a 0.2 μm micropore filter membrane.
3. Observe the particle size and ζ-potentials by Malvern Nano-ZAS 90 laser particle size analyzer.
4. The particle size and ζ-potentials are shown in Fig. 1c, d, respectively.

**Determination of Morphology by TEM**

1. Add copper grids coated with carbon films into micelles solution in order to absorb micelles particles.
2. Take out copper grids, then blot the grids with filter paper.
3. Float the grids in 1% uranyl acetate solution, then remove it.
4. Blot the grids with filter paper, then dry at room temperature overnight.
5. Observe with TEM at 120 kV as shown in Fig. 1b.

**Determination of Morphology by AFM**

1. Spread 10 μl micelles solution on silicon slice.
2. Dry at room temperature.
3. Observe with AFM.

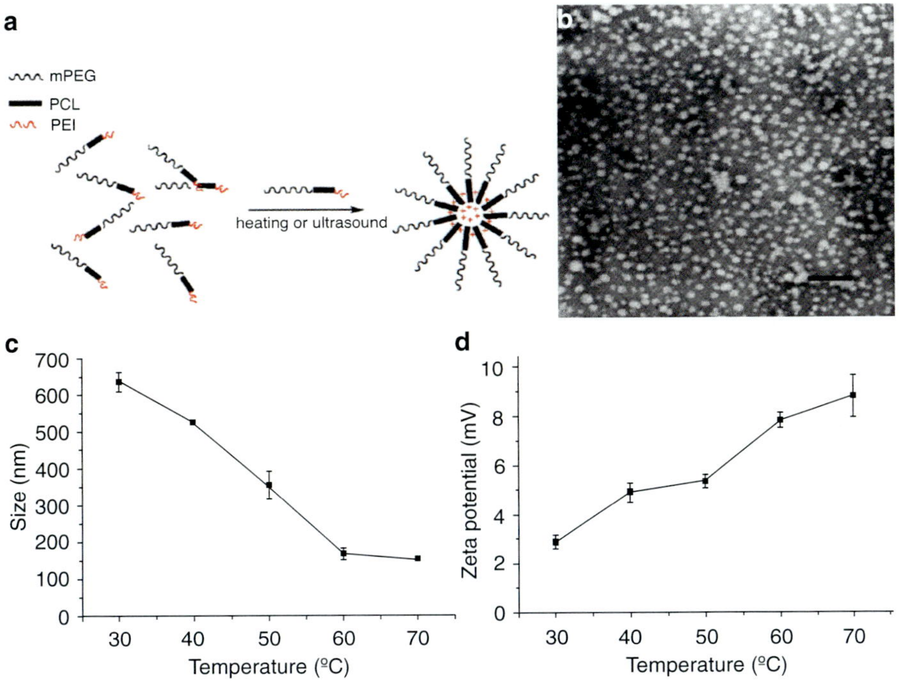


**Fig. 1** (**a**) Schematic illustration of MPEG-PCL-g-PEI micelles. (**b**) Morphology of MPEG-PCL-g-PEI micelles observed by TEM (scale bar: 100 nm). (**c**) Sizes of the micelles at different temperatures. (**d**) ζ-potentials of the micelles at different temperatures. (Adapted from Shi et al. (2010), with permission)

### 3.2.3 Cytotoxicity of Blank MPEG-PCL-g-PEI Micelles In Vitro

1. L929 and HEK293 cell lines are seeded in 96-well plates with $2 \times 10^4$ cells/well in 100 μL of growth medium and then incubated overnight.
2. Expose cells in a series of MPEG–PCL-g–PEI micelles at different concentrations.
3. Incubate for 24 h.
4. Observe cell viability by MTT assay, untreated cells are used as control group, absorbances are measured at 570 nm by Spectramax microplate reader (Molecular Devices, Sunnyvale, CA).

### 3.2.4 Preparation of pDNA/MPEG–PCL-g–PEI Complexes

1. Add pDNA solution into MPEG-PCL-g-PEI micelles solution and mix by pipetting.
2. Incubate for 30 min in room temperature.

### 3.2.5 Gel Retardation Assay of Blank MPEG-PCL-g-PEI Micelles

1. Add pDNA solution into MPEG-PCL-g-PEI micelles solution and mix by pipetting.
2. Incubate for 30 min in room temperature, then pDNA/MPEG–PCL-g–PEI complexes are electrophoresed with 1% agarose gel (100 V, 30 min).

### 3.2.6 Transfection Efficiency of Blank MPEG-PCL-g-PEI Micelles In Vitro

1. B16-F10 and 293 T cells are seeded in 6-well plates with $2 \times 10^5$ cells/well.
2. Incubate for 24 h, then remove the medium from each well.
3. Wash the cells once with Dulbecco's modified Eagle's medium without serum and antibiotic.
4. Add 900 μL of serum-free medium into each well.
5. Then add 100 μL of pDNA/micelle complex solution containing 2 μg green fluorescence protein reporter plasmid into each well.
6. Coculture with MPEG–PCL-g–PEI/plasmid DNA complexes for 6 h at 37 °C, discard the serum-free medium, and add fresh medium further culture.
7. Transfection efficiency of each well is examined by flow cytometry.

## 3.3 Preparation and Characterization of Doxorubicin and Msurvivin T34A Loaded MPEG-PCL-g-PEI Micelles

### 3.3.1 Preparation of Doxorubicin and Msurvivin T34A Loaded Micelles

1. Add 0.2 mL of phosphate-buffered saline (10×, pH 7.4) into 1 mL of MPEG-PCL-PEI micelles solution (20 mg/mL).
2. Add 0.8 mL of aqueous doxorubicin solution (2 mg/mL) into the micelles solution dropwise under moderate stirring.
3. Filter through a 0.2 μm micropore filter membrane.
4. Add Msurvivin T34A solution into doxorubicin loaded micelles solution and mix by pipetting.
5. Incubate for 30 min in room temperature.

### 3.3.2 Morphology of Doxorubicin and Msurvivin T34A Loaded Micelles

#### Determination of Morphology by Malvern Nano-ZAS 90 Laser Particle Size Analyzer

1. Dissolve MPEG-PCL-PEI copolymer in deionized water.
2. Filter with 0.2 μm micropore filter membrane.
3. Observe by Malvern Nano-ZAS 90 laser particle size analyzer as shown in Fig. 2.

#### Determination of Morphology by TEM

1. Copper grids coated with carbon films is used to absorb the micelles particles from the micelles solution.
2. Take out copper grids, then blot grids with filter paper.
3. Float the grids with 1% uranyl acetate solution, then remove it.
4. Blot grids with filter paper, then dry grids at room temperature overnight.
5. Observe with TEM at 120 kV.

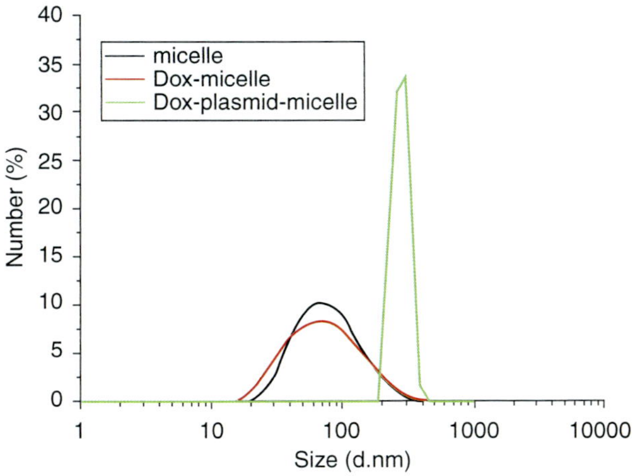


**Fig. 2** Size distribution spectrum of blank micelles, DOX loaded micelles, and DOX and DNA loaded micelles. (Adapted from Shi et al. (2014), with permission)

**Determination of Morphology by AFM**

1. Spread 10 μl micelles solution on silicon slice.
2. Dry at room temperature.
3. Observe with AFM.

### 3.3.3 Uptake of Doxorubicin Loaded Micelles In Vitro

1. B16-F10 cells are seeded into 6-well plates with cover slip in each well.
2. Incubate overnight, then replace growth medium with fresh growth medium containing doxorubicin loaded micelles.
3. Incubate at 37 °C for predetermined time.
4. Wash cells with phosphate-buffered saline (pH 7.4) for three times.
5. Observe uptake of doxorubicin loaded micelles by LSM 510 confocal laser scanning microscope (Leica, Germany).

### 3.3.4 Drug Release of Doxorubicin Loaded Micelles In Vitro

1. Transfer 1 mL doxorubicin loaded micelles (0.5 mg/mL) into dialysis bag (cut-off molecular weight, 3500 Da).
2. Place the bag in buffer solution (pH value, 6.8 and 5.5).
3. Collect the incubation samples at predetermined timepoints, the concentrations of samples are measured with high performance liquid chromatography instrument (Shimadzu LC-20 AD, Japan).
4. Equip solvent delivery system with column oven (CTO-20A) and plus auto-sampler (SIL-20 AC), phosphate buffer/acetonitrile (25 Mm, 75/25, v/v) is used as mobile phase with flow rate of 1 ml/min.
5. Detect with diode array detector (SPD-M20A). Chromatographic separations are performed with reversed phase C18 column (4.6 × 150 mm, 5 mm, zorbax eclipse XDB, Agilent, US).
6. Detection wavelength is 233 nm, retention time is 15 min.

### 3.3.5 Transfection Efficiency of Doxorubicin and Msurvivin T34A Loaded Micelles In Vitro

1. Nile red is used as model agent of hydrophobic drug.
2. Dissolve Nile red in acetone, then added into a bottle and dry it with nitrogen.
3. Add 1 mL of MPEG–PCL-g–PEI micelles (5 mg/mL) into the bottle, then load Nile red into micelles with ultrasonication.
4. Nile red loaded micelles are used to deliver green fluorescence protein in vitro (ratio of MPEG–PCL-g–PEI/DNA, 40).
5. Observe gene expression and cellular uptake of Nile red with Cellomics ArrayScan VTI 600 (Thermo Fisher Scientific, Waltham, MA).

## 3.4 Bio-distribution of Doxorubicin Loaded Micelles In Vivo

1. Tumor-bearing mice model is used to evaluate the bio-distribution of micelles in vivo. 2. Tumor-bearing mice model is prepared by subcutaneous injection of MCF-7 cells.
2. Two weeks later, the tumor-bearing mice are used for single-photon emission computerized tomography (short for SPECT) imaging at different timepoints.
3. To observe the distribution of doxorubicin loaded micelles in vivo, four mice are separately injected intravenously with 50 mBq/100 mL of 99Tc/DOX complexes and 99Tc/DOX loaded complex micelles.
4. The distribution of doxorubicin loaded micelles is shown in Fig. 3.

## 3.5 Effect of Doxorubicin and Msurvivin T34A Loaded Micelles in Lung Metastases Tumor Model

1. The effect of doxorubicin and Msurvivin T34A loaded micelles on cancer is investigated with B16-F10 tumor models.
2. C57 female mice (6 weeks old) are injected intravenously with $5 \times 10^5$ B16-F10 cells.
3. Randomly divide the mice into five groups (saline group, Msurvivin T34A loaded micelles group, free doxorubicin group, DOX loaded micelles group, Msurvivin T34A and DOX loaded micelles group, $n = 5$/group).
4. Each dose of 4 mg/kg DOX and (or) 5 mg/kg Msurvivin T34A plasmid are injected intravenously via tail vein every 2 days.
5. Mice of all groups are euthanized 1 week after administration.
6. After all mice are sacrificed, tumor nodules, heart, lung, spleen, liver, and kidney are used for subsequent experiment as shown in Fig. 4.

## 3.6 Effect of Doxorubicin and Msurvivin T34A Loaded Micelles in an Abdominal Cavity Metastases Tumor Model

1. The effect of doxorubicin and Msurvivin T34A loaded micelles on cancer is investigated with CT26 tumor models.
2. C57 female mice (6 weeks old) are injected intravenously with $5 \times 10^5$ CT26 cells.

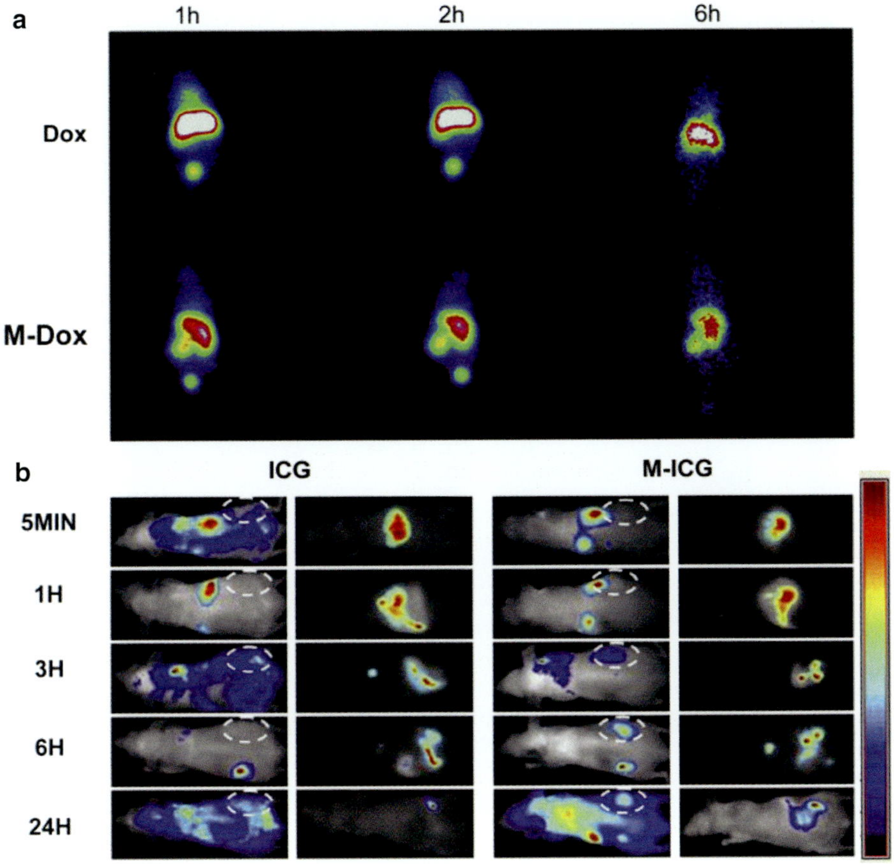


**Fig. 3** (**a**) SPECT images of mice injected with 99Tc/DOX complexes or 99Tc-labled micelles. Images were taken at 1, 2, and 6 h after 99Tc administrated. (**b**) Images of ICG-loaded MPEG-PCL-g-PEI micelles and free ICG (control group) injected intravenously in human breast tumor-bearing mice. (Adapted from Shi et al. (2014), with permission)

3. Randomly divide the mice into six groups (saline group, Msurvivin T34A loaded micelles group, free doxorubicin group, DOX loaded micelles group, Msurvivin T34A and DOX loaded micelles group, $n = 5$/group).
4. Each dose of 4 mg/kg DOX and (or) 5 mg/kg Msurvivin T34A plasmid are administered intravenously via tail vein every 2 days.
5. Mice of all groups are euthanized 1 week after administration.
6. After all mice are sacrificed, tumor nodules, heart, lung, spleen, liver, and kidney are used for subsequent experiment.
7. In order to observe the influence of micelles on mice, intraperitoneal tumor model is added an blank micelles is designed as one of treatment groups.
8. The treatment results are shown in Fig. 5.

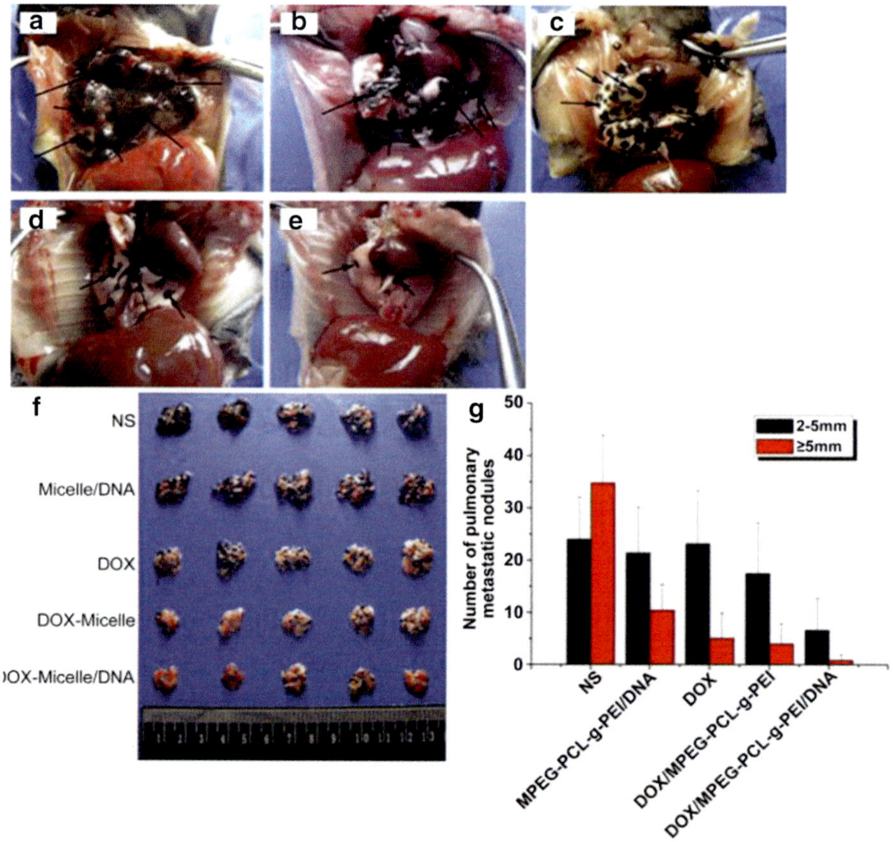


**Fig. 4** The images of lung from B16-F10 lung metastases tumor model after treatments of saline group (**a**), the gene therapy group (**b**), frees doxorubicin group (**c**), DOX-loaded micelles group (**d**), and the group of co-delivery of Msurvivin T34A and doxorubicin (**e**). (**f**) Image of the lung after treatment in B16-F10 lung metastases tumor model. (**g**) The statistics of tumor nodules in each group. (Adapted from Shi et al. (2014), with permission)

### 3.7 Effect of Doxorubicin and Msurvivin T34A Loaded Micelles in a Subcutaneous Tumor Model

1. The effect of doxorubicin and Msurvivin T34A loaded micelles on cancer is investigated with B16-F10 tumor models.
2. C57 female mice (6 weeks old) are injected subcutaneously with $5 \times 10^5$ B16-F10 cells.
3. Randomly divide the mice into five groups (saline group, Msurvivin T34A loaded micelles group, free doxorubicin group, DOX loaded micelles group, Msurvivin T34A and DOX loaded micelles group, $n = 5$/group).
4. Each dose of 4 mg/kg DOX and (or) 5 mg/kg Msurvivin T34A plasmid are administered intravenously via tail vein every 2 days.

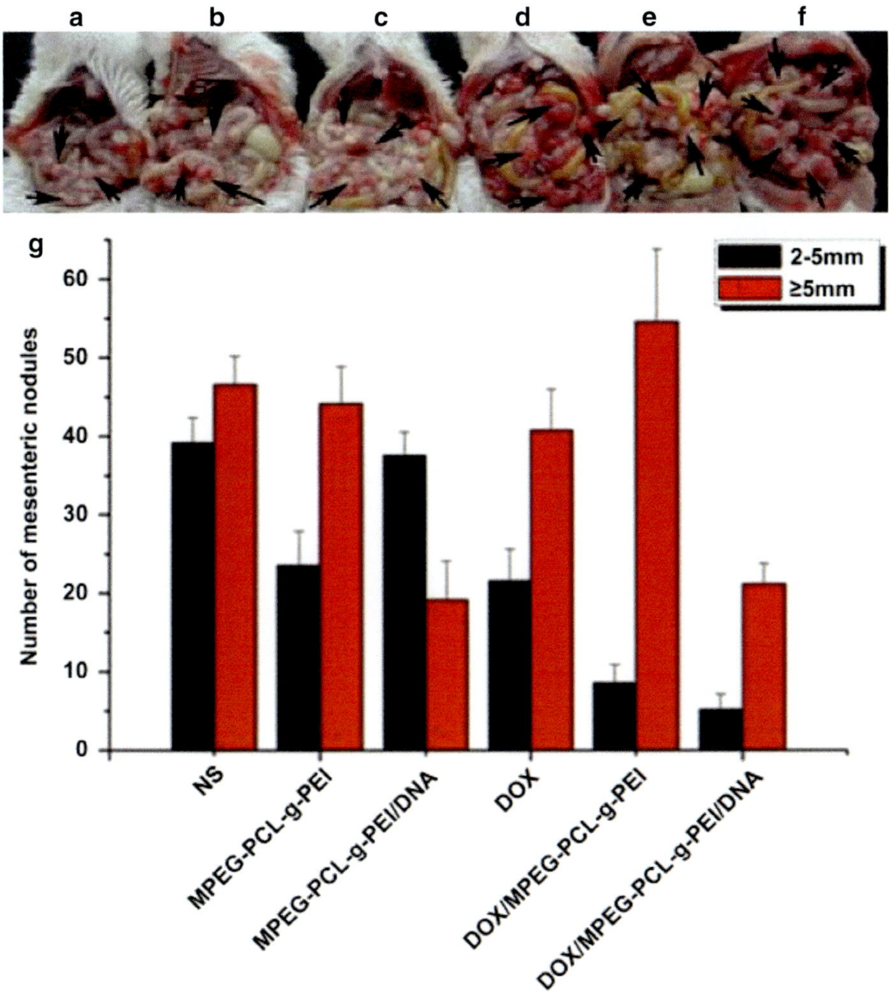


**Fig. 5** Representative images of abdominal metastatic nodes (arrows) after treated with (**a**) DOX/MPEG-PCL-g-PEI/DNA, (**b**) DOX/MPEG-PCL-g-PEI, (**c**) free DOX, (**d**) MPEG-PCL-g-PEI/DNA, (**e**) MPEG-PCL-g-PEI, (**f**) normal sodium, and (**g**) The statistics of abdominal metastatic nodes in each treatment group. (Adapted from Shi et al. (2014), with permission)

5. The tumor volume and body weight are recorded every 3 days; the tumor volume is calculated according to this formula:

   tumor volume $=$ length $\times$ width$^2$ $\times$ 0.52.
6. Mice are sacrificed once the tumor volume reach 3000 mm$^3$.
7. After all mice are sacrificed, the tumors, heart, lung, spleen, liver, and kidney are used for the subsequent experiment.
8. The treatment results are shown in Fig. 6.

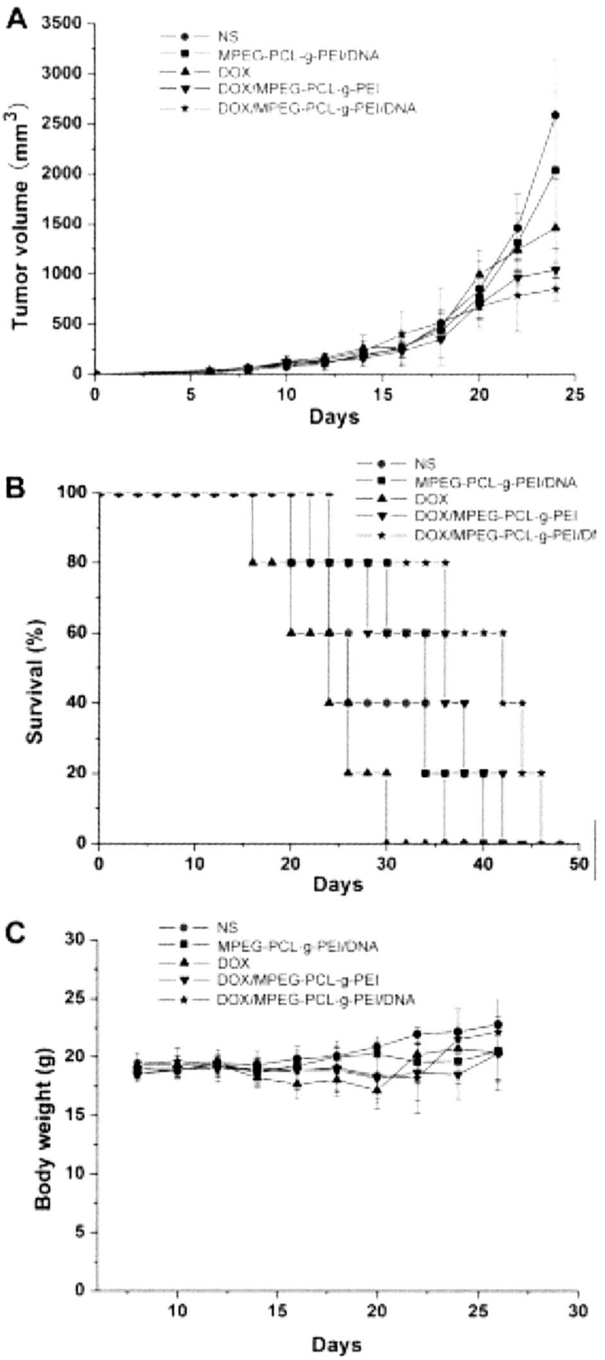


**Fig. 6** Tumor growth rate (**a**) after treatment, survival curves (**b**) of mice after treatment, and weight curves (**c**) of mice after treatment. (Adapted from Shi et al. (2014), with permission)

### 3.8 Statistical Analysis

1. Statistical analysis is performed with one-way analysis of variance (ANOVA) using SPSS software for comparison of individual experimental groups, and all data are expressed as the means with 95% confidence intervals.
2. Statistical significance is determined at $p > 0.05$.

## 4 Notes

1. The results of $^1$H-NMR spectrums of MPEG-PCL-g-PEI (Shi et al. 2012) indicate that three formations copolymers with MW at 5339.6, 8786.7, and 11,703 match the need of the original design ($MPEG_{2000}$-$PCL_{2000}$-g-$PEI_{2000}$; $MPEG_{5000}$-$PCL_{2000}$-g-$PEI_{2000}$; and $MPEG_{2000}$-$PCL_{6000}$-g-$PEI_{2000}$).
2. In consideration of transfection efficiency and toxicity, we chose the triblock $MPEG_{5000}$-$PCL_{2000}$-g-$PEI_{2000}$ as the vector in animal experiments.
3. The used parameters in SPECT are as follows: 100 kVp; matrix 128 $\times$ 256; field of view 25 $\times$ 43 mm; 256 projections; and 0.25 mA.

## 5 Discussion

The protocol presented a novel self-assembled micelle platform based on a triblock copolymer MPEG-PCL-PEI, which is designed to co-deliver doxorubicin and Msurvivin T34A plasmid for cancer therapy. These micelles could remarkably enhance the drug uptake efficiency and deliver therapeutic genes into cancer cells. The anticancer activity of doxorubicin and Msurvivin T34A loaded micelle platform was investigated in subcutaneous tumor model, lung metastasis model, and abdominal tumor model. Compared with free doxorubicin, the micelles platform had high anticancer activity, decreased systemic toxicity of doxorubicin.

## References

Aspe JR, Wall NR (2010) Survivin-T34A: molecular mechanism and therapeutic potential. Onco Targets Ther 3:247–254

Cai S, Thati S, Bagby TR, Diab H-M, Davies NM, Cohen MS et al (2010) Localized doxorubicin chemotherapy with a biopolymeric nanocarrier improves survival and reduces toxicity in xenografts of human breast cancer. J Control Release 146:212–218

Dobson J (2009) Nanomedicine for targeted drug delivery. J Mater Chem 19:6294–6307

Duan XM, Wang P, Men K, Gao X, Huang MJ, Gou ML et al (2012) Treating colon cancer with a suicide gene delivered by self-assembled cationic MPEG-PCL micelles. Nanoscale 4:2400–2407

Gong C, Deng S, Wu Q, Xiang M, Wei X, Li L et al (2012) Improving antiangiogenesis and anti-tumor activity of curcumin by biodegradable polymeric micelles. Biomaterials 34:1413–1432

Grossman D, Kim PJ, Schechner JS, Altieri DC (2001) Inhibition of melanoma tumor growth in vivo by survivin targeting. Proc Natl Acad Sci U S A 98:635–640

McKay TR, Bell S, Tenev T, Stoll V, Lopes R, Lemoine NR et al (2003) Procaspase 3 expression in ovarian carcinoma cells increases survivin transcription which can be countered with a dominant-negative mutant, survivin T34A; a combination gene therapy strategy. Oncogene 22:3539–3547

Rösler A, Vandermeulen GWM, Klok HA (2012) Advanced drug delivery devices via self-assembly of amphiphilic block copolymers. Adv Drug Deliv Rev 53:95–108

Shi S, Fan M, Wang X, Zhao C, Wang Y, Luo F et al (2010) Synthesis and characterization of mPEG-PCL-g-PEI and self-assembled nanoparticle uptake in vitro and in vivo. J Phys Chem C 114:21315–21321

Shi S, Zhu X, Guo QF, Wang Y, Zuo T, Luo F et al (2012) Self-assembled mPEG-PCL-g-PEI micelles for simultaneous codelivery of chemotherapeutic drugs and DNA: synthesis and characterization in vitro. Int J Nanomedicine 7:1749–1759

Shi S, Shi K, Tan LW, Qu Y, Shen GB et al (2014) The use of cationic MPEG-PCL-g-PEI micelles for co-delivery of Msurvivin T34A gene and doxorubicin. Biomaterials 35:4536–4547

Takemura G, Fujiwara H (2007) Doxorubicin-induced cardiomyopathy: from the cardiotoxic mechanisms to management. Prog Cardiovasc Dis 49(5):330–352

Venkataraman S, Hedrick JL, Ong ZY, Yang C, Ee PLR, Hammond PT et al (2011) The effects of polymeric nanostructure shape on drug delivery. Adv Drug Deliv Rev 63:1228–1246

Wang X, Yang L, Chen ZG, Shin DM (2008) Application of nanotechnology in cancer therapy and imaging. CA Cancer J Clin 58:97–110

Xue B, Wang Y, Tang XH, Xie P, Luo F, Wu C et al (2012) Biodegradable self assembled MPEG-PCL micelles for hydrophobic oridonin delivery in vitro. J Biomed Nanotechnol 8:80–89

# Preparation and Evaluation of Lipopeptides with Arginine-Rich Periphery for Gene Delivery

7

Xiaobing Chen, Rongrong Jin, and Yu Nie

## Contents



**Abstract**

Self-assemblies of arginine-containing dendritic lipopeptides provide remarkable benefits for gene delivery through the virus-inspired design and fabrication. The present protocol focuses on synthesis, preparation, characterization of the gene carriers, including gene transfection efficiency evaluation as well as intracellular tracking. The synthesis of dendritic lipopeptides with bio-reducible disulfide linkage and dual aliphatic chains was firstly described as the basic compound, followed by a series of integrated co-delivery modifications with hydrophobic drugs and fluorescent probe. The obtained results demonstrated that the fabricated nanovectors exhibited high gene transfection efficiency, specific turn-on fluorescence imaging in tumors, and fast drug release from the dendritic arginine peptide-prodrug conjugates.

X. Chen · R. Jin
National Engineering Research Center for Biomaterials, College of Biomedical Engineering, Sichuan University, Qingyang, Chengdu, Sichuan, P.R. China

Y. Nie (✉)
National Engineering Research Center for Biomaterials, College of Biomedical Engineering, Sichuan University, Qingyang, Chengdu, Sichuan, P.R. China

College of Biomedical Engineering, Sichuan University, Chengdu, Sichuan, China
e-mail: nie_yu@scu.edu.cn



H. Tian and X. Chen (eds.), *Gene Delivery*, Biomaterial Engineering,
https://doi.org/10.1007/978-981-16-5419-0_6

**Keywords**

Lipopeptides · Arginine-rich · Co-delivery · Theranostic vector

## 1 Introduction

Gene therapy has been hailed as a powerful therapeutic strategy and recognized as "magic bullets" to specifically repair or knockdown disease-causing genes, upregulate or enhance the therapeutic gene expression with various nucleic acids (including DNA, siRNA, miRNA and mRNA, etc.) (Swami et al. 2013). While the premise of successful gene therapy lies on sufficient nucleic acids transportation into targeted cells, which requires an efficient delivery vehicle (Wang et al. 2012). Viral vectors are recognized as the most effective natural transfection vehicles with high infectivity, but also with accumulating number of adverse events in clinical trials, such as immunogenicity and inflammatory response. Drawbacks in viral vectors lead to the exploitation of nonviral vectors (Thomas et al. 2003; Barrán-Berdón et al. 2014).

Powerful infection ability is the most appealing characteristic of virus, partly attributed to the cell-penetrating peptides (CPPs) decorated on viral envelope with positively charged amino acid clusters. In addition, virus could recognize the signs provided by the host cells and undergo stepwise disassembly according to the microenvironment changes, which ensure the release of viral genomes at proper time. Inspired by these ingenious virus gene delivery strategies, it is reasonable to introduce virus cell penetrating peptide structure and conditional genomes release behavior within the design of nonviral vectors to obtain high gene transfection efficiency (Yoo et al. 2011). Several synthetic arginine-rich molecules (including arginine-rich peptides, oligoarginines, and even arginine) for CPPs mimicking have been verified to greatly improve cell penetration and gene delivery (Walrant et al. 2012). Supramolecular self-assembly with microenvironment responsive linkers are being developed to achieve appropriate gene release. Accordingly, our group have developed a self-assembled nanovector composed of dendritic lipopeptides with arginine-rich periphery and dual hydrophobic tails, which showed efficient gene transfection and good biocompatibility (Xu et al. 2015; Jiang et al. 2016). Further, bio-reducible disulfide linkages were incorporated to promote nucleic acids release (Chen et al. 2017). And a series of arginine-rich dendritic molecules with different generations were continuously explored for better gene complexation, supramolecular assembly, and gene transfection (Liang et al. 2019).

However, gene therapy alone sometimes seems incapable to achieve satisfying therapeutic efficacy on major diseases, which possess multifactorial etiology and biological complexity. Combination with effective chemical drug by synergistic mechanism has been considered as a promising strategy to improve therapeutic outcome (Khan et al. 2012; Liu et al. 2016). For example, siRNA of drug efflux transporter was frequently employed for co-delivery system with anticancer drugs to overcome the multiple drug resistance. However, general physical blending or loading may lead to low encapsulation efficiency and unwanted interactions between therapeutics molecules. Thus, covalent conjugation with chemical drugs as "pro-drug" based gene vectors have been developed, combating the dilemma in gene/drug combination therapy. Accordingly, our group developed a series of co-delivery systems consisting of integrated dendritic peptide-prodrug conjugates, in which dendritic arginine was chosen as the hydrophilic part and low molecular chemical drugs (camptothecin and candesartan) (Jiang et al. 2019; Chen et al. 2021) acted as hydrophobic segment.

Besides, deep understanding of the in vivo fate of each component in delivery system is important. Gene delivery vector with real-time imaging capacity was intensively developed to visualize and quantify the pharmacokinetics of involved components at both cellular and tissue levels, facilitating the optimization and further development of vector design and synthesis. Theranostic nanomaterials with a specific "turn-on" feature offer an opportunity to reduce the background interference and improve the spatial resolution, for it could only switch from "OFF" to "ON" for selective molecules or events (Sheng et al. 2014). Recently, we also reported a novel platform rationally integrating indocyanine green analogues and an arginine-rich dendritic peptide with environment responsive linkers for selective and efficient gene delivery. Meanwhile, the platform displayed specific turn-on fluorescence imaging in tumors (Liang et al. 2020a, b).

Here, the protocol focuses on preparation and evaluation of lipopeptides with arginine-rich periphery for gene delivery. The synthesis of dendritic lipopeptides (RLS) with arginine-rich periphery and bio-reducible disulfide linkage was described. A series of co-delivery systems with chemical drugs or fluorescent probe were developed for combination therapy and theranostic vectors fabrication. The evaluation of gene transfection efficiency, intracellular tracking, and drug release from the carrier systems were introduced.

# 2 Protocol

## 2.1 Materials

### 2.1.1 Preparation of Dendritic Arginine-Containing Cationic Peptides

1. L-lysine methyl ester dihydrochloride
2. Boc-Arg(Pbf)-OH
3. Boc-Lys(Boc)-OH
4. N,N-diisopropylethylamine (DIEA)
5. N,N-dimethylformamide (DMF)
6. Dichloromethane (DCM)
7. Magnesium sulfate ($MgSO_4$)
8. Sodium bicarbonate ($NaHCO_3$)
9. Dilute hydrochloric acid
10. Saturated brine solution
11. Methanol

12. Sodium hydroxide (NaOH)
13. Trichloromethane
14. Rotary vacuum evaporator
15. Circulating water multipurpose vacuum pump
16. Magnetic stirrer

### 2.1.2 Preparation of Dendritic Arginine and Disulfide Bond-Containing Lipopeptides (RLS)

1. Oleyl acid (OA)
2. L-Lysine methyl ester dihydrochloride
3. 1-Hydroxybenzotriazole (HOBt)
4. 1-(3-Dimethylaminopropyl)-3-ethylcarbodiimide hydrochloride (EDCI)
5. DIEA
6. DCM
7. Ethyl acetate
8. $NaHCO_3$
9. $NaH_2PO_4$
10. $MgSO_4$
11. Methanol
12. NaOH
13. Hydrochloric acid
14. Boc-cystamine
15. Trifluoroacetic acid (TFA)
16. Rotary vacuum evaporator
17. Circulating water multipurpose vacuum pump
18. Magnetic stirrer

### 2.1.3 Synthesis of Low Molecular Drug Camptothecin and Candesartan as Hydrophobic Segment of Lipopeptides

1. Camptothecin (CPT)
2. Succinic anhydride
3. DCM
4. Dilute hydrochloric acid
5. Methanol
6. Boc-cystamine
7. HOBt
8. DMF
9. DIEA
10. TFA
11. Candesartan
12. $NaHCO_3$
13. Saturated brine solution
14. $MgSO_4$
15. Rotary vacuum evaporator

16. Circulating water multipurpose vacuum pump
17. Magnetic stirrer

#### 2.1.4 Synthesis of the Dendritic Arginine-Containing Cationic Peptides-Prodrug Conjugation

1. HOBt
2. DMF
3. DIEA
4. TFA
5. DCM
6. Rotary vacuum evaporator
7. Circulating water multipurpose vacuum pump
8. Magnetic stirrer

#### 2.1.5 Synthesis of Disulfide Bond-Modified Cyanine Dyes with Two Long Carbon Chains

1. 2, 3, 3-Trimethylindolenine
2. 1-Bromohexadecane
3. Toluene
4. Phosphorus oxychloride
5. DCM
6. Anhydrous DMF
7. Cyclohexanone
8. Sodium acetate anhydrous
9. Acetic anhydride
10. Saturated brine
11. Anhydrous $MgSO_4$
12. Dimethyl sulfoxide (DMSO)
13. Phloretic acid sodium salt
14. Hydrochloric acid
15. Boc-cystamine
16. DIEA
17. Diethyl ether

#### 2.1.6 Preparation of Assemblies and Gene Complexes and Characterization of Gene Complexes

1. Methanol
2. HBG solution (20 mM HEPES pH 7.4, 5% glucose)
3. Milli-Q water
4. Magnetic stirrer
5. Dynamic light scattering (DLS) analyzer (Malvern Zetasizer NanoZS)
6. Transmission electron microscope (JM-1011, JEOL)
7. 100-mesh copper grid coated with carbon
8. 1% Agarose gel

9. GelRed Nucleic Acid Gel Stain
10. Tris-acetate running buffer
11. 5 × Loading buffer
12. Molecular Imager ChemiDoc XRS+ (Bio-Rad, USA)

### 2.1.7 Drug Release from Cationic Assemblies

1. Glutathione (GSH)
2. Esterase
3. Amidase
4. Dialysis bag (MWCO 1000, Millipore)
5. Methanol
6. Shaker
7. High-performance liquid chromatography (HPLC)
8. Methanol (HPLC grade)
9. Water containing 1% phosphoric acid

### 2.1.8 Cell Culture and Gene Transfection

1. Hepatoma cell line (HepG2)
2. Human cervical carcinoma cell line (HeLa)
3. Dulbecco's modification of Eagle's medium (DMEM)
4. Fetal bovine serum
5. Streptomycin
6. Penicillin
7. 0.02% EDTA
8. 0.025% Trypsin
9. $CO_2$ incubator
10. Vertical flow clean bench
11. Optical microscope
12. Cell culture flask
13. 96-well tissue culture plates
14. 6-well tissue culture plates
15. pEGFP (enhanced green fluorescent protein plasmid)
16. pGL3 plasmid
17. Fluorescence microscope
18. Luciferase cell culture lysis reagent buffer
19. Luciferase reporter gene assay kit
20. Microplate reader
21. BCA protein assay kit

### 2.1.9 Intracellular Tracking of Gene Complexes

1. Confocal laser scanning microscope
2. 35 mm confocal dish ($\Phi = 15$ mm)
3. Cy3-labeled DNA
4. Hoechst 33342

## 2.2 Methods

### 2.2.1 Preparation of Dendritic Arginine-Containing Cationic Peptides (Fig. 1(I))

1. Dissolve L-lysine methyl ester dihydrochloride (1.5 g, 6.25 mmol), Boc-Arg (Pbf)-OH (7.5 g, 13.75 mmol), and HOBt (2.55 g, 18.75 mmol) in 50 mL of anhydrous DMF.
2. Add DIEA (2.38 g, 18.75 mmol) to the reaction system.
3. Stir at 30 °C under nitrogen atmosphere for 5 h.
4. Concentrate the mixture under reduced pressure to remove the residual DMF.
5. Dissolve the residue in 100 mL of DCM and then wash it with saturated $NaHCO_3$ (aq), diluted hydrochloric acid and saturated brine solution, sequentially.
6. Dry the obtained organic layer with $MgSO_4$.
7. Evaporate the solvents under reduced pressure by a rotary evaporator to obtain the crude product.
8. Purify the resultant residue by chromatography on silica gel (DCM: methanol = 15:1, v/v) to obtain a white powder.
9. Dissolve the obtained white powder (3 g, 2.5 mmol) in methanol (10 mL).
10. Add dropwise the same volume of 1 M NaOH solution.
11. Stir the mixture for 6 h.
12. Evaporate the solvent in the mixture under reduced pressure.
13. Redissolve the resultant residue in $H_2O$ (125 mL).
14. Adjust pH to 2 with 1 M hydrochloric acid.
15. Add 100 mL of trichloromethane and then wash the mixture with saturated brine.
16. Dry the organic phase with $MgSO_4$.
17. Remove the solvent by rotary evaporator to obtain G2(Pbf/Boc).

### 2.2.2 Preparation of Dendritic Arginine and Disulfide Bond-Containing Lipopeptides (RLS)

1. Dissolve OA (7.6 g, 27 mmol), HOBt (3.8 g, 28 mmol), EDCI (5.4 g, 28 mmol), and DIEA (5.3 g, 41 mmol) in anhydrous DCM (60 mL).
2. Stir the mixture under nitrogen atmosphere for 1 h at room temperature.
3. Add L-Lysine methyl ester dihydrochloride (3.1 g, 13 mmol) to the reaction mixture.
4. Stir the mixture for 12 h.
5. Concentrate the mixture under reduced pressure by a rotary evaporator.
6. Dissolve the resultant residue in ethyl acetate (60 mL).
7. Wash the organic solution with saturated $NaHCO_3$ (aq, 120 mL), saturated $NaH_2PO_4$ (aq, 120 mL) and saturated brine solution (60 mL) sequentially.
8. Dry the organic layer with $MgSO_4$.
9. Evaporate the solvent to obtain light yellow solid (8.3 g, yield: 90.2%).
10. Dissolve the obtained yellow solid in methanol.

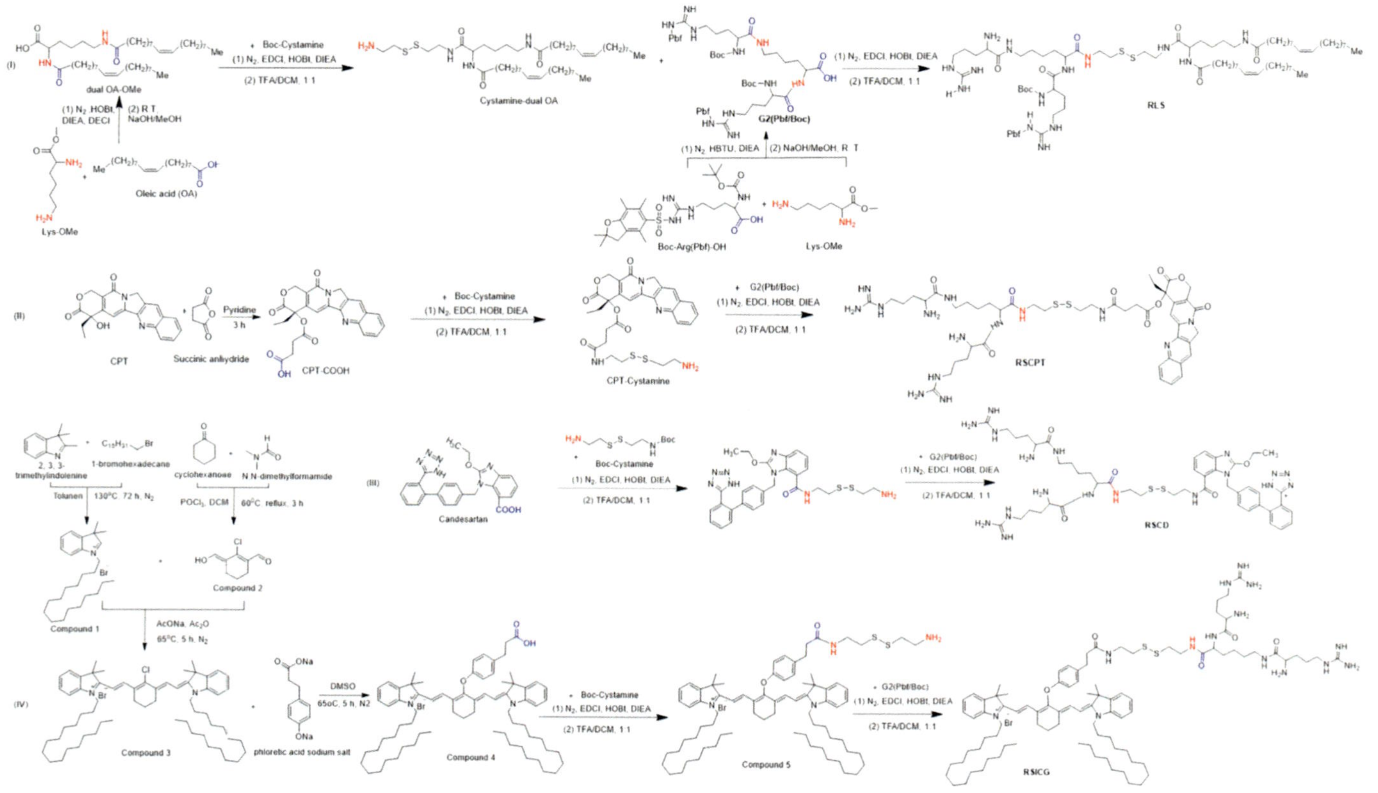

**Fig. 1** The synthesis route of dendritic arginine peptide-based conjugates as gene delivery vectors for combination therapy and theranostic vectors fabrication. (I) Synthesis of dendritic arginine and disulfide bond-containing lipopeptides (RLS). (II) and (III) Synthesis of the dendritic arginine-containing cationic peptides-prodrug conjugation. (IV) Synthesis of the dendritic arginine-containing cationic peptides-near-infrared fluorophore conjugation (RSICG)

11. Add dropwise 5 mL sodium hydroxide solution (0.1 g, 3 mmol) with ice bath.
12. Stir the mixture for 12 h.
13. Evaporate the organic solvent.
14. Dissolve the resultant residue in 50 mL $H_2O$.
15. Wash the mixture by ethyl acetate.
16. Adjust the aqueous phase to pH 2 by hydrochloric acid.
17. Extract by DCM.
18. Remove the organic solvent under reduced pressure to obtain dual OA-OMe (white powder).
19. Dissolve the obtained dual OA-OMe (1.7 g, 2.5 mmol), EDCI (0.6 g, 2.9 mmol), and HOBt (0.4 g, 2.9 mmol) in anhydrous DCM (15 mL).
20. Stir for 1 h under nitrogen atmosphere.
21. Add Boc-cystamine (0.6 g, 2.4 mmol) to the reaction system.
22. Stir the mixture for 12 h under $N_2$.
23. Evaporate the organic solvent.
24. Dissolve the resultant residue in ethyl acetate (35 mL).
25. Wash the organic solution with saturated $NaHCO_3$ (aq, 20 mL $\times$ 2), saturated $NaH_2PO_4$ (aq, 20 mL $\times$ 2), and saturated NaCl (aq, 20 mL), and then dry the product with $MgSO_4$.
26. Evaporate the solvent to obtain a light-yellow solid.
27. Dissolve the obtained light-yellow solid (1.2 g, 2.5 mmol) and TFA (1.5 g, 13 mmol) in anhydrous DCM (25 mL).
28. Stir the reaction mixture for 5 h.
29. Wash the mixture with saturated $NaHCO_3$ (aq, 25 mL), and then dry with $Na_2SO_4$.
30. Evaporate the solvent to obtain Cystamine-dual OA (light-yellow solid).
31. Dissolve G2(Pbf/Boc) and Cystamine-dual OA (0.6 g, 1 mmol), and HOBt (0.6 g, 4 mmol) in anhydrous DMF (25 mL).
32. Add dropwise DIEA (0.7 mL, 4 mmol) to the reaction system.
33. Stir the mixture in ice bath for 30 min and continue to stir at room temperature for 48 h under nitrogen atmosphere.
34. Remove the organic solvent under reduced pressure.
35. Dissolve the residue in ethyl acetate, and then wash it with saturated $NaHCO_3$(aq), diluted hydrochloric acid, and saturated brine sequentially.
36. Dry the obtained organic phase with $MgSO_4$ and concentrate the product under reduced pressure.
37. Recrystallize the residue by ethyl acetate and then dissolve it in DCM.
38. Add dropwise TFA (1.5 g, 13.2 mmol).
39. Stir the reaction mixture for 4 h and then remove the redundant solvents in vacuum.
40. Precipitate the obtained RLS product by diethyl ether.
41. Characterize all structures of compounds by $^1$H-NMR and ESI-MS.

### 2.2.3 Synthesis of Disulfide Bond-Modified Camptothecin and Candesartan Prodrug (Fig. 1(II), (III))

**Synthesis of Disulfide Bond-Modified Camptothecin**

1. Add camptothecin (CPT, 348.4 mg, 1.0 mmol) and succinic anhydride (300.3 mg, 3.0 mmol) to a 100 mL round-bottom flask and suspend the mixture with 30 mL of DCM.
2. Stir the reaction system for 4 h at room temperature and stop the reaction by 20 mL of water addition.
3. Acidize the mixture by 1% HCl solution.
4. Wash the collected yellow precipitate with 1% aqueous HCl solution and water thrice, and then add methanol for recrystallization.
5. Characterize the product (CPT-COOH) by nuclear magnetic resonance (NMR) spectrometry and electrospray ionization mass spectrometry (ESI-MS).
6. Dissolve CPT-COOH (440 mg, 0.1 mmol), Boc-cystamine (500 mg, 0.2 mmol), HOBt (54 mg, 0.4 mmol), and EDCI (83 mg, 0.4 mmol) in anhydrous DMF (50 mL).
7. Add DIEA (62 mg, 0.5 mmol) into the mixture, followed with stirring at room temperature for 48 h.
8. Filter the reaction mixture and concentrate the filtrate by a rotary evaporator.
9. Purify the resultant residue by column chromatography as a yellowish powder.
10. Dissolve the powder in TFA (50 mL) and DCM (20 mL) mixture for 24 h-deprotection with stirring at 0 °C.
11. Concentrate the solution by evaporation in vacuum and obtain CPT-cystamine (white powder) by precipitation in ether.

**Synthesis of Disulfide Bond-Modified Candesartan Prodrug**

1. Dissolve candesartan (440 mg, 1 mmol), the mixture of Boc-cystamine (275 mg, 1.1 mmol), and HOBt (270 mg, 2.0 mmol) in anhydrous DCM (50 mL).
2. Add DIEA (256 mg, 1.98 mmol) to the reaction solution.
3. Stir the reaction solution at room temperature overnight.
4. Concentrate the solvent by a rotary evaporator.
5. Dissolve the resultant residue in DCM and wash it with saturated $NaHCO_3$ (aq), dilute hydrochloric acid and saturated brine solution, sequentially.
6. Dry the collected organic layer with $MgSO_4$ and obtain the crude product after concentration.
7. Purify the crude product by column chromatography.
8. Dissolve the product in TFA (50 mL) and DCM (20 mL) mixture for 24 h-deprotection with stirring at room temperature.
9. Concentrate the organic solution under reduced pressure and obtain white powder after precipitation with ether.

### 2.2.4 Synthesis of the Dendritic Arginine-Containing Cationic Peptides-Prodrug Conjugation

1. Dissolve disulfide bond-modified prodrug (CPT prodrug 0.35 g, 0.6 mmol; candesartan prodrug 0.34 g, 0.6 mmol), G2(Pbf/Boc) (0.3 g, 0.5 mmol), HOBt (0.15 g, 1.1 mmol), and DIEA (0.12 g, 1.1 mmol) in anhydrous DMF (25 mL).
2. Stir the reaction system at room temperature for 48 h under nitrogen atmosphere.
3. Remove the organic solvent in vacuum.
4. Dissolve the resultant residue in DCM and wash it with saturated sodium bicarbonate, diluted hydrochloric acid, and saturated brine solution sequentially.
5. Dry the collected organic solution with $MgSO_4$ and concentrate it by a rotary evaporator.
6. Purify the crude products by column chromatography.
7. Dissolve the obtained crude products in TFA (50 mL) and DCM (20 mL), and stir the solution at room temperature to remove the N-tert-butoxycarbonyl group.
8. Concentrate the solution by evaporation in vacuum and obtain white powder by precipitation with ether.
9. Characterize the structures of compounds by nuclear magnetic resonance (NMR) spectrometry and mass spectrometry (MALDI-TOF MS).

### 2.2.5 Synthesis of Disulfide Bond-Modified Cyanine Dyes with Two Long Carbon Chains (Fig. 1(IV))

1. Dissolve 2,3,3-trimethylindolenine (5 g, 30 mmol) and 1-bromohexadecane (14.3 g, 47 mmol) in toluene (100 mL), followed by stirring at 130 °C for 72 h under nitrogen atmosphere.
2. Concentrate the solvent under reduced pressure to give the crude product.
3. Purify the crude product by silica column chromatography to yield compound **1**.
4. Dissolve phosphorus oxychloride (30.6 g, 200 mmol) and DMF (14.6 g, 200 mmol) in 8 mL DCM and slowly add the solution into anhydrous DMF (20 mL) with stirring in ice water bath.
5. Add cyclohexanone (5 g, 50 mmol) into the solution and reflux the mixture overnight under nitrogen atmosphere.
6. Cool and pour the mixture slowly into 100 mL ice-cold water.
7. Keep the solution in −20 °C to yield precipitation (compound **2**, yellow solid).
8. Dissolve a mixture of compound **1** (3 g, 6.4 mmol), compound **2** (0.44 g, 2.6 mmol), and sodium acetate anhydrous (0.79 g, 7.7 mmol) in 20 mL acetic anhydride.
9. Stir the reaction overnight at 65 °C under nitrogen atmosphere in dark.
10. Dissolve the mixture in 300 mL DCM and wash the mixture by saturated brine (3 × 50 mL).
11. Dry the organic phase with anhydrous magnesium sulfate and concentrate the organic solution in vacuum to give crude product.
12. Purify the crude product by silica column chromatography to yield compound **3** as green solid.

13. Dissolve compound **3** (1.4 g, 1.42 mmol) in 20 mL DMSO, followed with addition of the phloretic acid sodium salt (1.5 g, 7.14 mmol).
14. Heat the reaction to 65 °C for 5 h in dark.
15. Cool down the reaction to room temperature and add 100 mL DCM.
16. Wash the mixture by saturated brine and concentrate the organic phase in vacuum.
17. Redissolve the precipitate in methanol and adjust the pH to 2 with 1 M hydrochloric acid.
18. Add 100 mL DCM and wash the mixed solution twice by saturated brine.
19. Combine organic phase, dry it with anhydrous magnesium sulfate, and concentrate it by rotary evaporation.
20. Purify the obtained crude product by silica column chromatography to obtain compound **4** as green solid.
21. Dissolve Boc-cystamine (0.14 g, 0.54 mmol) and compound **4** (0.4 g, 0.36 mmol) in 10 mL anhydrous DMF.
22. Add HOBt (0.1 g, 0.72 mmol) and DIEA (0.09 g, 0.72 mmol) into the above solution.
23. Stir the mixture at 30 °C for 48 h under nitrogen atmosphere in dark.
24. Remove DMF in vacuum and add 100 mL DCM for redissolution.
25. Wash the mixture by saturated sodium bicarbonate, sodium dihydrogen phosphate, and brine, respectively.
26. Dry the combined organic phase with anhydrous magnesium sulfate and concentrate it by evaporation in vacuum.
27. Purify the crude product by silica column chromatography.
28. Dissolve the obtained product in 10 mL DCM together with the same volume of TFA.
29. Stir the mixture solution in ice water bath. And then stir the mixture at 30 °C for 5 h in dark.
30. Remove the redundant solvent in vacuum.
31. Precipitate the product by diethyl ether and obtain the sediment by centrifugation.
32. Remove the residual diethyl ether to obtain compound **5** as green solid.
33. The synthesis of the dendritic arginine-containing cationic peptides-near-infrared fluorophore conjugation (RSICG) is similar with the part 3.4.

### 2.2.6 Preparation of Assemblies and Gene Complexes and Characterization

1. Dissolve appropriate amphiphilic molecules in about 10 μL of methanol.
2. Drop the solution into 1 mL of fast stirring HBG solution (20 mM HEPES pH 7.4, 5% glucose) for gene transfection or Milli-Q water for the physical and chemical characterization.
3. Rapidly stir the solution for 0.5 h to form spontaneously cationic assemblies in the aqueous medium.

4. Mix DNA (100 ng/μL) and cationic lipid assembly (1 μg/μL) solution gently at different N/P ratios (in the range of 20–60) in HBG buffer and incubate at room temperature for 30 min before use.
5. Determine the particle size and zeta potential by dynamic light scattering, performing at 25 °C using a Malvern Zetasizer NanoZS with a 633 nm He/Ne Laser at a fixed scattering angle of 173°.
6. Prepare gene complexes solutions with 3 μg pDNA at varying N/P ratios and diluted to a final volume of 1 mL in Milli-Q water before measurement.
7. Observe the morphology of cationic assemblies by transmission electron microscopy (TEM, JM-1011, JEOL).
8. Drop 10 μL of cationic assemblies on a 100-mesh copper grid coated with carbon.
9. Dry the samples at room temperature and then put them into a desiccator for morphology observation by transmission electron microscopy.
10. Evaluate the gene compaction ability in complexes at various N/P ratios by gel retardation assay.
11. Load all samples containing 200 ng of gene onto 1% agarose gel for electrophoresis (85 V, 1 h) in tris-acetate running buffer.
12. Visualize the gel stained with GelRed and capture DNA bands by the Molecular Imager ChemiDoc XRS+ (Bio-Rad, USA).

#### 2.2.7 Release of Drug from Cationic Assemblies (Fig. 2)

1. Perform the in vitro release of CPT in these assemblies by dialysis against the release medium with 5 mM GSH, or 1 μM esterase, or a mix of the two in a time-course procedure.
2. Immerse a volume of 1 mL assemblies suspensions in dialysis bag (MWCO 1000, Millipore) in 50 mL of release medium.
3. Oscillate the suspensions with a shaker at 37 °C in a water bath at 100 rpm.
4. At predetermined time points, take out of aliquots (1 mL) and immediately replace it with equal volume of the medium after each sampling.
5. Mix the sample with 1 mL methanol to extract the released CPT.
6. Detect the CPT concentration in solution using HPLC equipped with a UV detector and a C18 column at 25 °C (Shimadzu, Japan).
7. The mobile phase is methanol and water (volume ratio 60: 40, Sigma, HPLC grade) at a flow rate of 1.0 mL/min and a UV detector at 254 nm wavelength.
8. Calculate the release percentage of CPT using the formula: Release percentage (%) = W1/W0 × 100%, where W1 is the weight of CPT in solution, W0 is the weight of total CPT in assemblies.
9. The in vitro release of candesartan is performed in PBS with 5 mM GSH and 10 μM amidase in a time-course procedure.
10. Measure the candesartan concentration in the solution by HPLC equipped with a UV detector at 256 nm wavelength. The mobile phase is methanol and water containing 1% phosphoric acid (volume ratio 66:34) at a flow rate of 1 mL/min.

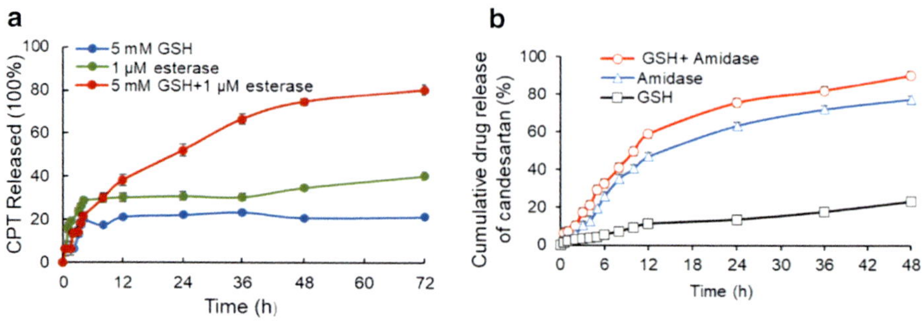


**Fig.2** (**a**) Quantitative release profiles of CPT from RSCPT with GSH and esterase at indicated concentrations. Reproduced from Ref. Jiang et al. 2019 with permission from the Royal Society of Chemistry. (**b**) Quantitative release profiles of candesartan from RSCD with GSH and amidase at indicated concentrations

### 2.2.8 Cell Culture and Gene Transfection (Fig. 3a)

#### Cell Culture

1. Culture HepG2 cells and HeLa cells in DMEM medium containing 10% (v/v) heat-inactivated fetal bovine serum, 100 μg/mL streptomycin, and 100 IU/mL penicillin.
2. Split the cells with 48 h after reaching full monolayer confluency in order to keep the cell in a healthy condition.
3. Maintain cells in an incubator with a humidified environment of 5% $CO_2$ and a constant temperature of 37 °C.

#### Gene Transfection

1. Seed cells at the density of $1 \times 10^4$ per well and culture to reach 70% cell confluence for reporter gene transfection.
2. Replace the medium in 96-well plates with 100 μl of fresh medium per well with or without 10% serum before transfection.
3. Add various gene complexes with 200 ng of pEGFP or pGL3 plasmid per well.
4. Incubate the transfected cells for 4 h at 37 °C in the incubator.
5. Replace the medium with fresh culture medium containing 10% serum.
6. Incubate the cells for an additional 44 h.
7. Visualize GFP-expressing cells using a fluorescence microscope (Leica, Germany).
8. Quantitatively measure pGL3 plasmid transfection efficiency using luciferase assay according to manufacturer's protocols.
9. Wash cells with cold PBS and lyse cells with luciferase cell culture lysis reagent buffer.
10. Measure relative light units (RLU) by the luciferase reporter gene assay kit on a microplate reader (Bio-Rad, model 550, USA).
11. Determine protein content of the lysed cell by BCA protein assay.

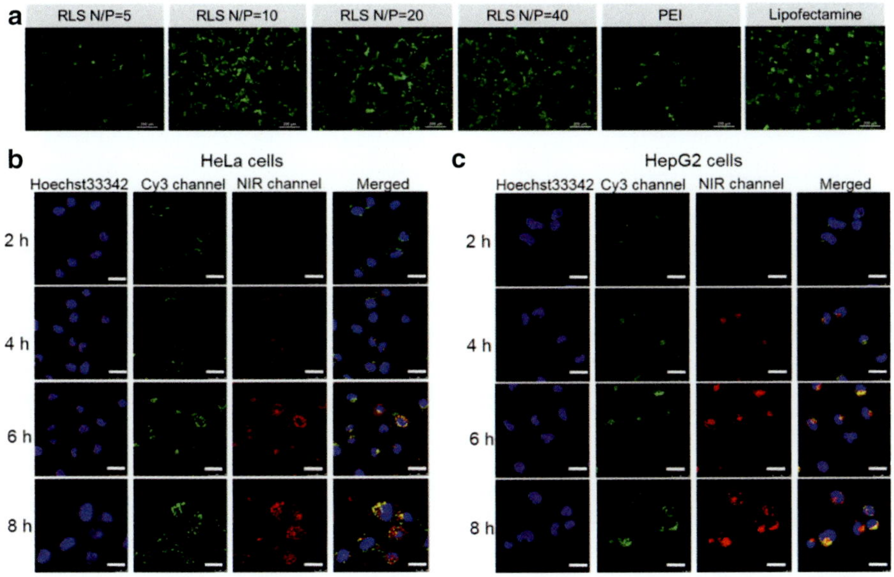


**Fig. 3** (**a**) Transfection efficiency of RLS complexes on HeLa cells. DNA of pEGFP was condensed by RLS assembly at varied N/P ratio. HeLa cells were incubated with RLS/DNA complexes for 4 h and captured by fluorescent microscope after 24 h continuous culture. PEI and lipofectamine served as control group. Reproduced from Ref. Chen et al. 2021 with permission from the Royal Society of Chemistry. (**b**) and (**c**). In vitro imaging for the disintegration of assemblies which investigated by confocal laser scanning microscope (CLSM). Cy3-labelled plasmid DNA were condensed by RSICG assemblies at N/P = 30 and then HeLa cells (**b**) and HepG2 cells (**c**) were incubated with the complexes for different time (2 ~ 8 h). The signal of Cy3 and NIR were marked as green and red, respectively. Green: fluorescent signal of Cy3. Red: fluorescent signal of NIR. Blue: fluorescent signal of Hoechst 33342 stained for nucleus

12. Calculate luciferase activity as the relative fluorescence intensity per mg protein (RLU/mg protein).

### 2.2.9 Intracellular Tracking of Gene Complexes (Fig. 3b, c)

1. Observe the intracellular distribution of gene complexes by confocal laser scanning microscope (CLSM).
2. Seed HeLa cells at a density of $1 \times 10^4$ cells per well in 35 mm confocal dish ($\Phi = 15$ mm) and culture overnight for attachment.
3. Remove the culture medium.
4. Add fresh complete culture medium containing RNS/DNA complexes with N/P = 30 (300 ng of Cy3-labeled pGL3).
5. Co-incubate the cells with complexes for different time (2, 4, 6, and 8 h) at 37 °C.
6. Wash the cells by cold PBS (pH = 7.4) twice to remove the assemblies which did not be taken.
7. Stain the nucleus by Hoechst 33342 for 15 min prior to observation.

8. Observe the modified NIR dyes containing gene complexes by excitation and emission wavelengths at 663 nm and 700 nm, respectively.
9. Observe the intracellular localization of DNA by laser excitation and emission wavelengths at 545 nm and 560 nm, respectively.
10. Observe the nucleus by Hoechst 33342 staining with the excitation and emission wavelengths of 350 nm and 461 nm, respectively.

## 3 Discussion

When following the above procedure, there are still some notes needing attention.

## 4 Notes

1. Nitrogen should be filled before covering or a balloon full of nitrogen is recommended to cover on top of the flask.
2. The assembly solution should be fresh and diluted enough before characterization using DLS and TEM.
3. Prepare calibration curves with known amounts of CPT or candesartan in the range of 1–1000 ng/ml. The retention time is ~3.9 min for CPT, and ~ 3.8 min for candesartan by HPLC method, respectively. The correlation coefficients of regression equations were all above 0.99. The limit of quantification was 0.5 ng/ml for tissue samples.
4. Warm up the culture medium and trypsin to 37 °C before using.
5. The cells must be mixed well when plated cells into the wells. It is essential to have cells uniformly suspended to ensure the consistent cell number be added into the wells.
6. Lipofectamine 2000 or polyethyleneimine (PEI) is chosen as positive control for gene transfection.
7. Store all samples after the addition of luciferase cell culture lysis reagent buffer at −80 °C overnight prior to analysis.

## 5 Conclusion

This protocol presents the synthesis and evaluation of a series of bioinspired cationic assemblies, which included an arginine-rich hydrophilic segment and a hydrophobic segment with oleic acid chains, hydrophobic low molecular drugs, or florescent probes. Hydrophilic part with arginine-rich corona could provide efficient cellular internalization, due to the bioactivity mimicking of viral cell-penetrating peptides. Meanwhile, rational integration of hydrophobic drugs as part of carrier could not only ensure high loading efficiency but also promote synergistic therapeutic effect. The ingenious fusion of the Y-shape florescent probe as the linker and hydrophobic part could simultaneously improve the accuracy and sensitivity of molecular imaging in vivo. All of the results demonstrate that the lipopeptides with arginine-rich periphery as gene carriers provide a promising platform for process, mechanism, and multi-therapy exploration.

## References


Barrán-Berdón AL, Misra SK, Datta S, Muñoz-beda M, Kondaiah P, Junquera E, Bhattacharya S, Aicart E (2014) Cationic gemini lipids containing polyoxyethylene spacers as improved transfecting agents of plasmid DNA in cancer cells. J Mater Chem B 2:4640–4652

Chen X, Yang J, Liang H, Jiang Q, Ke B, Nie Y (2017) Disulfide modified self-assembly of lipopeptides with arginine-rich periphery achieve excellent gene transfection efficiency at relatively low nitrogen to phosphorus ratios. J Mater Chem B 5:1482–1497

Chen X, Jin R, Jiang Q, Bi Q, He T, Song X, Barz M, Ai H, Shuai X, Nie Y (2021) Delivery of siHIF-1α to reconstruct tumor normoxic microenvironment for effective chemotherapeutic and photodynamic anticancer treatments. Small 17(25):e2100609

Jiang Q, Yue D, Nie Y, Xu X, He Y, Zhang S, Wagner E, Gu Z (2016) Specially-made lipid-based assemblies for improving transmembrane gene delivery: comparison of basic amino acid residue rich periphery. Mol Pharm 13:1809–1821

Jiang Q, Chen X, Liang H, Nie Y, Jin R, Barz M, Yue D, Gu Z (2019) Multistage rocket: integrational design of a prodrug-based siRNA delivery system with sequential release for enhanced antitumor efficacy. Nanoscale Advances 1:498–507

Khan M, Ong ZY, Wiradharma N, Attia ABE, Yang YY (2012) Advanced materials for co-delivery of drugs and genes in cancer therapy. Adv Healthc Mater 1:373–392

Liang H, Hu A, Chen X, Jin R, Wang K, Ke B, Nie Y (2019) Structure optimization of dendritic lipopeptide based gene vectors with the assistance from molecular dynamic simulation. J Mater Chem B 7:915–926

Liang H, Bi Q, Hu A, Chen X, Jin R, Song X, Ke B, Barz M, Nie Y (2020a) Nitroreductase and glutathione responsive nanoplatform for integration of gene delivery and near-infrared fluorescence imaging. Chem Commun 56:6949

Liang H, Chen X, Jin R, Ke B, Barz M, Ai H, Nie Y (2020b) Integration of indocyanine green analogs as near-infrared fluorescent carrier for precise imaging-guided gene delivery. Small 16: 1906538

Liu X, Wu M, Hu Q, Bai H, Zhang S, Shen Y, Tang G, Ping Y (2016) Redox-activated light-up nanomicelle for precise imaging-guided cancer therapy and real-time pharmacokinetic monitoring. ACS Nano 10:11385–11396

Sheng Z, Hu D, Zheng M, Zhao P, Liu H, Gao D, Gong P, Gao G, Zhang P, Ma Y, Cai L (2014) Smart human serum albumin-indocyanine green nanoparticles generated by programmed assembly for dual-modal imaging-guided cancer synergistic phototherapy. ACS Nano 8:12310–12322

Swami R, Singh I, Khan W, Ramakrishna S (2013) Diseases originate and terminate by genes: unraveling nonviral gene delivery. Drug Deliv Transl Res 3:593–610

Thomas CE, Ehrhardt A, Kay MA (2003) Progress and problems with the use of viral vectors for gene therapy. Nat Rev Genet 4:346–358

Walrant A, Bechara C, Alves ID, Sagan S (2012) Molecular partners for interaction and cell internalization of cell-penetrating peptides: how identical are they? Nanomedicine 7:133–143

Wang T, Upponi JR, Torchilin VP (2012) Design of multifunctional non-viral gene vectors to overcome physiological barriers: dilemmas and strategies. Int J Pharm 427:3–20

Xu X, Jiang Q, Zhang X, Nie Y, Zhang Z, Li Y, Cheng G, Gu Z (2015) Virus-inspired mimics: self-assembly of dendritic lipopeptides into arginine-rich nanovectors for improving gene delivery. J Mater Chem B 3:7006–7010

Yoo J-W, Irvine DJ, Discher DE, Mitragotri S (2011) Bio-inspired, bioengineered and biomimetic drug delivery carriers. Nat Rev Drug Discov 10:521–535

# Preparation and Evaluation of Multistage Delivery Nanoparticle for Efficient CRISPR Activation In Vivo

8

Q. Liu and Yang Liu

## Contents



Q. Liu · Y. Liu (✉)
Key Laboratory of Functional Polymer Materials of Ministry of Education, State Key Laboratory of Medicinal Chemical Biology, College of Chemistry, National Demonstration Center for Experimental Chemistry Education, Nankai University, Tianjin, China
e-mail: yliu@nankai.edu.cn



H. Tian and X. Chen (eds.), *Gene Delivery*, Biomaterial Engineering,
https://doi.org/10.1007/978-981-16-5419-0_5

**Abstract**

The clustered regularly interspaced short palindromic repeat (CRISPR)/nuclease-deactivated protein 9 (dCas9) system can modulate cancer-associated gene expression at the transcriptional level without causing damage to genomic DNA, providing a safer and natural tool to treat cancers. However, due to the conflicting surface requirements for different delivery stages, the development of drug delivery system for CRISPR/dCas9-based cancer gene therapy remains a great challenge. This protocol describes a multistage delivery nanoparticle (MDNP) that can present specific surface in response to its surrounding environment for efficient delivery of CRISPR/dCas9 system after systemic administration. This MDNP is fabricated by coating an acidity-responsive polymer shell on the surface of cationic polyplex core made of CRISPR/dCas9 plasmid (pDNA) and phenylboronic acid modified polyethyleneimine (PEI-PBA) via electrostatic interaction. The results demonstrated that PEGylated polymer shell significantly reduces nonspecific interaction at physiological condition. Furthermore, MDNP is capable of detaching polymer shell at tumor acidic microenvironment, facilitating the cellular internalization and tumor accumulation of CRISPR/dCas9 system. By loading a CRISPR/dCas9 pDNA that targeting miR-524, MDNP can effectively upregulate the expression of miR-524 in tumors and thus remarkably suppressed the tumor growth in vivo, providing a feasibility delivery platform to overcome multiple physiological barriers for effective CRISPR/dCas9-based cancer gene therapy.

**Keywords**

Multistage delivery · CRISPR/dCas9 system · Cancer gene therapy · Responsive polymer · Tumor microenvironment · miR-524

## 1 Overview

The clustered regularly interspaced short palindromic repeat (CRISPR)-associated protein 9 (Cas9) system, which derived from the RNA-based adaptable immune system of bacteria and archaea, has been a powerful and versatile genome-editing tool (Jinek et al. 2012; Ran et al. 2013). By inactivating the catalytic sites of Cas9 and fusing it with an effector domain (repressor or activator domain), CRISPR/nuclease-deactivated protein (dCas9) system can dominate the targeted gene regulation directed by a small guide RNA (sgRNA) without causing damage to genomic DNA (Bikard et al. 2013; Gilbert et al. 2014). Since cancers were characterized by dysregulation of oncogenes and cancer suppressor genes, CRISPR/dCas9 system can modulate cancer-associated gene expression at transcription level, providing a safer and natural tool to treat cancers (Hanahan and Weinberg 2011). To date, viral vectors such as lentivirus (LV), adenovirus (AV), and adeno-associated virus (AAV) have been successfully employed for delivery of CRISPR/dCas9 systems, especially in cell line-based studies (Joung et al. 2017). However, due to insertional mutagenesis, carcinogenesis, and immunogenicity, the clinical translation potential of viral vectors remains limited (Nault et al. 2015).

Benefit from low immunogenicity and high loading capability, nonviral vectors offered promising potentials for CRISPR/dCas9-based cancer gene therapies (Yin et al. 2014). Nowadays, several cationic materials such as cationic liposome (Wang et al. 2016), cationic polymers (Li et al. 2017), and cationic peptides (Ramakrishna et al. 2014) have been developed to deliver CRISPR plasmid DNA (pDNA) with high gene editing efficiency. However, these cationic materials usually fail to achieve satisfactory in vivo delivery of CRISPR systems (Kim et al. 2010). An important reason is strong nonspecific interaction between cationic complexes and anionic serum components, resulting in rapid clearance and undesirable side effects after systemic administration (Fischer et al. 2003; Jin et al. 2013). It is now realized that the successful delivery of CRISPR system would undergo following several stages. Stage 1: circulating in blood stream, Stage 2: accumulating in tumor tissues, Stage 3: internalizing by tumor cells, and Stage 4: escaping from endosomes/lysosomes and then entering nucleus (Eetezadi et al. 2015). Thus, it is necessary to develop a novel drug delivery system (DDS) to optimize its performance on these stages simultaneously, and eventually to enhance CRISPR/dCas9-based cancer gene therapy efficiency. However, in these stages, the requirements for the surface properties of DDS are often different, which poses a great challenge to the design of DDS.

As one of the most commonly used shielding strategy, PEGylated surface endows DDS with reduced nonspecific interaction in blood stream, thereby prolonging the blood circulation and enhancing tumor accumulation of DDS through enhanced permeation and retention (EPR) effects (Davis et al. 2008; Hatakeyama et al. 2011). However, PEGylation surface also hampers cellular internalization of DDS, which could decrease overall efficiency of DDS-based cancer therapy (Romberg et al. 2008). Thus, it is necessary to develop a novel delivery strategy to present specific surface in different delivery stages. Herein, the protocol describes a multistage delivery nanoparticle (MDNP) for efficient CRISPR/dCas9-based cancer gene therapy (Fig. 1). To transport the CRISPR/dCas9 system into cancer cells, CRISPR/dCas9 pDNA was first condensed with phenylboronic acid (PBA) modified low molecular weight polyethyleneimine (PEI-PBA) to form cationic polyplex via electrostatic interaction. For prolonging blood circulation and enhancing tumor accumulation, cationic polyplex was further encapsulated with an acidity-responsive polymer, 2,3-dimethylmaleic anhydride (DMMA)-modified poly(ethylene glycol)-*b*-polylysine (mPEG$_{113}$-*b*-PLys$_{100}$/DMMA) (Liu et al. 2019). After encapsulated with the polymer, MDNP can maintain a negatively charged and PEGylated surface during blood circulation after systemic administration. As reaching tumor

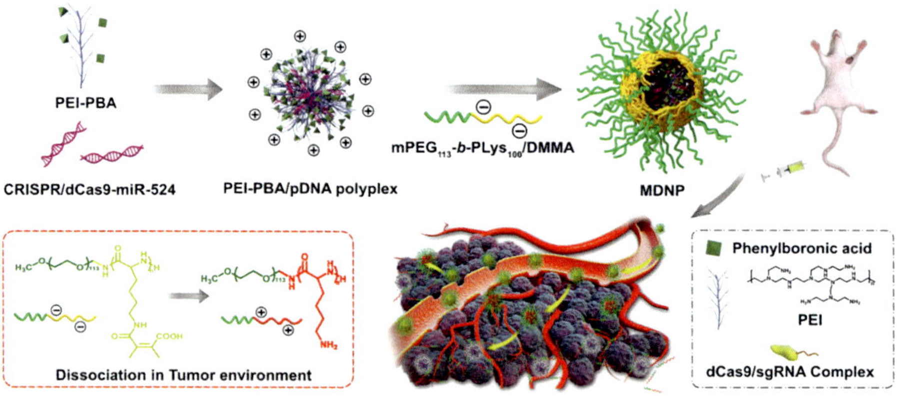


**Fig. 1** Scheme of the preparation of MDNP and the delivery process after injection. (Adapted from Liu et al. 2019, with permission)

tissues, the acidic microenvironment (pH 6.5) triggers the break of amide bond in DMMA, resulting in the rapid charge conversion of mPEG$_{113}$-*b*-PLys$_{100}$/DMMA to expose the cationic polyplex, which is then internalized by cancer cells eventually (Mintzer and Simanek 2009). Furthermore, the PBA groups on PEI can interact with sialic acid, which usually overexpressed on the surface of cancer cells (Deshayes et al. 2013; Zheng et al. 2019). Such cationic and PBA-rich surface would greatly enhance the cellular internalization efficiency. To evaluate the cancer treatment efficiency of MDNP, a pDNA encoding dCas9 activator and a single guide RNA (sgRNA) that targets the primary transcription content of miR-524 were employed for in vitro and in vivo antitumor experiments (Liu et al. 2019). For the better demonstration, a structurally similar but nonresponsive polymer, mPEG$_{113}$-*b*-PLys$_{100}$/SA, was employed to prepare a single-stage delivery nanoparticle (SDNP) for following studies.

## 2 Materials

### 2.1 Synthesis of PEI-PBA, mPEG$_{113}$-*b*-PLys$_{100}$, mPEG$_{113}$-*b*-PLys$_{100}$/DMMA, and mPEG$_{113}$-*b*-PLys$_{100}$/SA

1. Polyethylenimine (MW: 1800 Da, PEI$_{1.8K}$)
2. 2-bromomethylphenylboronic acid (PBA)
3. Methanol (analytical grade)
4. Ether (analytical grade)
5. N6-Carbobenzoxy-L-lysine N-carboxyanhydride (Lys(Z)-NCA)
6. Methoxypolyethylene glycol amine (MeO-PEG$_{113}$-NH$_2$) (Jinpan Biotech, Shanghai, China)

7. N, N-Dimethylformamide (analytical grade)
8. Trichloromethane (analytical grade)
9. Hydrobromic acid (analytical grade)
10. Trifluoroacetate (analytical grade)
11. 2, 3-dimethylmaleic anhydride (DMMA)
12. Sodium bicarbonate buffer (pH 8.5, 50 mM)
13. Phosphate buffered saline (PBS, pH 7.4, 10 mM)
14. Succinic anhydride (SA)
15. 100 mL pear-shaped flask
16. Vacuum drying oven
17. Rotary vacuum evaporator
18. Dialysis bag (molecular weight cut off: 3500 Da)
19. Lyophilizer
20. Constant temperature magnetic stirrer
21. Nuclear magnetic resonance spectrometer

## 2.2 Investigation on pH-Responsiveness of mPEG$_{113}$-*b*-PLys$_{100}$/DMMA

1. Deuterated phosphate buffer (pH 7.4, 10 mM)
2. Deuterium chloride (DCl)
3. Sodium deuteride oxide (NaOD)
4. Nuclear magnetic resonance spectrometer

## 2.3 Preparation of SDNP and MDNP

1. Pei-PBA
2. mPEG$_{113}$-*b*-PLys$_{100}$/DMMA
3. mPEG$_{113}$-*b*-PLys$_{100}$/SA
4. pDNA (Viewsolid Biotech, Beijing, China)
5. PBS (pH 7.4, 10 mM)

## 2.4 Characterization of MDNP and SDNP

1. Filter paper
2. 450 nm syringe filter
3. Distilled water
4. Carbon-coated copper grid (Zhongjingkeyi Technology, Beijing, China)
5. 1% uranyl acetate solution
6. Vacuum drying oven

7. Transmission electron microscopy (TEM)
8. Dynamic light scatterometer (DLS)

## 2.5 Fluorescence Resonance Energy Transfer (FRET) Assay

1. Cy3-NHS (Oukainasi Technology, Beijing, China)
2. Cy5-NHS (Oukainasi Technology, Beijing, China)
3. PBS (pH 7.4, 10 mM)
4. PBS (pH 6.5, 10 mM)
5. Dialysis bag (molecular weight cut off: 3500 Da)
6. Fluorescence spectrophotometer

## 2.6 Nonspecific Protein Adsorption Assay

1. Bovine serum albumin (BSA)
2. PBS (pH 7.4, 10 mM)
3. Ultrafiltration centrifuge tube (molecular weight cut off: 300 kDa)
4. BCA protein assay kit (Solarbio, Beijing, China)
5. NanoDrop

## 2.7 Cell Culture

1. Dulbecco's modification of Eagle's medium (DMEM) (Thermo Fisher, USA)
2. Heat-inactivated fetal bovine serum (FBS) (Thermo Fisher, USA)
3. Penicillin/streptomycin (Thermo Fisher, USA)
4. Trypsin (Thermo Fisher, USA)
5. Culture dish (55 $cm^2$)
6. Humidified incubator

## 2.8 Cellular Internalization and Endosome Escape

1. MDA-MB-231 cells
2. Confocal dish ($\Phi = 15$ mm)
3. YOYO-1 (Invitrogen, USA)
4. TOTO-3 (Invitrogen, USA)
5. 4% paraformaldehyde
6. LysoTracker Green (Beyotime Biotech, Shanghai, China)
7. 4, 6-diamino-2-phenyl indole (DAPI, Solarbio, Beijing, China)
8. Rhodamine phalloidin (Yeasen Biotech, Shanghai, China)
9. Confocal laser scanning microscope (CLSM)

10. Humidified incubator
11. Flow cytometry

## 2.9 Transfection Efficiency of MDNP in Cancer Cells

1. LN-229 cells
2. Polyethylenimine (MW: 25 kDa, $PEI_{25K}$)
3. 24-well plates
4. The pDNA encoding tdTomato fluorescent protein (Viewsolid Biotech, Beijing, China)
5. Humidified incubator
6. Fluorescence microscope
7. Flow cytometry

## 2.10 CRISPR Activation of miR-524 Expression with MDNP in Cancer Cells

1. MDA-MB-231 and LN-229 cells.
2. The pDNA expresses dCas9 activator (dCas9VP64) and a sgRNA (5'-GCAGTGA GCCAAGATCGGCGC-3′) that targets the Pri-miR-524 (dCas9-miR-524) (Viewsolid Biotech, Beijing, China).
3. The pDNA expresses dCas9 activator (dCas9VP64) and a nonfunctional sgRNA (dCa9-NC) (Viewsolid Biotech, Beijing, China).
4. 6-well plates.
5. TRIzol (Thermo Fisher, USA).
6. DEPC water.
7. Isopropanol (analytical grade).
8. Chloroform (analytical grade).
9. 75% ethanol.
10. PrimeScript RT reagent kit (TaKaRa, Tokyo, Japan).
11. Primer for Pri-miR-524 (Forward: 5'-GCTGTGACCCTACAAAGGGA-3′ and Reverse: 5'-AGCATCAACTTCAACGCTGC-3′) (GenePharma, Shanghai, China).
12. SYBR PremixExTaq (TaKaRa, Tokyo, Japan).
13. Humidified incubator.
14. Real-time PCR detection system.

## 2.11 In Vitro Antitumor Study

1. MDA-MB-231 and LN-229 cells
2. Cell counting kit-8 (CCK-8, Dojindo, Japan)
3. 96-well plates

4. Humidified incubator
5. Microplate reader

## 2.12 Tumor-Targeting Capability of MDNP in Mice

1. Female nude mice
2. MDA-MB-231 cells
3. TOTO-3 (Invitrogen, USA)
4. IVIS Lumina imaging system
5. 4% paraformaldehyde
6. Sucrose (Analytical grade)
7. DAPI (Solarbio, Beijing, China)
8. Optimal cutting temperature compound (OCT, Sakura, CA, USA)
9. Freezing microtome
10. Confocal laser scanning microscope

## 2.13 In Vivo Tumor Growth Inhibition

1. Female nude mice
2. MDA-MB-231 cells
3. Vernier caliper

## 2.14 Safety Evaluation

1. Kunming mice
2. Coagulant tube
3. Centrifuge
4. ELISA kits for mouse IL-6, IFN-γ, TNF-α, NF-kB, IgE, IgM, and IgG (Jianglai Biotech, Shanghai, China)
5. Microplate reader

# 3 Methods

## 3.1 Synthesis of PEI-PBA

1. Dissolve $PEI_{1.8K}$ (1.80 g, 1 mmol) and PBA (1.07 g, 5 mmol) with methanol in a 100 mL pear-shaped flask (**Note 1**).
2. Stir under reflux at 70 °C for 12 h.
3. Precipitate the reaction mixture in ether.
4. Dry the solid product under vacuum with vacuum drying oven.
5. The synthesis route of PEI-PBA is shown in Fig. 2, and the amount of PBA conjugated on each $PEI_{1.8K}$ in average is calculated by $^{1}H$ NMR (Fig. 3).

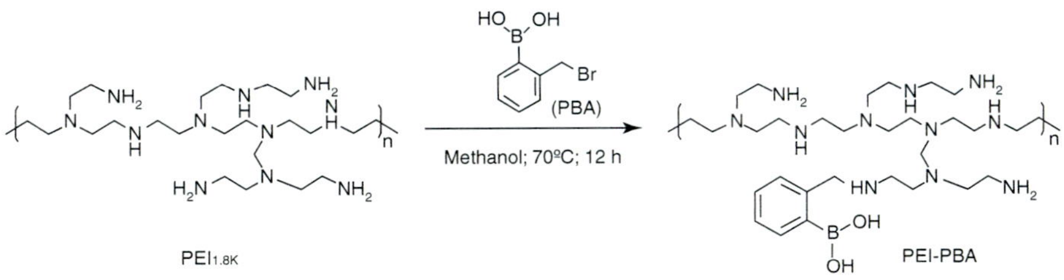


**Fig. 2** Synthesis route of PEI-PBA

**Fig. 3** $^1$H NMR spectra of PEI-PBA. (Adapted from Liu et al. 2019, with permission)

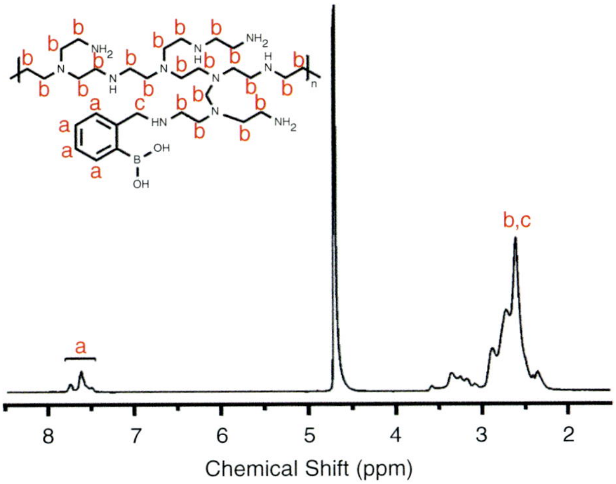


## 3.2 Synthesis of mPEG$_{113}$-*b*-PLys$_{100}$/DMMA and mPEG$_{113}$-*b*-PLys$_{100}$/SA

### 3.2.1 mPEG$_{113}$-*b*-PLys$_{100}$

1. Dissolve Lys(Z)-NCA (5.35 g, 17.4 mmol) in 30 mL DMF in a 100 mL pear-shaped flask (**Note 2**).
2. Add MeO-PEG$_{113}$-NH$_2$ (0.61 g, 0.123 mmol) into the Lys(Z)-NCA solution.
3. Stir at 35 °C for 72 h.
4. Evaporate the solvent with a rotary evaporator.
5. Dissolve the product in 10 mL $CHCl_3$.
6. Precipitate the reaction mixture in cold ether.
7. Dissolve the solid product in 10 mL $CF_3COOH$ and HBr (2:1, v/v).
8. Stir at 0 °C for 2 h.
9. Dissolve in 20 mL DMF and filter with 0.22 μm Millipore filter.
10. Precipitate the reaction mixture in cold ether again.
11. Dry the solid product under vacuum with vacuum drying oven.
12. Confirm the successful polymerization and calculate the degree of polymerization using $^1$H NMR.

13. The synthesis route of $mPEG_{113}$-*b*-$PLys_{100}$ was shown in Fig. 4, the degree of polymerization (DP) of lysine was estimated by comparing the integration of the peaks of the $-OCH_2CH_2-$ protons of PEG at 3.3–3.4 ppm and the $-NHCHCO-$ protons of lysine at 4.2–4.4 ppm (Fig. 5).

### 3.2.2 mPEG$_{113}$-*b*-PLys$_{100}$/DMMA and mPEG$_{113}$-*b*-PLys$_{100}$/SA

1. Dissolve 100 mg $mPEG_{113}$-*b*-$PLys_{100}$ (5.6 μmol) in 30 mL sodium bicarbonate buffer (pH 8.5, 50 mM) in a 100 mL pear-shaped flask.
2. Add 211.2 mg (1.67 mmol) DMMA and stir at 25 °C for 4 h (**Note 3**).
3. Maintain the pH of reaction solution in the range of 8.0–8.5 with 0.2 M NaOH (**Note 4**).
4. Remove unreacted DMMA by dialyzing the reaction solution against sodium bicarbonate buffer (pH 8.5, 5 mM) (**Note 5**).

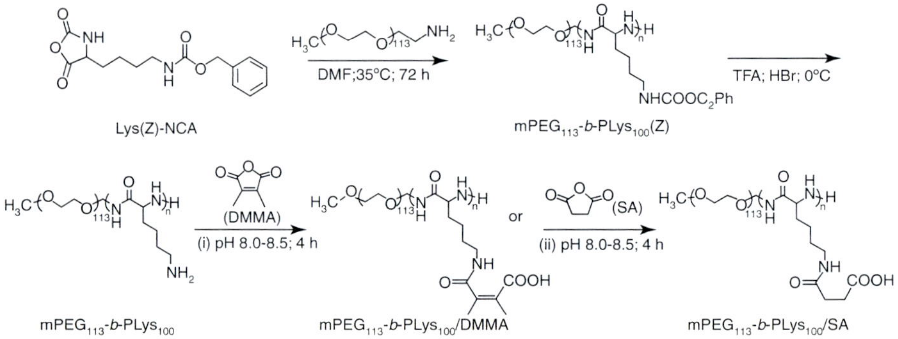


**Fig. 4** Synthesis routes of $mPEG_{113}$-*b*-$PLys_{100}$, $mPEG_{113}$-*b*-$PLys_{100}$/DMMA, and $mPEG_{113}$-*b*-$PLys_{100}$/SA

**Fig. 5** $^1$H NMR spectra of $mPEG_{113}$-*b*-$PLys_{100}$. (Adapted from Liu et al. 2019, with permission)

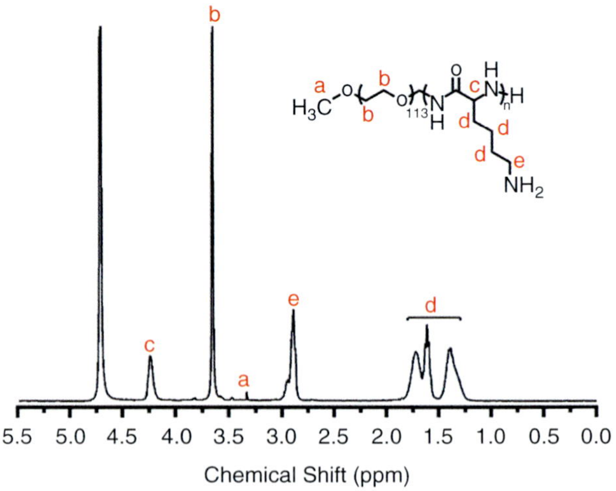

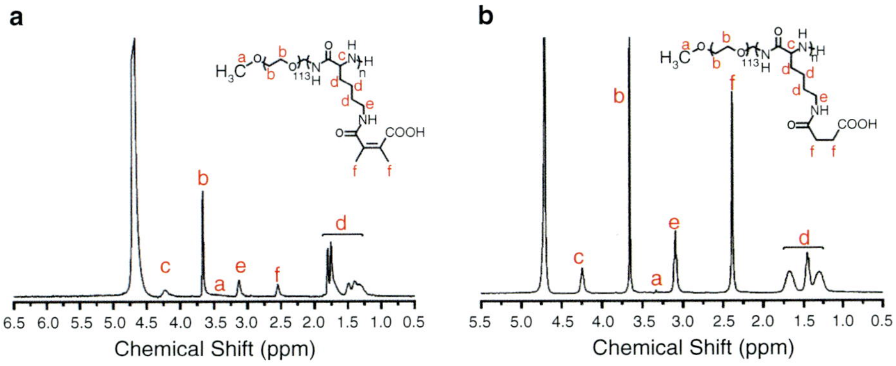


**Fig. 6** $^1$H NMR spectra of mPEG$_{113}$-*b*-PLys$_{100}$/DMMA and mPEG$_{113}$-*b*-PLys$_{100}$/SA. (Adapted from Liu et al. 2019, with permission)

5. Lyophilize the dialysate by a lyophilizer to obtain dry powder (mPEG$_{113}$-*b*-PLys$_{100}$/DMMA).
6. Synthesize mPEG$_{113}$-*b*-PLys$_{100}$/SA by replacing DMMA with SA (167.6 mg, 1.67 mmol) using the similar method.
7. The synthesis routes of mPEG$_{113}$-*b*-PLys$_{100}$/DMMA and mPEG$_{113}$-*b*-PLys$_{100}$/SA were shown in Fig. 4, and the successful conjugation of DMMA and SA was confirmed by $^1$H NMR (Fig. 6).

## 3.3 pH-Responsiveness of mPEG$_{113}$-*b*-PLys$_{100}$/DMMA

1. Adjust the pH of deuterated phosphate buffer (10 mM) from 7.4 to 6.5 using DCl and NaOD.
2. Dissolve 1 mg mPEG$_{113}$-*b*-PLys$_{100}$/DMMA in 1 mL deuterated phosphate buffer (pH 6.5, 10 mM).
3. Record the $^1$H NMR spectra at 0 min, 30 min, 60 min, 90 min, and 120 min at 25 °C (Fig. 7). Ha and Hb are assigned to the methylene protons adjacent to the amino group and amide bond, respectively.

## 3.4 Preparation and Characterization of MDNP and SDNP

### 3.4.1 Preparation of SDNP and MDNP

1. Dissolve pDNA, PEI-PBA, mPEG$_{113}$-*b*-PLys$_{100}$/DMMA, and mPEG$_{113}$-*b*-PLys$_{100}$/SA in PBS (pH 7.4, 10 mM) (**Note 6**).
2. Mix PEI-PBA (0.1 mL, 1.5 mg/mL) and pDNA (0.1 mL, 250 μg/mL) (**Note 7**).
3. Incubate the solution at 37 °C in water bath for 15 min to obtain PEI-PBA/pDNA polyplex.

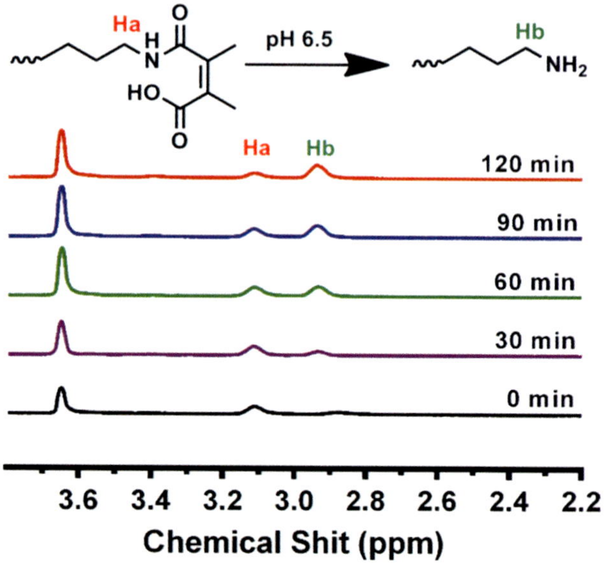


**Fig. 7** [1]H NMR characterization of mPEG$_{113}$-*b*-PLys$_{100}$/DMMA after incubating at pH 6.5 for different time. (Adapted from Liu et al. 2019, with permission)

4. Add mPEG$_{113}$-*b*-PLys$_{100}$/DMMA (0.1 mL, 3 mg/mL) into 0.1 mL PEI-PBA/pDNA polyplex and incubate at 37 °C for 15 min to obtain MDNP.
5. Add mPEG$_{113}$-*b*-PLys$_{100}$/SA (0.1 mL, 3 mg/mL) into 0.1 mL PEI-PBA/pDNA polyplex and incubate at 37 °C for 15 min to obtain SDNP.

### 3.4.2 Determination of Particle Size and Zeta Potential

1. Prepare PEI-PBA/pDNA, SDNP, and MDNP as described in section "Preparation of SDNP and MDNP," and then dilute in distilled water, pDNA is 10 μg/mL.
2. Filter the solution into sample bottles with 450 nm syringe filter.
3. Measure the particle sizes and zeta potentials of different formulations using DLS measurements (**Fig. 8**).
4. Drop 2 μL sample solution onto carbon-coated copper grids and incubate for 10 min at room temperature (**Note 8**).
5. Remove excess sample solution from the edges with filter paper.
6. Drop 5 μL 1% sodium uranyl acetate onto these grids for 90 s, remove with filter paper, and dry under vacuum with vacuum drying oven for 3 days.
7. Observe the morphology of SDNP and MDNP by TEM (**Fig. 8a** and **Fig. 8b**).

### 3.4.3 Zeta Potential Variation of MDNP and SDNP with pH Adjustment

1. Dilute the MDNP and SDNP in PBS (pH 8.0, 5 mM), pDNA is 10 μg/mL.
2. Adjust the pH of solution from pH 8.0 to 7.4, and then to 6.5.
3. Record the zeta potential of MDNP and SDNP during pH adjustment by DLS (Fig. 9).

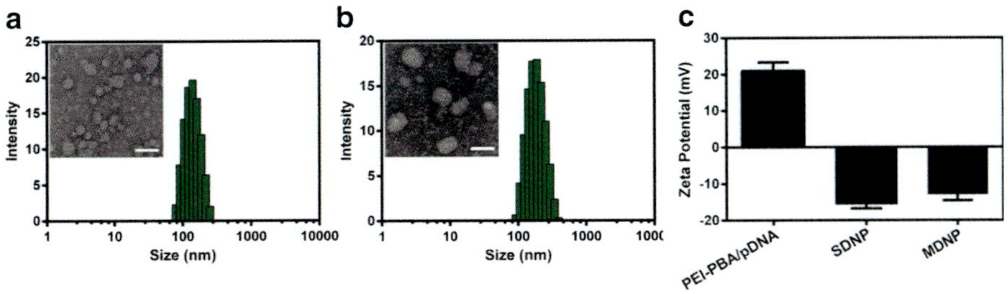


**Fig. 8** (**a**, **b**) TEM and DLS characterization of the PEI-PBA/pDNA polyplex (**a**) and MDNP (**b**) (scale bar: 100 nm). (**c**) Zeta potentials of PEI-PBA/pDNA polyplex, SDNP, and MDNP. Data in (**c**) is represented as mean ± s.d. (n = 3). (Adapted from Liu et al. 2019, with permission)

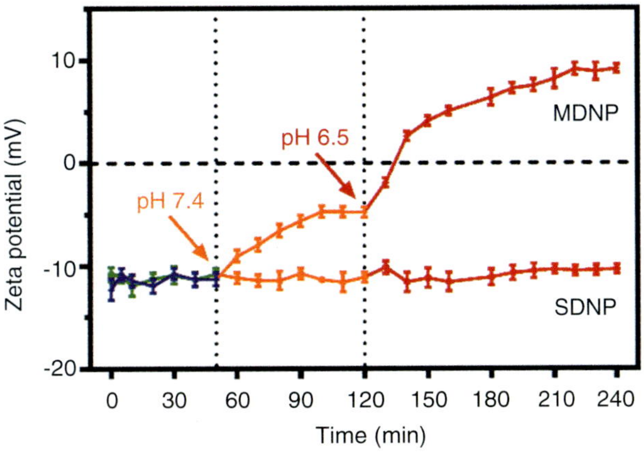


**Fig. 9** Zeta potential changes of MDNP and SDNP with pH adjustment from 8.0 to 6.5. Data is represented as mean ± s.d. (n = 3). (Adapted from Liu et al. 2019, with permission)

### 3.4.4 FRET Assay on SDNP and MDNP at Different pHs

1. Dissolve PEI-PBA, mPEG$_{113}$-*b*-PLys$_{100}$/DMMA, and mPEG$_{113}$-*b*-PLys$_{100}$/SA in PBS (pH 7.4, 10 mM).
2. Add Cy3-NHS and Cy5-NHS at molar ratio of 3:1 between fluorescent probe and polymer. PEI-PBA was labelled with Cy3 (Cy3-PEI-PBA), mPEG$_{113}$-*b*-PLys$_{100}$/DMMA, and mPEG$_{113}$-*b*-PLys$_{100}$/SA was labelled with Cy5 (Cy5-mPEG$_{113}$-*b*-PLys$_{100}$/DMMA, Cy5-mPEG$_{113}$-*b*-PLys$_{100}$/SA).
3. Stir at 4 °C in water bath for 2 h.
4. Remove the unconjugated fluorescent probe by dialysis against the PBS (pH 7.4, 10 mM) (**Note 9**).
5. Prepare the PEI-PBA/pDNA polyplex, SDNP, and MDNP using fluorescently labelled polymer as described in Sect. 3.4.1.
6. Dilute the PEI-PBA/pDNA polyplex, SDNP, and MDNP in PBS (pH 7.4, 10 mM) and detect the fluorescent emission spectra at the excitation wavelength of 515 nm, pDNA is 5 μg/mL.

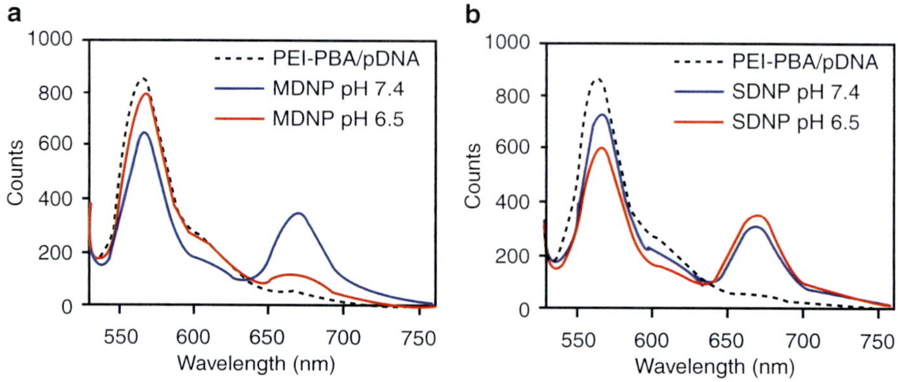


**Fig. 10** Fluorescence spectra of MDNP (a) and SDNP (b) at pH 7.4 and pH 6.5. (Adapted from Liu et al. 2019, with permission)

7. Adjust the pH from pH 7.4 to pH 6.5 and incubate at 37 °C for 2 h (**Note 10**).
8. Readjust the pH to 7.4 and detect the fluorescent emission spectra at the excitation wavelength of 515 nm (Fig. 10) (**Note 11**).

## 3.5 Quantification of Nonspecific Protein Adsorption

1. Dissolve BSA in PBS (pH 7.4, 10 mM).
2. Mix BSA (100 μL, 2 mg/mL) with PBS (100 μL, pH 7.4, 10 mM), PEI-PBA/pDNA polyplex (20 μg pDNA, 100 μL), and MDNP (20 μg pDNA, 100 μL).
3. Incubate at 37 °C in water bath for 2 h.
4. Remove free BSA by centrifugal filtration (5000 rpm, 5 min) for five times with ultrafiltration centrifuge tube (MWCO: 300 kDa), and PBS is used as the eluent (**Note 12**).
5. Determine the BSA content in effluent solution using BCA protein assay kit according to the manufacturer's instruction.
6. Measure the absorbance at 450 nm using NanoDrop.
7. Calculate the BSA adsorption according to the following formula: Adsorption (%) = (total content of BSA-BSA content in effluent solution)/total content of BSA × 100% (Fig. 11).

## 3.6 Cellular Internalization and Endosomal Escape

### 3.6.1 Cell Culture

1. Maintain LN-229 and MDA-MB-231 cells in DMEM supplemented with 10% (v/v) FBS, 100 units·$mL^{-1}$ penicillin, and 100 μg·$mL^{-1}$ streptomycin.
2. Culture all cells in 37 °C humidified incubator with 5% $CO_2$ atmosphere.

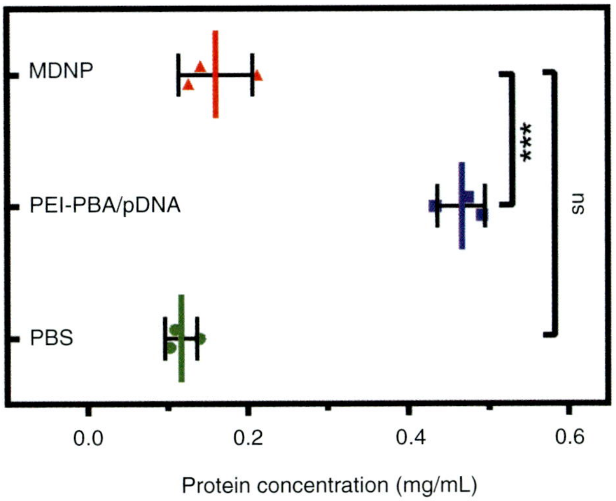


**Fig. 11** Quantitative measurements of BSA adsorption of PEI-PBA/pDNA polyplex and MDNP after incubated with BSA solution (1 mg/mL) for 1 h. Data is represented as mean ± s.d. (n = 3). The significance level is shown as ***$p < 0.001$. (Adapted from Liu et al. 2019, with permission)

3. Split the cells according to following steps after the cell confluence reaches 80%. Remove the culture medium, rinse the cells with 10 mL PBS (pH 7.4, 10 mM), add 1 mL trypsin to digest cells, add 1 mL culture medium to stop digestion, collect the cells by centrifugation (800 rpm, 5 min), and then divide the cells into culture dishes (**Note 13**).

### 3.6.2 Cellular Internalization

1. Seed MDA-MB-231 cells in a 35 mm confocal dish ($\Phi = 15$ mm) at density of $1 \times 10^4$ cells per well in 1 mL complete culture medium and incubate overnight for cell attachment.
2. Label pDNA with YOYO-1 according to manufacturer's instruction, and then prepare SDNP and MDNP using YOYO-1 labelled pDNA as described in Sect. 3.4.1.
3. Adjust pH of culture medium to pH 7.4 or pH 6.5 using HCl and NaOH (**Note 14**).
4. Replace the culture medium with 950 μL fresh medium (pH 7.4 or pH 6.5).
5. Add 50 μL MDNP and SDNP containing 1 μg pDNA per well and incubate for 2 h (**Note 15**).
6. Rinse the cells with 1 mL PBS (pH 7.4, 10 mM) for three times and fix the cells with 4% paraformaldehyde for 30 min at room temperature.
7. Stain the cell nucleus and F-actin using DAPI and rhodamine phalloidin following the manufacturer's instructions.
8. Observe the cells using CLSM (Fig. 12a).
9. Seed MDA-MB-231 cells in 6-well plates at density of $2 \times 10^5$ cells per well in 2 mL complete culture medium and incubate overnight for cell attachment.
10. Replace the culture medium with 1.9 mL fresh medium (pH 7.4 or pH 6.5).

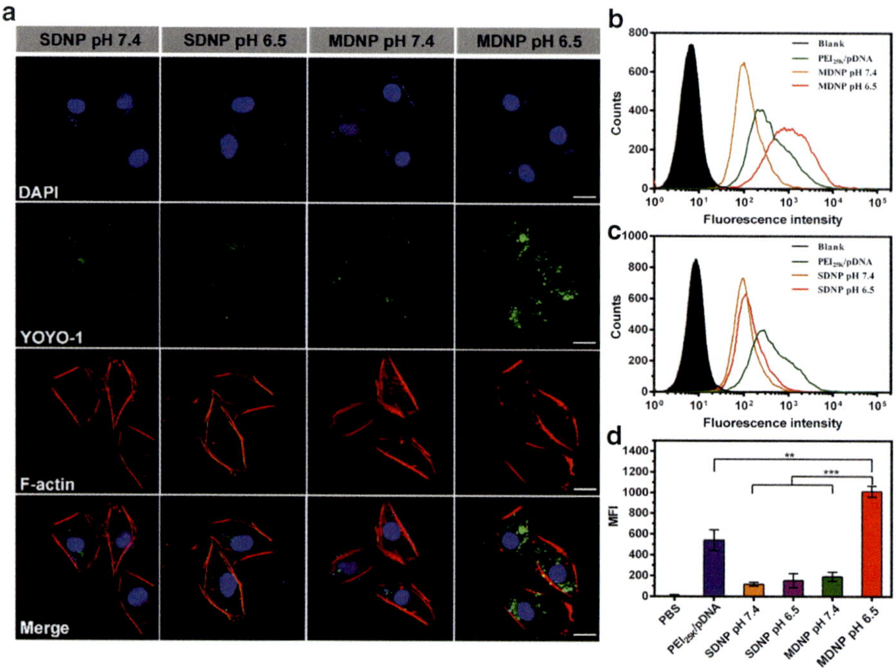


**Fig. 12** (**a**) CLSM images of MDA-MB-231 cells treated with SDNP and MDNP carrying YOYO-1 labeled pDNA (green) at different pHs. The scale bars are 20 μm. (**b**, **c**) Flow cytometry analyses of MDA-MB-231 cells treated with MDNP (**b**) and SDNP (**c**) carrying YOYO-1 labeled pDNA (green) at different pHs. (**d**) Quantification of cell internalization showing by mean fluorescence intensity (MFI). Data in (**d**) is represented as mean ± s.d. (n = 3). The significance levels are shown as $^{**}p < 0.01$ and $^{***}p < 0.001$. (Adapted from Liu et al. 2019, with permission)

11. Add 100 μL SDNP and MDNP containing 3 μg pDNA per well and incubate for 2 h at 37 °C in humidified incubator.
12. Rinse the cells with 2 mL PBS (pH 7.4, 10 mM) for three times, add 0.4 mL trypsin to detach cells, and collect the cells by centrifugation (800 rpm, 5 min).
13. Fix the cells with 4% paraformaldehyde for 30 min at room temperature and analyze with flow cytometry (Fig. 12b–d).

### 3.6.3 Endosomal Escape

1. Seed MDA-MB-231 cells in a 35 mm confocal dish (Φ = 15 mm) at density of $1 \times 10^4$ cells per well in 1 mL complete culture medium and incubate overnight for cell attachment.
2. Label pDNA with TOTO-3 according to manufacturer's instruction, and then prepare MDNP using TOTO-3 labelled pDNA as described in Sect. 3.4.1.
3. Replace the culture medium with 950 μL fresh medium (pH 6.5).
4. Add 50 μL MDNP containing 1 μg pDNA per well and incubate for 1, 2, and 4 h, respectively.

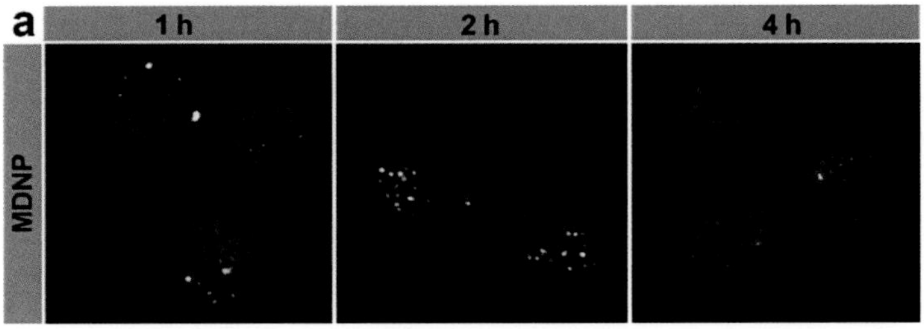


**Fig. 13** (**a**) Endosomal escape of MDNP containing TOTO-3 (red) labeled pDNA. Endosomes and lysosomes were stained with LysoTracker Green, and the nuclei were stained with DAPI (blue). (Adapted from Liu et al. 2019, with permission)

5. Add LysoTracker Green fluorescent probe to stain endosome/lysosomes according to manufacturer's instruction.
6. Rinse the cells with 1 mL PBS (pH 7.4, 10 mM) for three times, and then fix the cells with 4% paraformaldehyde for 30 min at room temperature.
7. Counterstain the nucleus using DAPI and observe using CLSM (Fig. 13) (**Note 16**).

## 3.7 In Vitro Gene Transfection

1. Seed LN-229 cells in 24-well plates at density of $5 \times 10^4$ cells per well in 0.5 mL complete culture medium and incubate overnight for cell attachment.
2. Replace the culture medium with 450 μL fresh medium (pH 7.4 or pH 6.5, containing 0% or 10% serum based on the purpose).
3. Add 50 μL MDNP and SDNP containing 1 μg pDNA encoding tdTomato and incubate for 4 h.
4. Replace the culture medium with 450 μL fresh medium for further 48 h incubation. $PEI_{25K}$/pDNA polyplex containing 1 μg pDNA encoding tdTomato is employed as positive control to perform the same studies.
5. Observe the tdTomato fluorescent protein expression (orange fluorescence) using fluorescence microscope (Fig. 14a) (**Note 17**).
6. Rinse the cells with 0.5 mL PBS (pH 7.4, 10 mM) for three times, add 0.2 mL trypsin to digest cells, and collect the cells by centrifugation (800 rpm, 5 min).
7. Fix the cells with 4% paraformaldehyde for 30 min at room temperature and quantify the transfection efficiency by flow cytometry (Fig. 14b).

## 3.8 In Vitro Cytotoxicity Analysis

### 3.8.1 In Vitro Cytotoxicity of Polymer

1. Seed MDA-MB-231 and LN-229 cells in 96-well plates at density of $5 \times 10^3$ cells per well in 0.1 mL complete culture medium and incubate overnight for cell attachment.

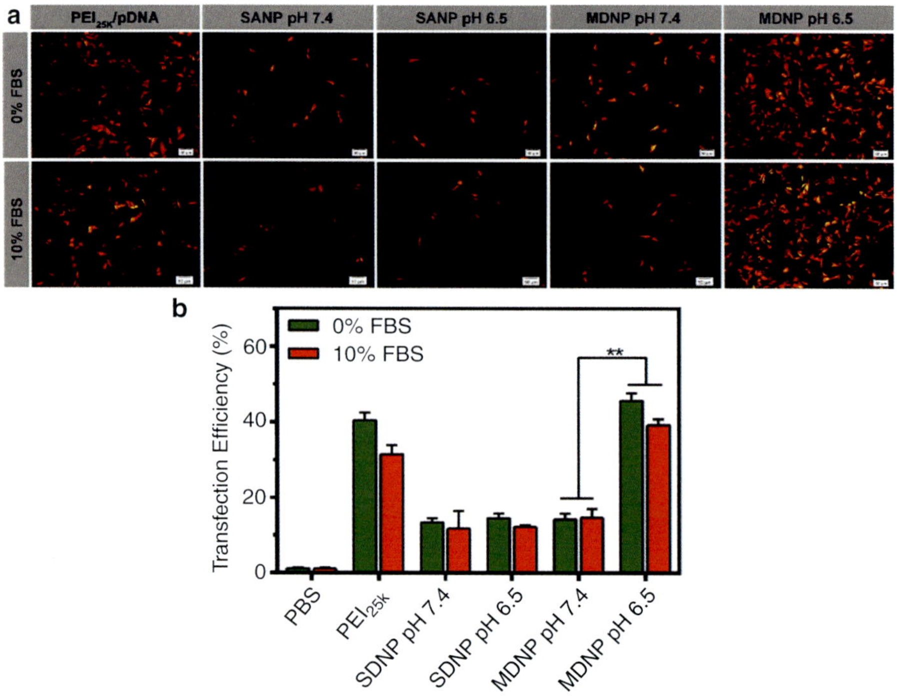


**Fig. 14** (**a**) Fluorescence microscope images of LN-229 cells treated with MDNP carrying pDNA encoding tdTomato fluorescent protein in culture medium with 0% or 10% serum, respectively. The scale bars are 50 μm. (**b**) Quantitative analysis results in (**a**) by flow cytometry. Data in (**b**) is represented as mean ± s.d. (n = 3). The significant level is shown as $^{**}p < 0.01$. (Adapted from Liu et al. 2019, with permission)

2. Replace the culture medium with 0.1 mL fresh medium containing different polymer at varied concentrations (6.25, 12.5, 25, 50, 100, and 200 μg/mL) for further 24 h incubation.
3. Mix CCK-8 reagent and fresh culture medium at a volume ratio of 1:9 to prepare CCK-8 working solution.
4. Rinse the cells with 0.1 mL PBS (pH 7.4, 10 mM), and then add 100 μL CCK-8 working solution for another 2 h incubation.
5. Measure the absorbance at 450 nm and 630 nm using microplate reader. Calculate the cell viability according to the following formula: Cell viability (%) = ($A_{450\ nm}$ of treated cells-$A_{630\ nm}$ of treated cells) / ($A_{450\ nm}$ of control cells- $A_{630\ nm}$ of control cells) × 100% (Fig. 15).

### 3.8.2 Activation of miR-524 Expression in Vitro

1. Prepare MDNP and SDNP with dCas9-miR-524 as described in Sect. 3.4.1 (denoted as MDNP/dCas9-miR-524 and SDNP/dCas9-miR-524, respectively).

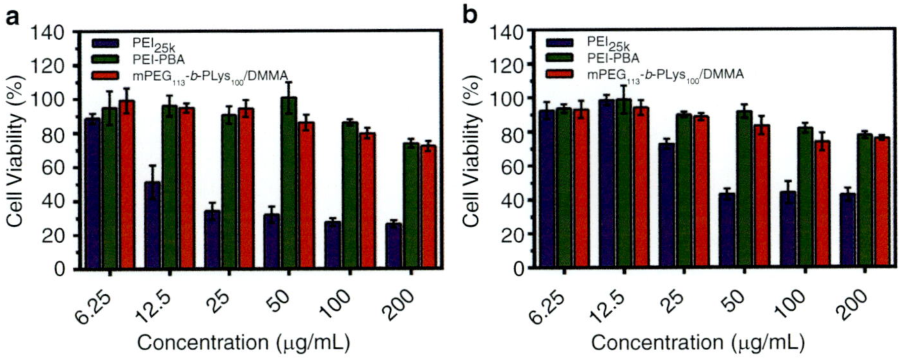


**Fig. 15** The cytotoxicity of $PEI_{25K}$, PEI-PBA, $mPEG_{113}$-*b*-$PLys_{100}$/DMMA to LN-229 (**a**) and MDA-MB-231 cancer cells (**b**) at various concentrations. Data are represented as mean ± s.d. (n = 3). (Adapted from Liu et al. 2019, with permission)

2. Seed MDA-MB-231 and LN-229 cells in 6-well plates at density of $2 \times 10^5$ cells per well in 2 mL complete culture medium and incubate overnight for cell attachment.
3. Replace the culture medium with 1.9 mL fresh medium (pH 7.4 or pH 6.5).
4. Add 100 μL MDNP/dCas9-miR-524 and SDNP/dCas9-miR-524 containing 3 μg pDNA and incubate for 4 h. MDNP carrying dCas9/NC (MDNP/dCas9-NC) was employed as control group to perform the same studies.
5. Replace the culture medium with fresh one for further 48 h incubation.
6. Rinse the cells with PBS (pH 7.4, 10 mM).
7. Add 100 μL TRIzol reagent and incubate for 10 min at room temperature.
8. Transfer to a 1.5 mL centrifuge tube, add 0.2 mL chloroform, shake for 15 s, and stand for 2 min.
9. Centrifuge at 12000 rpm for 15 min, take the supernatant.
10. Add 0.5 mL isopropanol, mix the liquid gently, and stand at room temperature for 10 min.
11. Centrifuge at 12000 rpm for 15 min, discard the supernatant.
12. Add 1 mL 75% ethanol to wash the precipitate, centrifuge at 7500 rpm for 5 min, discard the supernatant.
13. Dry in the air, dissolve in DEPC water, and then store at −20 °C for following experiments.
14. The miRNA is converted to cDNA using the PrimeScript RT reagent kit according to the manufacturer's protocol.
15. The cDNAs are quantified by real-time quantitative PCR instrument. Expression of U6 is employed as endogenous control. Fold changes for the expression levels of Pri-miR-524 are calculated using the comparative cycle threshold (CT) method ($2^{-\Delta\Delta CT}$) (Fig. 16).

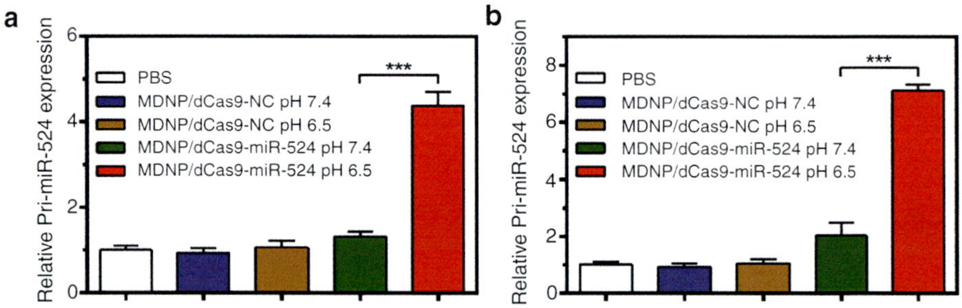


**Fig. 16** Relative expression levels of Pri-miR-524 in MDA-MB-231 (**a**) and LN-229 (**b**) cells treated with MDNP/dCas9-NC and MDNP/dCas9-miR-524 at different pHs. Data in (**a**) and (**b**) are represented as mean ± s.d. (n = 3). The significance level is shown as ***$p < 0.001$. (Adapted from Liu et al. 2019, with permission)

### 3.8.3 In Vitro Antitumor Effect of MDNP

1. Seed MDA-MB-231 and LN-229 cells in 96-well plates at density of $5 \times 10^3$ cells per well in 0.1 mL complete culture medium and incubate overnight for cell attachment.
2. Replace the culture medium with 90 μL fresh medium (pH 7.4 or pH 6.5).
3. Add 10 μL MDNP/dCas9-miR-524, and SDNP/dCas9-miR-524 containing 200 ng pDNA per well and incubate for 4 h at 37 °C. MDNP/dCas9-NC is employed as the control group.
4. Refresh the culture medium and further incubate for 24 h, 48 h, and 72 h.
5. Mix CCK-8 reagent and fresh culture medium at a volume ratio of 1:9 to prepare CCK-8 working solution.
6. Rinse the cells with PBS, and then add 100 μL CCK-8 working solution for another 2 h incubation.
7. Measure the absorbance at 450 nm and 630 nm using a microplate reader. Calculate the cell viability according to the formula in Sect. 3.4.1 (Fig. 17).

## 3.9 In Vivo Distribution of MDNP

1. Establish tumor-bearing mice by subcutaneously injecting MDA-MB-231 cells ($5 \times 10^6$ cells per mouse) in the mammary fat pad.
2. Divide tumor-bearing mice into three groups randomly (three mice per group), when tumor volume is around 400 $mm^3$. Calculate the tumor volume using the following formula: Volume ($mm^3$) = 0.5 × length × $width^2$.
3. Label pDNA with TOTO-3, and then prepare $PEI_{25K}$/pDNA polyplex, SDNP, and MDNP using TOTO-3 labelled pDNA as described in Sect. 3.4.1.
4. Inject 100 μL $PEI_{25K}$/pDNA polyplex, SDNP, and MDNP containing 10 μg TOTO-3 labeled pDNA via tail vein, respectively.

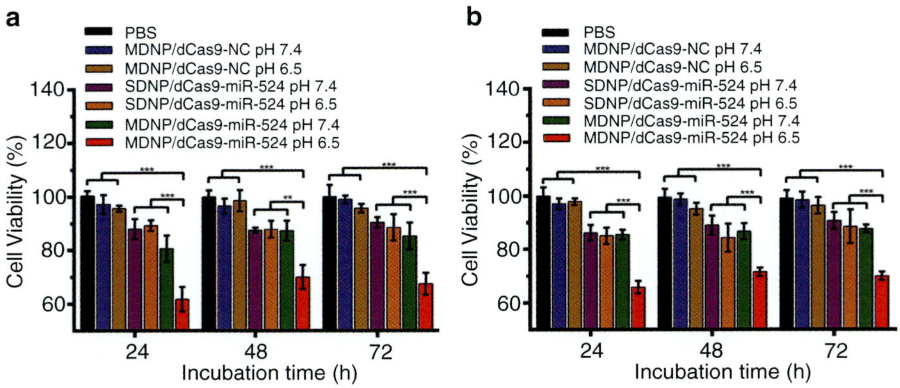


**Fig. 17** Cell viability of MDA-MB-231 (**a**) and LN-229 (**b**) cells treated with MDNP/dCas9-NC, SDNP/dCas9-miR-524, and MDNP/dCas9-miR-524 at different pHs for 24 h, 48 h, and 72 h incubation. Data in (**a**) and (**b**) are represented mean ± s.d. (n = 3). The significance levels are shown as $^{**}p < 0.01$ and $^{***}p < 0.001$. (Adapted from Liu et al. 2019, with permission)

5. Sacrifice mice and collect tumors and major organs at 1 h, 6 h, and 24 h postinjection.
6. Ex vivo imaging tumors and major organs using IVIS, and then analyze these images with Living Image 3.1 (**Note 18**).
7. Fix the tumors by 4% paraformaldehyde at 4 °C for 12 h, and then dehydrate with different concentrations of sucrose solution (10%, 20%, and 30%, w/w), 6 h each concentration.
8. Embed the tumors in OCT and freeze at −80 °C for 2 h.
9. Prepare the 8 μm slices and counterstain with DAPI for CLSM observation (Fig. 18) (**Note 19**).

## 3.10 Tumor Growth Inhibition

1. Establish tumor-bearing mice by subcutaneously injecting MDA-MB-231 cells ($5 \times 10^6$ cells per mouse) in the mammary fat pad.
2. Divided tumor-bearing mice into three groups randomly (five mice per group), when tumor volume was around 25 $mm^3$. Calculate the tumor volume as described in Sect. 3.9.
3. Inject 100 μL $PEI_{25K}$/pDNA polyplex, SDNP/dCas9-miR-524 and MDNP/dCas9-miR-524 containing 10 μg pDNA per mouse via tail vein every 3 days for 20 days, respectively. MDNP/dCas9-NC is employed as comparative group.
4. Monitor the tumor volumes using Vernier caliper during the treatment (Fig. 19).

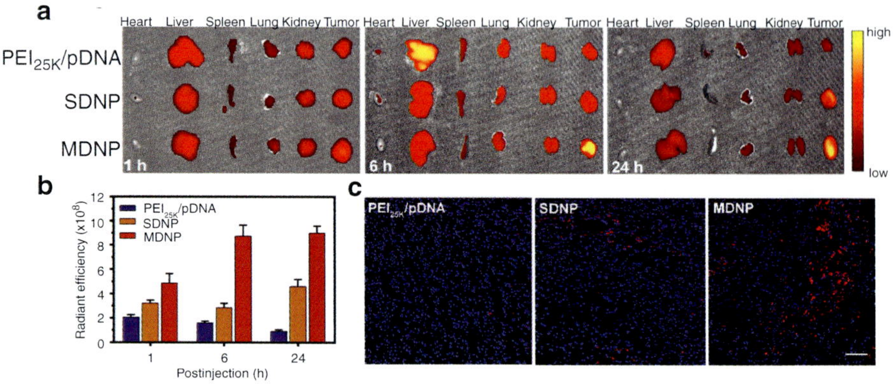


**Fig. 18** (**a**) Ex vivo fluorescence images of isolated tissues from the MDA-MB-231 tumor-bearing mice after intravenous injection of $PEI_{25K}$/pDNA, SDNP and MDNP carrying TOTO-3 labeled pDNA (red) at 1 h, 6 h, and 24 h postinjection. (**b**) Quantitative analysis of the tumor accumulation of the pDNA based on the fluorescence intensity in (**a**). (**c**) CLSM images of the tumor sections from the mice treated with different formations. The scale bar is 100 μm. Data in (**b**) is represented as mean ± s.d. (n = 3). (Adapted from Liu et al. 2019, with permission)

**Fig. 19** Tumor growth curves of the mice treated with PBS, MDNP/dCas9-NC, $PEI_{25K}$/dCas9-miR-524, SDNP/dCas9-miR-524, MDNP/dCas9-miR-524, respectively. Data is represented as mean ± s.d. (n = 5). (Adapted from Liu et al. 2019, with permission)

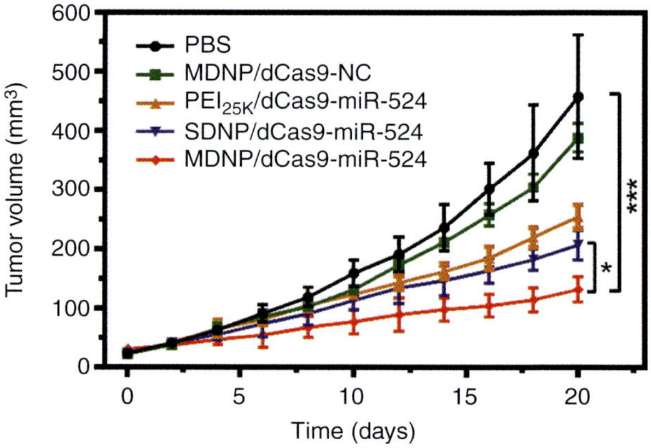


## 3.11 Analysis of the Activation of miR-524 Expression in Mice

1. Collect tumors and normal organs (heart, liver, spleen, lung, kidney) after treatment.
2. Freeze tissues (100 mg) with liquid nitrogen, and grind into powder.
3. Transfer to a 1.5 mL centrifuge tube, add 100 μL TRIzol reagent, and incubate for 10 min at room temperature.
4. Add 0.2 mL chloroform, shake for 15 s, and stand for 2 min.
5. Centrifuge at 12000 rpm for 15 min, take the supernatant.

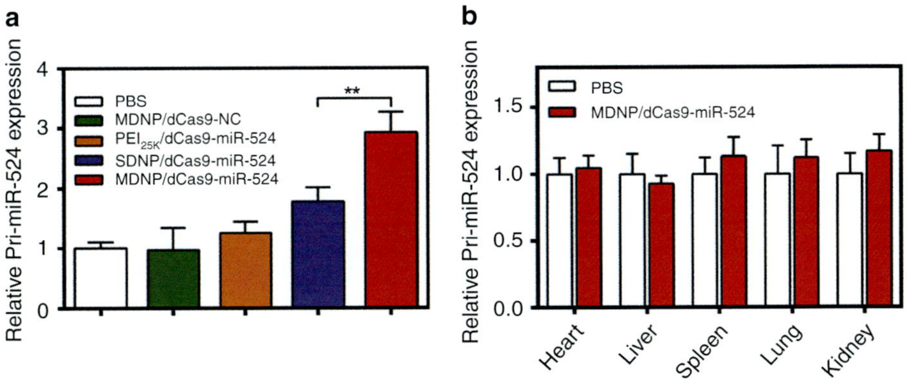


**Fig. 20** Relative expression levels of Pri-miR-524 in tumors (**a**) and non-targeted organs (**b**) from the mice treated with MDNP/dCas9-miR-524 and PBS, respectively. All data in (**a**) and (**b**) are represented as mean ± s.d. (n = 3). The significant level is shown as ** $p < 0.01$. (Adapted from Liu et al. 2019, with permission)

6. Add 0.5 mL isopropanol, mix the liquid gently, and stand at room temperature for 10 min.
7. Centrifuge at 12000 rpm for 15 min, discard the supernatant.
8. Add 1 mL 75% ethanol to wash the precipitate, centrifuge at 7500 rpm for 5 min, and then discard the supernatant.
9. Dry in the air, and then dissolve in DEPC water.
10. The miRNA was converted to cDNA using the PrimeScript RT reagent kit according to the manufacturer's protocol.
11. The cDNAs were quantified by real-time quantitative PCR instrument. Expression of U6 was employed as endogenous control. Fold changes for the expression levels of Pri-miR-524 were calculated using the comparative cycle threshold (CT) method ($2^{-\Delta\Delta CT}$) (Fig. 20).

## 3.12 Safety Evaluation of MDNP

1. Divide Kunming mice into two groups randomly (six mice per group).
2. Inject 100 μL PBS and MDNP containing 10 μg pDNA per mouse via tail vein every 5 days for 15 days, respectively.
3. Collect the blood samples using coagulant tube.
4. Centrifuge at 2000 rpm for 20 min to obtain supernatant.
5. Analyze levels of IL-6, IFN-γ, TNF-α, NF-kB, IgE, IgM, and IgG in supernatant by mouse IL-6, IFN-γ, TNF-α, NF-kB, IgE, IgM, and IgG ELISA kits following the protocol provided by the manufacture (**Note 20**).
6. Determine the concentrations of inflammatory cytokine and immune globulin (Ig) using a microplate reader (Fig. 21).

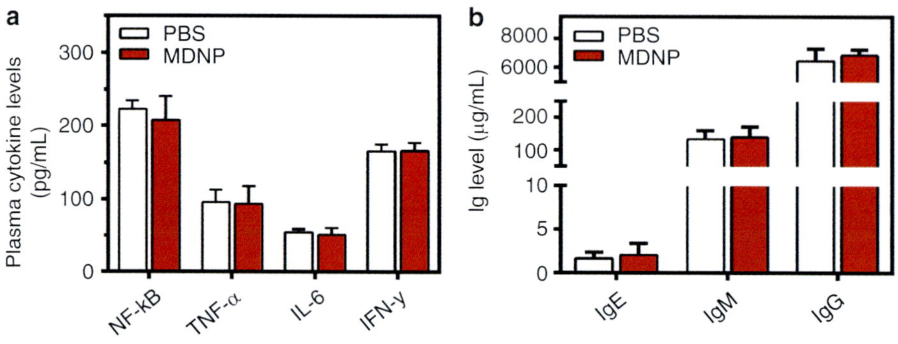


**Fig. 21** Plasma cytokine levels after the injection of MDNP. PBS was used as control. All data in (**a**) and (**b**) are represented as mean ± s.d. (n = 6). (Adapted from Liu et al. 2019, with permission)

### 3.13 Statistical Analysis

All statistical analyses were carried out using GraphPad Prism 5.0. Data were expressed as mean ± s.d., and specific differences were performed using student's t-test and one-way with Dunnett post-test. The significant levels are shown as $^*p < 0.05$, $^{**}p < 0.01$, and $^{***}$ $p < 0.001$.

## 4 Notes

1. The PBA can bind with sialic acid, which usually overexpressed in cancer cells. Thus, $PEI_{1.8K}$ modified with PBA can significantly enhance cellular internalization. However, excessive PBA modification would reduce the positive charge density of $PEI_{1.8K}$, and then decrease its transfection efficiency eventually (Peng et al. 2010). It is recommended that the number of PBAs conjugated on each $PEI_{1.8K}$ does not exceed 3.5.
2. To increase the degree of polymerization, ultradry DMF should be used in polymerization of Lys(Z)-NCA.
3. DMMA would gradually hydrolyze in water. To improve the modification ratio of DMMA onto $mPEG_{113}$-*b*-$PLys_{100}$, DMMA could be added in batches.
4. Due to the acid sensitivity of DMMA-derived amide bonds, the pH value of reaction solution should be continuously monitored during the DMMA modification.
5. To quickly and thoroughly remove the unreacted DMMA, replace the sodium bicarbonate buffer (pH 8.5, 5 mM) every 3 h.
6. Incubate at 60 °C for 1 h to fully dissolve PEI-PBA before using.
7. Add PEI-PBA solution into pDNA solution.
8. Dilute PEI-PBA/pDNA polyplex and MDNP solution to different concentrations before preparation of TEM samples.

9. It is recommended to keep in the dark during the reaction and dialysis. The pH of reaction solution should maintain in the range of 8.0–8.5.
10. After adjusting the pH from 7.4 to 6.5, the concentration of MDNP and SDNP should remain unchanged.
11. When the emission spectrum of the donor fluorescent molecule overlaps with the absorption spectrum of the acceptor fluorescent molecule, and the distance between the donor and acceptor fluorescent molecules is very close (< 10 nm), FRET signal can be observed, which reduces the fluorescence intensity of the donor and significantly enhances the fluorescence intensity of the acceptor (Liu et al. 2013; Selvin 2000). In this protocol, FRET assay is employed to evaluate the detachment of polymer shell from PEI-PBA/pDNA polyplex, Cy3 and Cy5 were selected as donor-acceptor fluorescent molecules.
12. It is recommended to collect free protein by multiple centrifugal filtration, and then dilute the eluent to a uniform volume.
13. Culture medium and trypsin were incubated at 37 °C in water bath for 15 min before using.
14. The pH of adjusted culture medium is measured with pH meter, and then filter with 450 nm syringe filter before using.
15. Mix MDNP and SDNP solution with culture medium.
16. The overlap coefficient between endosome/lysosomes (green) and pDNA (red) could be calculated by image J.
17. For clear observation, replace the culture medium with PBS (pH 7.4, 10 mM) before imaging using fluorescence microscope.
18. Before ex vivo imaging, remove residual blood in tumors and organs using PBS (pH 7.4, 10 mM).
19. For CLSM observation, the abovementioned process should be carried out as soon as possible under dark conditions.
20. Dilute the serum to the measurable concentration range of the ELISA kit according to manufacturer's instruction, and then set different dilution times in this measurement. The correlation coefficients of the standard curves of these samples should exceed 0.99.

## 5 Conclusion

This protocol presented a multistage delivery nanoparticle (MDNP) to overcome multiple physiological barriers for tumor-targeted delivery of CRISPR/dCas9 system. MDNP was synthesized with a positively charged core made from PEI-PBA and CRISPR/dCas9 pDNA, and an acid-responsive polymer shell. With this multistage delivery strategy, MDNP successfully delivered CRISPR/dCas9-miR-524 system to tumors and effectively inhibited the growth of tumors eventually (Liu et al. 2019). More importantly, such strategy could also be applied to deliver any other forms of nucleic acid-based therapeutics (e.g., sgRNA, siRNA, mRNA, etc.), providing a universal platform for developing novel cancer gene therapies.

## References

Bikard D, Jiang W, Samai P et al (2013) Programmable repression and activation of bacterial gene expression using an engineered CRISPR-Cas system. Nucleic Acids Res 41(15):7429–7437
Davis ME, Chen Z, Shin DM (2008) Nanoparticle therapeutics: an emerging treatment modality for cancer. Nat Rev Drug Discov 7(9):771–782
Deshayes S, Cabral H, Ishii T et al (2013) Phenylboronic acid-installed polymeric micelles for targeting Sialylated epitopes in solid tumors. J Am Chem Soc 135(41):15501–15507
Eetezadi S, Ekdawi SN, Allen C (2015) The challenges facing block copolymer micelles for cancer therapy: in vivo barriers and clinical translation. Adv Drug Deliv Rev 91:7–22
Fischer D, Li YX, Ahlemeyer B et al (2003) In vitro cytotoxicity testing of polycations: influence of polymer structure on cell viability and hemolysis. Biomaterials 24(7):1121–1131
Gilbert LA, Horlbeck MA, Adamson B et al (2014) Genome-scale CRISPR-mediated control of gene repression and activation. Cell 159(3):647–661
Hanahan D, Weinberg RA (2011) Hallmarks of cancer: the next generation. Cell 144(5):646–674
Hatakeyama H, Akita H, Harashima H (2011) A multifunctional envelope type nano device (MEND) for gene delivery to tumours based on the EPR effect: a strategy for overcoming the PEG dilemma. Adv Drug Deliv Rev 63(3):152–160
Jin E, Zhang B, Sun X et al (2013) Acid-active cell-penetrating peptides for in vivo tumor-targeted drug delivery. J Am Chem Soc 135(2):933–940
Jinek M, Chylinski K, Fonfara I et al (2012) A programmable dual-RNA-guided DNA endonuclease in adaptive bacterial immunity. Science 337(6096):816–821
Joung J, Konermann S, Gootenberg JS et al (2017) Genome-scale CRISPR-Cas9 knockout and transcriptional activation screening. Nat Protoc 12(4):828–863
Kim HJ, Ishii A, Miyata K et al (2010) Introduction of stearoyl moieties into a biocompatible cationic polyaspartamide derivative, PAsp(DET), with endosomal escaping function for enhanced siRNA-mediated gene knockdown. J Control Release 145(2):141–148
Li L, Song L, Liu X et al (2017) Artificial virus delivers CRISPR-Cas9 system for genome editing of cells in mice. ACS Nano 11(1):95–111
Liu Y, Du J, Yan M et al (2013) Biomimetic enzyme nanocomplexes and their use as antidotes and preventive measures for alcohol intoxication. Nat Nanotechnol 8(3):187–192
Liu Q, Zhao K, Wang C et al (2019) Multistage delivery nanoparticle facilitates efficient CRISPR/dCas9 activation and tumor growth suppression in vivo. Adv Sci 6(1):1801423
Mintzer MA, Simanek EE (2009) Nonviral vectors for gene delivery. Chem Rev 109(2):259–302
Nault J-C, Datta S, Imbeaud S et al (2015) Recurrent AAV2-related insertional mutagenesis in human hepatocellular carcinomas. Nat Genet 47(10):1187–1193
Peng Q, Chen F, Zhong Z et al (2010) Enhanced gene transfection capability of polyethylenimine by incorporating boronic acid groups. Chem Commun 46(32):5888–5890
Ramakrishna S, Dad A-BK, Beloor J et al (2014) Gene disruption by cell-penetrating peptide-mediated delivery of Cas9 protein and guide RNA. Genome Res 24(6):1020–1027
Ran FA, Hsu PD, Wright J et al (2013) Genome engineering using the CRISPR-Cas9 system. Nat Protoc 8(11):2281–2308
Romberg B, Hennink WE, Storm G (2008) Sheddable coatings for long-circulating nanoparticles. Pharm Res 25(1):55–71
Selvin PR (2000) The renaissance of fluorescence resonance energy transfer. Nat Struct Biol 7(9): 730–734
Wang M, Zuris JA, Meng F et al (2016) Efficient delivery of genome-editing proteins using bioreducible lipid nanoparticles. Proc Natl Acad Sci U S A 113(11):2868–2873
Yin H, Kanasty RL, Eltoukhy AA et al (2014) Non-viral vectors for gene-based therapy. Nat Rev Genet 15(8):541–555
Zheng C, Wang Q, Wang Y et al (2019) In situ modification of the tumor cell surface with immunomodulating nanoparticles for effective suppression of tumor growth in mice. Adv Mater 31(32):1902542

# Preparation and Evaluation of Rationally Designed Polymers for Efficient Endosomal Escape of siRNA

9

Chunhui Li, Yuhua Weng, Anjie Dong, Xing-Jie Liang, and Yuanyu Huang

## Contents



C. Li · Y. Weng · Y. Huang (✉)
School of Life Science, Advanced Research Institute of Multidisciplinary Science, and Institute of Engineering Medicine, Key Laboratory of Molecular Medicine and Biotherapy, Beijing Institute of Technology, Beijing, China
e-mail: yyhuang@bit.edu.cn

A. Dong
Department of Polymer Science and Technology, School of Chemical Engineering and Technology, Key Laboratory of Systems Bioengineering of the Ministry of Education, Tianjin University, Tianjin, China

X.-J. Liang (✉)
Chinese Academy of Sciences (CAS) Key Laboratory for Biomedical Effects of Nanomaterials and Nanosafety, CAS Center for Excellence in Nanoscience, National Center for Nanoscience and Technology of China, Beijing, China
e-mail: liangxj@nanoctr.cn



H. Tian and X. Chen (eds.), *Gene Delivery*, Biomaterial Engineering,
https://doi.org/10.1007/978-981-16-5419-0_4

**Abstract**

Small interfering RNA (siRNA) showed promising prospect in the fields of basic research and drug development due to its capability in inhibition of the expression of any interest gene. However, delivery is the most complicated and challenging process that hampers the wide application of siRNA. Rapid and efficient escape of siRNA from endosome to cytoplasm constitutes a determinant factor for gene silencing. In this chapter, we provide a detailed protocol of rationally designed pH-sensitive polymeric nanomicelles with high endosomal escape efficiency that can facilitate the cytosolic release of internalized siRNA. We elaborately described the synthesis of the polymer, preparation, and characterization of the siRNA-loaded nanoparticles, the process of internalization and intracellular trafficking of nanoparticles, as well as *in vitro* and *in vivo* gene silencing and cancer treatment effects of proposed organic nanoformulation.

**Keywords**

siRNA · Endosomal escape · pH-sensitive · Polymeric nanomicelle · Gene therapy

## 1 Overview

The development of gene therapy technology supplies a promising technique for the treatment of numerous life-threatening diseases (Weng et al. 2019; Cheng et al. 2020). Among them, RNA interference (RNAi) refers to the sequence-specific degradation induced by endogenously produced or exogenously synthesized siRNA through complementary pairing with homologous mRNA, resulting in post-transcriptional gene silencing of the target gene. After several years of research, the stability and off-target effect of siRNA, to a great extent, have been solved via state-of-the-art chemical modification, but how to achieve efficient siRNA delivery is a major challenge for its clinical transformation. Nonviral vectors, considered to be the most potential siRNA delivery system, have shown excellent therapeutic effects and safety profiles in recent clinical studies (Zhou et al. 2016; Zhang et al. 2018). However, the lack of safe and efficient siRNA delivery system still restricts the development of RNAi therapy. The siRNA delivery vectors need to overcome obstacles including endocytosis and endosomal escape in order to achieve robust gene silencing. Improving cell endocytosis, such as increasing the electrostatic interaction between the carrier and the negatively charged cytoplasmic membrane, or employing receptor-mediated endocytosis, is the most common strategy to improve delivery efficiency. However, increasing research indicates that intracellular release is considered to be a key determinant of affecting gene silencing, and only 3.5% (or even less than 1%) of siRNA can be released to cytoplasm, highlighting the demands of developing a carrier with the ability of efficient endosomal escape (Wittrup et al. 2015). pH-sensitive cationic polymers, which can load negatively charged siRNA through electrostatic interaction and promote endosomal escape by responding to changes in endosome pH, have been applied to deliver siRNA (Xu et al. 2016; Li et al. 2014a; Yu et al. 2011). Nevertheless, there is a lack of clear and definite guidance for the design of vectors to promote endosomal escape, since high-efficiency siRNA delivery systems are always accompanied with high endocytosis, it is hard to distinguish the contribution of endocytosis and endosomal escape to siRNA delivery efficiency (Li et al. 2014b; Du et al. 2018). Consequently, we designed a series of pH-responsive polymers termed $PEG_{2k}$-P($DPA_x$-*co*-$DMAEMA_y$)-PT (PDDT). The PDDT polycation composed of polyethylene glycol ($PEG_{2k}$), the pH-sensitive copolymer of poly (dimethylaminoethyl methacrylate-*co*-diisopropylethyl methacrylate) (P($DPA_x$-*co*-$DMAEMA_y$)), and poly (N, N, N-trimethyl ammonium ethyl methacrylate) (PTDMAEMA, PT). The hydrophilic polymer $PEG_{2k}$ is widely utilized as drug carriers by virtue of their extensively investigated mechanisms and notable safety profile. It shows many merits such as forming the hydrophilic shell to stabilize the nanomicelles, resisting nonspecific adherence of serum albumin, prolonging blood circulating time, shielding positive charge, and reducing cell uptake and toxicity (Li et al. 2014b; Yuan et al. 2012; Qingguo Xu et al. 2015). PT provides a positive charge, which enables the carrier to adsorb siRNA via electrostatic charge (Cheng et al. 2013; Zhang et al. 2007). DPA with pKa value of approximate 6.0 is hydrophobic at physiological conditions. Tuning the molar ratio of DPA and DMAEMA could regulate the disassembles behavior of the cationic polymeric nanomicelles in the varied pH environment, thus can obtain optimal endosomal release and achieve the efficient delivery of siRNA *in vitro* and *in vivo* (Zhou et al. 2016). The addition of PT and $PEG_{2k}$ supplies a clean background, which will not affect endosomal escape, so as to specifically investigate the influence of pH-responsive hydrophobic core on endosomal escape and intracellular trafficking of siRNA.

## 2 Protocol

### 2.1 The Synthesis of CTAm, mPEG$_{2k}$-CTAm, and TDMAEMA

1. Dodecyl mercaptan
2. Tetrabutylammonium bisulfate
3. Acetone
4. Carbon disulfide
5. Chloroform
6. HCl
7. NaOH

8. Dichloromethane (DCM)
9. 4-Dimethylaminopyridine (DMAP)
10. N, N′-Dicyclohexylcarbodiimide (DCC)
11. N, N-dimethylaminoethyl methacrylate (DMAEMA)
12. Tetrahydrofuran (THF)
13. Methyl iodide
14. Ether
15. Methoxy poly(ethylene glycol) ($mPEG_{2k}$)

### 2.2 The Synthesis of $mPEG_{2k}$-P($DPA_x$-*co*-$DMAEMA_y$)-PT (PDDT) Polymers

1. 2-diisopropylaminoethyl methacrylate (DPA)
2. N, N-dimethylaminoethyl methacrylate (DMAEMA)
3. N, N-dimethylformamide (DMF)
4. $D_2O$
5. Azobisisobutyronitrile (AIBN)
6. Trifluoroethanol

### 2.3 The pH-Sensitivity and the pH-Dependence of PDDT-Ms

1. 2,2,2-trifluoroethyl alcohol
2. pH 8.0 phosphate buffer
3. Nile red
4. HCl
5. NaOH

### 2.4 siRNA Transfection *In Vitro*

1. Fetal bovine serum (FBS)
2. Dulbecco's modified Eagle's medium (DMEM)
3. Lipofectamine 2000 (Lipo 2000)
4. Trypsin
5. Opti-MEM
6. Penicillin-streptomycin
7. Agarose
8. Ethidium bromide (EB)
9. 3-[4,5-dimethylthiazol-2-thiazolyl]-2,5-diphenyltetrazolium bromide (MTT)
10. Dimethyl sulfoxide (DMSO)
11. Lysotracker Green DND-26
12. Hoechst 33342

13. Chloroquine
14. Bafilomycin A1

# 3 Method

## 3.1 The Synthesis of mPEG$_{2k}$-P(DPA$_x$-*co*-DMAEMA$_y$)-PT$_n$ (PDDT) Polymers

The polymers of mPEG$_{2k}$-P(DPA$_x$-*co*-DMAEMA$_y$)-PT$_n$ (PDDT polycations) are synthesized by RAFT (reversible addition fragmentation chain transfer) reaction (Fig. 1).

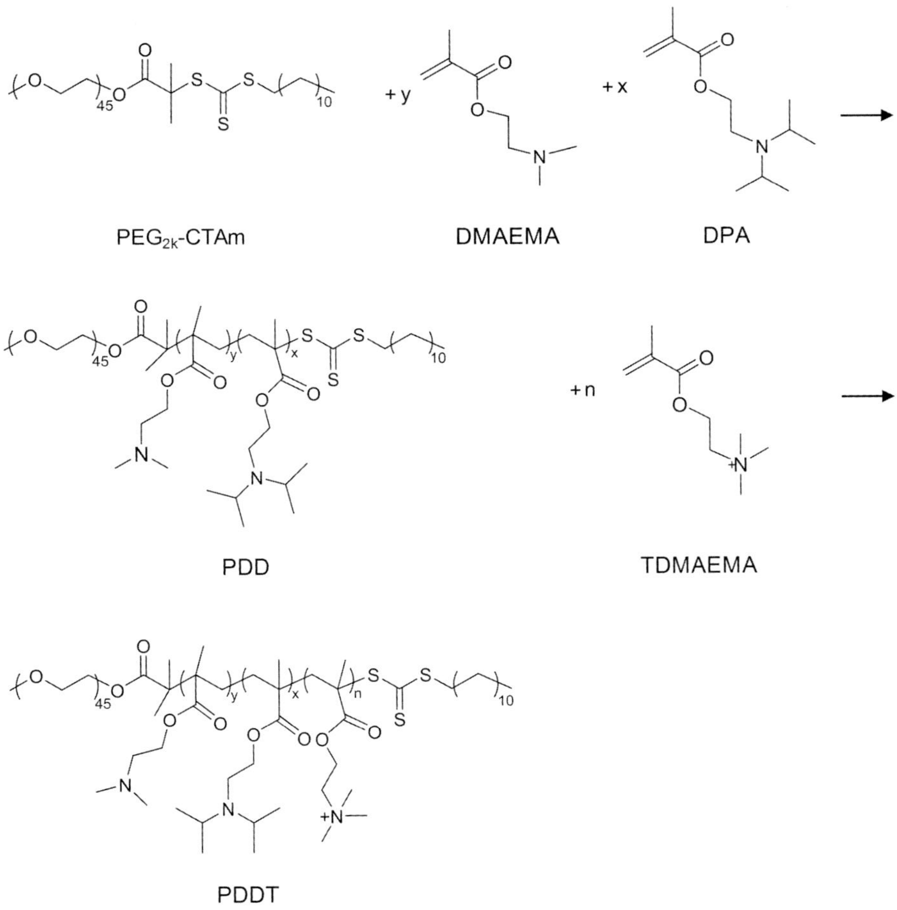


**Fig. 1** The synthesis process of PDDT polymers. Copyright American Chemical Society 2021

### 3.1.1 The Synthesis of $PEG_{2k}$-CTAm

1. Firstly, the chain transfer agent S-1-dodecyl-S-($\alpha$, $\alpha'$-dimethyl-$\alpha''$-acetic acid) trithiocarbonate (CTAm) (Convertine et al. 2006; Lin et al. 2013) is synthesized according to the protocol described in ***note 1*** (*see* **Note 1**).
2. Then, CTAm (365 mg, 1 mmol), $mPEG_{2k}$ (1 g, 0.5 mmol) are dissolved in 50 mL anhydrous DCM.
3. Subsequently, the catalyzer of DMAP (6.1 mg, 0.05 mmol) and the dehydrating agent of DCC (206 mg, 1 mmol) are added into the above solution, followed by stirring for 72 h at room temperature.
4. The resulting solution is filtered to obtain the yellow filtrate, accompanied with rotary evaporation to remove the DCM.
5. Lastly, the remaining solution is dropped into 200 mL ice ether and then filtered three times to obtain the final product $mPEG_{2k}$-CTAm.

### 3.1.2 The Synthesis of TDMAEMA

1. DMAEMA (3.9 g, 25 mmol) dissolved in 50 mL THF is added into a 100 mL round-bottom flask in ice water bath.
2. Afterwards, methyl iodide (3.5 g, 25 mmol) in 10 mL THF is added dropwise to the flask and reacted overnight at room temperature.
3. After the reaction, the Buchner funnel is applied for suction filtration to obtain white powder followed by washing three times with THF.
4. Afterwards, the resulting product is dried to obtain TDMAEMA.

### 3.1.3 The Synthesis of PDDT

1. $mPEG_{2k}$-CTAm is employed as the chain transfer agent to synthesize a small library of PDDT polycations. Tailoring the addition ratio of DPA and DMAEMA could control the constitution of hydrophobic core to achieve the switchable hydrophilicity-hydrophobicity, thus can regulate their pH-responsive properties. The ratios of x to y varied from approximate 1:9, 2:8, 5:5, 7:3, 8:2, 9:1, and 10:0. Eventually, the leading polymer of $mPEG_{2k}$-P($DPA_{50}$-*co*-$DMAEMA_{56}$)-$PTMAEMA_{53}$ (PDDT) is screened out via comprehensive comparison, such as the pH-responsive property, particle disassembling feature under different pH environment, siRNA binding ability, and gene silencing.
2. Taking $mPEG_{2k}$-P($DPA_{50}$-*co*-$DMAEMA_{56}$)-$PTMAEMA_{53}$ (PDDT) for example. $mPEG_{2k}$-CTAm (200 mg, 0.085 mmol), DMAEMA (480 mg, 3.06 mmol) and DPA (435 mg, 2.06 mmol) all are dissolved in 5 mL anhydrous DMF. Meanwhile, AIBN (6.56 mg, 0.04 mmol) is as the initiator added to solution in aims of supporting the polymerization accompanied with three freeze-pump-thaw cycles.
3. Then the solution is placed in a thermostatic oil bath at 70 °C for 24 h in argon atmosphere and dialyzed and lyophilized to obtain intermediate product $mPEG_{2k}$-P($DPA_x$-*co*-$DMA_y$) polymer.
4. TDMAEMA dissolved in 5 mL anhydrous DMF is added into the resulting $mPEG_{2k}$-P($DPA_x$-*co*-$DMA_y$) followed by adding AIBN (3.8 mg, 0.015 mmol) with degassing via three freeze-pump-thaw cycles three times.

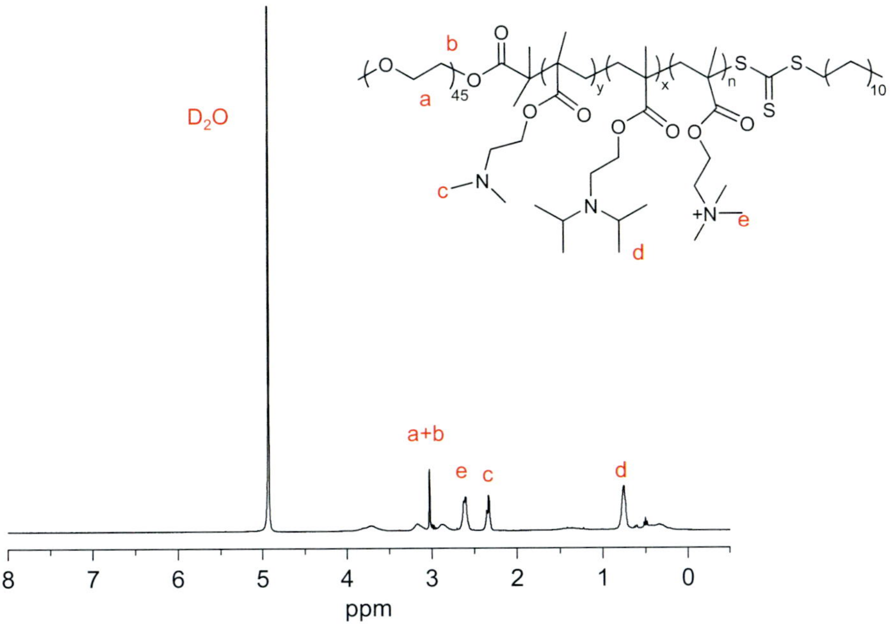


**Fig. 2** The [1]H-NMR spectra of PDDT polymers. Copyright American Chemical Society 2021

5. Finally, the mixture solution is placed in a thermostatic oil bath at 70 °C for 24 h, followed by dialysis and lyophilization to obtain the final product mPEG$_{2k}$-P (DPA$_x$-*co*-DMA$_y$)-PT$_{53}$. In addition, the structure of PDDT is confirmed by $^1$H-NMR (Fig. 2).
6. The PDDT nanomicelles (PDDT-Ms) are prepared by nanoprecipitation. In detail, the PDDT (10 mg) is dissolved in 1 mL trifluoroethanol and dropped into 10 mL water at 0.5 mL/h. Then, trifluoroethanol is removed via dialysis in water overnight to obtain PDDT-Ms.

## 3.2 The pH-Sensitivity and Characterization of PDDT-Ms/siRNA Nanomicelles

### 3.2.1 The pH-Sensitivity of PDDT-Ms Assessed with Nile Red

1. The PDDT polymer (20 mg) is dissolved in 1 mL 2,2,2-trifluoroethyl alcohol that containing 20 μg Nile red dye to obtain PDDT micelles, termed PDDT-Ms (*see* **Note 2**).
2. The resulting solution is slowly added to 20 mL buffer solution with pH = 8.0 to acquire Nile red-loaded micelles.
3. Then the micelles solution is regulated with 0.01 mol/L HCl to obtain the solutions with pH = 8.0, 7.8, 7.4, 7.2, 7.0, 6.8, 6.5, 6.3, 6.0, and 5.4.

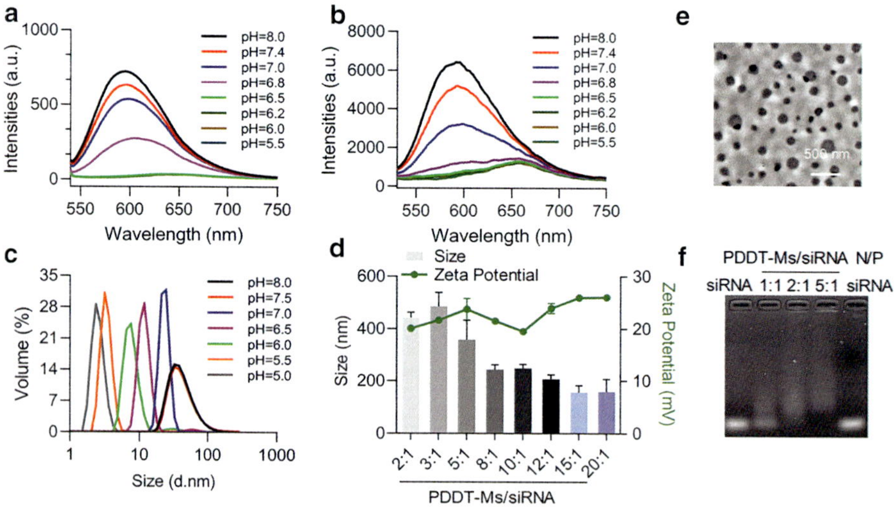


**Fig. 3** Characterization of the physicochemical properties of PDDT and PDDT /siRNA complexes *in vitro*. (**a** and **b**) The assemble and disassemble behaviors of (**a**) PDDT and (**b**) PDDT /siRNA complexes in various pH environments by using Nile red dye. (**c**) DLS is used to record the size changes of PDDT-Ms polycations under varying pH conditions. (**d**) The size and zeta potential of the PDDT/siRNA complexes at various N/P ratios. (**e**) The TEM of PDDT/siRNA complexes. (**f**) Gel retardation measurement of PDDT-Ms/siRNA complexes. Copyright American Chemical Society 2021

4. After 2 h, the fluorescence intensity of the treated solution is measured via Varian fluorescence spectrophotometer (Fig. 3a).
5. Furthermore, the pH-sensitivity of PDDT-Ms/siRNA polyplexes is also examined. Briefly, PDDT micelles loaded with Nile red is incubated with siRNA for 20 min at room temperature to obtain the Nile red and siRNA co-loaded polyplexes.
6. Then the evaluation is carried out according to the same protocol of PDDT-Ms/ Nile red formulation (Fig. 3b).

### 3.2.2 pH-Responsive Dissociation of PDDT-Ms Examined with DLS

1. The polymer of PDDT (20 mg) is dissolved in 1 mL 2,2,2-trifluoroethyl alcohol, and 1 mg/mL nanoparticles are prepared by dropping the solution into pH 8.0 phosphate buffer (50 mL).
2. The pH of the PDDT-Ms solution is adjusted at pHs 8.0, 7.8, 7.6, 7.4, 7.2, 7.0, 6.8, 6.5, 6.0, and 5.4.
3. The size changes of PDDT-Ms in various solutions at different pH are analyzed by DLS (dynamic light scattering) (Zetasizer Nano ZS, Malvern, UK) (Fig. 3c).

### 3.2.3 The Size and Morphology of Polyplexes

1. DLS is also applied to verify the size distributions and zeta potentials of polymeric nanoparticles with various N/P ratios at neutral pH. The siRNA (0.67 μg)

and PDDT-Ms with various N/P ratios are prepared and incubated at room temperature for 20 min. The N/P ratio refers to the ratio of the number of cationic amine groups of the polymer to the number of phosphate groups of the siRNA.

2. Then the volume of PDDT /siRNA complexes is adjusted to 1 mL using DEPC water and detected at a constant angle of 173° with wavelength of 633 nm (Fig. 3d).
3. Meanwhile, transmission electron microscopy (TEM) (Tecnai G2 20 STWIN transmission electron microscope, Philips, Netherlands) is used to characterize the size and morphology of polyplexes. The siRNA (0.40 μg) and PDDT-Ms at N/P = 5 are incubated at room temperature for 20 min. The volume of the PDDT-Ms/siRNA is approximately 10 μL.
4. After that, 10 μL of PDDT-Ms/siRNA is dipped onto a carbon-coated copper grid and air-dried at room temperature. The images are acquired with 200 kV acceleration voltage (Fig. 3e).

#### 3.2.4 Gel Retardation Assay

A gel retardation assay is performed to determine the mass ratio between PDDT-Ms and siRNA at which the copolymers can completely load siRNA.

1. The complexes containing 400 ng siRNA and PDDT-Ms are prepared and cultured at room temperature for 20 min with various N/P ratios of 1:1, 2:1, and 5:1. Naked siRNA is included as a control.
2. Then 6 × loading buffer is added to the complexes solution.
3. The mixture is totally added into the 2% (w/w) agarose gel containing ethidium bromide of 5 μg/mL.
4. At last, electrophoresis is carried out in 1 × TAE buffer at 120 V and kept for 20 min. The gel is detected at UV light wavelength of 254 nm by image master VDS thermal imaging system (Bio-Rad, Hercules, CA). The analysis of siRNA retardation is expressed via the location of the siRNA in the gel (Fig. 3f).

### 3.3 The Evaluation of PDDT-Ms/siRNA Polyplexes *In Vitro*

#### 3.3.1 Cell Transfection

1. On the day before transfection, cells are counted and seeded into 6-well plates, or 24-well plates, or 96 well plates.
2. Take the 6-well plate as an example, approximately $2 \times 10^5$ cells are seeded in each well of 6-well plates. Twenty-four hours later, the transfection is carried out when the cell density reaches approximate 40–50%.
3. Firstly, the DMEM is replaced with 2 mL Opti-MEM. Opti-MEM is also used to prepare the transfection solution containing siRNA and polymer. PDDT-Ms/siRNA with various N/P ratios are prepared and incubated at room temperature for 20 min.
4. Opti-MEM is applied to adjusted the volume of the complexes to 400 μL after incubating, and the polymer/siRNA complexes are added into the well of 6-well plates evenly. The transfection concentration of siRNA is 50 nM.

5. Then the cells are cultured at 37 °C in a humidified atmosphere of 5% $CO_2$ for 4–6 h.
6. Finally, all the media are replaced with fresh complete DMEM and further cultured for 20 h.

### 3.3.2 Cellular Uptake of Complexes

In order to evaluate whether the carrier can deliver Cy5-labeled siRNA into cells, flow cytometry is applied to record the endocytosis of the complexes (*see* **Note 3, 4**).

1. The HepG2-Luc cells, a liver cancer cell line stably expressing firefly luciferase, are seeded in 6-well plates and transfected with PDDT-Ms/siRNA complexes at N/P ratio of 5:1 and siRNA concentration of 50 nM (three replicates).
2. Four hours later, the solution is removed and the treated cells are washed with PBS.
3. Then 200 μL trypsin is added to each well for digestion at 37 °C for about 2 min, and then 1 mL DMEM is added to the well, followed by centrifuging at 800 rpm for 5 min at 4 °C.
4. Next, the supernatant is carefully removed, and the cells are washed with PBS for three times to remove the medium.
5. At last, the cells are suspended in 400 μL PBS and introduced into a BD FACSCalibur flow cytometer (Becton Dickinson, San Jose, CA, USA) for detection (Fig. 4a, b).

### 3.3.3 Cytotoxicity Assessment

In order to assess the cytotoxicity of the PDDT-Ms/siRNA complexes *in vitro*, MTT (3-(4,5-dimethyl-2-thiazolyl)-2,5-diphenyl-2-H-tetrazolium bromide) is applied.

1. The HepG2-Luc cells are seeded in 96-well plates (six replicates).
2. After the transfection for 24 h, the medium is removed gently and 100 μL of fresh DMEM containing 2 μL MTT solution (5 mg/mL in PBS) is added into each well. Then the cells are cultured for another 4 h.
3. After that, the solution of each well is replaced with 50 μL DMSO and the cells are further incubated for 15–20 min at 37 °C to completely dissolve formazan.
4. Finally, the absorbance at 540 nm is measured with a reference wavelength of 650 nm (Fig. 4c) (*see* **Note 3, 5**).

$$\text{Cell viability}(\%) = \frac{OD_{540(\text{Sample})} - OD_{650(\text{Sample})}}{OD_{540(\text{Mock})} - OD_{650(\text{Mock})}} \times 100$$

### 3.3.4 Quantitative Real-Time PCR

1. The HepG2-Luc cells, Hek-293A cells, and MCF7 cells (a human breast adenocarcinoma cell line) are seeded in 6-well plates, respectively.
2. Twenty-four hours later, the transfection is performed with PDDT-Ms/siRNA complexes at N/P ratio of 5:1 and siRNA concentration of 50 nM (*see* **Note 4, 6**).

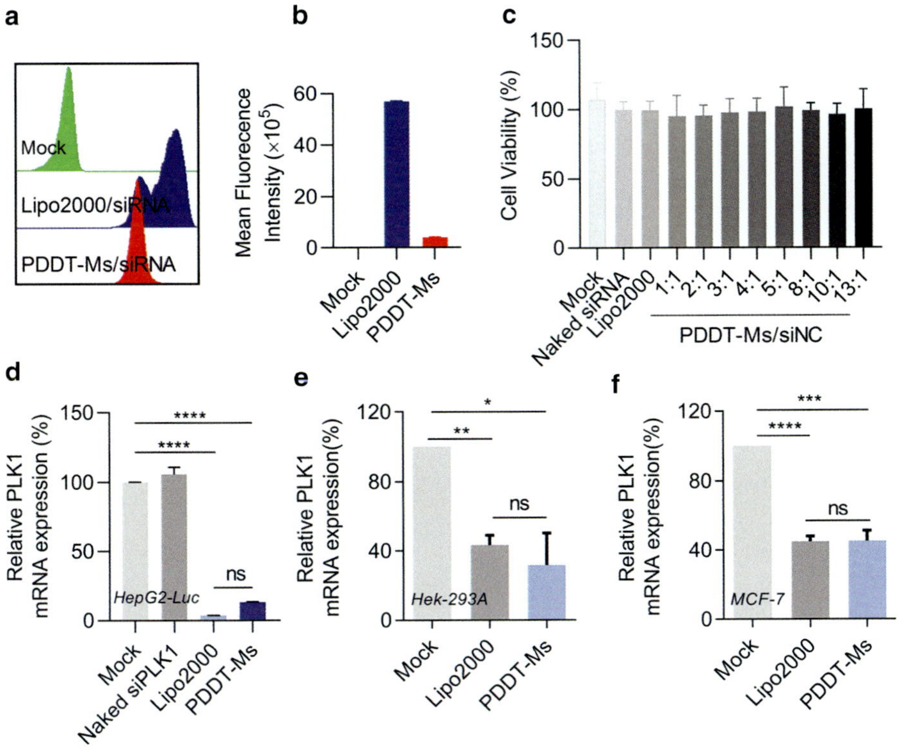


**Fig. 4** Transfection performances of PDDT-Ms/siRNA complexes *in vitro*. (**a**) Cellular uptake efficiency of PDDT-Ms/Cy5-siRNA complexes in HepG2-Luc cells at N/P = 5:1 evaluated by flow cytometry. (**b**) Quantitative analysis of the cellular uptake showed in (**a**). (**c**) The cytotoxicity of PDDT-MS/siRNA complexes (N/P = 1:1, 2:1, 3:1, 4:1, 5:1, 8:1, 10:1, 13:1). The transfection concentration of siRNA is 50 nM. (**d–f**) Gene silencing efficiencies recorded in (**d**) HepG2-Luc cells, (**e**) Hek-293A cells, and (**f**) MCF7 cells. *$P < 0.05$; **$P < 0.01$; ***$P < 0.001$, ****$P < 0.0001$. "ns," no statistical difference. Copyright American Chemical Society 2021

3. Twenty-four hours after transfection, the cells are collected and total RNA is extracted with TRIzol reagent.
4. Then reverse transcription is carried out by using 1 μg total RNA to prepare cDNA.
5. At last, quantitative real-time PCR is performed to evaluate gene silencing efficiency (Fig. 4d–f) (*see* **Note 7, 8**).

### 3.4 The Endosomal Escape of PDDT-Ms/siRNA Polyplexes *In Vitro*

In order to evaluate whether the polyplexes can escape from the endosome efficiently, confocal laser scanning microscopy (CLSM) is applied to observe the subcellular localization and intracellular trafficking of PDDT-Ms/siRNA complexes *in vitro*.

### 3.4.1 Cell Transfection in HepG2-Luc Cell

1. Firstly, $1 \times 10^5$ HepG2-Luc cells are seeded into 20 mm dishes.
2. Twenty-four hours later, the transfection is performed with PDDT-Ms/Cy5-siRNA complexes at N/P ratio of 5:1 and Cy5-siRNA concentration of 50 nM. Commercial lipofectamine 2000 (Lipo 2000) is included as a control.
3. The HepG2-Luc cells are washed with $1 \times$ PBS for three times to remove residual free complexes after transfected for 1, 3, 5, 8, or 10 h, respectively.
4. Subsequently, 1 mL of $1 \times$ PBS containing Lysotracker Green DNA-26 (0.3 μL) and Hoechst 33342 (1 μL) are added into each dish to stain the endosome/lysosome organelles and nucleus for 15 min, respectively. Then the cells are observed with CLSM (Fig. 5a).
5. The colocalization of siRNA and lysosome/endosome, as well as the MFIs are analyzed with Nikon NIS-Elements analysis software (Fig. 5b, c).

### 3.4.2 The Influence of Chloroquine and Bafilomycin A1 on Transfection

1. In addition, the influence of chloroquine (100 μM) and bafilomycin A1 (200 nM) on the internalization and intracellular trafficking of PDDT-Ms/Cy5-siRNA complexes are explored in HepG2-Luc cells in parallel (*see* **Note 9**).
2. Firstly, chloroquine (100 μM) and bafilomycin A1 (200 nM) are added to the cells 1 h before transfection.
3. Then, the cells pre-treated with chloroquine are transfected with PDDT-Ms/Cy5-siRNA and chloroquine (100 μM) for 4 h, and the cells pre-treated with bafilomycin A1 are transfected with PDDT-Ms/Cy5-siRNA for 4 h.
4. The CLSM observation and analysis are performed according to the above-mentioned procedures employed in assays without adding chloroquine or bafilomycin A1 (Fig. 5d–f).

## 3.5 Antitumor Activity of PDDT-Ms/siPLK1 Complexes

The antitumor efficacy of PDDT-Ms/siPLK1 is evaluated on hepatocellular carcinoma patient-derived xenograft (PDX) model (*see* **Note 10**).

1. The tumor tissues are cut into fragments and are inoculated to the right flank of BALB/c nude mice weighting 16–18 g.
2. Treatments are started when the average tumor volume reaches approximate 100–200 $mm^3$. The animals are randomly divided into four groups (nine mice per group) and received the treatments of (1) PBS, (2) Sorafenib, (3) PDDT-Ms/siNC, and (4) PDDT-Ms/siPLK1 every 2 days, respectively (*see* **Note 11**). Sorafenib was orally dosed at 30 mg/kg, and siRNA was intratumorally injected at 1 mg/kg.

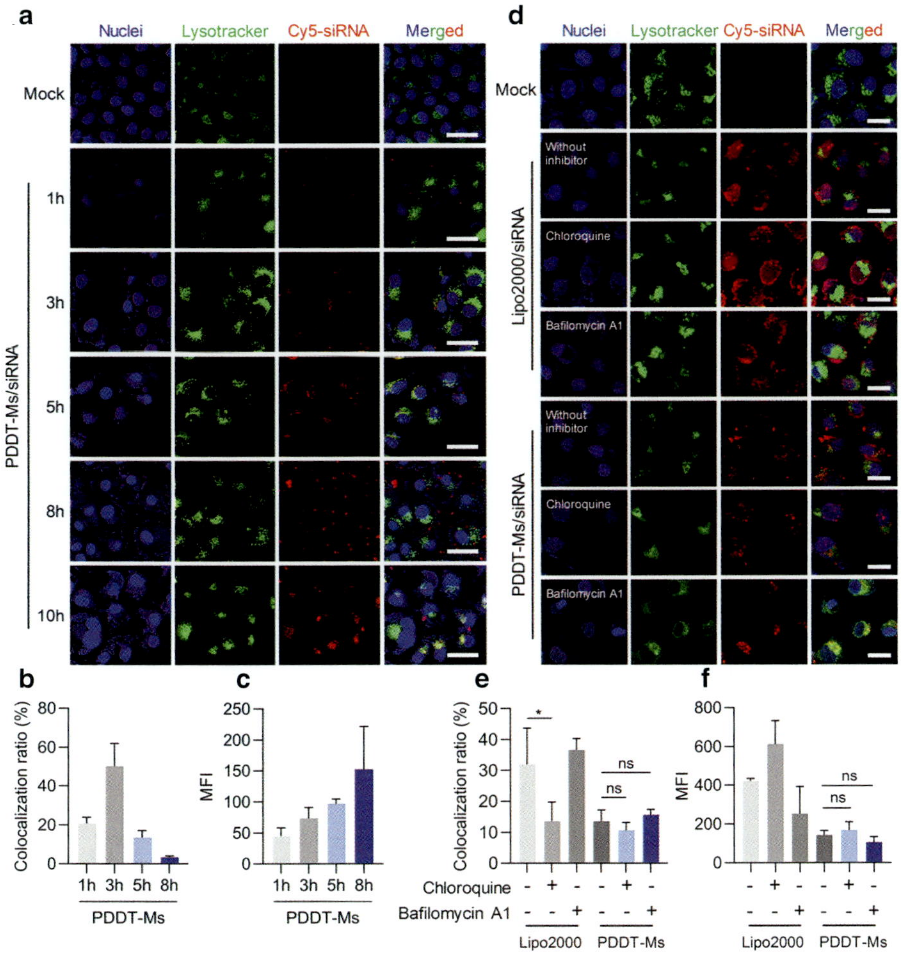


**Fig. 5** Endosomal escape and colocalization analysis of PDDT-Ms/siRNA polyplexes in cells. (**a**) The subcellular localization and intracellular trafficking of PDDT-Ms/Cy5-siRNA complexes in HepG2-Luc cells at different transfection time points. Scale bar, 40 μm. (**b**) The colocalization analysis of Lysotracker Green-stained endosomes and Cy5-siRNA. (**c**) The mean fluorescence intensities (MFIs) of PDDT-Ms/Cy5-siRNA complexes in HepG2-Luc cells at different transfection time points. (**d**) Influence of chloroquine and bafilomycin A1 on transfection of PDDT-Ms/Cy5-siRNA complexes in HepG2-Luc cells. Scale bar, 20 μm. (**e**) The colocalization analysis of Lysotracker Green-stained endosomes and Cy5-siRNA. (**f**) The MFIs of PDDT-Ms/Cy5-siRNA complexes in HepG2-Luc cells 4 h after transfection. "ns," no statistical difference. Copyright American Chemical Society 2021

3. Tumor volume and animal survival are recorded throughout the treatment course. The tumor volume ($mm^3$) $= 0.5 \times$ length $\times$ width$^2$. At the end of the experiment, isolated tumor tissues are weighted and optically imaged (Fig. 6).

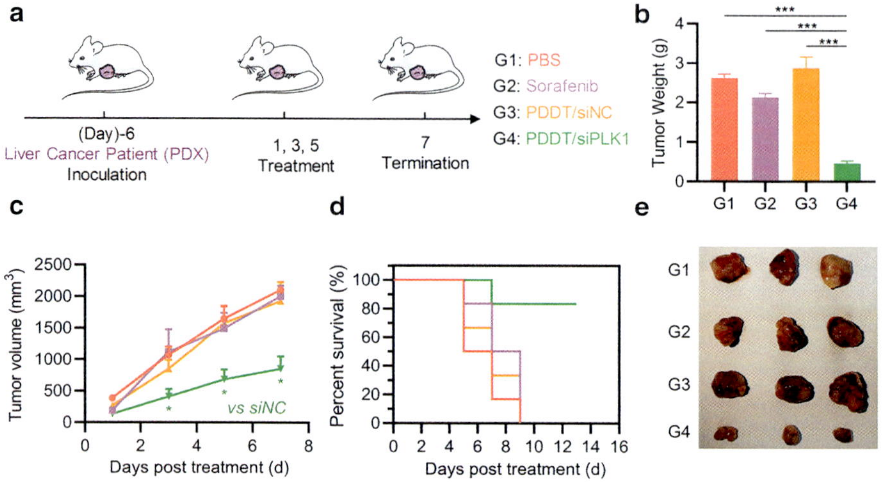


**Fig. 6** Antitumor efficacy of PDDT-Ms/siPLK1 complexes in liver cancer patient-derived xenograft model. (**a**) Treatment schedule and grouping information ($n = 9$). (**b**) Tumor weights recorded at the end time point of treatment. (**c**) Tumor growth curves of mice receiving various treatment during the entire treatment course. (**d**) Survival curves. (**e**) Optical images of isolated tumor tissues. $^*P < 0.05$, $^{***}P < 0.001$. Copyright American Chemical Society 2021

## 4 Notes

1. Dodecyl mercaptan (80.76 g) and tetrabutylammonium bisulfate (6.49 g) are dissolved in 240 mL acetone and cooled in ice water bath for 20 min under a nitrogen atmosphere. Then, 17 mL sodium hydroxide solution (50%) is added to mixture over 15 min, 24 mL carbon disulfide in 50 mL acetone are added for an additional 10 min. Next, adding 50% sodium hydroxide solution (8 mL) into 47 mL chloroform by dropwise, which are stirred overnight. After that, 100 mL HCl dissolved in 600 mL double-distilled water ($ddH_2O$) are added with rapid stirring to remove acetone under the protection of nitrogen. The reaction solution is filtered and dissolved in 1 L propanol later to exclude the undissolved products by filter. The target compound is recrystallized from hexane for three times to obtain molecular chain transfer agent, termed CTAm.
2. Nile red is a hydrophobic fluorescent fuel, which can be encapsulated in the hydrophobic core of PDDT-Ms by hydrophobic interaction. As the pH value decreases gradually, the hydrophobic nucleus of PDDT-Ms is protonated and mediates the pH-triggered disassembly. Consequently, Nile red is released from the hydrophobic core of PDDT-MS that fluorescence signal is gradually weakened until it cannot be detected.
3. The group of mock represents the cells without any treatment. Lipofectamine 2000 is used as a positive control. The transfection concentration of siRNA is

50 nM. Four microliters of Lipofectamine 2000 were used for transfection in 6-well plate.

4. Cy5-labeled siRNA (Cy5-siRNA), siNC, and siPLK1 are supplied by Suzhou Ribo Life Science Co., Ltd. (Suzhou, Jiangsu Province, China). Chemical modifications, such as 2′-OMe, 2′-F, and phosphorothioate, are placed at certain sites of both strands of siRNA to enhance siRNA's stability and specificity. The detailed sequences are as follows:
   (1) Cy5-siRNA: sense strand, 5′-Cy5-CCUUGAGGCAUACUUCAAAdTdT-3′, antisense, 5′-UUUGAAGUAUGCCUCAAGGdTdT-3′.
   (2) siNC: sense strand, 5′-CCUUGAGGCAUACUUCAAAdTdT-3′, antisense strand, 5′-UUUGAAGUAUGCCUCAAGGdTdT-3′.
   (3) siPLK1: sense strand, 5′-UGAAGAAGAUCACCCUCCUUAdTdT-3′, antisense strand, 5′-UAAGGAGGGUGAUCUUCUUCAdTdT-3′.
5. siNC is a scramble siRNA without any target sequence in the transcripts of human beings, monkey, rat, and mouse.
6. Anti-PLK1 siRNA (siPLK1) targets polo-like kinase 1 (PLK1) gene that usually is highly expressed in cancer cells.
7. Glyceraldehyde 3-phosphate dehydrogenase (GAPDH) is used as an internal control.
8. The sequences of primer sets are as follows: (1) primer set for human GAPDH, forward: 5′-AGAAGGCTGGGGCTCATTTG-3′, reverse: 5-′-AGGGGCCATCCACAGTCTTC-3′; (2) primer set for human PLK1, forward: 5′-GCCCCTCACAGTCCTCAATA-3′, reverse: 5-′-TACCCAAGGCCGTACTTGTC-3′.
9. Chloroquine is a lysosomal disruptor that promotes endosomal escape of PDDT-Ms, whereas bafilomycin A1 prevents the acidification of endosomes and thus can inhibit the endosomal escape of PDDT-Ms.
10. Tumor tissue is provided by the Chinese People's Liberation Army (PLA) General Hospital and kept by Institute of Chemistry, Chinese Academy of Sciences. The human tissue used in this study is approved by the hospital's ethics committee and complied with all relevant ethical regulations.
11. Sorafenib, a clinically employed anticancer drug, is included as a control in this assay.

## 5 Discussion

In this chapter, we introduce a series of pH-sensitive polymers that can facilitate endosomal escape of siRNA in cells. The leading polymer termed PDDT is synthesized by RAFT reaction. PDDT/siRNA polymeric nanomicelles can dissociate in endosomal pH environment, leading to efficient cytosolic release of siRNA. As a result, PDDT/siRNA exhibits robust gene silencing activity both *in vitro* and *in vivo*. It paves a simple and feasible way for the siRNA delivery and cancer treatment.

**Acknowledgments** This work is supported by the National Natural Science Foundation of China (31871003, 31901053, 31671021, and 31971306), the Beijing Nova Program from Beijing Municipal Science & Technology Commission (Z201100006820005), the Beijing-Tianjin-Hebei Basic Research Cooperation Project (19JCZDJC64100), the National Key R&D Program of China (2021YFE0106900), the Natural Science Foundation of Guangdong Province (2019A1515010776), and the Young Elite Scientist Sponsorship Program of Beijing Association for Science and Technology (2020–2022). We thank Biological & Medical Engineering Core Facilities (Beijing Institute of Technology) for providing advanced equipment and help.

## References

Cheng Q, Huang Y, Zheng H, Wei T, Zheng S, Huo S, Wang X, Du Q, Zhang X, Zhang HY, Liang XJ, Wang C, Tang R, Liang Z (2013) The effect of guanidinylation of PEGylated poly (2-aminoethyl methacrylate) on the systemic delivery of siRNA. Biomaterials 34(12):3120–3131

Cheng Q, Wei T, Farbiak L, Johnson LT, Dilliard SA, Siegwart DJ (2020) Selective organ targeting (SORT) nanoparticles for tissue-specific mRNA delivery and CRISPR-Cas gene editing. Nat Nanotechnol 15:313

Convertine AJ, Lokitz BS, Vasileva Y, Myrick LJ, Scales CW, Lowe AB, McCormick CL (2006) Direct synthesis of thermally responsive DMA/NIPAM diblock and DMA/NIPAM/DMA tri-block copolymers via aqueous, room temperature RAFT polymerization. Macromolecules 39: 1724–1730

Du L, Wang C, Meng L, Cheng Q, Zhou J, Wang X, Zhao D, Zhang J, Deng L, Liang Z, Dong A, Cao H (2018) The study of relationships between pKa value and siRNA delivery efficiency based on tri-block copolymers. Biomaterials 176:84–93

Li J, Yu X, Wang Y, Yuan Y, Xiao H, Cheng D, Shuai X (2014a) A reduction and pH dual-sensitive polymeric vector for long-circulating and tumor-targeted siRNA delivery. Adv Mater 26(48): 8217–8224

Li Y, Cheng Q, Jiang Q, Huang Y, Liu H, Zhao Y, Cao W, Ma G, Dai F, Liang X, Liang Z, Zhang X (2014b) Enhanced endosomal/lysosomal escape by distearoyl phosphoethanolamine-polycarboxybetaine lipid for systemic delivery of siRNA. J Control Release 176:104–114

Lin D, Jiang Q, Cheng Q, Huang Y, Huang P, Han S, Guo S, Liang Z, Dong A (2013) Polycation-detachable nanoparticles self-assembled from mPEG-PCL-g-SS-PDMAEMA for in vitro and in vivo siRNA delivery. Acta Biomater 9(8):7746–7757

Qingguo Xu LME, Boylan NJ, Schön A, Gong X, Yang J-C, Lamb NW, Cai S, Yu T, Freire E, Hanes J (2015) Impact of surface polyethylene glycol (PEG) density on biodegradable nano-particle transport in mucus ex vivo and distribution in vivo. ACS Nano 9(9):9217–9227

Weng Y, Xiao H, Zhang J, Liang XJ, Huang Y (2019) RNAi therapeutic and its innovative biotechnological evolution. Biotechnol Adv 37(5):801–825

Wittrup A, Ai A, Liu X, Hamar P, Trifonova R, Charisse K, Manoharan M, Kirchhausen T, Lieberman J (2015) Visualizing lipid-formulated siRNA release from endosomes and target gene knockdown. Nat Biotechnol 33(8):870–876

Xu X, Wu J, Liu Y, Yu M, Zhao L, Zhu X, Bhasin S, Li Q, Ha E, Shi J, Farokhzad OC (2016) Ultra-pH-responsive and tumor-penetrating nanoplatform for targeted siRNA delivery with robust anti-cancer efficacy. Angew Chem Int Ed Engl 55(25):7091–7094

Yu H, Zou Y, Wang Y, Huang X, Huang G, Sumer BD, Boothman DA, Gao J (2011) Overcoming endosomal barrier by amphotericin B-loaded dual pH-responsive PDMA-b-PDPA micelleplexes for siRNA delivery. ACS Nano 5(11):9246–9255

Yuan Y-Y, Mao C-Q, Du X-J, Du J-Z, Wang F, Wang J (2012) Surface charge switchable nanoparticles based on zwitterionic polymer for enhanced drug delivery to tumor. Adv Mater 24(40):5476–5480

Zhang B, Ji W, Liu W, Yao K (2007) Guanidinylated allylamine-N-isopropylacrylamide copolymer nonviral transgene vectors. Int J Pharm 331(1):116–122

Zhang T, Huang Y, Ma X, Gong N, Liu X, Liu L, Ye X, Hu B, Li C, Tian JH, Magrini A, Zhang J, Guo W, Xing JF, Bottini M, Liang XJ (2018) Fluorinated oligoethylenimine nanoassemblies for efficient siRNA-mediated gene silencing in serum-containing media by effective endosomal escape. Nano Lett 18(10):6301–6311

Zhou J, Wu Y, Wang C, Cheng Q, Han S, Wang X, Zhang J, Deng L, Zhao D, Du L, Cao H, Liang Z, Huang Y, Dong A (2016) pH-sensitive nanomicelles for high-efficiency siRNA delivery in vitro and in vivo: an insight into the design of polycations with robust cytosolic release. Nano Lett 16 (11):6916–6923

# Molecular and Supramolecular Construction of Arginine-Rich Nanohybrids for Visible Gene Delivery

# 10

Xianghui Xu

## Contents



**Abstract**

Supramolecular construction emerges as a robust and an efficient tactic for the fabrication of sophisticated nanostructures with multiple functionabilities. In this section, we demonstrated a molecular and supramolecular approach of arginine-rich nanohybrids (ARNHs) based on coassembly of low-generation dendrimers

X. Xu (✉)
Department of Pharmacy, College of Biology, Hunan University, Changsha, Hunan, China
e-mail: xianghui.xu@hnu.edu.cn



H. Tian and X. Chen (eds.), *Gene Delivery*, Biomaterial Engineering,
https://doi.org/10.1007/978-981-16-5419-0_3

and inorganic nanoparticles for visible gene delivery. Arginine-rich corona of ARNHs provided efficient DNA-binding ability, high internalization, and intracellular and nuclear delivery for efficient gene transfection efficiency, and inorganic cores of quantum dots were able to track gene delivery and monitor protein expression. In vitro and in vivo results demonstrated that the ARNHs exhibited high gene transfection efficiency, good biocompatibility, facile fabrication, and real-time bioimaging capabilities.

**Keywords**

Bio-inspired nanomaterials · Supramolecular hybrid dendrimers · Gene delivery · Arginine-rich nanohybrids

## 1 Overview

Cationic polymers are widely regarded as an excellent candidate for developing advanced gene delivery systems, owing to inherent potency on nucleic acid condensation and protection (Pack et al. 2005). Notably, cationic dendrimers attracted much attention as versatile vectors because of their unique properties such as perfect macromolecular structures, highly branched architectures, and 3D nanostructures (Zhang et al. 2015a, b, 2018a, b). However, gene delivery efficiency of dendrimers greatly depends on large molecular weight and high density of positive charge, like other cationic polymers. First, high-generation dendrimers with high delivery efficiency often show serious toxicity to targeted cells. Second, high-generation dendrimers are very difficult to be manufactured, industrialized, and commercialized, accompanying with high cost. As a result, how to address the contradictions between transfection efficiency and high cytotoxicity remains a great challenging work for designing satisfactory gene vectors.

Supramolecular self-assembly of low-generation dendrimers provided a novel strategy on the construction of high-efficiency gene delivery systems (Xu et al. 2012, 2015). Low-generation dendrimers usually have low cytotoxicity and poor efficiency, but supramolecular assembly can endow the low-generation dendrimers with high gene delivery efficiency. Hybrid supramolecular assembly based on organic and inorganic components is expected to gain the most promising gene delivery systems with improved physiochemical and biological properties (Zhao et al. 2019). Diverse inorganic components have many advantages on photothermal, optical, and magnetic properties for disease diagnosis and treatment (Li et al. 2018; Xu et al. 2014; Yang et al. 2014; Zhao et al. 2017). Therefore, hybrid supramolecular strategy on dendrimer-based delivery systems is expected to construct multifunctional nanoplatforms for improving gene transfection.

In this section, a supramolecular hybrid strategy on coassembly of peptide dendrimers and inorganic nanoparticles will be demonstrated to build arginine-rich nanohybrids (ARNHs) for visible gene delivery. Low-generation peptide dendrons

(PD) are completely functionalized with arginine as peripheral units, and their cores were modified with lipoic acid (LA) with coordinating potentials. Guanidinium groups on arginine-rich dendrons not only can interact with nucleic acid for gene condensation, but also can mimic the components of cell-penetrating peptides for enhancing internalization and endosomal escape. On the other hand, quantum dots (QDs) were used as model inorganic nanoparticles due to their good fluorescent properties for both *in vitro* detection and *in vivo* fluorescence imaging. According to recent studies, UV irradiation can activate in situ reduction of the LA groups (functionalized core of PDs) into dihydrolipoic acid. Then the dual-functionalized PDs could spontaneously coordinate onto the surface of QDs to generate a single bioinspired arginine-rich nanohybrid. These arginine-rich nanohybrids have well-defined nanostructure and uniform small size. ARNHs showed highly efficient gene delivery but low cytotoxicity, as compared with positive control of PEI 25K. ARNHs provide inherent fluorescence for tracking intracellular pathways including internalization, endosomal escape, and gene delivery. And ARNHs also serve as an alternative reference for monitoring DNA-encoded protein expression. Meanwhile, *in vivo* animal experiments suggest that ARNHs provide high gene delivery efficiency and real-time bioimaging. This construction strategy and prepare protocol can be applied to fabricate more multifunctional arginine-rich nanohybrids for gene delivery.

## 2 Materials

### 2.1 Synthesis of Arginine-Terminal PDs

1. H-Lys-OMe.HCl
2. Boc-Lys(Boc)-OH
3. Boc-Arg(Pbf)-OH
4. N-(tert-butoxycarbonyl) ethylenediamine
5. Lipoic acid (LA)
6. 1-Ethyl-3-(3-dimethylaminopropyl)carbodiimide hydrochloride (EDC.HCl)
7. 1-Hydroxybenzotriazole (HOBt)
8. N,N-Diisopropylethylamine (DIPEA)
9. Benzotriazol-1-yl-oxytripyrrolidino-phosphonium Hexafluorophosphate (PyBOP)
10. Trifluoroacetic acid (TFA)
11. Dichloromethane ($CH_2Cl_2$)
12. Anhydrous ether
13. Sodium chloride (NaCl)
14. Sodium bisulfate ($NaHSO_4$)
15. Sodium bicarbonate ($NaHCO_3$)
16. Magnetic stirrer
17. Rotary evaporator

## 2.2 Preparation of ARNHs

1. Tetramethylammonium hydroxide (TMAH)
2. n-Hexane
3. CdSe/ZnS QDs-605 (QDs)
4. Alcohol
5. Ultrasonic apparatus

## 2.3 Preparation and Characterizations of ARNHS/DNA Complex

1. Plasmids pEGFP-C1
2. Diethyl pyrocarbonate (DEPC) water
3. Tris-acetate-EDTA (TAE) buffer
4. Agarose
5. GoldView
6. UV illuminator
7. Dynamic light scattering (DLS)
8. Transmission electron microscopy (TEM)
9. Thermal gravimetric analysis (TGA)

## 2.4 Investigation of In Vitro Gene Transfection

1. Dulbecco's Modified Eagle (DMEM) media
2. Fetal bovine serum (FBS)
3. Penicillin-Streptomycin (10,000 U/mL)
4. Phosphate buffer saline (PBS)
5. Reporter lysis buffer
6. Luciferase substrate
7. BCA protein assay kit
8. Polyethylenimine 25 k (PEI)
9. Microplate reader

## 2.5 Cytotoxicity and Intracellular Tracking

1. CCK-8
2. IT Cy5 nucleic acid labeling kit
3. Phosphate buffered saline (PBS)
4. LysoTracker Blue DND-22
5. 0.5% Glutaraldehyde
6. 3% Glutaraldehyde
7. Acetone
8. Eponate812 (Epon812)

9. Uranyl acetate
10. Microplate reader
11. TEM
12. Confocal laser scanning microscope (CLSM)
13. Live cell imaging system (LCIS)

## 2.6 In Vivo Gene Transfection

1. BALB/c nude mice
2. BALB/c mice
3. pCMV-β-gal DNA
4. pGL3-Luc DNA
5. pCMV-p53 DNA
6. β-Galactosidase reporter gene assay kit
7. RIPA lysis buffer
8. BCA assay kit

## 2.7 In Vivo Imaging

1. BALB/c nude mice
2. BALB/c mice
3. *In vivo* fluorescence imaging system

# 3 Protocol

## 3.1 Synthesis of Arginine-Terminal PDs

### 3.1.1 Synthesis of Arginine-Terminal Dendrons

1. Fig. 1 shows the synthesis route of arginine-terminal dendrons. Dissolve H-Lys-OMe.HCl (5 mmol) and Boc-Lys(Boc)-OH (15 mmol) with EDC (15 mmol), HOBT (15 mmol), and DIPEA (40 mmol) in 60 mL of $CH_2Cl_2$ under a nitrogen atmosphere, and stir the reaction system at room temperature for 24 h. Monitor the reaction by thin layer chromatography.
2. Evaporate $CH_2Cl_2$ and dissolve the mixture in 300 mL $CHCl_3$. Wash the solution with saturated NaCl, $NaHSO_4$, and $NaHCO_3$ solution 3 times, separately. Dry the final organic solution by anhydrous $Na_2SO_4$ overnight.
3. Concentrate the dried solution, and purify the raw product by silica gel column chromatography ($CH_2Cl_2$: $CH_3OH$ = 10:1) to afford **Compound 1**.
4. Treat the Compound 1 with TFA/$CH_2CH_2$ (Boc groups: TFA = 1:10, mol/mol) for 4 h to deprotect Boc groups.
5. Evaporate $CH_2Cl_2$ and TFA, and precipitate the product in anhydrous diethyl ether under stirring. Remove the anhydrous diethyl ether to obtain **Compound 2**.

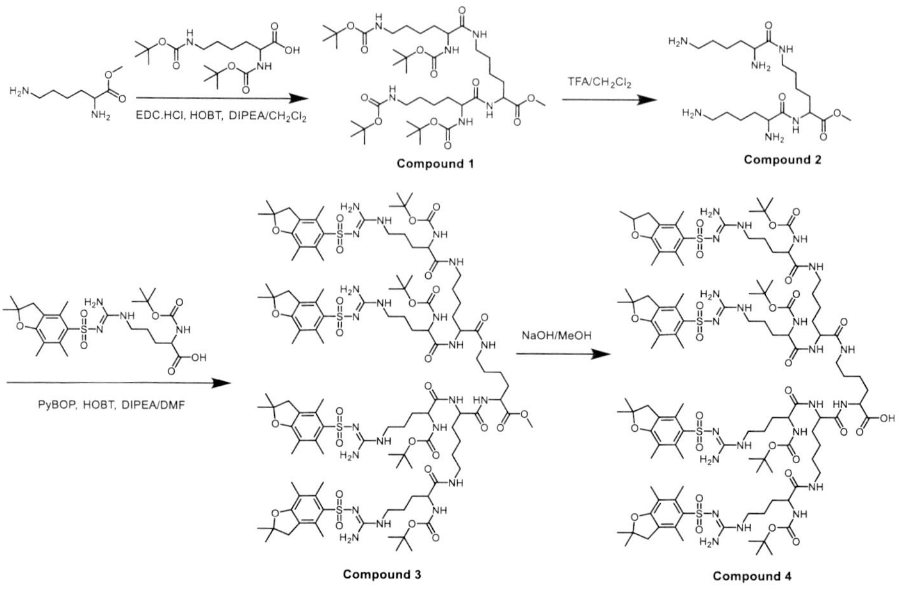


**Fig. 1** Synthesis route of arginine-terminal dendrons (Compound 4)

6. Dissolve Compound 2 (3 mmol), Boc-Arg(Pbf)-OH (18 mmol), HBTU (18 mmol), HOBT (18 mmol), and DIPEA (48 mmol) in 50 mL $CH_2Cl_2$ under a nitrogen atmosphere. Stir the reaction system at room temperature for 48 h. According to Step 2 in Sect. 3.1.1, Wash and purify the reaction solution to obtain **Compound 3**.
7. Treat **Compound 4** with NaOH/MeOH solution (1 M) to remove methyl ester (OMe) group (OMe: NaOH = 1:10, mol/mol). Carry out this reaction overnight at room temperature.
8. Evaporate the MeOH and add $CH_2Cl_2$ to dissolve the residues. Adjust the pH value to 2–3 by HCl (1 M) to extract the product into organic phase. Dry the organic solution by anhydrous $Na_2SO_4$ overnight, filter $Na_2SO_4$, and remove $CH_2Cl_2$ to obtain **Compound 4**.

### 3.1.2 Decoration of Lipoic Acid

1. Fig. 2 shows the synthesis route of lipoic acid derivative. Dissolve N-(tert-butoxycarbonyl) ethylenediamine (28.8 mmol), lipoic acid (24.0 mmol), EDC (36.0 mmol), HOBT (36.0 mmol), and DIPEA (96 mmol) in 50 mL $CH_2Cl_2$, and stir at room temperature under nitrogen atmosphere for 24 h.
2. Wash the mixture by saturated NaCl, $NaHSO_4$, and $NaHCO_3$ solution 3 times, separately. Dry the final organic solution by anhydrous $Na_2SO_4$ overnight.
3. Evaporate the solvent, and purify the rude product by silica gel column chromatography (ethyl acetate: petroleum ether = 1:1) to afford **Compound 5**.

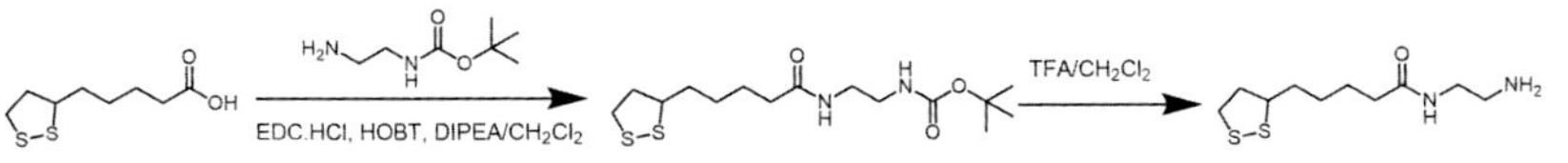


**Fig. 2** Synthesis route of lipoic acid derivative (Compound 6)

4. Treat the **Compound 6** with TFA/$CH_2CH_2$ (Boc groups: TFA = 1:10, mol/mol) for 4 h to deprotect Boc groups.
5. Remove $CH_2CH_2$ and TFA, and precipitate the product in anhydrous diethyl ether under stirring. Remove the anhydrous diethyl ether to obtain **Compound 6**.

### 3.1.3 Synthesis of PDs

1. Fig. 3 shows the synthesis route of PDs. Dissolve Compound 5 (1.5 mmol), Compound 7 (1.8 mmol), PyBOP (1.8 mmol), HOBT (1.8 mmol), and DIPEA (6.0 mmol) in 40 mL DMF and stir for 48 h at room temperature under nitrogen atmosphere.
2. Remove DMF and dissolve raw product in $CH_2Cl_2$ and wash with saturated $NaHCO_3$, $NaHSO_4$, and NaCl solutions 3 times. Dry the organic phase by $Na_2SO_4$ overnight. Concentrate the solution, and purify the product by silica gel column chromatography ($CH_2Cl_2$: $CH_3OH$ = 10:1) to obtain **Compound 7**.
3. Treat Compound 8 with TFA/$CH_2CH_2$ (Boc groups: TFA = 1:10, mol/mol) for 4 h to deprotect Boc groups. Dialyze and lyophilize the precipitate to obtain **Compound 8**.

### 3.1.4 Characterization of Compounds

Confirm the molecular structure from **Compound 1** to **Compound 9** with mass spectrum and $^1$H NMR.

## 3.2 Self-Assembly of PDs into ARNHs

1. Fig. 4 shows the self-assembly of ARNHs. Add PDs aqueous solution (20 mg $mL^{-1}$, 500 μL) in a vial and adjust to pH 7–8 with TMAH. Add QDs *n*-hexane solution (1.6 μmol $L^{-1}$, 100 μL) to PDs solution and stir vigorously for 2 h with UV-irradiation (λ = 365 nm). During this process, PDs can spontaneously self-assemble onto QDs to replace the original ligand via coordination interactions to generate ARNHs, and ARNHs gradually transferred into water-phase.
2. Remove the *n*-hexane. Precipitate ARNHs by alcohol and purify by centrifuge at 10,000 rpm for 5 min. Dissolve the precipitation in water. Dialyze and lyophilize the solution to obtain solid ARNHs.

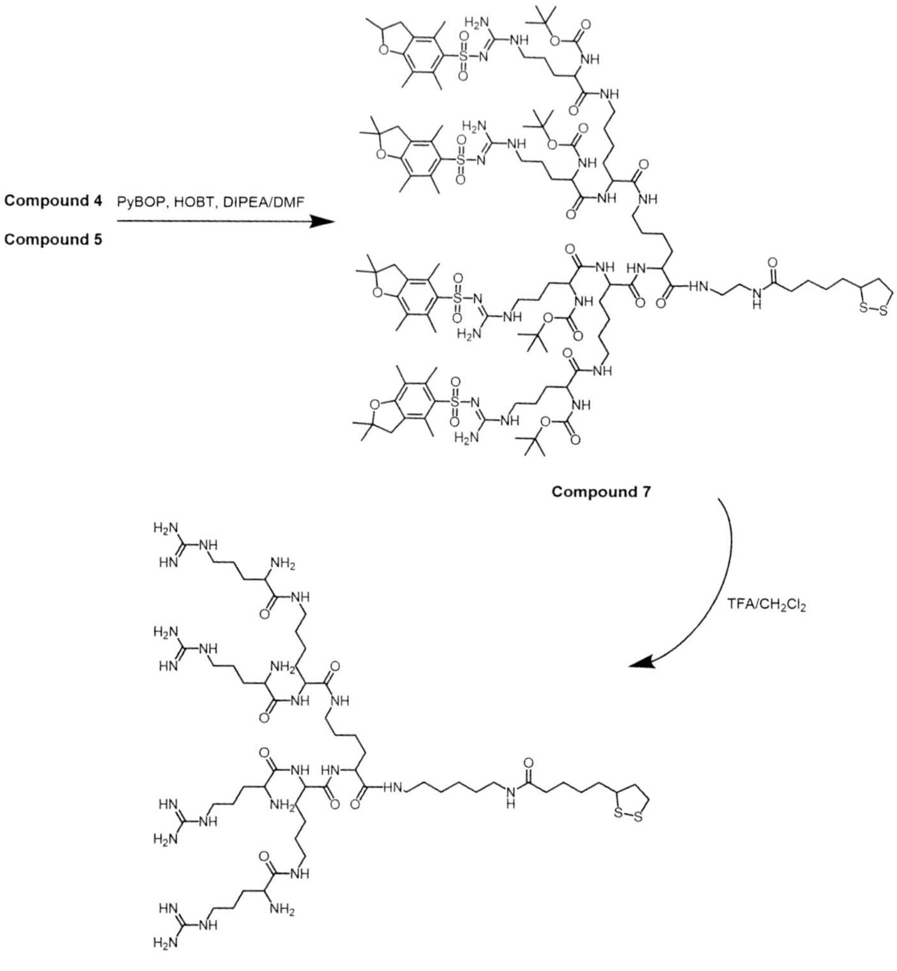


**Fig. 3** Synthesis route of PDs (Compound 8)

## 3.3 Preparation of the ARNHS/DNA Complex and DNA Condensation Assay

1. Mix 400 ng DNA and ARNHs in DEPC water with different arginine (R) in ARNHs to DNA phosphate groups (R/P) ratios and incubate at 37 °C for 30 min.
2. Determine DNA condensation ability of ARNHs by gel electrophoresis method. Prepare 1% (w/v) agarose gel with TAE buffer. Load the samples on the gel and electrophorese at 100 V for 60 min.
3. Stain the gel with GoldView.
4. Image the gel by UV illuminator and analyze by Image Lab software (Fig. 5).

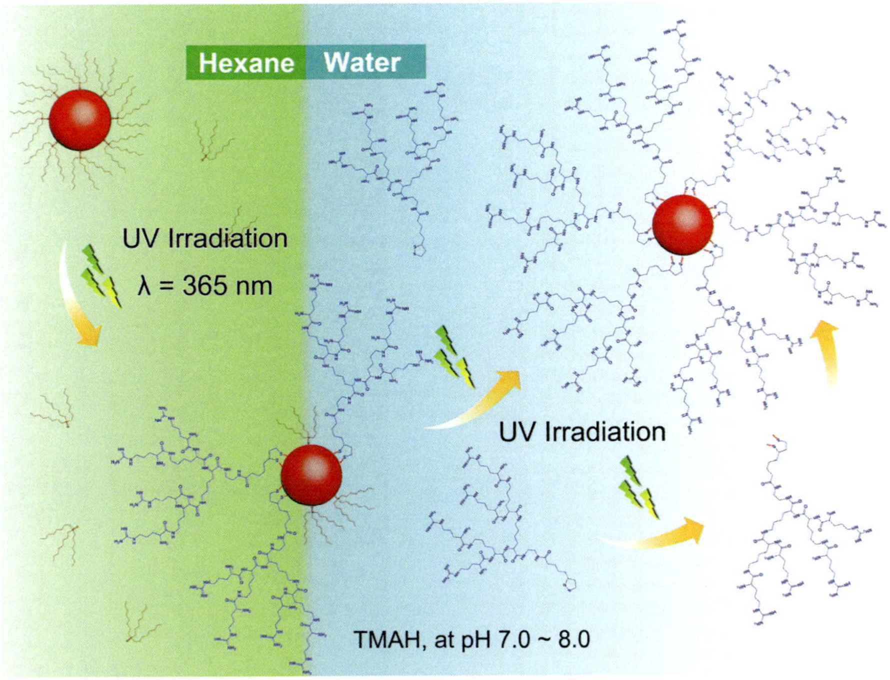


**Fig. 4** Illustration for self-assembly of ARNHs

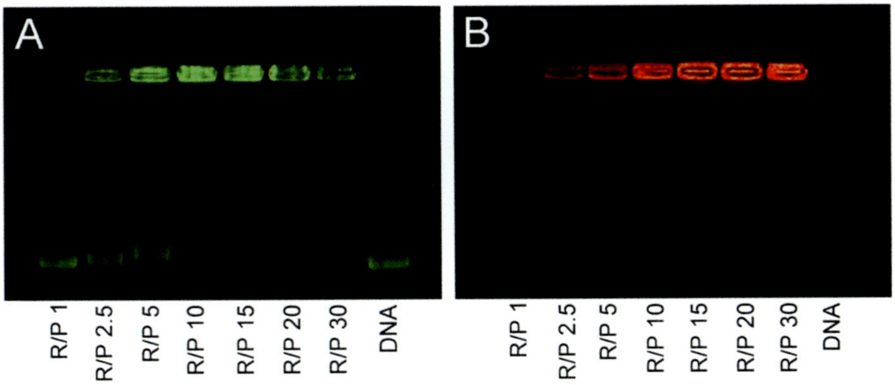


**Fig. 5** Gel electrophoresis assay of ARNHS/DNA for fluorescence images of (**a**) ARNHs and (**b**) DNA

DNA binding ability of ARNHs was determined by agarose gel retention assay. The ARNHs was showed with red fluorescence and DNA with green fluorescence. As shown in Fig. 5, the DNA was completely retarded by ARNHs at the R/P ratio of 10, indicating the appropriate DNA binding ability of ARNHs.

## 3.4 Characterizations of ARNHs

### 3.4.1 Thermal Gravimetric Analysis

Analysize the composite ratio of ARNHs by thermal gravimetric analysis under flowing air with a ramp rate of 10 °C $min^{-1}$ as shown in Fig. 6.

As shown in Fig. 6, TGA curves revealed that the PDs content in ARNHs was 40.51 wt%. It suggested that abundant PDs are attached into a single ARNH. And functional groups of low-generation PDs were amplified on the surface of ARNHs via supramolecular effects.

### 3.4.2 Size and Zeta Potential of ARNHs and ARNHS/DNA Complex

1. Disperse ARNHs in water and filter by 0.02 μm filter to prepare 2.0 mg $mL^{-1}$ solution.
2. Mix ARNHs solution and DNA at 20 arginine/P (A/P) ratio and incubate at room temperature for 30 min.
3. Measure the ARNHs and ARNHs/DNA solution by a dynamic light scattering (DLS, NANO ZSPO, Malvern) at 25 °C three times as shown in Fig. 7.

### 3.4.3 Morphology of ARNHS/DNA Complex

1. Prepare ARNHS/DNA complex as "Size and Zeta Potential of ARNHs and ARNHS/DNA Complex."
2. Drop the ARNHS/DNA complex on copper grid and adsorb for 5 min.
3. Remove the excess solution by filter paper. Dry the copper grid with infrared lamp.
4. Image ARNHS/DNA complex by TEM to analyze the nanostructure (Fig. 8).

The TEM results revealed that the ARNHs with positive charge and the DNA with negative charge could assemble into a compact nanoparticle with an average size of 143.33 ± 8.79 nm in aqueous solution (Figs. 7 and 8).

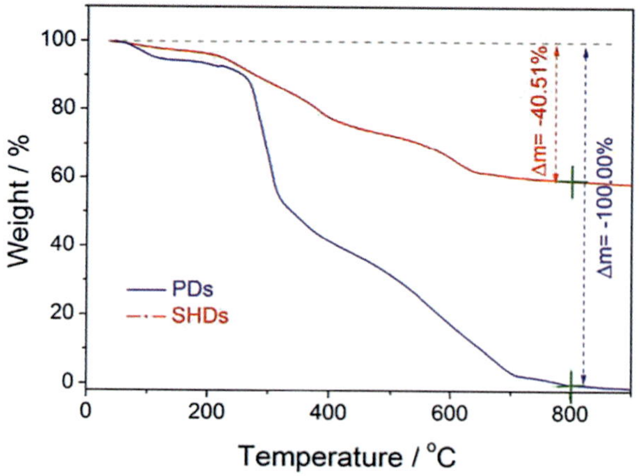


**Fig. 6** TGA profiles of PDs and ARNHs

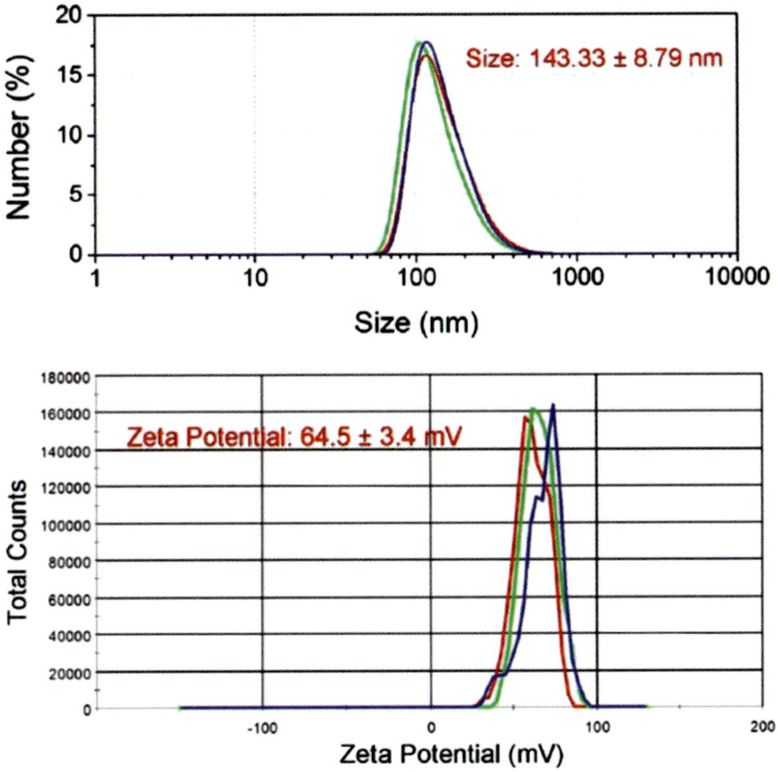


**Fig. 7** Size and zeta potential of ARNHS/DNA complex

**Fig. 8** TEM images of ARNHS/DNA complex

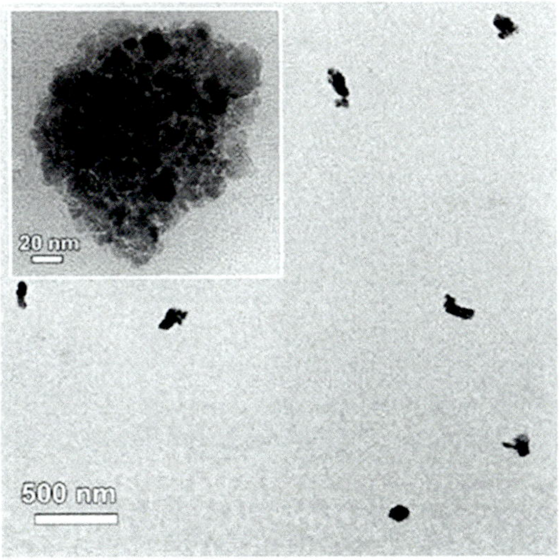

## 3.5 Investigation of In Vitro Gene Transfection Effect

### 3.5.1 In Vitro Luciferase Activity Assay

1. Cell Culture

   HepG2 cells were cultured DMEM media with 10% FBS, 100 U/mL streptomycin, and 100 U/mL penicillin at 37 °C in 5% $CO_2$ humidified atmosphere.
2. Seed HepG2 cells ($1.2 \times 10^4$ cells/well) in 96-well plates and culture for 24 h. Add ARNH/pGL-3 (pGL-3 DNA: 200 ng) complex with R/P ratio of 2.5, 5, 10, 15, and 20.
3. After 48 h, remove the media and wash with PBS three times. Add 70 μL reporter lysis buffer to each well with multigelation. Mix 20 μL cell lysates and 50 μL luciferase substrates, then detect light emission by microplate reader.
4. Determine protein concentration of the cell extracts by BCA protein assay kit.
5. Relative light units (RLU) were calculated as follows: RLU = light emission value/total protein concentrates. The results are shown in Fig. 9.

pGL3-Luc delivery efficiency was quantitatively analyzed in HepG2 cell line. The results indicated that the supramolecular strategy could fabricate highly efficient gene delivery system by low-generation PDs. The gene transfection efficiency of pGL3-Luc was enhanced approximately 50,000-fold as compared to single PDs at the same R/P ratio of 20. In the presence of FBS, luciferase gene transfection of ARNHs (R/P 20) was much more efficient than that of PEI, which is still 30-fold higher than that of PEI/pGL3 complex without FBS. Such an excellent transfection efficiency should take advantage of the dendritic peptide coatings with plenty of arginine groups which simulate the components and structure of viral capsids.

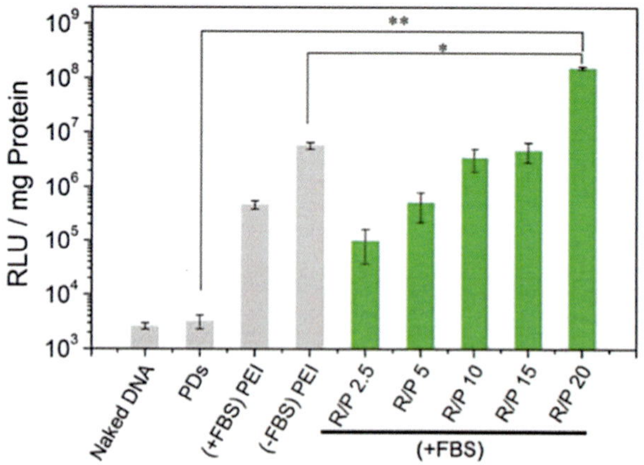


**Fig. 9** Luciferase expression in HepG2 cells after treatment with ARNH/pGL3 complex at different R/P ratios

### 3.5.2 GFP Expression

1. Seed HepG2 cells (1 × $10^5$ cells/well) in 12-well plate and culture for 24 h.
2. Treat the cells with ARNH/pEGFP (2 μg pEGFP DNA) complex at different ratio of 2.5, 5, 10, 15, and 20 for 48 h.
3. Wash the cells 3 times and image with fluorescence microscopy (Leica DMI4000B).
4. Treat HepG2 cells as above. Collect and resuspend in PBS. Measure the GFP fluorescence by FACS with 488 nm excitation. PEI/DNA complex with N/P ratio of 10 was set as positive control.

As shown in Fig. 10, ~75% of HepG2 cells were internalized ARNH/pEGFP complex at 12 h, but only ~15% cells expressed GFP (Fig. 10a). And the mean fluorescence intensity (MFI) of ARNHs was much higher than GFP. At 12 h, ARNH-positive cells and MFI of ARNHs kept stable to 60 h. Notably, the GFP-positive cells and MFI of GFP increased over three- and fivefold, respectively. Afterward, GFP expression increased along with the amount of ARNHs.

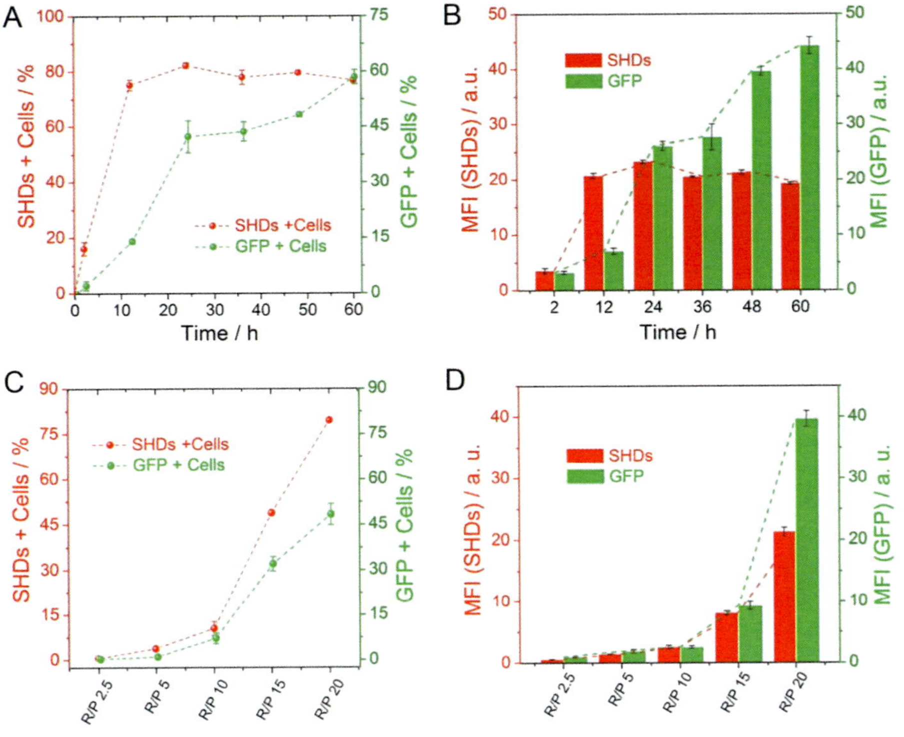


**Fig. 10** (**a**) ARNHs and GFP-positive cells; (**b**) MFI of ARNHs and GFP after incubation for different times; (**c**) ARNHs and GFP-positive cells; and (**d**) MFI of ARNHs and GFP after incubation with ARNH/pEGFP complex at different R/P ratios

## 3.6 Cytotoxicity and Intracellular Tracking in HepG2 Cells

### 3.6.1 Cytotoxicity of ARNHS/DNA Complex

1. Seed HepG2 cells in 96-well plate and culture 24 h. Replace the culture media with ARNHS/DNA complex solutions at different R/P ratios and incubate for 48 h.
2. Remove the media and wash the cells with PBS 3 times.
3. Prepare CCK-8 working solution by ten times dilution with fresh culture media. Add 100 μL CCK-8 working solution and incubate for 2 h.
4. Measure absorbance (OD) of each well at 450 nm. Calculate cell viability with the following formula:

$$\text{Cell viability} = \left(OD_{\text{sample}} - OD_{blank}\right) / \left(OD_{control} - OD_{blank}\right) \times 100\%$$

$OD_{\text{sample}}$: OD value of treated cells; $OD_{\text{control}}$: OD value of untreated cells; and $OD_{\text{blank}}$: OD value of CCK-8 solution.

As shown in Fig. 11, there was no obvious cytotoxicity to HepG2 cells of ARNHs (R/P 2.5 to R/P 20). However, the PEI/DNA showed significant cytotoxicity (less than ~50% cell survival) for the inherent cytotoxicity of cationic polymer.

### 3.6.2 Intracellular Tracking

1. Seed HepG2 cells ($1 \times 10^4$ cells) in glass-bottomed dishes and culture for 24 h.
2. Treat the cells with ARNH/pGL-3 (300 ng/dish, R/P is 20) containing 33% Cy5-labeled pGL-3 DNA for 1, 3, 8, and 18 h.
3. Remove the media and wash the cells with PBS three times.
4. Prepare a lysosome-staining solution: 75 nM LysoTracker Blue DND-22 in culture media. Stain the cells in 37 °C incubator for 1 h. Wash the cells with PBS three times.

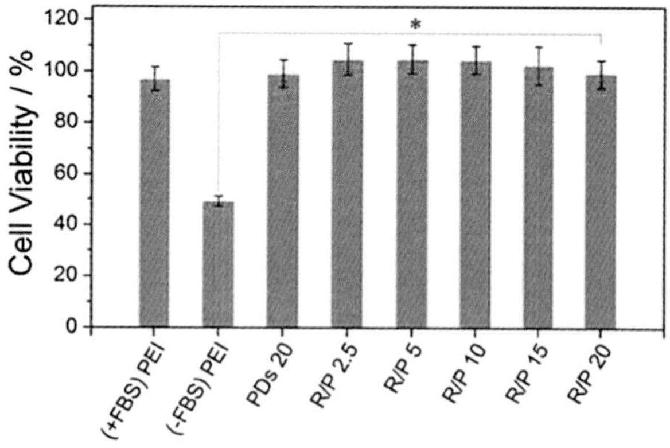


**Fig. 11** Cell viability of HepG2 cells after treatment with PEI and ARNHS/DNA complex

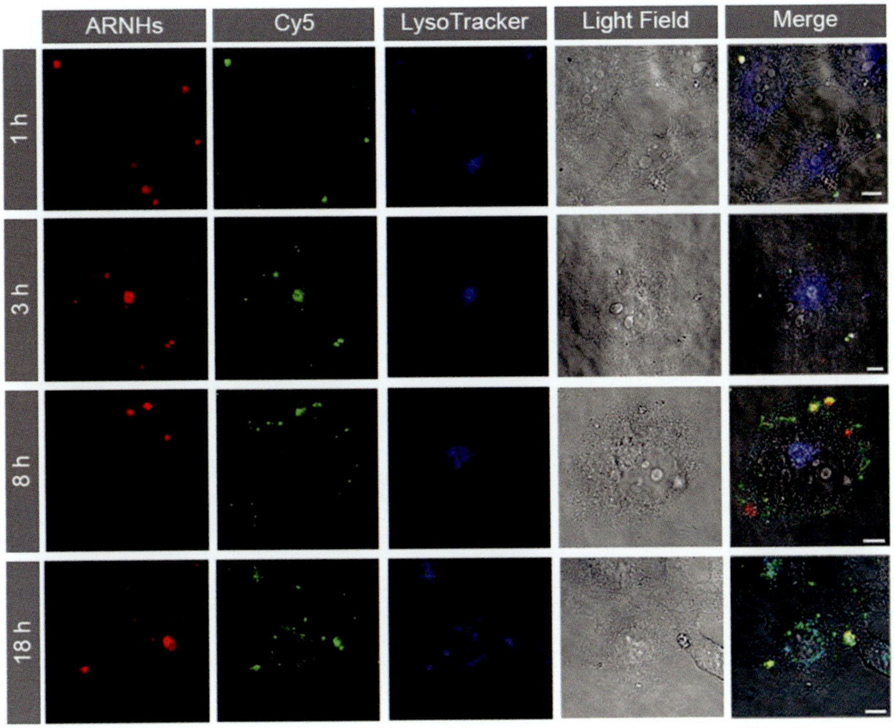


**Fig. 12** CLSM images of HepG2 cells after incubation with ARNHS/DNA complex at different time points (Red: ARNHs, Green: Cy5-labeled DNA, and Blue: lysosome). The scale bars correspond to 10 μm

5. Image the cells by confocal laser-scanning microscope (Leica TCS SP5). Condition: $\lambda_{ex} = 488$ nm for QDs; $\lambda_{ex} = 633$ nm for Cy5 (Fig. 12).

The intracellular delivery pathway of ARNHs/DNA complex was revealed by CLSM. At first, ARNHS/DNA complex was located on the cell membrane and internalized into cell quickly. After incubation for 3 h, the ARNHS/DNA complex was located in subcellular organelles (endosomes and lysosomes). At 8 h incubation, ARNHs and DNA escaped from lysosomes as the separation of blue and red/green fluorescence. Finally, DNA was distributed into the nucleus.

### 3.6.3 Live Cell Imaging System (LCIS) Observation

1. Seed cells ($1 \times 10^4$ cells) glass-bottomed dishes and culture for 24 h.
2. Treat the cells with ARNHS/DNA complex. Observe in real time the cells by LCIS and culture at 37 °C with 5% $CO_2$ humidified atmosphere for 1 day. Capture a fluorescence image every 5 min.

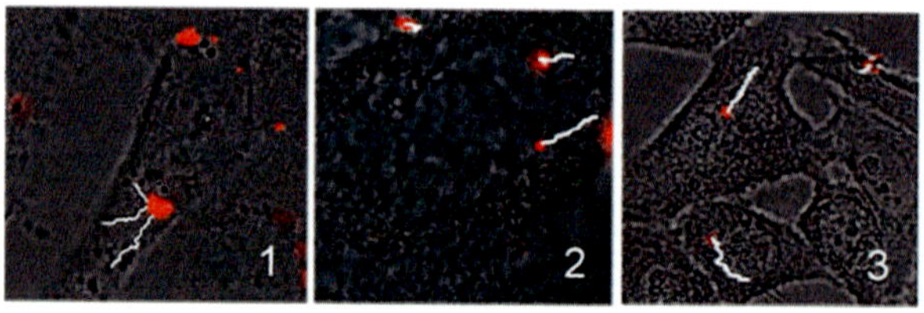


**Fig. 13** LCIS imaging of ARNHS/DNA complex in HepG2 cells (white lines: motion trails of ARNHS/DNA complex)

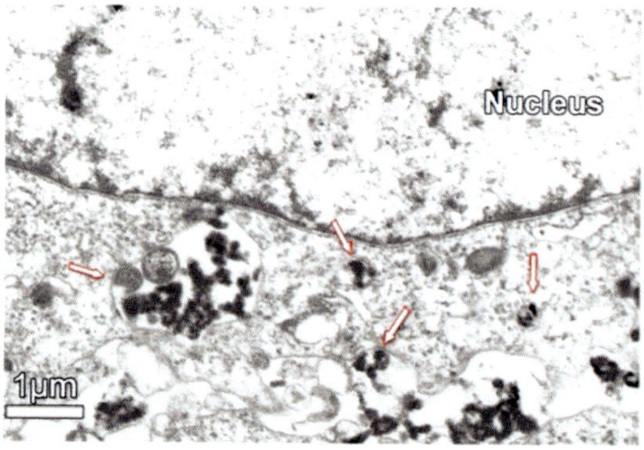


**Fig. 14** TEM image of HepG2 cells incubation with ARNHS/DNA complex

HepG2 cells' treatment with ARNHS/DNA complex was imaged in real time by LCIS (Fig. 13). ARNHS/DNA complex was delivered into cell and entrapped into endosome or lysosome. The motion trails of ARNHS/DNA complex indicated the complex trend to move toward nucleus and located around the nucleus within 4 h.

### 3.6.4 Transmission Electron Microscope Imaging

1. Seed HepG2 cells in 6-well plate and culture for 24 h.
2. Remove the culture media. Treat the cells with ARNHS/DNA complex for 24 h.
3. Collect the cells and fix in 0.5% glutaraldehyde for 15 min at 4 °C. Centrifuge the cells at $1 \times 10^4$ rpm for 15 min. Treat the cells with 3% glutaraldehyde for 15 min at 4 °C.
4. Dehydrate by 30%, 50%, 70%, 90%, and 100% acetone (5 min for each step).
5. Embed the cells in Epon812 and cut into sections. Stain the sections with lead citrate and uranyl acetate.
6. Image the cells with transmission electron microscope (Hitachi H-600IV).

As shown in Fig. 14, intracellular distribution of ARNHS/DNA complex was analyzed by TEM. ARNHS/DNA complex was entrapped into multivesicular structures such as endosomes and lysosomes, and some of the complex was located in the cytosol.

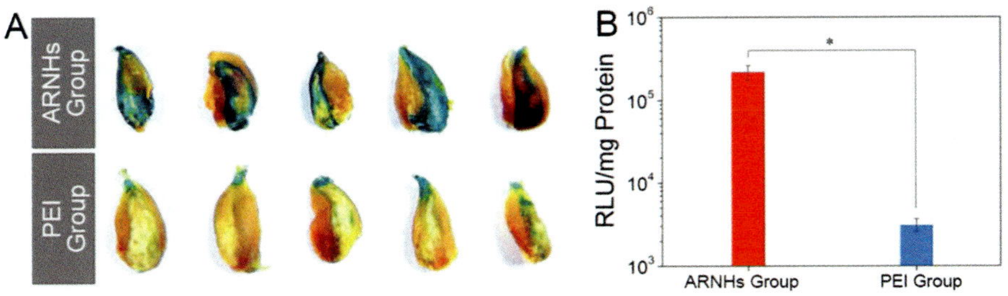


**Fig. 15** (**a**) pCMV-β-gal expression, and (**b**) luciferase activity in mouse muscles after administration with ARNHS/DNA complex and PEI complex for 4 days

## 3.7 In Vivo Gene Transfection

### 3.7.1 Tumor Model

1. House BALB/c nude mice under standard condition.
2. Inject subcutaneously 100 μL HepG2 cell suspension ($3 \times 10^6$ cells in PBS) on the right back area.

### 3.7.2 pCMV-β-gal Transfection in Mouse Muscles

1. Inject ARNH/pCMV-β-gal complex (R/P 20, 10 μg of pCMV-β-gal) into the tibialis anterior muscles of Balb/c mice.
2. Harvest the muscles at 4 days postinjection. Measure the β-galactosidase expression by the β-galactosidase reporter gene assay kit.

### 3.7.3 Luciferase Activity in Mouse Muscles

1. Inject ARNH/pGL3-Luc complex (R/P 20, 10 μg of pGL3-Luc) into the tibialis anterior muscles of Balb/c mice.
2. Harvest the muscles at 4 days postinjection. Quantify the gene transfection efficiency by luciferase activity in RLU/mg protein.

pCMV-β-gal expression and luciferase assays were used to investigate in vivo gene transfection of ARNHs. The muscular tissue turns into blue after β-galactosidase expression. Large dark blue was observed after ARNHs/DNA was administrated, indicating the high-gene transfection efficiency of ARNHs (Fig. 15a). In contrast, blue color was barely observed in PEI group. Similarly, ARNHs mediated optimal pGL3-Luc transfection ($2.2 \times 10^5$ RLU/mg of protein, R/P 20) with much higher luciferase activity than that of PEI ($3.1 \times 10^3$ RLU/mg of protein) with 70-fold increase.

### 3.7.4 p-53 Gene Expression in Tumor Tissues

1. Inject ARNH/pCMV-p53 complex (R/P 20, 20 μg pCMV-p53) into tumors of HepG2 tumor-bearing nude mice.
2. After 2 days, harvest tumor tissues and lyse. Quantify the total protein by BCA assay kit.
3. Analyze the p-53 content by western blot assay as shown in Fig. 16.

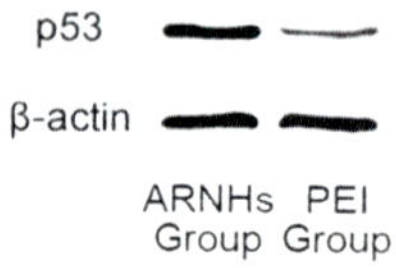


**Fig. 16** p53 expression in HepG2 tumor tissue

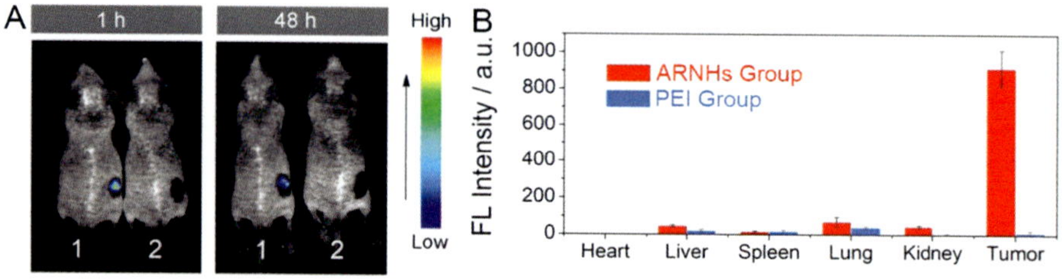


**Fig. 17** (**a**) Fluorescence images of HepG2 tumor-bearing mice administration with ARNHs/DNA and PEI/DNA; (**b**) fluorescence intensity of organs and tumor tissues

p53 as an important tumor-suppression gene was used to investigate the transfection efficiency of ARNHs for therapeutic gene. As shown in the western blot analysis, significant higher expression of p53 protein was detected in the HepG2 tumor tissue with treatment of ARNHs/pCMV-p53 complex versus the PEI/pCMV-p53 complex.

### 3.8 In Vivo Imaging

1. Inject ARNHS/DNA complex (R/P 20) into muscle or a tumor xenograft.
2. Anesthetize the mice and image at 1 and 48 h with in vivo fluorescence imaging system (excitation: 450 nm, emission: 605 nm).
3. Measure the fluorescence intensity of organs by *in vivo* fluorescence imaging system.

The *in vivo* fluorescence images revealed ARNHs could be located in tumor tissue generating significant fluorescence signal even at 48 h (Fig. 17a). The fluorescence intensity of organs indicated most of the ARNHs distributed in tumor tissue (Fig. 17b).

## 4 Discussion

The protocol presents a supramolecular dendritic system based on arginine-rich nanohybrids for efficient *in vitro*- and *in vivo*-visible gene delivery. This strategy successfully drives the assembly of peptide dendrons onto inorganic nanoparticles to generate multifunctional nanohybrids. The arginine-rich corona of ARNHs contributes to strong DNA binding, high internalization, intracellular delivery, and satisfactory gene transfection. This hybrid tactic endows unique features to ARNHs for intracellular tracking and *in vivo* imaging. Following this strategy, many multifunctional supramolecular nanohybrids can be fabricated for biomedical applications, such as arginine-rich gold nanorods and arginine-rich upconversion nanoparticles. In summary, the sophisticated design of supramolecular nanohybrids holds great potential in the development of advanced gene delivery systems.

## References

Li Y, Zhang X, Zhang Z, Wu H, Xu X, Zhongwei G (2018) Tumor-adapting and tumor-remodeling AuNR@dendrimer-assembly nanohybrids overcome impermeable multidrug-resistant cancer. Mater Horiz 5:1047–1057

Pack DW, Hoffman AS, Pun S, Stayton PS (2005) Design and development of polymers for gene delivery. Nat Rev Drug Discov 4:581–593

Xu X, Yuan H, Chang J, He B, Zhongwei G (2012) Cooperative hierarchical self-assembly of peptide dendrimers and linear polypeptides into nanoarchitectures mimicking viral capsids. Angew Chem Int Ed 51:3130–3133

Xu X, Jian Y, Li Y, Zhang X, Zhaoxu T, Zhongwei G (2014) Bio-inspired supramolecular hybrid dendrimers self-assembled from low-generation peptide dendrons for highly efficient gene delivery and biological tracking. ACS Nano 8:9255–9264

Xu X, Jiang Q, Zhang X, Yu N, Zhang Z, Li Y, Cheng G, Zhongwei G (2015) Virus-inspired mimics: self-assembly of dendritic lipopeptides into arginine-rich nanovectors for improving gene delivery. J Mater Chem B 3:7006–7010

Yang X, Zhao N, Fu-Jian X (2014) Biocleavable graphene oxide based-nanohybrids synthesized via ATRP for gene/drug delivery. Nanoscale 6:6141–6150

Zhang X, Zhang Z, Xu X, Li Y, Li Y, Jian Y, Zhongwei G (2015a) Bioinspired therapeutic dendrimers as efficient peptide drugs based on supramolecular interactions for tumor inhibition. Angew Chem Int Ed 54:4289–4294

Zhang Z, Zhang X, Xu X, Li Y, Li Y, Zhong D, He Y, Zhongwei G (2015b) Virus-inspired mimics based on dendritic lipopeptides for efficient tumor-specific infection and systemic drug delivery. Adv Funct Mater 25:5250–5260

Zhang X, Li Y, Hu C, Wu Y, Zhong D, Xu X, Zhongwei G (2018a) Engineering anticancer amphipathic peptide-dendronized compounds for highly-efficient plasma/organelle membrane perturbation and multidrug resistance reversal. ACS Appl Mater Interfaces 10:30952–30962

Zhang X, Xu X, Li Y, Hu C, Zhang Z, Zhongwei G (2018b) Virion-like membrane-breaking nanoparticles with tumor-activated cell-and-tissue dual-penetration conquer impermeable cancer. Adv Mater 30:1707240

Zhao H, Ding R, Zhao X, Li Y, Liangliang Q, Pei H, Yildirimer L, Wu Z, Zhang W (2017) Graphene-based nanomaterials for drug and/or gene delivery, bioimaging, and tissue engineering. Drug Discov Today 22:1302–1317

Zhao N, Yan L, Zhao X, Chen X, Li A, Zheng D, Zhou X, Dai X, Fu-Jian X (2019) Versatile types of organic/inorganic nanohybrids: from strategic design to biomedical applications. Chem Rev 119:1666–1762

# Bioinspired Fabrication of Peptide-Based Capsid-Like Nanoparticles for Gene Delivery

# 11

Yachao Li and Xianghui Xu

## Contents



**Abstract**

Biomimetic nanomaterials have shown great potentials for improving therapeutic delivery. This chapter describes a novel macromolecular and supramolecular strategy to drive the assembly of peptide dendrimers and polypeptides into capsid-like nanoparticles (CLNs) for gene delivery. Low-generation poly (L-lysine) dendrimers and glutamic acid-functionalized polypeptides can assemble into dendritic supramolecular amphiphiles via supramolecular interactions in a common solvent. These supramolecular amphiphiles are able to further assemble in well-defined nanoparticles in an aqueous solution. These nanoparticles

Y. Li · X. Xu (✉)
Department of Pharmacy, College of Biology, Hunan University, Changsha, Hunan, China
e-mail: xianghui.xu@hnu.edu.cn





H. Tian and X. Chen (eds.), *Gene Delivery*, Biomaterial Engineering,
https://doi.org/10.1007/978-981-16-5419-0_2

have capsid-like nanostructures, ordered secondary structures and biofunctions for molecular delivery. CLNs are capable of serving as biocompatible, biosafety, and efficient gene vectors. The following section will describe the typical protocols for fabricating the peptide-based capsid-like nanoparticles for gene delivery.

**Keywords**

Capsid-like nanoparticles · Hierarchical self-assembly · Peptide dendrimers · Gene delivery

## 1 Overview

Over the past decades, wonderful natural systems have constantly stimulated scientists to create advanced materials through mimicking biological structures and functions (Wegst et al. 2015; Zan and Wu 2016). Virus, as one of the simplest organisms in nature, have been widely developed as virus-based vectors for therapeutic delivery owing to their robust infection on host cells (Davidson and Breakefield 2003; Kotterman and Schaffer 2014; Li and Xu 2020). However, the adverse events of virus-based delivery systems hamper their biomedical applications, such as toxicity, immunogenicity, and mutagenesis. Many researchers devote to fabricating artificial viruses for efficient and safe therapeutic delivery (Mastrobattista et al. 2006; Pack et al. 2005; Li and Xu 2020; Zhang et al. 2018a, b). With modern molecular and supramolecular engineering, the dream of synthesizing artificial viruses with man-made building blocks is becoming a reality.

Among many artificial building blocks, peptide dendrimers are considered as an excellent macromolecule mimicking the natural proteins because of their biomimetic components, precise molecular structure, globular shape, and 3D nanostructures (Li et al. 2016; Xu et al. 2012, 2014a, b, 2015; Zhang et al. 2015). And viral capsids are often made up of globular proteins, which provides outstanding biological functions on protecting and delivering viral genome. For these reasons, supramolecular assembly of peptide dendrimers is expected to construct capsid-like nanostructure and biofunctions (Li et al. 2016; Xu et al. 2015; Zhang et al. 2018b). However, globular dendrimers having same peripheral groups are always monodisperse in the water, and how to drive assembly of dendrimers into well-organized nanostructures remains a great challenge. This section introduces a new approach to fabricate capsid-like nanoparticles (CLNs) through supramolecular construction of peptide dendrimers. Low-generation (Generation 2), biocompatible and affordable poly(L-lysine) dendrimers (G2-Lys) are synthesized for capsid construction. In the first step, hydrophobic and end-functionalized polypeptides with carboxyl groups are utilized to first assemble with amino groups on G2-Lys, forming dendritic supramolecular amphiphiles via electrostatic interactions and/or hydrogen bond. When these supramolecular amphiphiles are added into an aqueous solution, these amphiphiles can assemble into peptide-based CLNs with polypeptide-based hydrophobic cores and G2-Lys-based shells. The CLNs possess well-defined and hierarchical nanostructures, and their size and morphology can be regulated by ratios between polypeptides and G2-Lys. The well-organized secondary structures of CLNs are also confirmed by circular dichroism spectrum. CLNs provide inner core to harbor hydrophobic drugs, and supramolecular aggregation of low-generation peptide dendrimers generates high performance for nucleic acid condensation via non-covalent interactions. Based on inherent properties of peptide-based materials, supramolecular interactions within supramolecular amphiphiles would disappear when pH condition is close to isoelectric point (pI) of polypeptides or G2-Lys, leading to disassembly of CLNs for molecular release. CLNs show high delivery efficiency of plasmid DNA, which is comparable to positive PEI 25 K. Altogether, CLNs show great potentials as biocompatible, biosafety, and efficient bioinspired nanocarriers for gene delivery.

## 2 Materials

### 2.1 Synthesis of Poly(L-lysine) Dendrimers

1. (3-aminopropyl)-triethoxysilane
2. Hydrochloric acid (HCl)
3. O(7Azabenzotriazol1yl) N,N,N′,N′-tetramethyluronium hexafluorophosphate (HBTU)
4. 1-Hydroxybenzotriazole (HOBt)
5. Dimethylformamide (DMF)
6. Boc-Lys(Boc)-OH
7. N,N-diisopropylethylamine (DIPEA)
8. Sodium bicarbonate ($NaHCO_3$)
9. Sodium bisulfate ($NaHSO_4$)
10. Sodium chloride (NaCl)
11. Magnesium sulfate ($MgSO_4$)
12. Trifluoroacetic acid (TFA)
13. Acetonitrile
14. Ninhydrin staining solution (0.5% w/v ethanol solution)
15. Thin layer chromatography (TLC) plate
16. Ultraviolet analyzer

### 2.2 Synthesis of Poly(L-leucine)

1. Cbz-Leu
2. Tetrahydrofuran (THF)
3. Thionyl chloride ($SOCl_2$)
4. Anhydrous hexane
5. Glutamic acid

### 2.3 Preparation of Capsid-Like Nanoparticles (CLNs)

1. N,N-Dimethylformamide (DMF)
2. Dynamic light scattering (DLS)
3. High precision pH meter
4. Atomic force microscope (AFM)
5. Transmission electron microscope (TEM)
6. Scanning electron microscopy (SEM)
7. Carbon film coated copper grids
8. Silicon wafer
9. Mica plate

### 2.4 pH Responsive Properties of CLNs

1. Pyrene
2. Acetone
3. Sodium carbonate ($Na_2CO_3$)
4. $D_2O$
5. $CF_3COOD$
6. Nuclear magnetic resonance (NMR) spectrometer
7. High precision pH meter
8. Fluorescence spectrophotometer
9. AFM
10. TEM

### 2.5 In Vitro Gene Condensation of CLNs

1. Luciferase encoding plasmid DNA
2. Diethyl pyrocarbonate (DEPC) water
3. Agarose
4. Tris-acetate (TAE)
5. Gel loading buffer
6. GelView™
7. UV illuminator

### 2.6 In Vitro Gene Transfection Investigation of CLNs

1. HEK 293 cells
2. Dulbecco's Modified Eagle (DMEM) media
3. Fetal bovine serum (FBS)
4. Penicillin-Streptomycin solution (10,000 U/mL)
5. DEPC water

6. Inverted fluorescence microscopy
7. Flow cytometry

# 3 Protocol

## 3.1 Synthesis of Poly(L-lysine) Dendrimers

### 3.1.1 Synthesis of Octa(3-Aminopropyl)Silsesquioxane (OAS) Hydrochloride

1. Fig. 1 shows the synthetic route of poly(L-lysine) dendrimers. Dissolve (3-aminopropyl)-triethoxysilane (13.28 g, 60 mmol) and hydrochloric acid (12 M, 30 mL) in methanol and stir for 3 days.
2. Filter the rude product and recrystallize in hot methanol to obtain white solid.

### 3.1.2 Synthesis of Generation 2 OAS-poly(L-lysine) (G2-Lys) Dendrimers

1. Dissolve OAS (1.76 g, 2 mmol), HBTU (9.10 g, 24 mmol), and HOBt (3.24 g, 24 mmol) in DMF and stir at ice bath and $N_2$ atmosphere.
2. Add Boc-Lys(Boc)-OH (11.09 g, 32 mmol) DMF solution and DIPEA (10.6 mL, 64 mmol) into the reaction mixture and stir for 3 days at room temperature.
3. Remove DMF by rotary-evaporator and add chloroform to the mixture. Wash the mixture with saturated $NaHCO_3$, $NaHSO_4$, and NaCl solution several times. Analyze the solution by TLC plate with ultraviolet analyzer and ninhydrin staining.
4. Dry the solution with $MgSO_4$ overnight. Remove chloroform and recrystallize in cold acetonitrile to obtain a white solid G1-Lys-$Boc_{16}$.
5. Treat G1-Lys-$Boc_{16}$ with TFA (10 equiv. to Boc groups, 80% DCM solution) in ice bath at $N_2$ atmosphere for 30 min. Remove the ice bath and react at room temperature for 12 h to remove Boc groups.
6. Remove the solvent and TFA by rotary-evaporator. Precipitate the mixture with anhydrous diethyl ether for three times to obtain solid G1-Lys.
7. Dissolve G1-Lys (3.22 g, 2 mmol), HBTU (18.20 g, 48 mmol), HOBT (6.49 g, 48 mmol), and Boc-Lys(Boc)-OH (22.17 g, 64 mmol) in DMF and protect with $N_2$. Stir the mixture at ice bath.
8. Add DIPEA into the solution and stir at ice bath for 30 min. Remove the ice bath and react for 72 h.
9. Concentrate the solution by rotary-evaporator. Dissolve the mixture with chloroform.
10. Wash the solution with saturated $NaHCO_3$, $NaHSO_4$, and NaCl solution several times. Analyze the solution by TLC plate with ultraviolet analyzer and ninhydrin staining.
11. Remove the chloroform. Precipitate in cold acetonitrile to obtain solid G2-Lys-$Boc_{32}$.

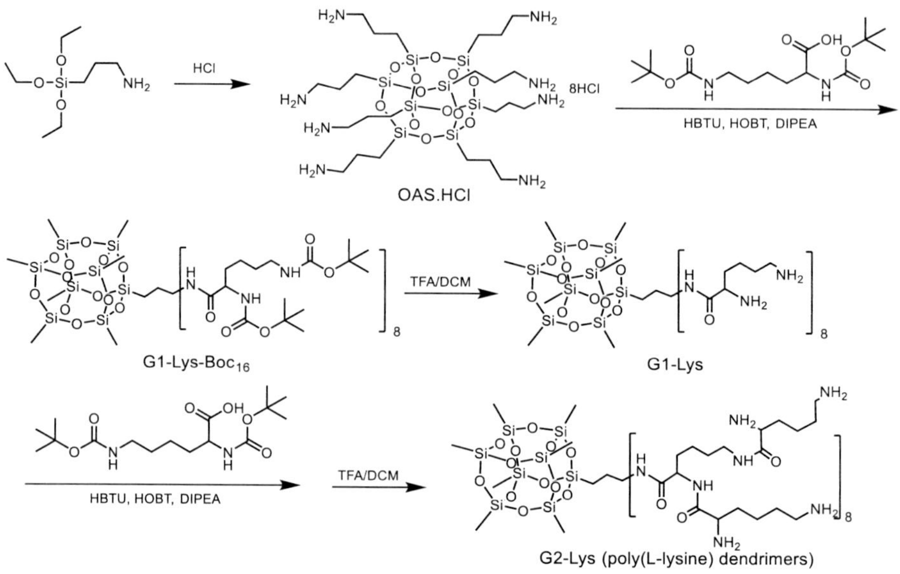


**Fig. 1** Synthesis route of poly(L-lysine) dendrimers

12. Treat the G2-Lys-Boc$_{32}$ with TFA (10 equiv. to Boc groups, 80% DCM solution) at ice bath for 30 min. Remove the ice bath and stir for 12 h to deprotect the Boc groups.
13. Remove TFA and DCM by rotary-evaporator. Precipitate the residue by anhydrous diethyl ether for three times.
14. Dissolve the precipitate in water and purify with dialysis membrane (MWCO 2000). Afterwards, freeze-dry the solution to obtain solid G2-Lys (Fig. 1).

## 3.2 Synthesis of Poly(L-leucine)

### 3.2.1 Synthesis of L-leucine N-carboxyanhydride (NCA-Leu)

1. Fig. 2 shows the synthetic route of poly(L-leucine). Dissolve Cbz-Leu in THF at 40 °C in $N_2$ atmosphere. Add $SOCl_2$ into the mixture and stir for 4 h.
2. Add excess anhydrous hexane into the reaction mixture and keep at 40 °C for 12 h.
3. Filter to obtain the white precipitate. And dissolve the precipitate in anhydrous ethyl acetate and recrystallize with hexane to obtain NCA-Leu.

### 3.2.2 Synthesis of Poly(L-leucine) with Terminal Group of Double Carboxyl

1. Dissolve glutamic acid (initiator) in DMF with anhydrous conditions in $N_2$ atmosphere.

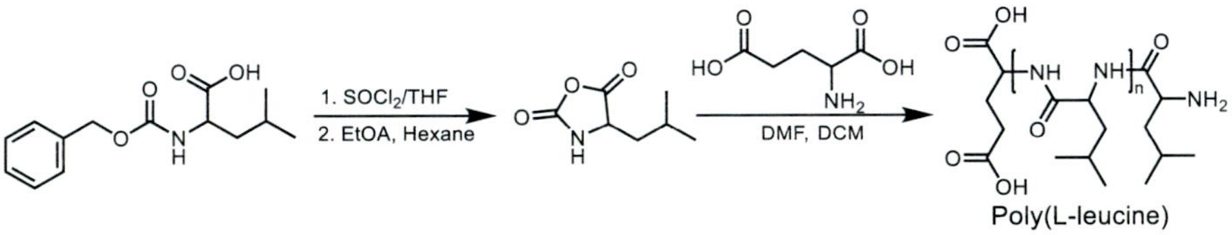


**Fig. 2** Synthesis route of poly(L-leucine)

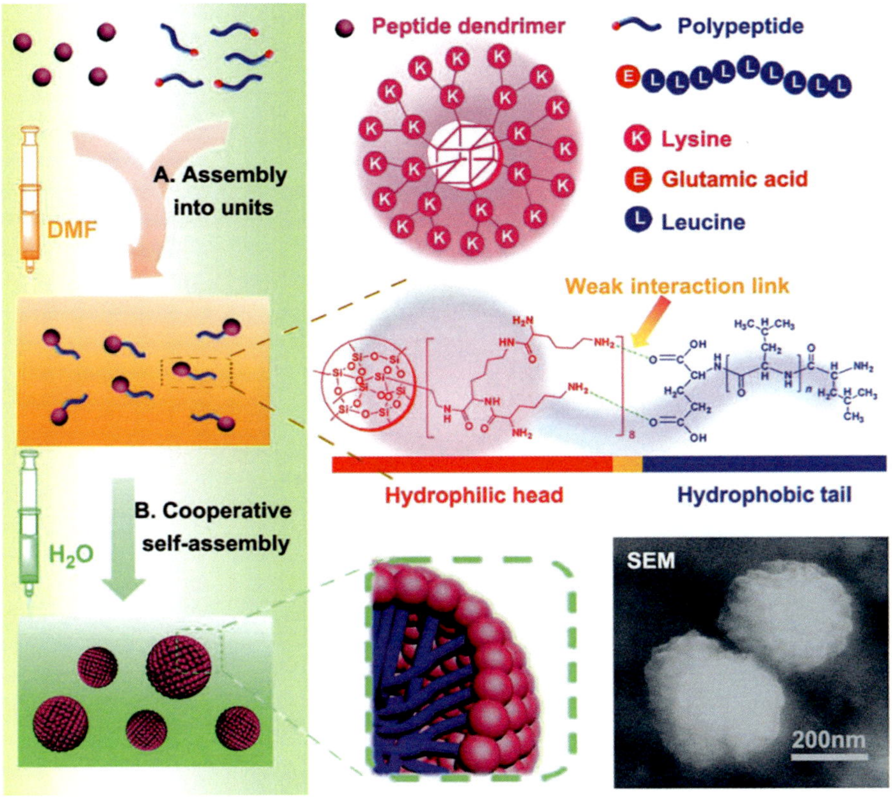


**Fig. 3** Scheme of self-assembly of peptide dendrimers and polypeptides

2. Add NCA-Leu in DCM solution into the reaction and stir for 48 h at room temperature.
3. Purify the poly(L-leucine) with MeOH, $H_2O$, and DCM in order (Fig. 2).

## 3.3 Preparation of Capsid-Like Nanoparticles (CLNs)

1. Dissolve poly(L-lysine) dendrimers and poly(L-leucine) in DMF (common solution) with appropriate concentrations, respectively (Fig. 3).

2. Mix the poly(L-lysine) dendrimers and poly(L-leucine) solution with different poly(L-lysine) dendrimers and poly(L-leucine) ratios of 50:1, 40:1, 30:1, 20:1, 10:1, 5:1, 1:1, 1:5, and 1:10.
3. Determine the average size of CLNs by DLS, and observe their nanostructures by TEM.
4. Drop the mix solution into water (poor solvent) dropwise to self-assemble into nanoparticles.
5. Dialyze and freeze-dry the solution to obtain solid CLNs.
6. Drop the CLNs solution (50 μL) on carbon film coated copper grids and adsorb for 5 min. Remove the excess solution by filter paper and dry with infrared lamp. Observe the copper grid with TEM.
7. Drop the CLNs solution (10 μL) on mica plate. Dry the solution at room temperature. Then observe the nanostructure of CLNs by AFM.
8. Drop the CLNs solution (10 μL) on silicon wafer. Dry the solution at room temperature. Then observe the nanostructure of CLNs by SEM.

The cooperative self-assembly of CLNs were investigated. In the TEM image (Fig. 4a), CLNs demonstrate viral capsid-like nanostructure with a size of about 250 nm. Also, many small spherical dendrimers could be observed on the shell of CLNs. Consistently, the AFM and SEM images showed the similar nanostructure with TEM image. As shown in Fig. 4c, the zoom images (c1 and c2) exhibited the detailed surface pattern of CLNs, which were similar to those of viral capsids.

As shown in Fig. 5, the nanostructure of CLNs could be controlled by changing the concentration and ratios between peptide dendrimers and linear polypeptides. With the ratio of peptide dendrimers to linear polypeptides decreased from 10:1 to 1:5 (w/w, 100 μg $mL^{-1}$ totally), the size of nanoparticles changed from 300 to 800 nm. In addition, the nanostructure of CLNs varied from spherical to fusiform. Figure 4d shows the size of the nanoparticles at different total concentrations. At the same concentration, the nanoparticles size increased along with the increasing portion of linear polypeptide. The nanoparticles size was increased at a higher concentration.

## 3.4 pH Responsive Properties of CLNs

### 3.4.1 Fluorescence Analysis

1. Prepare pyrene acetone solution (3 mg $mL^{-1}$). Added 1 mL pyrene solution into 500 mL volumetric flask. After the solution dried, add 500 mL water into the volumetric flask to prepare 6 mg $L^{-1}$ pyrene solution. Treat the solution with ultrasound to disperse pyrene sufficiently.
2. Prepare CLNs solutions (100 μg $mL^{-1}$) using pyrene solution with different pH. Measure the fluorescence spectrum of CLNs solutions ($\lambda_{em} = 395$ nm) and calculate intensity ratio of $I_{338}$ and $I_{334}$ (Fig. 6).

Pyrene is a polarity probe that change its fluorescence property in different polarity of the local environment. The $I_{338}/I_{334}$ ratio of pyrene at pH 7.4 and pH 6.2 reduced

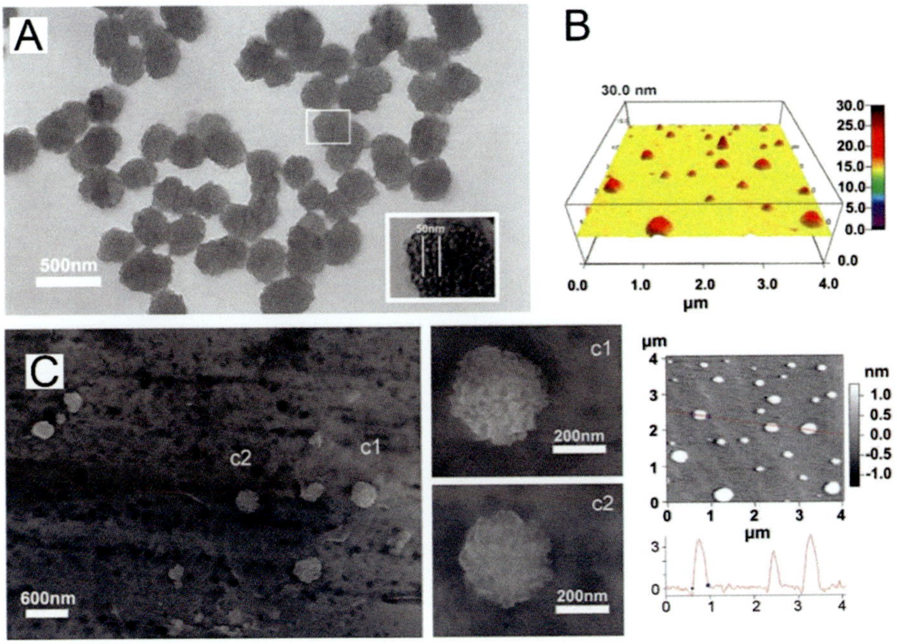


**Fig. 4** (**a**) TEM image, (**b**) AFM images (top: 3D view, middle: top view and bottom: the size profile along the red line), and (**c**) SEM image of CLNs

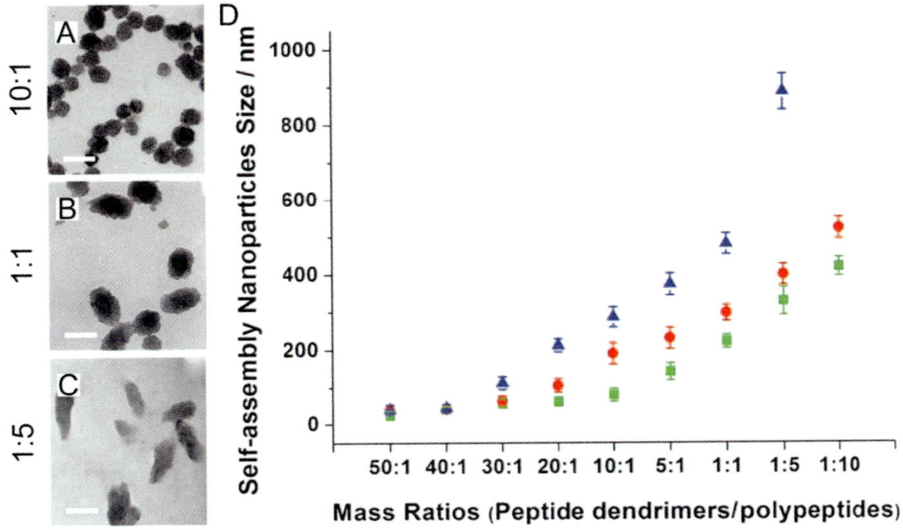


**Fig. 5** TEM images of CLNs with peptide dendrimers/linear polypeptides ratios (w/w) of (**a**) 10:1, (**b**) 1:1, (**c**) 1:5. (**d**) Size of CLNs against the ratios of peptide dendrimers/linear polypeptides at total mass concentrations of 10 (green squares), 50 (red circles), and 100 mg mL-1 (blue triangles)

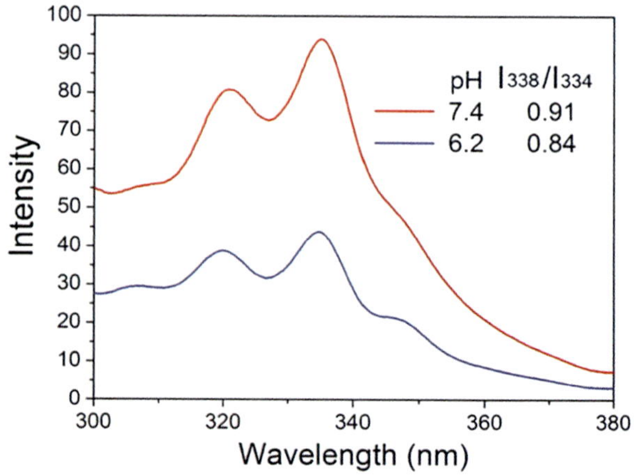


**Fig. 6** Fluorescence spectra of pyrene with the same concentration of CLNs at different pH values

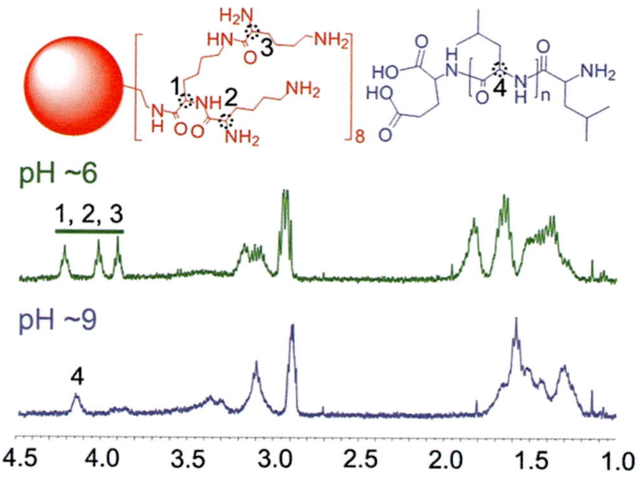


**Fig. 7** $^1$H-NMR spectrum of CLNs in different pH

from 0.91 to 0.84 with the same concentration of CLNs, suggesting pyrene released from nonpolar hydrophobic pockets of CLNs to polar aqueous environment due to the pH-triggered disassembly (Fig. 6).

### 3.4.2 NMR Analysis of CLNs at Different pH Conditions

1. Dissolve CLNs in 2 mL $D_2O$. Adjust the solution to pH 6 and 9 using $CF_3COOD$ and $Na_2CO_3$, respectively.
2. Analysis the solutions by an NMR spectrometer at 400 MHz (Fig. 7).

$^1$H-NMR spectra of CLNs at pH 6 and 9 was analyzed to reveal the mechanism of pH responsible feature. At pH value close to the pI of poly(L-leucine), poly(L-leucine) was insoluble and uncharged (pH 6.2), showing no signal in $^1$H-NMR. But the signals of the α-H on poly(L-lysine) dendrimers appeared at 3.5–4.5 ppm for the strong solubility from the protonated groups ($-NH_3^+$). With pH value increased to pKa of poly(L-lysine) dendrimers (pH 9), the amino groups ($-NH_2$) on peptide dendrimers were deprotonated, which further led to the lowered solubility of peptide dendrimers. Therefore, $^1$H-NMR signals of peptide dendrimers were barely detected when the pH values around the pKa of peptide dendrimers. However, the $^1$H-NMR signals of α-H on poly(L-leucine) appeared significantly at 3.5–4.5 ppm because the pH value was away from the pI of poly(L-leucine) with carboxyl groups ionized. As a result, the pH could largely influence the supramolecular interactions between poly (L-lysine) dendrimers and poly(L-leucine). At weakly alkaline conditions (such as, pH 7.4 and 7.9), the carboxyl groups ($-COO^-$) on poly(L-leucine) specifically interacted with protonated groups ($-NH_3^+$) on poly(L-lysine) dendrimers to generate CLNs.

### 3.4.3 Nanostructure Changes of CLNs at Different pH Conditions

1. Dissolve CLNs in water with different pH conditions.
2. Drop the solutions on copper grid and adsorb for 3 ~ 5 min. Remove the solutions and dry the copper grid at room temperature. Then, observe the nanoparticles by TEM.
3. Drop 10 μL solutions on mica plate and dry at room temperature. Then, observe the nanoparticles by AFM.

TEM images and AFM images showed CLNs formed well-defined nanoparticles at pH 7.4 (Figs. 8 and 9). This was according to previous results which showed that CLNs self-assembled into core-shell nanostructures in deionized water. However, CLNs presented irregular nanostructure at pH 6.2.

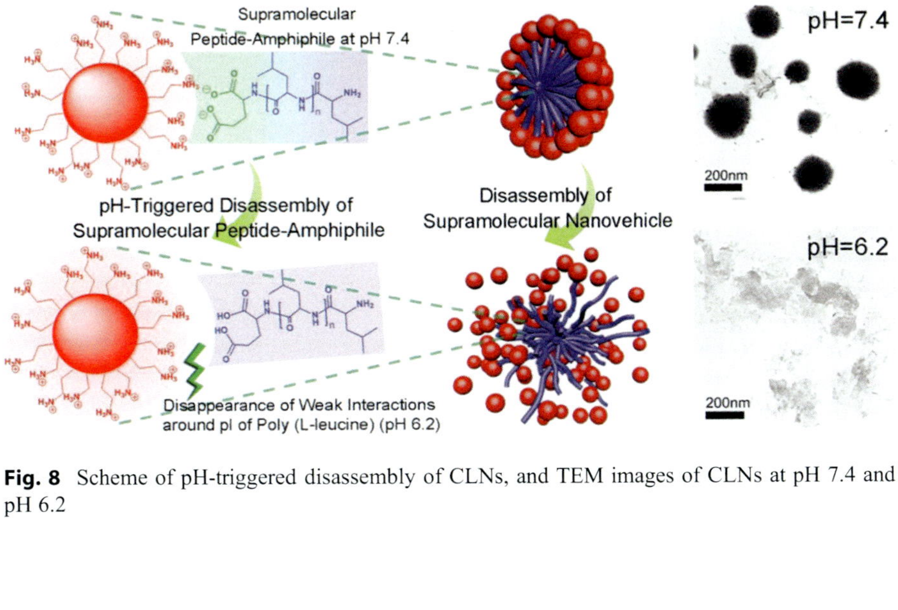


**Fig. 8** Scheme of pH-triggered disassembly of CLNs, and TEM images of CLNs at pH 7.4 and pH 6.2

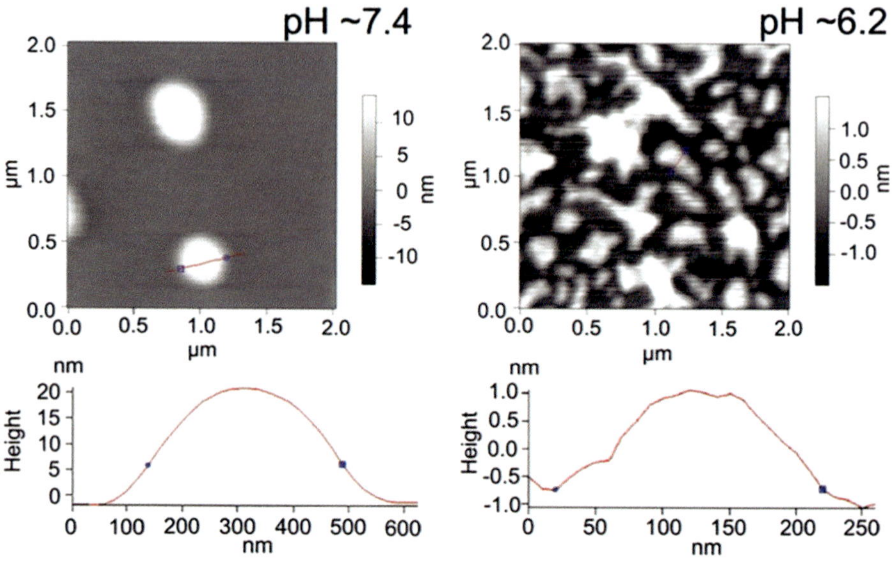


**Fig. 9** AFM images and profiles of CLNs at pH 7.4 and pH 6.2

## 3.5 In Vitro Gene Condensation of CLNs

### 3.5.1 Gel Retardation Assay

1. Prepare CLNs solution (1 mg $mL^{-1}$) in PBS (1 mM, pH 7.4).
2. Prepare luciferase encoding plasmid DNA solution with a concentration of 800 ng $mL^{-1}$ using nuclease-free water.
3. Mix DNA (400 ng) with different volume of CLNs solution to prepare CLNs and DNA complex with N/P ratio ranging from 1 to 30. Incubate the complexes at 37 °C for 30 min.
4. Mix the complexes with gel loading buffer and load the mixture on 1% (w/v) agarose gel in TAE running buffer. (80 V, 70 min.) Stain the DNA with GelView™ and visualize by a UV illuminator.

The positively charged CLNs could interact with negatively charged DNA by electrostatic interaction. And the DNA was retarded totally at N/P ratio of 10, indicating the gene transfection potential of CLNs (Fig. 10).

## 3.6 In Vitro Gene Transfection Investigation of CLNs

1. Seed HEK 293 cells on 24-well plate with $8 \times 10^4$ cells per well and culture overnight.
2. Prepare CLNs and DNA complexes containing 800 ng DNA per well using fresh DMEM culture media with N/P ratio of 35, 45, and 55 (3.5 Step 1 and 2).

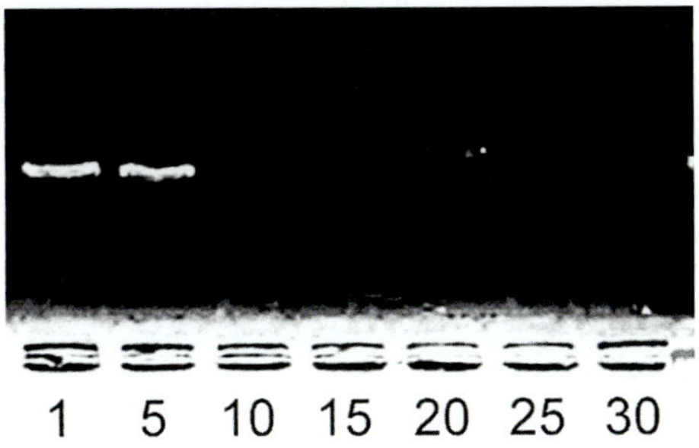


**Fig. 10** Gel retardation assay of CLNs and DNA complexes at N/P ratio of 1, 5, 10, 15, 20, 25, and 30

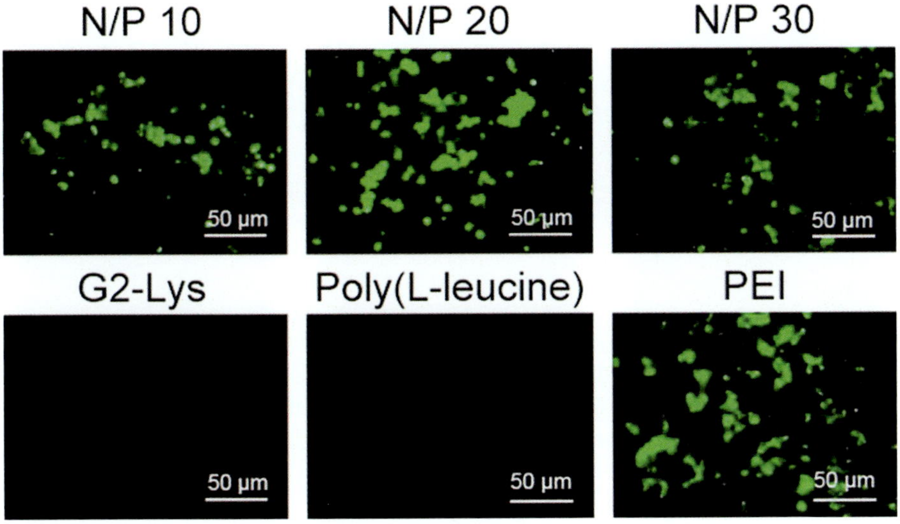


**Fig. 11** Fluorescence images of HEK 293 cells after incubation with G2-Lys, Poly(L-leucine), and CLNs (Scale bar = 50 μm)

3. Incubate the complexes with cells for 4 h at 37 °C. Then, replace the culture media with fresh DMEM media containing 10%FBS and culture for 48 h.
4. Image the cells by inverted fluorescence microscopy to analyze the GFP expression.
5. Analyze the cells treated as above by flow cytometer to quantify the gene transfection effect.

GFP gene was used to investigate the gene transfection efficiency of CLNs. The GFP gene expression was analyzed by invert fluorescence microscope and flow cytometer (Figs. 11 and 12). After incubation with CLNs/GFP complex, strong GFP fluorescence was observed and comparable with positive control of PEI group.

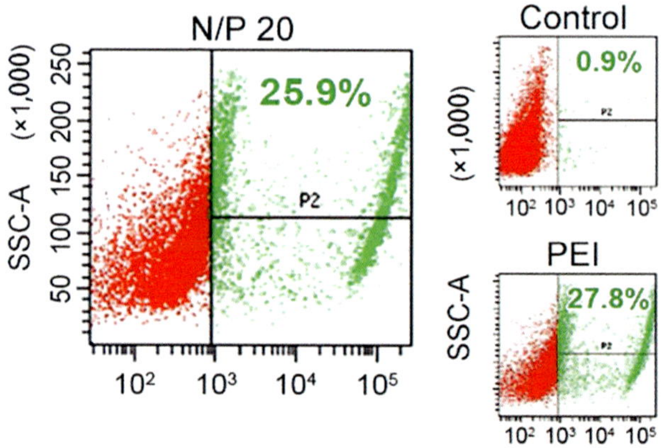


**Fig. 12** GFP expression of HEK 293 cells after treatment with PEI and DNA/CLNs complex

## 4 Discussion

In this section, a versatile strategy on cooperative assembly of peptide dendrimers and linear polypeptides into capsid-like nanoparticles is proposed for developing advanced gene delivery vectors. These supramolecular dendrimeric systems possess a capsid-like nanoarchitecture, which could be regulated by changing concentration and ratio of peptide dendrimer and linear polymer. In addition, these CLNs exhibited pH dependent features of assembly and disassembly for smart molecular delivery. As expected, CLNs can be used as a safe and efficient gene delivery system. Bioinspired fabrication of peptide-based CLNs may be a promising strategy for development of a new generation of smart nanocarriers for gene delivery.

## References

Davidson BL, Breakefield XO (2003) Viral vectors for gene delivery to the nervous system. Nat Rev Neurosci 4:353–364

Kotterman MA, Schaffer DV (2014) Engineering adeno-associated viruses for clinical gene therapy. Nat Rev Genet 15:445–451

Li Y, Xu X (2020) Nanomedicine solutions to intricate physiological-pathological barriers and molecular mechanisms of tumor multidrug resistance. J Control Release 323:483–501

Li Y, Lai Y, Xu X, Zhang X, Wu Y, Hu C, Zhongwei Gu MS (2016) Capsid-like supramolecular dendritic systems as pH-responsive nanocarriers for drug penetration and site-specific delivery. Nanomedicine 12:355–364

Mastrobattista E, van der Aa MAEM, Hennink WE, Crommelin DJA (2006) Artificial viruses: a nanotechnological approach to gene delivery. Nat Rev Drug Discov 5:115–121

Pack DW, Hoffman AS, Pun S, Stayton PS (2005) Design and development of polymers for gene delivery. Nat Rev Drug Discov 4:581–593

Wegst UGK, Bai H, Saiz E, Tomsia AP, Ritchie RO (2015) Bioinspired structural materials. Nat Mater 14:23–36

Xu X, Yuan H, Chang J, He B, Zhongwei G (2012) Cooperative hierarchical self-assembly of peptide dendrimers and linear polypeptides into nanoarchitectures mimicking viral capsids. Angew Chem Int Ed 51:3130–3133

Xu X, Jian Y, Li Y, Zhang X, Zhaoxu T, Zhongwei G (2014a) Bio-inspired supramolecular hybrid dendrimers self-assembled from low-generation peptide dendrons for highly efficient gene delivery and biological tracking. ACS Nano 8:9255–9264

Xu X, Li Y, Li H, Liu R, Sheng M, He B, Zhongwei G (2014b) Smart nanovehicles based on pH-triggered disassembly of supramolecular peptide-amphiphiles for efficient intracellular drug delivery. Small 10:1133–1140

Xu X, Jiang Q, Zhang X, Yu N, Zhang Z, Li Y, Cheng G, Zhongwei G (2015) Virus-inspired mimics: self-assembly of dendritic lipopeptides into arginine-rich nanovectors for improving gene delivery. J Mater Chem B 3:7006–7010

Zan G, Wu Q (2016) Biomimetic and bioinspired synthesis of nanomaterials/nanostructures. Adv Mater 28:2099–2147

Zhang X, Zhang Z, Xu X, Li Y, Li Y, Jian Y, Zhongwei G (2015) Bioinspired therapeutic dendrimers as efficient peptide drugs based on supramolecular interactions for tumor inhibition. Angew Chem Int Ed 54:4289–4294

Zhang X, Li Y, Hu C, Wu Y, Zhong D, Xu X, Zhongwei G (2018a) Engineering anticancer amphipathic peptide-dendronized compounds for highly-efficient plasma/organelle membrane perturbation and multidrug resistance reversal. ACS Appl Mater Interfaces 10:30952–30962

Zhang X, Xu X, Li Y, Hu C, Zhang Z, Zhongwei G (2018b) Virion-like membrane-breaking nanoparticles with tumor-activated cell-and-tissue dual-penetration conquer impermeable cancer. Adv Mater 30:1707240

# Peptide-Modified Polycations with Acid-Triggered Lytic Activity for Efficient Gene Delivery

12

Yilong Cheng

## Contents



**Abstract**

Gene therapy has been regarded as the potent way to treat a series of acquired or congenital diseases in highly specific manner. The applications of nucleic acid–based therapeutics, including plasmid DNA (pDNA), small interfering RNA (siRNA), messenger RNA (mRNA), micro-RNA (miRNA), and CRISPR/Cas, have entered different phases of clinical trials. However, in vivo delivery of this class of drugs has encountered various obstacles, especially endo/lysosome entrapment. Previous studies showed that endosomal release is the rate-limiting

Y. Cheng (✉)
School of Chemistry, Xi'an Jiaotong University, Xi'an, Shaanxi, China
e-mail: yilongcheng@mail.xjtu.edu.cn



H. Tian and X. Chen (eds.), *Gene Delivery*, Biomaterial Engineering,
https://doi.org/10.1007/978-981-16-5419-0_1

step for gene transfection in mitotic cells, and lysosomal degradation may happen if egress does not occur. Therefore, "proton sponge effect," incorporation of membrane-active peptides, hydrophobic domains, and photosensitizer with aggregation-induced emission (AIE) characteristics have been utilized to endow synthetic polycations with the capability to facilitate efficient endo/lysosome release. Among them, peptides with membrane-lytic activity has attracted increasing attention due to the facile modified method and potent membrane-active capability as well as promising gene delivery efficiency. Until now, several peptides, such as melittin, C6M3, sHGP, CMA-2, FL-20, and MEP-2, have been incorporated with polycations to construct a series of nonviral vector to mediate efficient endo/lysosomal release and successful gene delivery. However, due to nonselective membrane lysis behavior, these functional polycations usually accompany with serious safety concerns. Hence, to simultaneously realize good biocompatibility and high transfection efficiency by lytic peptide modified polycations is on demand. In the chapter, the preparation methods and experimental details for the peptide-modified polycations will be discussed, and the possible way to balance the membrane-lytic activity and safety concerns will be proposed.

**Keywords**

Gene delivery, Polycations, Lytic peptide, Membrane lysis, pH sensitive, Endosome escape

## 1 Overview

Due to the instability and membrane impermeability of nucleic acids, successful gene delivery and further gene therapy need the assistant of potent gene carriers to transfer therapeutic genes into targeting cell (Naldini 2015; Yin et al. 2014; Molla and Levkin 2016). In the past decades, researchers have made great effort to explore different types of gene vectors, including viral and nonviral vectors. Viruses possess the natural ability to infect cells, and thus they can efficiently pass various physiological barriers and deliver therapeutic genes into targeting cells to realize gene therapy. However, due to high cost and potential safety concerns, such as immunogenicity, inflammation, and mutation, the broad applications of viral vectors in gene transfer may be limited (Thomas et al. 2003). As an alternative way, nonviral vector, especially for polycations, has attracted increasing attention owing to the good biocompatibility and facile preparation with low cost (Lachelt and Wagner 2015). With the development of various polymerization methods, polycations with well-defined structures and functionalities have been explored, and great progresses have been made in vitro and in vivo gene delivery (Xu and Yang 2011; Freitag and Wagner 2021; Ahmed and Narain 2013). However, the delivery efficiency mediated by polycations is usually orders of magnitude lower than their viral counterparts (Freitag and Wagner 2021; Peng and Wagner 2019). Hence, the design of polymeric gene vectors with high delivery efficiency as virus but low cost and high safety is on demand for gene therapy.

Successful gene delivery using cationic polymers needs to meet these following requirements: gene condensation, good stability in blood circulation, cell uptake, endo/lysosome escape, effective release in cytoplasm, and delivery into nucleus and gene expression (Miyata et al. 2012). In the past two decades, researchers have introduced shielding systems, targeting groups and stimuli-sensitive linkers to modify polycations to realize long blood circulation time, accumulation in targeting tissue, efficient cell uptake, and fast gene release intracellularly, which have made great progress for in vivo gene delivery (Yang et al. 2014; Li et al. 2014; Christie et al. 2012; Liu et al. 2016; Sun et al. 2015; Guan et al. 2016). However, the therapeutic effect is far from expectation. It is reported that the limiting step for the low efficiency by polycations is the endo/lysosomal entrapment (Pei and Buyanova 2019; Arnold et al. 2017). If the complexes formed by polycations and genes are restricted in endosome, they will be routed into lysosomal degradation, leading to the failed delivery (Varga et al. 2005; Varkouhi et al. 2011). Hence, endowing the cationic polymers with inherent endosomal escape capability is crucial for nonviral vectors–based gene delivery.

In order to address the issue of endo/lysosome entrapment for the complexes, great effort has been made to design polycations with enhanced endo/lysosome release capability, including buffering in acidic pH ("proton sponge effect") (Bus et al. 2018; Degors et al. 2019), functionalization with alkylated carboxylic acid (Jones et al. 2003; Convertine et al. 2009), fluorination of polycations (Wang et al. 2014a; Wang et al. 2016; Ge et al. 2020), and incorporation of photosensitizer with aggregation-induced emission (AIE) characteristics into polycations (Nishiyama et al. 2006; Yuan et al. 2015). These approaches showed enhanced endo/lysosome release in cultured cells through different mechanisms, but may be not easily translated for in vivo applications. The proton sponge effect is the widely used method for polycation-mediated endosomal release (Akinc et al. 2005). For example, poly(2-dimethylaminoethyl methacrylate) (PDMAEMA), a widely used polycation as gene vector, could enable osmotic swelling, membrane destabilization, and endosomal rupture in some cell types, but the efficiency was pretty low due to the pendant tertiary amine groups. Additionally, to realize successful endo/lysosome release in vivo, there needs a large amount of polymer accumulation in the endo/lysosome, which may raise serious safety concerns. As an alternative way, Liu and coworkers reported a polymeric gene vector composed of a tetraphenylethylene derivative and oligoethylenimine (OEI), by which the generated reactive oxygen species (ROS) upon visible light irradiation could disrupt the endo/lysosome membrane and enable the cytoplasm transfer of the cargoes (Yuan et al. 2015). Although promising in vitro, this approach is hard to be applied in vivo, which was due to the penetrating limitation of visible lights.

Peptides with membrane-lytic activity, such as melittin, Tat, C6M3, CMA-2, FL-20, MEP-2, and hemagglutinin, have been employed to modify nonviral gene delivery vectors to improve the endo/lysosome escape capability (Brooks et al. 2005; Chen et al. 2006; Boeckle et al. 2006; Peeler et al. 2019; Chen et al. 2017a; Jafari et al. 2012; Cerovsky et al. 2008; Rudolph et al. 2003; Zhang et al. 2001). For example, Pun and coworkers incorporated sHGP, a peptide derived from HIV gp41, into oligolysine-based polycations to improve the gene delivery efficiency (Kwon et al. 2008; Schellinger et al. 2013a). It was found that compared to the parent polycations, the hemolysis ratio mediated by sHGP functionalized polymer was around 80% when the polymer concentration was 40 ug/mL, which led to significantly high expression of luciferase in HeLa cells. In the followed work, melittin, a 26-amino acid membrane-lytic peptide derived from the venom of honey bee, was introduced into the same polycations to improve the gene transfer efficiency (Schellinger et al. 2013b). In vitro hemolysis results showed that obvious membrane lysis was observed when the polymer concentration was as low as 4 ug/mL, indicating the potent lytic activity by melittin. However, serious cytotoxicity was also detected due to the off-site lysis, by which the cell viability was even lower than 30% when the amine-to-phophate (N/P) ratio was 5 for in vitro transfection study. To address the issue of safety versus transfection efficiency, Wagner and coworkers masked melittin with maleic anhydride derivatives to prepare a pH-sensitive polycation, by which the lytic activity was deactivated at neutral pH and activated at endosomal pH due to the hydrolysis of the anhydride capping groups (Meyer et al. 2008). The masked melittin polycations mediated efficient siRNA delivery in vitro compared to polylysine and polyethylenimine (PEI) with acceptable biocompatibility. While effective, the anhydride protecting group is susceptible to hydrolysis even at physiological pH, which reduces the stability and shelf life of the materials and may result in safety concerns during applications.

Although lytic peptides usually show nonselective membrane lysis and induce serious safety concerns, it is undoubted that the introduction of lytic peptides into polymer design could obviously improve gene transfection efficiency through fast endo/lysosome escape. In this chapter, two methods are proposed to balance the cytotoxicity and endo/lysosome release in polycations-based gene delivery. In the first method, a functional polymer, (P(OEGMA-DMAEMA)-b- P(DIPAMA-(PDSEMA-melittin))), composed of poly(oligo(ethylene glycol) monomethyl ether methacrylate)-co-poly(2-(dimethylamino)ethyl methacrylate) (P(OEGMA-DMAEMA)) as polycations to protect genes and poly(2-diisopropylaminoethyl methacrylate)-co-poly(pyridyl disulfide ethyl methacrylate) (P(DIPAMA-PDSEMA)) to enable modification with thiol-containing lytic peptides through disulfide exchange reactions, was prepared to realize selective membrane lysis for safe and efficient gene transfer (Fig. 1a). P(OEGMA-DMAEMA)-b-P(DIPAMA-

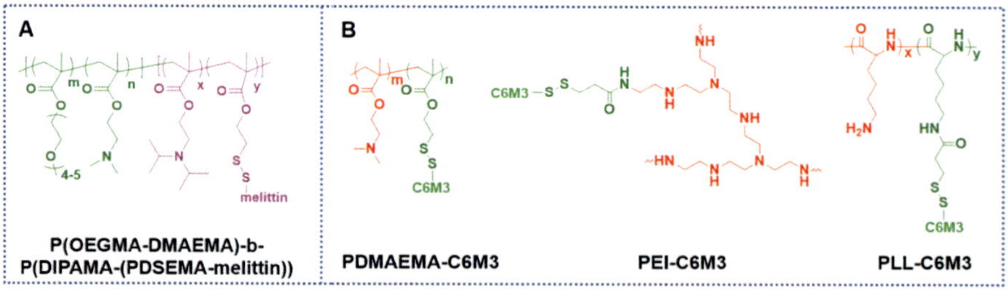


**Fig. 1** Structures of peptide-modified polycations

(PDSEMA-melittin)) was designed to self-assemble into micelles at physiological pH with melittin buried within the hydrophobic core of PDIPAMA. After endocytosis, the acidic endosomal environment triggers a hydrophilic transition of the PDIPAMA block, unveiling the melittin peptide, which can then facilitate endosomal release by disruption of the endo/lysosome membrane. In another method, C6M3 peptide (a peptide derived from C6) was incorporated with three widely used polycations, poly(2-dimethylaminoethyl methacrylate (PDMAEMA), poly (L-lysine) (PLL), and branched polyethylenimine (PEI 25 kDa), to afford the synthesis of peptide-modified polycations (PDMAEMA-C6M3, PLL-C6M3 and PEI-C6M3) (Fig. 1b). C6M3 shows pH-triggered lytic activity, and promising membrane lysis was observed under endo/lysosomal acidic conditions rather than at a normal pH value, by which the peptide-modified polycations can achieve selective membrane lysis and improve gene transfection efficiency as well as acceptable biocompatibility. The principle of polymer synthesis, manipulation of polyplexes preparation, in vitro transfection, and experimental details are discussed in this chapter.

## 2 Protocol

### 2.1 Materials

The materials used for the preparation of P(OEGMA-DMAEMA)-b-P(DIPAMA-(PDSEMA-melittin)) are shown as follows: 2-(dimethylamino)ethyl methacrylate (DMAEMA) and oligo(ethylene glycol) monomethyl ether methacrylate (OEGMA, $M_n = 300$ and pendent EO units DP 4 ~ 5) were purchased from Sigma-Aldrich, and the monomers were purified by passing through a column filled with basic alumina to remove the inhibitor prior to polymerization; RAFT CTA 4-cyanopentanoic acid dithiobenzoate (CPADB), N,N′-azobisisobutyronitrile (AIBN), anhydrous N,N-′-dimethylacetamide (DMAc, HPLC, 99.9%), and dioxane were purchased from Sigma-Aldrich and used without further purification; pyridyl disulfide ethyl methacrylate was synthesized as described previously (Song et al. 2015); 2-diisopropylaminoethyl methacrylate (DIPAMA) was purchased from Scientific Polymer Products Company and purified by passing through a basic alumina; cysteine-melittin (Mel-cys; NH2-GIGAVLKVLTTGLPALISWIKRKRQQCCONH2) was purchased from GL Biochem Ltd. (Shanghai, China); endotoxin-free plasmid pCMV-Luc (photinuspyralis luciferase under control of the cytomegalovirus (CMV) enhancer/promoter) was produced with the Qiagen Plasmid Giga kit (Qiagen, Hilden, Germany) according to the manufacturer's recommendations; and YOYO-1 iodide and lipofectamine 2000 (LF) were purchased from Invitrogen (Carlsbad, CA). HeLa cells (ATCC CCL-2™) and KB cells (ATCC CCL-17) were maintained in minimum essential medium (MEM) supplemented with 10% fetal bovine serum (FBS) and antibiotics/antimyotics (AbAm) (100 IU of penicillin, 100 ug/mL of streptomycin, and 0.25 ug/mL of amphotericin B). A549 cells (ATCC CCL-185) were maintained in F-12 K medium supplemented with 10% fetal bovine serum (FBS) and antibiotics/antimyotics (AbAm)

(100 IU of penicillin, 100 ug/mL of streptomycin, and 0.25 ug/mL of amphotericin B). Z310 cells were donated by Prof. Wei Zheng (Purdue) and cultured in Dulbecco's minimum essential medium (DMEM) supplemented with 10% heat-inactivated FBS, 10% penicillin/streptomycin, 40 mg/mL gentamicin, and 10 ng/mL nerve growth factor (NGF).

The materials used for the preparation of PDMAEMA-C6M3, PLL-C6M3, and PEI-C6M3 are shown as follows: triphosgene, $N_{\varepsilon}$-carbobenzoxy-L-lysine, 4-cyano-4-(phenylcarbonothioylthio)pentanoic acid (CPADB), 2,2′-dithiodipyridine, 3-mercaptopropionic, hexylamine, and methacryloyl chloride were purchased from Aladdin. Branched polyethylenimine (PEI, 25 kDa, Sigma) was dissolved in PBS with a concentration of 10 mg/mL followed by the pH adjustment using 1 M HCl to ~6, and it was diluted with water to get the final concentration for experiments; pyridyl disulfide ethyl methacrylate (PDSEMA) was synthesized as described previously (Song et al. 2015); cysteine-C6M3 ($NH_2$-RLWHLLWRLWRRLHRLLRCCONH$_2$) was purchased from GL Biochem Ltd. (Shanghai, China).

## 2.2 Methods

### 2.2.1 Synthesis of P(OEGMA-DMAEMA)-b-P(DIPAMA-(PDSEMA-Melittin))

#### Synthesis of P(OEGMA-DMAEMA)

P(OEGMA-DMAEMA) was prepared by reversible addition-fragmentation chain transfer polymerization (RAFT). In brief, OEGMA (1.0 g, 3.44 mmol), DMAEMA (2.7 g, 17.2 mmol), AIBN (9.5 mg, 0.058 mmol), and CPADB (80 mg, 0.29 mmol) were dissolved in 5 mL dioxane. After purging with argon for 10 min, the reaction mixture was stirred in an oil bath at 60 °C for 18 h to complete the polymerization. Afterward, the polymerization was quenched by immersing the reaction flask in liquid nitrogen. After thawing, the solution was precipitated in ether. The polymer was separated by centrifugation and further purified by redissoving/reprecipitating with DCM/ether three times.

#### Synthesis of P(OEGMA-DMAEMA)-b-P(DIPAMA-PDSEMA)

The same polymerization method was used to synthesize the block copolymer. P(OEGMA-DMAEMA)-b-P(DIPAMA-PDSEMA) was prepared using P(OEGMA-DMAEMA) as macro-CTA. Detailedly, P(OEGMA$_{11}$-DMAEMA$_{56}$) (80 mg, 0.0066 mmol), DIPAMA (282 mg, 1.32 mmol), PDSEMA (17 mg, 0.066 mmol), and AIBN (0.36 mg, 0.0022 mmol) were first dissolved in 1.32 mL DMAc. After purging with argon for 5 min, the reaction solution was immersed in an oil bath at 60 °C. After 30 min, the polymerization was quenched using liquid nitrogen. The polymer was purified by the dialysis against methanol for two days followed by evaporation of the solvent.

**Conjugation of Cys-Melittin to P(OEGMA-DMAEMA)-*b*-P(DIPAMA-PDSEMA)**
Cys-melittin was conjugated to the block copolymer through disulfide exchange reaction described as the previous work (Schellinger et al. 2013b). P(OEGMA-DMAEMA)-*b*-P(DIPAMA-PDSEMA) (20 mg, 0.001 mmol PDS groups) was dissolved in 2 mL PB buffer (0.2 M, pH 5.7) in a 10 mL flask. Then, 6.1 mg (0.002 mmol, 2 equiv. relative to PDS groups) of cys-melittin was added into the flask and allowed to stir under argon at room temperature. The reaction was monitored by UV at 340 nm for the release of 2-thio-pyridine. After 20 h, the absorption was saturated and the reaction mixture was passed through a PD-10 column to remove the side product and unreacted peptide followed by lyophilization.

### 2.2.2 Synthesis of PDMAEMA-C6M3, PLL-C6M3, and PEI-C6M3

**Synthesis of PDMAEMA-Co-PDSEMA**
PDMAEMA-co-PDSEMA was prepared by RAFT polymerization. In brief, pyridyl disulfide ethyl methacrylate (PDSEMA) (9.14 mg, 7.2 mmol), 2-(dimethylamino)-ethyl methacrylate (DMAEMA) (557 mg, 64.5 mmol), N,N-azobisisobutyronitrile (AIBN) (3.92 mg, 0.072 mmol), and 4-cyanopentanoic acid dithio-benzoate (CPADB) (10 mg, 0.072 mmol) were dissolved in dioxane (896 μL). After purging with nitrogen for 30 min, the polymerization was initiated in an oil bath at 70 °C and the mixture was stirred for 24 h. The monomer conversion was monitored by $^{1}$H NMR spectrum. The polymerization was quenched by immersing the reaction flask in liquid nitrogen. The polymer, PDMAEMA-co-PDSEMA, was collected by three cycles of dissolving/precipitating with dichloromethane/hexane.

**Synthesis of PLL-SPDP**
PLL was synthesized by ring-opening polymerization and 3-(pyridin-2-yldisulfanyl) propanoic acid (PDSPA) was prepared according to the previous work (Schellinger et al. 2013b; Chen et al. 2017b). PDSPA (0.039 g, 0.18 mmol) was first dissolved in the mixture of DMSO and water (1 mL) followed the addition of by 1-(3-dimethylaminopropyl)-3-ethylcarbodiimide hydrochloride (EDC•HCl) (0.036 g, 0.19 mmol) and N-hydroxysuccinimide (NHS) (0.022 g, 0.19 mmol). The reaction was stirred at room temperature for 0.5 h to obtain 3-(2-pyridyldithio)propionic acid N-hydroxysuccinimide ester (SPDP). Afterward, the solution of SPDP was slowly added to PLL (500 mg, 0.09 mmol) dissolved in the mixture of DMSO and water (2 mL), and the reaction was stirred at room temperature for additional 72 h. PLL-SPDP was obtained by dialysis and lyophilization.

**Synthesis of PEI-SPDP**
The conjugation of PDSPA to PEI was similar to that for PLL as shown above, and PEI-SPDP was obtained by dialysis and lyophilization.

**Synthesis of C6M3-Modified Polycations**
Cys-C6M3 was conjugated to the polycations through a disulfide exchange reaction. For example, PDMAEMA-co-PDSEMA (7.5 mg, 0.001 mmol PDS groups) was

dissolved in 2 mL phosphate buffer (PB buffer, 0.2 M, pH 5.7) in a 10 mL flask. Then, 6.1 mg (0.002 mmol, 2 equiv. relative to PDS groups) of cys-C6M3 was added into the flask and allowed to stir under nitrogen at room temperature. The reaction was monitored by the UV spectrum at 340 nm for the release of 2-thio-pyridine. After 24 h, the absorption was saturated and the reaction mixture was passed through a PD-10 column to remove the side product and unreacted peptide followed by lyophilization. The conjugations of C6M3 to PLL-SPDP and PEI-SPDP were performed as the same procedure. The peptide-modified polycations were denoted as PDMAEMA-C6M3, PLL-C6M3, and PEI-C6M3.

### 2.2.3 Hemolysis of Polymers

Hemolysis assay was used to evaluate the acid-triggered membrane-lytic activity of the synthetic materials at pH 7.4 (extracellular pH) and 5.7 (endosomal pH), respectively. Briefly, plasma from human blood was removed by centrifugation. The red blood cells were then washed three times with 150 mM NaCl, and resuspended into phosphate buffer (PB) at pH 7.4 or 5.7. The polymers at various concentrations and 1% Triton X-100 as control were added to the red blood cell suspensions in a 96-well conical plate and was allowed to incubate for 1 h at 37 °C. After centrifugation, the released hemoglobin within the supernatant was measured by UV at 541 nm. Percent hemolysis was calculated relative to Triton X-100. Experiments were performed in triplicate.

### 2.2.4 Preparation and Characterization of DNA Polyplexes

The polymer/DNA polyplexes was formed by adding polymer to DNA solution followed by 30 min incubation at room temperature. For the gel retardation study, the polyplexes with various N/P ratios were loaded onto a 1% agarose gel containing TAE buffer (40 μmM tris-acetate, 1 mM EDTA) and 5 mg/mL ethidium bromide, and were electrophoresed at 100 V for 40 min. The plasmid DNA was then visualized using a Kodak (Rochester, NK) UV transilluminator (laser-excited fluorescence gel scanner).

The size and surface charge of the polyplexes formed by polycations and DNA were tested on a ZetaPLUS instrument (Brookhaven Instruments Corporation, Holtsvile, NY). The samples were prepared by mixing polyplexes (1 μg DNA, 20 μL solution) with 800 μL dd$H_2O$. The measurements were performed in triplicate.

The morphology of the polyplexes formed by different polymers and luciferase plasmid in dried state was imaged on a JEOL 1140 TEM at an acceleration voltage of 100 kV. The polyplexes solutions (10 μL) were deposited on the top of the 400-mesh formvar/copper grids and incubated at room temperature for 30 min. After staining with uranyl acetate, the grids were allowed to air-dry overnight.

### 2.2.5 Endosomal Escape of Polyplexes by Confocal Microscope

To evaluate the endosomal escape ability of melittin-polymer-based polyplexes, DNA was first labeled with YOYO-1. The cells were incubated with polyplexes for 4 h. The acidic vesicles and the nuclei of cells were stained with LysoTracker

Red, DND-99, and 4′,6-diamidino-2-phenylindole (DAPI), respectively. To quantify the endosomal escape ratio of polyplexes, the colocalization ratio between DNA and LysoTracker Red was quantified as follows using Image J software:

Colocalization ratio (%) = $(\text{YOYO-1 pixels})_{\text{colocalization}}/(\text{YOYO-1 pixels})_{\text{total}} \times 100\%$.

where YOYO-1 $\text{pixels}_{\text{colocalization}}$ represent the number of YOYO-1 pixels colocalizing with Lysotracker Red, and YOYO-1 $\text{pixels}_{\text{total}}$ represent the number of all YOYO-1 pixels in the confocal images. Results were presented as the mean of 15 individual cells.

### 2.2.6 Polyplex Uptake Assay

Cellular uptake of polyplexes was evaluated via flow cytometry using fluorescently labeled DNA. HeLa cells were seeded at 25,000 cells per well in 24-well plate and incubated for 20 h at 37 °C. pCMV-Luc2 plasmid was mixed with the bis-intercalating dye YOYO-1 iodide at a dye/base pair ratio of 1:100 and incubated at room temperature for 1 h. Polyplexes were prepared at N/P ratio 5 using 0.5 μg of pCMV-Luc2 plasmid DNA in 10 μL total volume. Each sample was diluted to 200 μL with complete cell culture medium. Cells were washed once with PBS and incubated with polyplexes solution for 4 h at 37 °C. Then cells were washed twice with PBS, detached by treatment with trypsin, pelleted, and then resuspended in 300 μL PBS (containing 0.5% BSA), kept on ice and analyzed using flow cytometry, MACSQuant Analyzer (Miltenyi Biotec Inc., Auburn, CA).

### 2.2.7 In Vitro Transfection

HeLa cells were seeded at a density of 25,000 cells/well in complete cell culture medium in a 24-well plate. Cells were first incubated at 37 °C, 5% $CO_2$ for 20 h. Polyplexes were prepared at different N/P ratios using 0.5 or 1.0 μg of luciferase plasmid in 10 μL total volume. Each sample was diluted to 200 μL with complete cell culture medium or OptiMEM medium. The cells were rinsed once with PBS, followed by the addition of transfection solution. After incubation for 2 and 4 h, cells were washed with PBS twice and the polyplexes solution was replaced with complete cell culture medium. After additional 22 or 44 h incubation, luciferase activity was quantified with a luciferase assay kit (Promega Corp, Fitchburg, WI) according to the manufacturer's instruction, except that a freeze-thaw cycle at −80 °C was included after the addition of the lysis buffer to ensure complete cell lysis. Luminescence intensity was measured on the plate reader with integration for 1 s. The total protein content in each well was measured by a BCA protein assay kit (Thermo Scientific, Rockford, IL) according to the manufacturer's instruction so that the luciferase activity was normalized to the total protein content in each well. Each sample was tested with a sample size (n) = 3.

The transfection with GFP (green fluorescence protein) plasmid was the same as that with luciferase plasmid. For analysis, cells were washed with PBS, trypsinized, and pelleted at 300 × g for 5 min at 4 °C. The pellet was resuspended in 0.3 mL propidium iodide (PI) solution (1 μg/mL in 0.5% BSA in PBS), kept on ice and analyzed using flow cytometry. All experiments were conducted in triplicate.

# 3 Discussion

## 3.1 Optimization of P(OEGMA-DMAEMA)-b-P(DIPAMA-(PDSEMA-Melittin)) Synthesis

Melittin was introduced into the polymers through disulfide exchange reaction. Since the molecular weight of melittin is around 3000, it is difficult to purify the peptide functional polycations through dissolution-precipitation process. It is suggested to use the spin-column (PD-10) to purify the polymer, by which the column can retain the small molecules with molecular weight lower than 3000. But it should be noted that a small amount of melittin may be collected with the peptide-modified polymer. Hence, it is recommended that the purification should be processed twice. On the other hand, the polymer should be dissolved in PB buffer with pH lower than 6 before passing through the column. If the polymer was dissolved in neutral media, part of the free melittin may be entrapped in the core of the micelles, which can result in serious toxicity in transfection study.

The ratio of OEGMA and DMAEMA in the polymerization process is of importance for the gene condensation and colloidal stability. Usually, PDMAEMA with degree of polymerization (DP) around 50 is sufficient for genes condensation and protection, but higher DP may raise safety concerns due to excess positive charge. For OEGMA, its ratio to DMAEMA should be in the range of 0.2–0.4, which can enable efficient gene protection and good stability of polycation/gene complexes. PDIPAMA is a widely used pH-sensitive polymers with pKa around 6.3, which has been exploited in drug delivery and diagnose (Wang et al. 2014b; Yu et al. 2011; Wang et al. 2017; Xu et al. 2016). Although the DP of DIPAMA does not obviously affect the hydrophobic to hydrophilic transition, it shows DP-dependent shielding and release of lytic peptide. It is supposed that there is one melittin in the sidechain of PDIPAMA. When the DP of DIPAMA is lower than 15, the molecular weight is 3200 kDa, and it is slightly higher than the molecular weight of melittin (2950 kDa), which cannot completely shield the lytic peptide under physiological condition. Therefore, serious cytotoxicity was observed in cell transfection. It is found that DIPAMA with DP higher than 25 could deactivate the lytic activity of melittin under normal condition. However, for in vitro transfection, when the DP of PDIPAMA was higher than 40, the transfection efficiency was declined, probably due to the slow dissociation of the micellar structure under endo/lysome acidic condition. Hence, the DP of DIPAMA should be in the range of 25–40 with one melittin in the polymer sidechain. Due to the potent lytic activity of melittin, the introduction of more meliitin into PDIPAMA may require the higher DP of DIPAMA to realize efficient encapsulation. For example, the DP of DIPAMA should be as high as 50 if two melittin are incorporated into the polymers. Based on the above discussion, the structure transition of DIPAMA is limited, and thus the in vitro transfection efficiency is low. And also high content of melittin may raise safety concerns to cells. Hence, to balance the safety and lytic activity, it is suggested that the DP of DIPAMA should be in the range of 25–40 with one melittin decorated in the sidechains.

### 3.2 Preparation of P(OEGMA-DMAEMA)-b-P(DIPAMA-(PDSEMA-Melittin)) Micelles

Due to the hydrophobic nature of PDIPAMA at pH 7.4, P(OEGMA-DMAEMA)-b-P (DIPAMA-(PDSEMA-melittin)) micelles can self-assemble into micellar structure in aqueous solution. Three methods were employed to form melittin-buried nano-assemblies. For the first one, the amphiphilic polymer was directly dissolved in buffer solution (PB buffer with pH 7.4). It was found that the distribution of the micellar size by the functional polymer was not uniform, and large aggregation was detected by DLS testing. This may be attributed to the aggregative trends of PDIPAMA block in aqueous solution. Moreover, the hemolysis testing at pH 7.4 revealed that around 30% hemolysis was observed when the concentration of the polymer was higher than 120 ug/mL, and cytotoxicity was also detected in gene transfection study. Since melittin can be dissolved in water, the lytic peptide may be exposed outside the hydrophobic core of PDIPAMA block, which can directly interact with cell membrane to induce cell death. Hence, this method is not recommended for the preparation of the micelles formed by P(OEGMA-DMAEMA)-b-P(DIPAMA-(PDSEMA-melittin).

For the second one, the assemblies can be formed by nanoprecipitation method. P (OEGMA-DMAEMA)-b-P(DIPAMA-(PDSEMA-melittin)) was first dissolved in organic solvent, such as dimethyl sulfoxide (DMSO), and the uniform solution was added dropwise into water to form melittin-buried micelles with vigorous stirring. This way can efficiently deactivate melittin under physiological condition, but there are still some issues. The organic solvent should be removed for the in vitro and in vivo application. However, due to the high boiling point, DMSO is difficult to evaporate from the solution of the micellar system. Although the dialysis method can be used for the exchange of organic solvent with water, it may lead to the loss of the block copolymer during dialysis and lyophilization process, which can result in the inaccurate nitrogen-to-phosphate ratio for gene delivery. Besides, it is found that the solubility of P(OEGMA-DMAEMA)-b-P(DIPAMA-(PDSEMA-melittin)) is lower than its parent polymer, P(OEGMA-DMAEMA)-b-P(DIPAMA-PDSEMA), which also raises the issue for the preparation of micellar stock solution with high concentrations for in vivo applications.

A neutralization method is recommended for the preparation the micelles formed by P(OEGMA-DMAEMA)-b-P(DIPAMA-(PDSEMA-melittin). The functional polymer can be first dissolved in 0.2 M monobasic sodium phosphate solution with pH around 4.5, in which DIPAMA is completely ionized and mellitin is exposed. Then the solution of dibasic sodium phosphate (0.2 M) with relative volume was added to adjust the pH of the above solution to pH 7.4, and PDIPAMA block was deprotonated to undergo the hydrophilic to hydrophobic transition, by which melittin was completely encapsulated in the core of PDIPAMA. Hemolysis study demonstrated that negligible membrane lysis with human red blood cells was detected for the formed micelles at pH 7.4, which was similar as that by the parent polymer, demonstrating the acceptable biocompatibility. On the other hand, the release of hemoglobin with lysis ratio higher than 90% was observed at pH 5.7, indicating the selective shielding and release of the lytic peptide. Moreover, the same trend of hemolysis was found for the complexes formed by P(OEGMA-DMAEMA)-b-P(DIPAMA-(PDSEMA-melittin)) and plasmids, and the formation of polyplexes did not take any effect on the lytic activity. In vitro cell transfection showed that the delivery efficiency of luciferase and GFP plasmid by P(OEGMA-DMAEMA)-b-P(DIPAMA-(PDSEMA-melittin)) was much higher than that by P(OEGMA-DMAEMA)-b-P(DIPAMA-PDSEMA), which was even superior to the "gold standard" PEI 25 k. This method can not only address the issue of off-site lysis, but also realize facile preparation and timesaving without the use of organic solvent.

## 3.3 Endo/Lysosome Release of the Polyplexes

The endo/lysosome escape of the polyplexes formed by lytic peptide modified polymer and the parent polymer was tracked by triple fluorescence confocal microscopy, in which DNA was labeled by YOYO-1 with green fluorescence and the lysosome was stained with red fluorescence. It was found that most of the green fluorescence (YOYO-1 DNA) from the polyplexes formed by melittin-functionalized polycations was separated from the red fluorescence (LysoTracker Red), indicating efficient endo/lysosomal escape. On the other hand, nearly complete colocalization (yellow) of green and red fluorescence was observed in cells treated with polyplexes formed by the parent polycations. Moreover, the colocalization ratio of polyplexes including lytic peptide with lysosomes was only 9.4% compared with 72.2% for melittin absented group, which was consistent with the observation by confocal microscopy. Usually, PEI polyplexes show similar intracellular distribution profiles as the polyplexes formed by parent polymer and plasmid DNA. These results confirmed the efficient endo/lysosome release of the polyplexes mediated by melittin-modified polycations.

## 3.4 In Vitro Transfection by P(OEGMA-DMAEMA)-b-P(DIPAMA-(PDSEMA-Melittin))

Due to positive charge nature of polycations, these polymers may interact with negative charged biomacromolecules (bovine serum in the cell culture medium) to result in the unpacking of the payloads in transfection. Hence, optiMEM is commonly used to dilute the polyplexes formed by polycations and genes for in vitro transfection. However, incubating cells with optiMEM may be not beneficial to the proliferation of cells. Hence, it is recommended to use complete culture medium for the preparation of the transfection solution in this system. It should be noted that the presence of bovine serum in the transfection media did not affect the delivery efficiency.

For cell transfection, the incubation time of polyplexes with cells is related with transfection efficiency and cytotoxicity. In the most of the reported work, the polyplexes were usually contacted with cells for 4 h before medium renewal, by which enough polycations can be endocytosed by cells to mediate endo/lysosome release through "proton sponge effect," such as PEI, PDMAEMA-mediated gene transfection. For P(OEGMA-DMAEMA)-b-P(DIPAMA-(PDSEMA-melittin)), the potent membrane lysis activity by melittin could enable fast escape of the formed complexes from endo/lysosome entrapment with less polymers, and thus the incubation was shortened. It was found that the percentage of YOYO-1 positive cells was around 100% after 2 h incubation of the polyplexes formed by melittin-modified block copolymer and YOYO-1-labeled DNA with HeLa cells, indicating that efficient uptake was achieved. Hence, in this system, the incubation time of 2 h is recommended. On the other hand, the gene dose for transfection is also of importance. For the "gold standard" PEI polycation, the dose of 1 ug DNA per well (24-well plate with cell density of 25,000 cells/well) can obtain the best transfection. To realize the efficient protection of genes, there needs more polycations if the gene dose is higher, which may lead to potential cytotoxicity by the excess polycations. It is found that 0.5 ug DNA per well (24-well plate with cell density of 25,000 cells/well) is sufficient to achieve high gene transfection efficiency. Through the optimization of these conditions, the luciferase expression mediated by P(OEGMA-DMAEMA)-b-P(DIPAMA-(PDSEMA-melittin) was orders of magnitude higher than that by PEI 25 k in various cell lines (HeLa and KB cervical carcinomas, A549 lung carcinoma, and Z310 choroidal epithelial cells), and the percentage of GFP positive cells was in the range of 36–77%, which was 11- to 46-fold of PEI 25 k. In the HeLa and KB cells, it was also found that the transfection efficiency was even higher than the commercial transfection reagent, lipofectamine 2000.

### 3.5 Optimization of the Synthesis of PDMAEMA-C6M3, PEI-C6M3, and PLL-C6M3

It is reported that the EC50 (the concentration of free peptide for 50% hemolysis) of C6M3 (6 uM) is similar as that by meliitin (5 uM) at pH 5.5, demonstrating their potent membrane lysis activity in endo/lysosome. However, at pH 7.4, the EC50 of C6M3 (100 uM) is much higher than that by melittin (6 uM), indicating the acceptable biocompatibility extracellularly. Hence, modification of polycations with this pH-sensitive lytic peptide is expected to address the dilemma of safety concerns and transfection efficiency. However, It is found that the hemolysis mediated by PDMAEMA-C6M3, PEI-C6M3, and PLL-C6M3 was lower than 60% even the concentration of the functional polycations was higher than 100 ug/mL, by which there were 2, 1.2, and 0.9 C6M3 for PDMAEMA, PLL, and PEI, respectively. Therefore, it is recommended that more than 2 C6M3 are required to be incorporated with the polycations.

## 3.6 Polyplexes Formation by PDMAEMA-C6M3, PEI-C6M3, and PLL-C6M3 and Plasmid DNA

For the preparation of polyplexes in this system, the pH of the polymer solution is recommended to be around 6, by which the polycations can efficiently condense plasmids into nanostructure. Besides, at pH 7.4, C6M3 is relatively hydrophobic, and thus the size of the formed polyplexes by PDMAEMA-C6M3, PEI-C6M3, and PLL-C6M3 was slight bigger than that by the parent polycations. Besides, due to the hydrophobic shielding of C6M3, the zeta potential of the polyplexes was also reduced.

## 3.7 In Vitro Transfection by PDMAEMA-C6M3, PEI-C6M3, and PLL-C6M3

For the complexes formed by PDMAEMA-C6M3, PEI-C6M3, PLL-C6M3, and DNA, due to the lack of the structure to maintain the colloidal stability, these formations are not stable in the presence of negative-charged biomacromolecules (e.g., bovine serum in cell culture media). Hence, for the transfection study, it is recommended to use optiMEM instead of complete cell culture media. The DNA dose and incubation time of cells with transfection solution are 1 ug DNA per well (24-well plate with cell density of 25,000 cells/well) and 4 h followed previous studies, respectively. It is found that the luciferase expression in HeLa cells mediated by PDMAEMA-C6M3, PEI-C6M3, and PLL-C6M3 with the nitrogen-to-phosphate ratio of 5 was around 5.7, 3.1, and 7.8 times higher than that by PDMAEMA, PEI, and PLL, respectively. When GFP plasmid was used, PDMAEMA-C6M3 and PEI-C6M3 can transfected 22% and 29% cells, which were much higher than those mediated by the parent PDMAEMA and PEI (7.0% and 16.3%). However, for PLL-C6M3, the transfection efficiency was pretty low, which may be attributed to the hard unpackaging of the payloads in the cytoplasm. Although the higher transfection efficiency was achieved when the nitrogen-to-phosphate ratio was elevated to 7, the cell viability was lower than 80%. Hence, the nitrogen-to-phosphate ratio of 5 is recommended for in vitro transfection study in this system.

Although the in vitro transfection efficiency by C6M3-modified polycations was effective, it is far from the expectation. As mentioned above, the EC50 of C6M3 and melittin is similar under endo/lysosome acidic condition, and thus the in vitro transfection should be in the same level. But it was found that the transfection efficiency was much lower in this system. The probable reason is that the stability of the polyplexes is poor even in optiMEM. On the other hand, the cell biocompatibility of PDMAEMA-C6M3, PEI-C6M3, and PLL-C6M3 was improved compared with melittin-modified polycations. When the nitrogen-to-phosphate ratio was 5 in the transfection, the cell viability mediated by PDMAEMA-C6M3, PEI-C6M3, and PLL-C6M3 was higher than 80%, which was reduced to around 30% for melittin-functionalized oligo-lysine (Zhang et al. 2001).

## 4 Conclusion

Tremendous efforts have been made to address the issues of polycations-based gene vectors for gene therapy. While effective, they still face various challenges during the delivery process, especially endo/lysosome entrapment. As a potent membrane-lytic agent, peptides, such as mellitin and C6M3, could disrupt the membrane structures of endo/lysosomes, followed by successful cytoplasm delivery of the payloads. However, due to nonselective lytic behavior, promising gene transfection usually accompanies with serious safety concerns by the peptides modified polycations. To address this dilemma, the lytic peptides can be shielded by stimuli-triggered structure transformation or modified with revisable chemical linkages to realize selective membrane-lytic activity. In this chapter, pH-sensitive polymer, PDIPAMA with pKa of 6.3, was selected to shield melittin at physiological pH and unveil its natural membrane-lytic activity under endo/lysosome acidic condition to realize the acceptable biocompatibility and efficient endo/lysosome escape; C6M3 peptide featuring pH-triggered lytic activity was used to modified polycations (PLL, PDMAEMA, and PEI) to achieve the balance of off-site membrane lysis and improved gene transfection. Through the utilization of the intracellular stimuli, the undesired cytotoxicity by lytic peptides can be minimized and the gene delivery efficiency can be enhanced. However, due to the lack of tissue and cell targeting capability, the peptide-modified polycations presented in this chapter were not easily translated into in vivo applications. Hence, further studies may focus on the optimization of the lytic peptide functionalized polycations with the capability of long circulation time in blood and targeting tissues accumulation.

## References


Ahmed M, Narain R (2013) Progress of RAFT based polymers in gene delivery. Prog Polym Sci 38 (5):767–790

Akinc A, Thomas M, Klibanov AM, Langer R (2005) Exploring polyethylenimine-mediated DNA transfection and the proton sponge hypothesis. J Gene Med 7(5):657–663

Arnold AE, Czupiel P, Shoichet M (2017) Engineered polymeric nanoparticles to guide the cellular internalization and trafficking of small interfering ribonucleic acids. J Control Release 259:3–15

Boeckle S, Fahrmeir J, Roedl W, Ogris M, Wagner E (2006) Melittin analogs with high lytic activity at endosomal pH enhance transfection with purified targeted PEI polyplexes. J Control Release 112(2):240–248

Brooks H, Lebleu B, Vives E (2005) Tat peptide-mediated cellular delivery: back to basics. Adv Drug Deliver Rev 57(4):559–577

Bus T, Traeger A, Schubert US (2018) The great escape: how cationic polyplexes overcome the endosomal barrier. J Mater Chem B 6(43)

Cerovsky V, Hovorka O, Cvacka J, Voburka Z, Bednarova L, Borovickova L, Slaninova J, Fucik V (2008) Melectin: a novel antimicrobial peptide from the venom of the cleptoparasitic bee Melecta albifrons. Chembiochem 9(17):2815–2821

Chen CP, Kim JS, Steenblock E, Liu DJ, Rice KG (2006) Gene transfer with poly-melittin peptides. Bioconjug Chem 17(4):1057–1062

Chen BL, Yoo K, Xu W, Pan R, Han XX, Chen P (2017a) Characterization and evaluation of a peptide-based siRNA delivery system in vitro. Drug Deliv Transl Re 7(4):507–515

Chen JJ, Ding JX, Wang YC, Cheng JJ, Ji SX, Zhuang XL, Chen XS (2017b) Sequentially responsive shell-stacked nanoparticles for deep penetration into solid tumors. Adv Mater 29(32)

Christie RJ, Matsumoto Y, Miyata K, Nomoto T, Fukushima S, Osada K, Halnaut J, Pittella F, Kim HJ, Nishiyama N, Kataoka K (2012) Targeted polymeric micelles for siRNA treatment of experimental cancer by intravenous injection. ACS Nano 6(6):5174–5189

Convertine AJ, Benoit DSW, Duvall CL, Hoffman AS, Stayton PS (2009) Development of a novel endosomolytic diblock copolymer for siRNA delivery. J Control Release 133(3):221–229

Degors IMS, Wang CF, Rehman ZU, Zuhorn IS (2019) Carriers break barriers in drug delivery: endocytosis and endosomal escape of gene delivery vectors. Acc Chem Res 52(7):1750–1760

Freitag F, Wagner E (2021) Optimizing synthetic nucleic acid and protein nanocarriers: the chemical evolution approach. Adv Drug Deliver Rev 168:30–54

Ge CL, Yang JD, Duan SZ, Liu Y, Meng FH, Yin LC (2020) Fluorinated alpha-helical polypeptides synchronize mucus permeation and cell penetration toward highly efficient pulmonary siRNA delivery against acute lung injury. Nano Lett 20(3):1738–1746

Guan XW, Guo ZP, Lin L, Chen J, Tian HY, Chen XS (2016) Ultrasensitive pH triggered charge/size dual-rebound gene delivery system. Nano Lett 16(11):6823–6831

Jafari M, Xu W, Naahidi S, Chen BL, Chen P (2012) A new amphipathic, Amino-Acid-Pairing (AAP) peptide as siRNA delivery carrier: physicochemical characterization and in vitro uptake. J Phys Chem B 116(44):13183–13191

Jones RA, Cheung CY, Black FE, Zia JK, Stayton PS, Hoffman AS, Wilson MR (2003) Poly (2-alkylacrylic acid) polymers deliver molecules to the cytosol by pH-sensitive disruption of endosomal vesicles. Biochem J 372:65–75

Kwon EJ, Bergen JM, Pun SH (2008) Application of an HIV gp41-derived peptide for enhanced intracellular trafficking of synthetic gene and siRNA delivery vehicles. Bioconjug Chem 19(4): 920–927

Lachelt U, Wagner E (2015) Nucleic acid therapeutics using polyplexes: a journey of 50 years (and beyond). Chem Rev 115(19):11043–11078

Li JG, Yu XS, Wang Y, Yuan YY, Xiao H, Cheng D, Shuai XT (2014) A reduction and pH dual-sensitive polymeric vector for long-circulating and tumor-targeted siRNA delivery. Adv Mater 26(48):8217–8224

Liu X, Xiang JJ, Zhu DC, Jiang LM, Zhou ZX, Tang JB, Liu XR, Huang YZ, Shen YQ (2016) Fusogenic reactive oxygen species triggered charge-reversal vector for effective gene delivery. Adv Mater 28(9):1743–1752

Meyer M, Philipp A, Oskuee R, Schmidt C, Wagner E (2008) Breathing life into polycations: functionalization with pH-responsive endosomolytic peptides and polyethylene glycol enables siRNA delivery. J Am Chem Soc 130(11):3272–3273

Miyata K, Nishiyama N, Kataoka K (2012) Rational design of smart supramolecular assemblies for gene delivery: chemical challenges in the creation of artificial viruses. Chem Soc Rev 41(7): 2562–2574

Molla MR, Levkin PA (2016) Combinatorial approach to nanoarchitectonics for nonviral delivery of nucleic acids. Adv Mater 28(6):1159–1175

Naldini L (2015) Gene therapy returns to centre stage. Nature 526(7573):351–360

Nishiyama N, Arnida, Jang WD, Date K, Miyata K, Kataoka K (2006) Photochemical enhancement of transgene expression by polymeric micelles incorporating plasmid DNA and dendrimer-based photosensitizer. J Drug Target 14(6):413–424

Peeler DJ, Thai SN, Cheng YL, Horner PJ, Sellers DL, Pun SH (2019) pH-sensitive polymer micelles provide selective and potentiated lytic capacity to venom peptides for effective intracellular delivery. Biomaterials 192:235–244

Pei DH, Buyanova M (2019) Overcoming endosomal entrapment in drug delivery. Bioconjug Chem 30(2):273–283

Peng L, Wagner E (2019) Polymeric carriers for nucleic acid delivery: current designs and future directions. Biomacromolecules 20(10):3613–3626

Rudolph C, Plank C, Lausier J, Schillinger U, Muller RH, Rosenecker J (2003) Oligomers of the arginine-rich motif of the HIV-1 TAT protein are capable of transferring plasmid DNA into cells. J Biol Chem 278(13):11411–11418
Schellinger JG, Pahang JA, Shi JL, Pun SH (2013a) Block copolymers containing a hydrophobic domain of membrane-lytic peptides form micellar structures and are effective gene delivery agents. ACS Macro Lett 2(8):725–730
Schellinger JG, Pahang JA, Johnson RN, Chu DSH, Sellers DL, Maris DO, Convertine AJ, Stayton PS, Horner PJ, Pun SH (2013b) Melittin-grafted HPMA-oligolysine based copolymers for gene delivery. Biomaterials 34(9):2318–2326
Song CF, Li LY, Dai LZ, Thayumanavan S (2015) Responsive single-chain polymer nanoparticles with host-guest features. Polym Chem-UK 6(26):4828–4834
Sun CY, Shen S, Xu CF, Li HJ, Liu Y, Cao ZT, Yang XZ, Xia JX, Wang J (2015) Tumor acidity-sensitive polymeric vector for active targeted siRNA delivery. J Am Chem Soc 137(48):15217–15224
Thomas CE, Ehrhardt A, Kay MA (2003) Progress and problems with the use of viral vectors for gene therapy. Nat Rev Genet 4(5):346–358
Varga CM, Tedford NC, Thomas M, Klibanov AM, Griffith LG, Lauffenburger DA (2005) Quantitative comparison of polyethylenimine formulations and adenoviral vectors in terms of intracellular gene delivery processes. Gene Ther 12(13):1023–1032
Varkouhi AK, Scholte M, Storm G, Haisma HJ (2011) Endosomal escape pathways for delivery of biologicals. J Control Release 151(3):220–228
Wang MM, Liu HM, Li L, Cheng YY (2014a) A fluorinated dendrimer achieves excellent gene transfection efficacy at extremely low nitrogen to phosphorus ratios. Nat Commun 5
Wang YG, Zhou KJ, Huang G, Hensley C, Huang XN, Ma XP, Zhao T, Sumer BD, DeBerardinis RJ, Gao JM (2014b) A nanoparticle-based strategy for the imaging of a broad range of tumours by nonlinear amplification of microenvironment signals. Nat Mater 13(2):204–212
Wang LH, Wu DC, Xu HX, You YZ (2016) High DNA-binding affinity and gene-transfection efficacy of bioreducible cationic nanomicelles with a fluorinated core. Angew Chem Int Edit 55 (2):755–759
Wang YG, Wang CS, Li Y, Huang G, Zhao T, Ma XP, Wang ZH, Sumer BD, White MA, Gao JM (2017) Digitization of endocytic pH by hybrid ultra-pH-sensitive nanoprobes at single-organelle resolution. Adv Mater 29(1)
Xu FJ, Yang WT (2011) Polymer vectors via controlled/living radical polymerization for gene delivery. Prog Polym Sci 36(9):1099–1131
Xu XD, Wu J, Liu YL, Yu MY, Zhao LL, Zhu X, Bhasin S, Li Q, Ha E, Shi JJ, Farokhzad OC (2016) Ultra-pH-responsive and tumor-penetrating nanoplatform for targeted siRNA delivery with robust anti-cancer efficacy. Angew Chem Int Edit 55(25):7091–7094
Yang XC, Niu YL, Zhao NN, Mao C, Xu FJ (2014) A biocleavable pullulan-based vector via ATRP for liver cell-targeting gene delivery. Biomaterials 35(12):3873–3884
Yin H, Kanasty RL, Eltoukhy AA, Vegas AJ, Dorkin JR, Anderson DG (2014) Non-viral vectors for gene-based therapy. Nat Rev Genet 15(8):541–555
Yu HJ, Zou YL, Wang YG, Huang XN, Huang G, Sumer BD, Boothman DA, Gao JM (2011) Overcoming endosomal barrier by amphotericin B-loaded dual pH-responsive PDMA-b-PDPA micelleplexes for siRNA delivery. ACS Nano 5(11):9246–9255
Yuan YY, Zhang CJ, Liu B (2015) A photoactivatable AIE polymer for light-controlled gene delivery: concurrent endo/lysosomal escape and DNA unpacking. Angew Chem Int Edit 54 (39):11419–11423
Zhang XH, Collins L, Fabre JW (2001) A powerful cooperative interaction between a fusogenic peptide and lipofectamine for the enhancement of receptor-targeted, non-viral gene delivery via integrin receptors. J Gene Med 3(6):560–568

# Preparation and Evaluation of Supramolecular Hydrogels for Localized Sustained Gene Delivery

# 13

Lingjie Ke, Yun-Long Wu, and Huayu Tian

## Contents



**Abstract**

Multidrug resistance is one of the biggest challenges in cancer therapy which makes less therapeutic effect. Studies have shown that drug resistance in most tumor cells is caused by overexpression of Bcl-2 protein. Orphan nuclear receptor Nur77/ΔDBD which lacks DNA-binding domain can combine in the middle of BH3 and BH4 domain of Bcl-2 protein to reverse Bcl-2 protein function from anti-apoptosis to promoting apoptosis. Therefore, cancer gene therapy based on Nur77/ΔDBD is expected to be another effective strategy for treating multidrug resistance of tumors. For this, gene therapy system needs an effective gene delivery system to realize the genetic modification of tumor cells. Compared with viral vectors with high immunogenicity in vivo, highly biocompatible cationic polymeric nonviral vectors become popular for gene delivery due to their good biocompatibility and high affinity. Amphiphilic MPEG-PCL-PEI

L. Ke · Y.-L. Wu (✉)
Fujian Provincial Key Laboratory of Innovative Drug Target Research and State Key Laboratory of Cellular Stress Biology, School of Pharmaceutical Sciences, Xiamen University, Xiamen, China
e-mail: wuyl@xmu.edu.cn

H. Tian (✉)
Key Laboratory of Polymer Ecomaterials, Changchun Institute of Applied Chemistry, Chinese Academy of Sciences, Changchun, China
e-mail: thy@ciac.ac.cn



H. Tian and X. Chen (eds.), *Gene Delivery*, Biomaterial Engineering,
https://doi.org/10.1007/978-981-16-5419-0_13

(PPP) tri-block cationic polymer have been designed to deliver Nur77/ΔDBD gene with high transfection efficiency, which consisted of methoxy-poly(ethylene glycol) (MPEG), polycaprolactone (PCL), and positively charged poly-ethyleneimine (PEI). In order to further maintain long-lasting gene therapy, we introduced α-CD to form a supramolecular hydrogel with polymer by host-guest interaction, achieving a sustained gene release up to 7 days, which might indicate the importance of sustained gene delivery systems.

**Keywords**

Multidrug resistance; Gene delivery; Cationic polymer; Supramolecular hydrogel; Sustained release

## 1 Overview

Cancer is still one of highest mortality rate diseases in the world and the morbidity of cancer is rising year by year (Barta et al. 2019; Mattiuzzi and Lippi 2019; Wu et al. 2019). Chemotherapy has a great effect in the treatment of cancer, but long-term drug treatment will cause the tumor cells to develop their own drug resistance, which will gradually lose the effectiveness of therapy (Nikolaou et al. 2018; Sarmento-Ribeiro et al. 2019; Vasan et al. 2019). In general treatment, a large number of patients will develop drug resistance after taking the same chemotherapy drug (Freimund et al. 2018; O'Donnell et al. 2019). In this case, the approach to solve the problem of drug resistance is a key to conquer tumor treatment. There are many proteins that regulate the apoptosis of tumor cells, among which the B-cell lymphoma-2 (Bcl-2) protein family plays important role and is mainly divided into two categories: pro-apoptotic proteins and anti-apoptotic proteins (Ashkenazi et al. 2017; Knight et al. 2019). Among them, anti-apoptotic proteins of Bcl-2 mainly refer to Bcl-$X_L$ and Bcl-2, while the pro-apoptotic proteins mainly include Bid and Bax (Tsujimoto 1998; Huang et al. 2019). The manner to exert anti-apoptotic or pro-apoptotic effects mainly depends on the expression of BH3 domain of Bcl-2 protein. As the multidrug resistance of tumor cells is mainly due to the occlusion of BH3 domain by other proteins, a Bcl-2 analogue containing BH3 domain might reverse the anti-apoptotic effect of Bcl-2 protein (Cyrille et al. 2018; Tutusaus et al. 2018). A number of reports have shown that the orphan nuclear receptors Nur77 without deoxyribonucleic acid (DNA) binding domain (Nur77/ΔDBD) under the stimulus of different death signals might locate on the mitochondria and insert between BH3 and BH4 structure domains of Bcl-2 protein family. In this case, conformation heterogeneous of Bcl-2 might cause the BH3 domain structure exposure, thus Bcl-2 anti-apoptotic mechanisms will be reversed for pro-apoptosis mechanism (Sun et al. 2012; Cheng et al. 2018).

Owing to genetic instability and degradation characteristics, rational design of efficient gene delivery vector with intra-nucleus Nur77/ΔDBD gene delivery ability might be useful to reverse Bcl-2 anti-apoptotic mechanisms and to reverse tumor multidrug resistance (Wang et al. 2017). In the long-term research of gene therapy, there are two primary gene delivery vector, viral vector and nonviral vector (Ayen et al. 2018; Ke et al. 2020). Because of obvious immune toxicity, viral vectors might be gradually replaced by nonviral vectors (Kesharwani et al. 2018; Patil et al. 2019). Cationic polymer vector is one of the most important nonviral vectors, which mainly relies on its own large amount of positive charge to complexing and wrapping genes through electrostatic interaction, forming nanoparticles of dozens to hundreds particle sizes (Guan et al. 2016). Cationic polymers are widely used for gene delivery due to their high biosafety, high stability, and easy modification (Fang et al. 2018; Li et al. 2018; Liu et al. 2019). Polyethyleneimine (PEI) is the most typical cationic polymer, whose high positive property makes its gene delivery efficiency greatly increased, but its toxicity in vivo also increases at the same time (Zakeri et al. 2018; Jiang et al. 2019).

Cationic polymer micelle structure can achieve good transfection efficiency, but the action time is very short, while supramolecular hydrogel can greatly extend the gene expression efficiency and enhance the effect of gene therapy due to its high loading efficiency and controllable sustained-release ability. Here, methoxy-poly (ethylene glycol) (MPEG) and biodegradable polycaprolactone (PCL) are modified on the basis of PEI to form amphiphilic tri-block copolymer MPEG-PCL-PEI (PPP), which can be complexed with genes to form micelle structure, with high stability, transfection efficiency, and safety (Liu et al. 2017). It is worth mentioning that by adding α-cyclodextrin (α-CD) ring polymer, the long MPEG chain of PPP can assemble with α-CD to form polyrotaxane supramolecular hydrogel structure through host-guest interaction. In this protocol, we have summarized detailed preparation procedure of PPP/Nur77 polyplex loading gene and PPP/α-CD/Nur77 supramolecular hydrogel, and further elaborated sustained releasing experiment process of hydrogel, in vitro gene transfection experiment process, drug-resistant cell line construction method, and in vitro toxicity experiment method.

# 2 Protocol

## 2.1 Materials

### 2.1.1 Synthesis and Characterization of Positively Charged Amphiphilic PPP Copolymer

1. Methoxy-poly(ethylene glycol) (MPEG)
2. ε-Caprolactone (ε-CL)
3. $N_2$
4. Polyethyleneimine (PEI)
5. Stannous octoate [$Sn(Oct)_2$]
6. Toluene
7. Diethyl ether
8. Dimethyl sulfoxide (DMSO)
9. Dimethylformamide (DMF)

10. 1,1′-carbonyldiimidazole (CDI)
11. MeOD
12. Spectrum dialysis membrane (molecular weight cut-off or MWCO, 10 k)
13. Deionized water
14. Magnetic stirrer
15. Lyophilizer
16. Nuclear magnetic resonance (NMR, Bruker AV600, Bruker)
17. Fourier transform infrared spectrometer (FITR, Nicolet 380, Thermo Electron)
18. Gel permeation chromatography (GPC, Tosoh EcoSEC)

#### 2.1.2 Preparation of PPP/Nur77 Polyplex

1. Nur77/ΔDBD plasmid deoxyribonucleic acid or pDNA
2. Double distilled water

#### 2.1.3 Gel Retardation Assay of PPP/Nur77 Polyplex

1. 1× Tris-acetic acid-EDTA (TAE)
2. GelRed
3. Agarose
4. Deionized water
5. 6× Loading buffer
6. DNA Marker (2500 bp)
7. Horizontal electrophoresis apparatus
8. Gel imager (Tanon-2500B, Tanon)

#### 2.1.4 Particle Size and Potential Measurement of PPP/Nur77 Polyplex

1. Dynamic light scattering zetasizer (DLS) (Nano S90, Malvern)

#### 2.1.5 Preparation of PPP/α-CD/Nur77 Supramolecular Hydrogels

1. α-Cyclodextrin (α-CD)
2. Double distilled water
3. Magnetic stirrer

#### 2.1.6 Sustained Gene Release Assay of Supramolecular Hydrogels

1. Phosphate buffered solution (PBS)
2. Nano Droper 1000 Micro-Ultraviolet Spectrophotometer

#### 2.1.7 Cell Culture

1. Dulbecco's Modified Eagle's Medium (DMEM)
2. Penicillin
3. Streptomycin
4. Trypsin-EDTA
5. Fetal bovine serum (FBS)
6. $CO_2$ incubator
7. Vertical flow clean bench
8. Optical microscope

### 2.1.8 In Vitro Gene Delivery Efficiency Assessment of PPP/Nur77 Polyplex

1. 12-well cell culture plates
2. Renilla luciferase reporter gene assay kit
3. Multifunctional microplate reader

### 2.1.9 Construction of HepG2/Bcl-2 Hepatocellular Carcinoma Cell Lines Overexpressing Bcl-2

1. HEK-293 cells
2. pCDH-GFP-Bcl-2 viral plasmid
3. Lentiviruses packing auxiliary plasmid I (vsvg)
4. Lentiviruses packing auxiliary plasmid II (Δ8.91
5. Polybrene
6. Confocal microscope (LSM5 EXCITER, Zeiss)

### 2.1.10 Cytotoxicity Verification of PPP/Nur77 Polyplex for Tumor-Resistant Cells

1. Thiazolyl blue (MTT)
2. DMSO
3. Multifunctional microplate reader

## 2.2 Methods

### 2.2.1 Preparation of Positively Charged Amphiphilic PPP Copolymer (Note 1, 2)

#### Synthesis Method of MPEG-PCL-OH

1. A certain amount of MPEG and ε-CL (molar ratio, 1:15) was respectively measured and put into the dryer, which was stirred and mixed well under the protection of $N_2$.
2. $Sn(Oct)_2$ catalyst was added and reacted in toluene at 120 °C for 48 h.
3. Prepare the precooled diethyl ether and precipitate the reactant in the ice diethyl ether twice.
4. The obtained MPEG-PCL-OH products were dried under vacuum at 60 °C.

#### Synthesis Method for MPEG-PCL-Imidazole

1. Prepare MPEG-PCL-OH (0.9 g) solution in DMSO solvent (5 mL), and 0.5 g CDI was dissolved in anhydrous DMF (5 mL), and the two were mixed and stirred overnight under the protection of $N_2$.
2. Prepare the precooled diethyl ether and precipitate the reactant in the ice diethyl ether twice, and the reaction product MPEG-PCL-imidazole was precipitated.

**Synthesis Method for PPP**

1. Prepare MPEG-PCL-imidazole (0.9 g) solution in DMSO solvent (5 mL), and 1.5 g PEI was dissolved in DMSO (5 mL) too.
2. MPEG-PCL-imidazole solution was added to the PEI solution and the reaction stirred slowly for 36 h at room temperature.
3. PPP copolymer products was purified by dialysis bag (MWCO, 10 kDa) to remove the unbranched PEI.
4. PPP dry products was obtained by freeze-drying (Fig. 1).

### 2.2.2 Characterization of PPP Cationic Polymer

1. $^1$H-NMR: 5 mg PPP solid was dissolved in 1 mL MeOD. NMR was used to detect the NMR hydrogen spectra of MPEG, MPEG-PCL, and PPP, respectively (Fig. 2).

2. GPC: The Tosoh EcoSEC GPC system was used to determine the molecular mass, PDI, and critical micelle concentration of the polymer, thus determining the molecular ratio of grafting.

3. FTIR: FTIR was used to detect the FTIR spectra of MPEG-PCL and PPP polymer (Fig. 3).

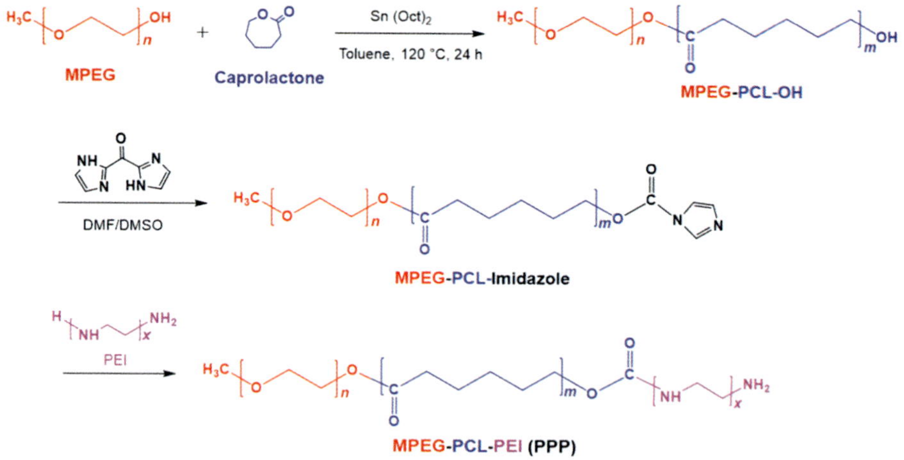


**Fig. 1** Synthesis route of positively charged amphiphilic PPP copolymer. (Adapted from Liu et al. (2017), with permission, Copyright Wiley VCH)

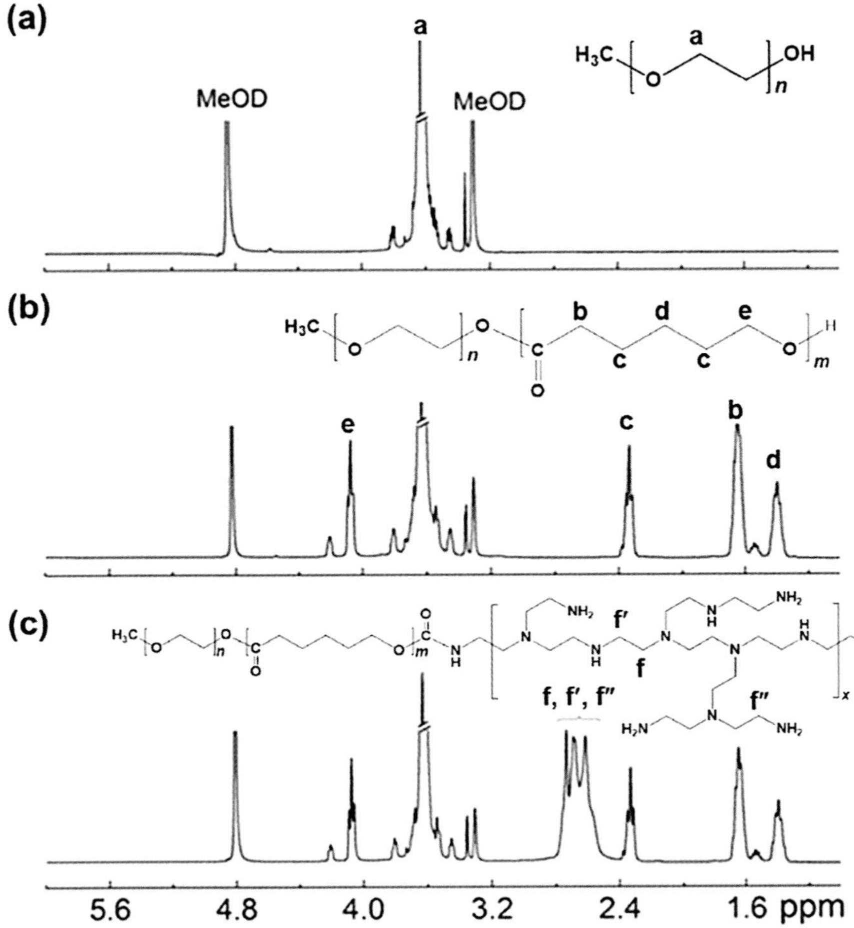


**Fig. 2** [1]H-NMR spectra of (**a**) MPEG, (**b**) MPEG-PCL, and (**c**) PPP, respectively (solvent, MeOD). (Adapted from Liu et al. (2017), with permission, Copyright Wiley VCH)

### 2.2.3 Preparation of PPP/Nur77 Polyplex (Note 3)

1. 0.5 mg PPP was dissolved in 1 mL water for 0.5 mg/mL.
2. Nur77/ΔDBD pDNA was added to the above cationic polymer aqueous solution according to the gradient polymer/DNA weight ratios and incubated for 30 min at room temperature.

### 2.2.4 Gene Binding Capacity Characterization of PPP Polymer (Note 4)

#### Gel Retardation Assay

1. The cationic polymer PPP was prepared into an aqueous solution with a concentration of 5 mg/mL as the mother liquor.

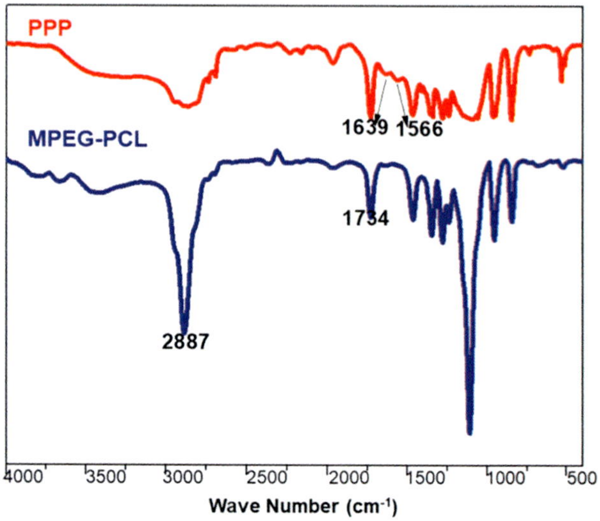


**Fig. 3** FTIR spectra of MPEG-PCL and PPP, respectively. (Adapted from Liu et al. (2017), with permission, Copyright Wiley VCH)

2. The cationic polymer aqueous solution and 0.5 mg/mL Nur77/ΔDBD plasmid aqueous solution with different weight ratios (polymer/plasmid = 0.05, 0.1, 0.5, 1, 1.5, 2, 5, 10) mixed (consistent DNA amount, fixed in 400 ng), incubation for 30 min at room temperature. A branching PEI with molecular weight of 25 kDa was used as control to prepare complexes with different weight ratios under the same conditions.
3. Weigh 1.2 g agarose with 1× TAE solution (60 mL) in a 300 mL conical flask and then was heated to boil in a microwave oven; take out the conical flask and shake fully. Reheat and boil the solution 2–3 times until it is completely clear and transparent. When the solution was cooled to about 60 °C at room temperature, add 6 μL 30,000× GelRedTM, mix it thoroughly, and pour it into the assembled gel electrophoresis module to solidify completely at room temperature.
4. The solidified agarose gel was placed in a horizontal electrophoresis apparatus and sufficient amount of 1× TAE electrophoretic solution was added until the gel was completely submerged.
5. A certain amount of DNA loading buffer was added to PPP/Nur77 solution. Then mixture and 5000 bp DNA marker were successively added into the sample slot. After 40 min of electrophoresis under constant pressure of 110 V, the gel retardation results were observed in the gel imager (Fig. 4).

### Particle Size and Potential Detection

1. A series of PPP/Nur77 polyplex with concentration gradient were prepared and diluted with double distilled water to polymer's concentration of 50 μg/mL.
2. The particle size and potential of PPP/Nur77 polyplex were detected by dynamic light scattering zetasizer (Fig. 5).

**Fig. 4** Gel retardation assay of PPP/Nur77 polyplex at different weight ratios. (Adapted from Liu et al. (2017), with permission, Copyright Wiley VCH)

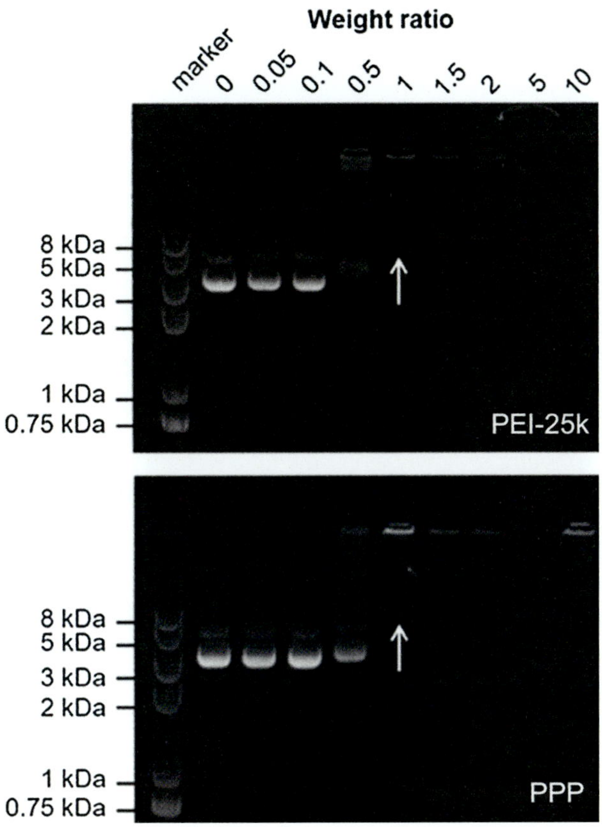


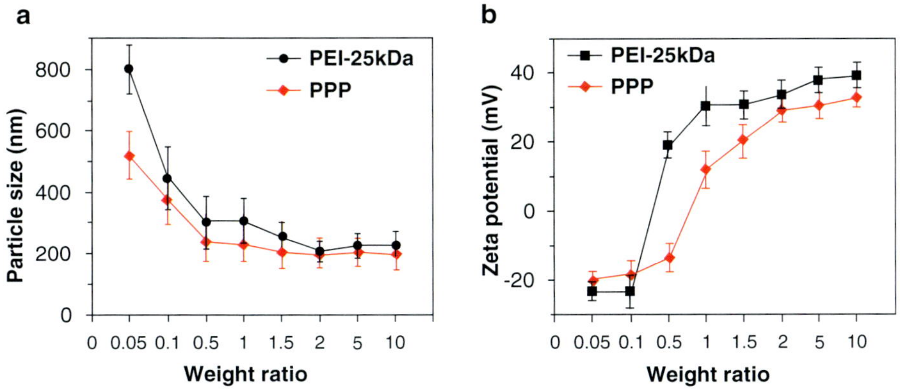


**Fig. 5** Characteristics of PPP/Nur77 polyplex. (a) Particle size and (b) potential of PPP/Nur77 polyplex at different weight ratios by dynamic light scattering. (Adapted from Liu et al. (2017), with permission, Copyright Wiley VCH)

### 2.2.5 Preparation of Supramolecular Hydrogels (Note 5)

1. The cationic polymer PPP was mixed with Nur77/ΔDBD plasmid at a certain weight ratio and incubated at normal temperature for another 30 min.
2. PEG was weighed and added to the above PPP/pDNA complex solution to achieve 1% (w/v) final concentration of PEG, mixed and incubated for another 10 min.
3. α-CD solution was added above solution to bring the final concentration to 8% (w/v).
4. At 4 °C overnight, PPP/α-CD/Nur77 white hydrogel was formed.

### 2.2.6 Evaluation of Sustained Release of Supramolecular Hydrogels in Vitro

1. 400 μL supramolecular hydrogel was prepared in a 2 mL EP tube, and the hydrogel was formed overnight in a refrigerator at 4 °C.
2. Equal volume PBS solution as the release medium was added to the upper layer of hydrogel slowly along the tube wall.
3. EP tubes were placed vertically in a constant temperature shaker and the genes were released at 37 °C and 50 rpm.
4. The supernatant PBS release medium was extracted on 0, 1, 2, 3, 4, 5, 6, 7 days, respectively, and fresh PBS was supplemented in time.
5. The Nur77/ΔDBD plasmid concentration released was determined with Nano Droper 1000 Micro-Ultraviolet Spectrophotometer (Fig. 6).

### 2.2.7 In Vitro Gene Transfection Evaluation of PPP Polymer (Note 6, 7)

1. The luciferin reporter gene system was utilized to determine the gene transfection capacity of cationic polymers.
2. HEK 293 cells were cultured in DMEM medium containing 10% FBS, 100 U/mL penicillin-streptomycin at 37 °C, 5% $CO_2$.

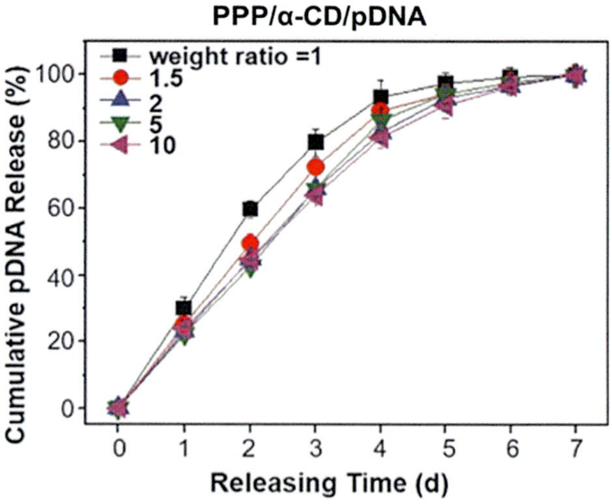


**Fig. 6** Cumulative Nur77/ΔDBD plasmid release curves of PPP/α-CD/Nur77 hydrogels at different weight ratios. (Adapted from Liu et al. (2017), with permission, Copyright Wiley VCH)

3. When the cells were in good condition, HEK 293 cells were spread in 48-well plates, and the density of cells was $5 \times 10^4$ cells/well.
4. PPP/pDNA polyplex was prepared using fresh medium according to the weight ratio of 1, 1.5, 2, 5, and 10 (polymer/luciferin reporter gene), gene transfection amount of each well in the 24-well plate was 500 ng, then place polyplex incubate at normal temperature for 30 min.
5. Before transfection, the cell culture medium in the 48-well plates was absorbed and replaced with the medium solution of PPP/pDNA polyplex with different weight ratios. Each group was set with at least 3 multiple wells and continued to be cultured in the incubator for 4–6 h.
6. The medium was siphoned and 100 μL of cell lysate was added to each well for incubating half an hour on the ice.
7. The lysed cells were transferred to a 96-well all-white plate, and 100 μL diluted sea kidney luciferase substrate was added in the dark. The fluorescence intensity was measured with a multifunctional microplate reader. Also, fluorescence was observed by inverted fluorescence microscope (Fig. 7).

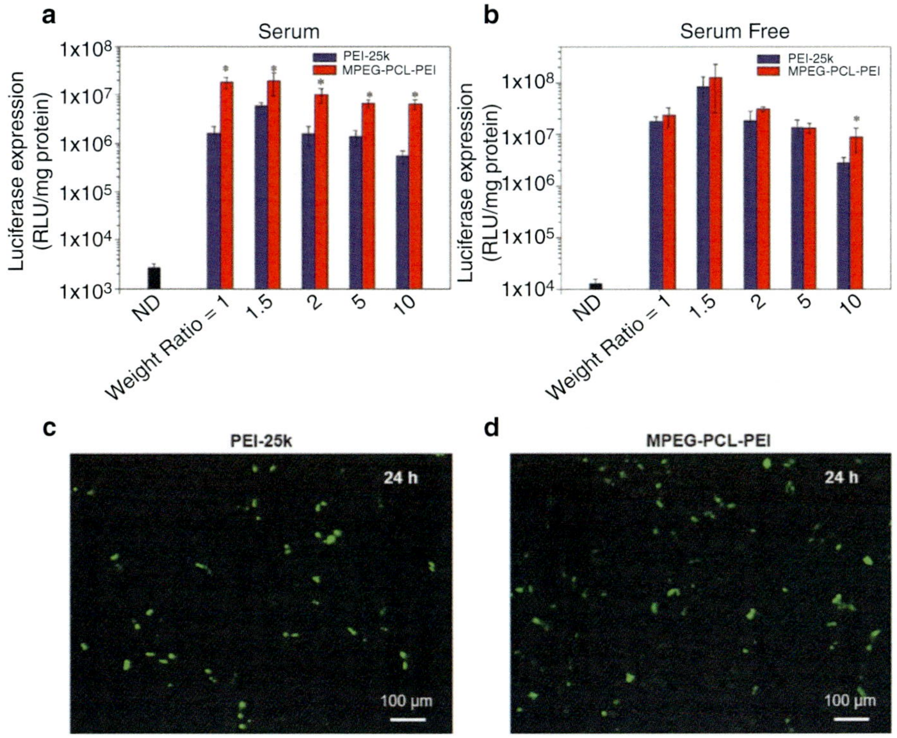


**Fig. 7** (**a**, **b**) In vitro gene transfection efficiency of cationic polymer PPP with serum and without serum. (**c**, **d**) The fluorescence expression of PPP under inverted fluorescence microscope was compared with the gold standard PEI. (Adapted from Liu et al. (2017), with permission, Copyright Wiley VCH)

### 2.2.8 Construction Method of Bcl-2 Overexpressed Tumor Cells (Note 8)

1. The density of HEK 293 cells reached about 70%, and the cells were cultured in serum-free DMEM medium at 37 °C for half an hour.
2. pCDH-GFP-Bcl-2 lentiviral plasmids containing Bcl-2 fragments, vsvg, and Δ8.91 helper plasmids (weight ratio, 5:2:3) were diluted in serum-free DMEM medium, mixed with PEI solution, and incubated for 30 min.
3. The mixed solution was transferred to HEK 293 cells and cultured at 37 °C for 4–6 h.
4. The culture medium was replaced with fresh DMEM medium containing 10% FBS.
5. The virus particles were collected by centrifuging at 3000 rpm for 15 min after culturing for 48–72 h.
6. Culture medium containing virus venom, 10% FBS, and 0.1% polybrene was transferred to HepG2 cells with a cell density of 50%.
7. The cells were passed on every 1–2 days, during which the cells were repeatedly infected with the virus venom for 3–4 times.
8. The fluorescence ratio of GFP was observed by inverted fluorescence microscope (Fig. 8).

### 2.2.9 Therapeutic Effect Evaluation of PPP/Nur77 Polyplex on Bcl-2 Drug-Resistant Tumor Cells

1. HepG2/Bcl-2 cells were seeded in a 96-well plate at a cell density of $1 \times 10^4$.
2. According to the results of reporter gene transfection, keep transfection weight ratio consistent, and PPP/Nur77 polyplex containing different plasmid concentrations was prepared. After incubation at room temperature for 30 min, PPP/Nur77 polyplex was added into the 96-well plate.
3. The original polyplex solution was replaced with fresh medium after 4–6 h culture in an incubator, then keep culturing for another 24 h.
4. 10 μL 5 mg/mL MTT solution was added to 96-well plate, and 150 μL DMSO was added after 3–4 h culture.
5. Ultraviolet absorption at 492 nm was detected by a multifunctional microplate reader (Fig. 9).

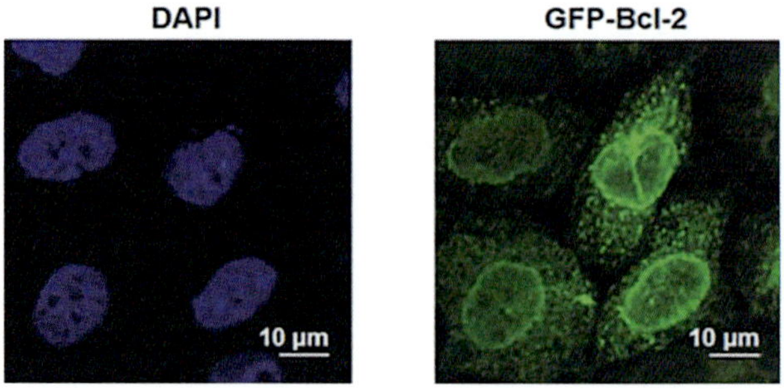


**Fig. 8** Fluorescence expression of GFP in Bcl-2 overexpressed HepG2 drug-resistant tumor cells by confocal microscope. (Adapted from Liu et al. (2017), with permission, Copyright Wiley VCH)

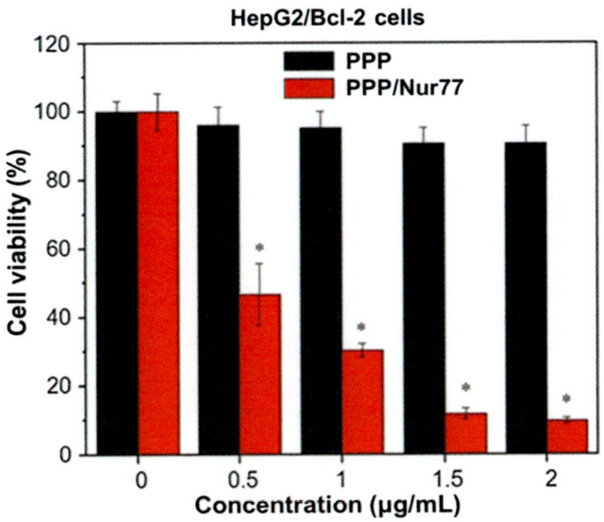


**Fig. 9** In vitro growth inhibition effect of PPP/Nur77 polyplex on HepG2/Bcl-2 cells. (Adapted from Liu et al. (2017), with permission, Copyright Wiley VCH)

## 3 Discussion

1. The synthesis of MPEG-PCL-OH was mainly formed by the ring-opening reaction of the caprolactone ester bond with the MPEG terminal hydroxyl group, and $Sn(Oct)_2$ as catalyst.
2. MPEG-PCL-imidazole is an intermediate for the synthesis of PPP, which is obtained mainly by activating the terminal hydroxyl group of MPEG-PCL-OH through CDI activator. Subsequently, a large number of amino groups on PEI can be used to replace the active group imidazole on MPEG-PCL-imidazole to obtain PPP tri-block copolymer through substitution reaction.
3. It can be seen from Table 1 that CMC of PPP copolymer is 23.4 μg/mL, which indicates that micelle structure can be formed when the polymer concentration is higher than 23.4 μg/mL.
4. PPP mainly depends on positively charged PEI structure to condense gene. When the gene is bound by the polymer through electrostatic interactions, the band of the gene will be blocked in the injection port of agarose gel. And the complexation between polymer and gene will change the particle size and potential of the polymer.
5. Cyclodextrins are widely used for encapsulating compound molecule due to their large hydrophobic cavities and hydrophilic shells in the middle, which can also be inserted by long-chain polymers to form polyrotaxane supramolecular hydrogels through molecular recognition and self-assembly (Xu et al. 2019).

**Table 1** Comparison table of molecular characterization of MPEG-OH, MPEG-PCL-OH, and PPP

| Samples | Copolymer composition (Da)[a] | | | $[M_n]$/kDa[a] | PDI[a] | N%[b] | CMC (μg/mL)[c] |
|---|---|---|---|---|---|---|---|
| | PEG | PCL | PEI/FE | | | | |
| MPEG-OH | 4900 | – | – | 4.9 | 1.1 | – | –[d] |
| MPEG-PCL-OH | 4900 | 1300 | – | 6.2 | 1.2 | – | 12.1 |
| MPEG-PCL-PEI | 4900 | 1300 | 11,500 | 17.7 | 1.6 | 12.8 | 23.4 |

[a]Determined by gel permeation chromatography (GPC)
[b]Nitrogen weight content was evaluated from elemental analyses (EA)
[c]Critical micellization concentration (CMC) was determined using dye solubilization method
[d]Not determined
Adapted from Liu et al. (2017), with permission, Copyright Wiley VCH

6. Luciferin reporter gene system is often used to detect the expression efficiency of polymer vector or virus vector delivering genes to nucleus. In addition, HEK 293 cells are often used as transfected cells due to its easy transfection.
7. PEI exhibits excellent gene load capacity and gene transfection efficiency due to its high cationic charge, but high charge is also associated with high toxicity. Grafting hydrophilic and hydrophobic fragments with high biocompatibility has been shown to effectively reduce the toxicity of PEI and even improve the transfection efficiency of genes (Huang et al. 2018; Li et al. 2019).
8. The construction of Bcl-2 overexpressed tumor cells is based on lentivirus packaging procedure, which mainly includes: (1) Construction of viral shuttle plasmids containing Bcl-2 target genes; (2) Co-transfection of shuttle plasmids and helper plasmids into HEK 293 cells to express virus particles; (3) The virus particles containing Bcl-2 expressing genes were transfected into host cells to express Bcl-2 proteins.

## 4 Conclusion

The chapter presents a variety of typical gene delivery vector, cationic polymer PPP, modified with hydrophilic MPEG and hydrophobic PCL fragment on the basis of PEI, which was used for drug-resistance Nur77/ΔDBD gene delivery. In terms of gold standard PEI, PPP has greatly increased the safety and efficiency of in vitro gene delivery. Cationic polymer is complexed with genes by electrostatic interaction. Furthermore, polymer/gene polyplex can be loaded with α-CD to form polyrotaxane supramolecular hydrogel structure. Due to its solid gel properties, gene loading rate of polymer is increased substantially, and the sustained time of gene release can be achieved for up to 7 days. The gene encapsulation capacity, gene release, particle size, potential, and transfection efficiency of cationic polymer have all been characterized. In general, the results show that the supramolecular cationic hydrogel system can slowly release genes, achieve efficient gene transfection, and also have a high pro-apoptotic effect on drug-resistant cells, suggesting polymer gene delivery system has a great prospect in the field of gene therapy.

## References

Ashkenazi A, Fairbrother WJ, Leverson JD et al (2017) From basic apoptosis discoveries to advanced selective BCL-2 family inhibitors. Nat Rev Drug Discov 16(4):273–284

Ayen A, Jimenez Martinez Y, Marchal JA et al (2018) Recent progress in gene therapy for ovarian cancer. Int J Mol Sci 19(7):e1930

Barta JA, Powell CA, Wisnivesky JP (2019) Global epidemiology of lung cancer. Ann Glob Health 85(1):1–16

Cheng H, Wu Z, Wu C et al (2018) Overcoming STC2 mediated drug resistance through drug and gene co-delivery by PHB-PDMAEMA cationic polyester in liver cancer cells. Mater Sci Eng C Mater Biol Appl 83:210–217

Cyrille T, Paulo M, Martine A et al (2018) Targeting Bcl-2 for the treatment of multiple myeloma. Leukemia 32:1899–1907

Fang H, Guo Z, Lin L et al (2018) Molecular strings significantly improved the gene transfection efficiency of polycations. J Am Chem Soc 140(38):11992–12000

Freimund AE, Beach JA, Christie EL et al (2018) Mechanisms of drug resistance in high-grade serous ovarian cancer. Hematol Oncol Clin North Am 32(6):983–996

Guan X, Guo Z, Lin L et al (2016) Ultrasensitive pH triggered charge/size dual-rebound gene delivery system. Nano Lett 16(11):6823–6831

Huang Q, Li S, Ding YF et al (2018) Macrocycle-wrapped polyethylenimine for gene delivery with reduced cytotoxicity. Biomater Sci 6(5):1031–1039

Huang K, O'Neill KL, Li J et al (2019) BH3-only proteins target BCL-xL/MCL-1, not BAX/BAK, to initiate apoptosis. Cell Res 29(11):942–952

Jiang C, Chen J, Li Z et al (2019) Recent advances in the development of polyethylenimine-based gene vectors for safe and efficient gene delivery. Int J Mol Sci 16(4):1–14

Ke L, Cai P, Wu YL et al (2020) Polymeric nonviral gene delivery systems for cancer immunotherapy. Adv Ther 3(6):e1900213

Kesharwani SS, Kaur S, Tummala H et al (2018) Overcoming multiple drug resistance in cancer using polymeric micelles. Expert Opin Drug Delivery 15(11):1127–1142

Knight T, Luedtke D, Edwards H et al (2019) A delicate balance-the BCL-2 family and its role in apoptosis, oncogenesis, and cancer therapeutics. Biochem Pharmacol 162:250–261

Li L, Hu S, Chen X (2018) Non-viral delivery systems for CRISPR/Cas9-based genome editing: challenges and opportunities. Biomaterials 171:207–218

Li Y, Zhang K, Liu P et al (2019) Encapsulation of plasmid DNA by nanoscale metal-organic frameworks for efficient gene transportation and expression. Adv Mater 31(29):e1901570

Liu X, Chen X, Chua MX et al (2017) Injectable supramolecular hydrogels as delivery agents of Bcl-2 conversion gene for the effective shrinkage of therapeutic resistance tumors. Adv Healthc Mater 6(11):e1700159

Liu X, Li Z, Loh XJ et al (2019) Targeted and sustained corelease of chemotherapeutics and gene by injectable supramolecular hydrogel for drug-resistant cancer therapy. Macromol Rapid Commun 40(5):e1800117

Mattiuzzi C, Lippi G (2019) Current cancer epidemiology. J Epidemiol Glob Health 9(4):217–222

Nikolaou M, Pavlopoulou A, Georgakilas AG et al (2018) The challenge of drug resistance in cancer treatment: a current overview. Clin Exp Metastasis 35(4):309–318

O'Donnell JS, Teng MWL, Smyth MJ (2019) Cancer immunoediting and resistance to T cell-based immunotherapy. Nat Rev Clin Oncol 16(3):151–167

Patil S, Gao YG, Lin X et al (2019) The development of functional non-viral vectors for gene delivery. Int J Mol Sci 20(21):e5491

Sarmento-Ribeiro AB, Scorilas A, Goncalves AC et al (2019) The emergence of drug resistance to targeted cancer therapies: clinical evidence. Drug Resist Updat 47:e100646

Sun Z, Cao X, Jiang MM et al (2012) Inhibition of beta-catenin signaling by nongenomic action of orphan nuclear receptor Nur77. Oncogene 31(21):2653–2667

Tsujimoto Y (1998) Role of Bcl-2 family proteins in apoptosis apoptosomes or mitochondri? Genes Cells 3:697–707

Tutusaus A, Stefanovic M, Boix L et al (2018) Antiapoptotic BCL-2 proteins determine sorafenib regorafenib resistance and BH3-mimetic efficacy in hepatocellular carcinoma. Oncotarget 9(24):16701–16717
Vasan N, Baselga J, Hyman DM (2019) A view on drug resistance in cancer. Nature 575(7782): 299–309
Wang X, Liow SS, Wu Q et al (2017) Codelivery for paclitaxel and Bcl-2 conversion gene by PHB-PDMAEMA amphiphilic cationic copolymer for effective drug resistant cancer therapy. Macromol Biosci 17(11):e1700186
Wu C, Li M, Meng H et al (2019) Analysis of status and countermeasures of cancer incidence and mortality in China. Sci China Life Sci 62(5):640–647
Xu C, Wu Y-L, Li Z et al (2019) Cyclodextrin-based sustained gene release systems: a supramolecular solution towards clinical applications. Mater Chem Front 3(2):181–192
Zakeri A, Kouhbanani MAJ, Beheshtkhoo N et al (2018) Polyethylenimine-based nanocarriers in co-delivery of drug and gene: a developing horizon. Nano Rev Exp 9(1):e1488497

# MRI-Visible Nanocarrier for Synergistic MicroRNA Therapy in Liver Fibrotic Rat

14

Jinsheng Huang and Du Cheng

## Contents



**Abstract**

Liver fibrosis, characterized by the extracellular matrix (ECM) accumulation as a result of the activation of hepatic stellate cells (HSCs), is a major cause of liver-associated morbidity and mortality. However, there is no potent anti-fibrotic therapeutic drug yet. The microRNA-29b (miR-29b) and microRNA-122 (miR-122) could regulate the pro-fibrotic genes of HSCs, thus showing great potential in the treatment of liver fibrosis. The development of HSC-targeting miRNAs delivery nanosystem in a noninvasively trackable manner was essential. Therefore, a vitamin A (VA)-tailed and pH-sensitive cationic copolymer **VA–poly(ethylene glycol)–poly (ethyleneimine)–poly(*N*-(*N'*,*N'*-diisopropylaminoethyl)-*co*-benzylamino) aspar tamide** (VA-PEG-bPEI-PAsp(DIP-BzA), T-PBP) **has been synthesized. The** T-PBP amphiphilic copolymer was then assembled to encapsulate the magnetic r esonance imaging (MRI) contrast superparamagnetic iron oxide (SPIO) via a hydr ophobic interaction and to complex both miR-29b and miR-122 via an electrostatic interaction. The miRNA- and SPIO-encapsulating micelle was named

J. Huang
School of Materials Science and Engineering, Sun Yat-sen University, Guangzhou, China

Department of Urology, The Seventh Affiliated Hospital of Sun Yat-sen University, Shenzhen, China

D. Cheng (✉)
School of Materials Science and Engineering, Sun Yat-sen University, Guangzhou, China
e-mail: chengdu@mail.sysu.edu.cn



H. Tian and X. Chen (eds.), *Gene Delivery*, Biomaterial Engineering,
https://doi.org/10.1007/978-981-16-5419-0_14

T-PBP@miRNA/SPIO which specifically delivered the miRNA-29b and miRNA-122 into the HSCs in an MRI-monitorable manner, leading to a synergistic anti-fibr osis outcome via the downregulation of pro-fibrotic protein such as collagen I (COL1A1), $\alpha$-smooth muscle actin ($\alpha$-SMA), and tissue inhibitor of metallopr oteinase I (TIMP1). The strategy of synergistic microRNA therapy using HSC-tar geting and pH-sensitive polymeric nanocarrier greatly improved liver function and r elieved hepatic fibrosis.

**Keywords**

MRI-visibility · Polymeric nanocarrier · Synergistic microRNA therapy · Treatment of liver fibrosis

## 1 Overview

Liver fibrosis, characterized by the accumulation of collagen fibers in the extracellular matrix (ECM), is a major liver disease and may progress into the cirrhosis, liver failure, and even liver cancer, which caused significant damage to human health (Koyama and Brenner 2017). Many pathogenic factors, such as hepatitis virus, alcohol, autoimmune diseases, jaundice hepatitis, bile duct ligation, and non-alcoholic fatty liver, would induce liver fibrosis. Although clinical studies have shown that the early liver fibrosis can be slowly recovered after removal of pathogenic factors, a long-term treatment is required for the advanced liver fibrosis (stage 3 or 4 fibrosis) (Seki and Schwabe 2015). Nowadays, the anti-fibrosis drugs in clinic and clinical trial include the anti-inflammatory drugs (e.g., cenicriviroc and pirfenidone), antioxidants (e.g., N-acetylcysteine and vitamin E), and antivirals (e.g., entecavir and interferon-$\gamma$), but limited efficacy and side effects hindered their wide application (Hauff et al. 2015; Wang et al. 2016). Therefore, there is an urgent need to develop a potent drug for the effective treatment of liver fibrosis.

The activation of hepatic stellate cells (HSCs) plays a key role in the development of liver fibrosis (Schuppan and Kim 2013; Trautwein et al. 2015). After the liver was damaged by the pathogenic factors, the static HSCs are activated to proliferate massively and transform into the myofibroblast-like cells with high expression of $\alpha$-smooth muscle actin ($\alpha$-SMA). In addition, the activated HSCs (aHSCs) secrete not only the abundant type I collagen $\alpha$1 protein (COL1A1) to increase collagen fiber but also the tissue inhibitors of metalloproteinases (TIMPs) to inhibit the activity of metalloproteinases (MMPs) responsible for the degradation of ECM, leading to an excessive deposition of ECM and atrophy of liver tissue (Hernandez-Gea and Friedman 2011). Therefore, inhibition of the activation of HSCs is an ideal strategy for the development of potent anti-fibrosis drug.

The microRNA (miRNA) molecule, about 22 nucleotides long and noncoding RNA, can bind to the 3'-UTR of targeted mRNAs and induce the degradation of the targeted mRNAs, thus has emerged as a promising alternative to conventional drug for multiple diseases (Szabo and Bala 2013; Abba et al. 2017). In fact, the upregulated expressions of miR-199a, miR-21, miR-125-5p, miR-221, and miR-302c but the downregulated expressions of miR-29, miR-122, miR-19, and miR-139-5p were found in activated HSCs during liver fibrosis (Szabo and Bala 2013; Murakami and Kawada 2017). Among these miRNAs, miR-122 is the most abundant miRNA in liver and participates in the development of nonalcoholic steatohepatitis, hepatocellular carcinoma, and liver fibrosis (Murakami and Kawada 2017). Upregulation of miR-122 not only inhibited the proliferation of HSCs, but also reduced the collagen secretion via inhibition of TGF-$\beta$-miR-122-FN1/SRF signaling cascade and the collagen maturation via suppression of P4HA1 (Li et al. 2013; Zeng et al. 2015). In addition, miRNA-29b regulated the expression of various fibrosis-related genes in HSCs and has gained many attentions in the treatment of liver fibrosis (Roderburg et al. 2011). The COL1A1 has been suppressed by the miRNA-29b via directly binding to the COL1A1 mRNA,(Roderburg et al. 2011) and indirectly inhibiting the TGF-β1/Smad3, PI3K/AKT, or hedgehog (Hh) pathway (Murakami and Kawada 2017). Moreover, both miRNA-29b and miR-122 could not only suppress the activation and proliferation of HSCs but also induce the apoptosis of HSCs via inhibiting the expression of Bcl-w and IGFR1, and the PI3K/Akt signaling pathway (Li et al. 2013; Zhang et al. 2014; Zeng et al. 2015). Given that the HSCs may develop compensatory signaling pathways to promote collagen synthesis, a combination of miRNA-29b and miRNA-122 is expected to achieve a synergistic anti-liver fibrosis outcome via acting on different targets. In fact, the combination of two or multiple miRNAs has shown a synergistic effect in the treatment of cancer and cardiovascular disease (Hashimoto et al. 2013; Zhu et al. 2013; Esposito et al. 2016).

Carrier is needed for miRNA-based gene therapy, because the miRNA is easy degraded by nucleases in vivo and hardly crosses the cell membrane. Cationic polymeric nanocarriers such as chitosan (CS), PAMMA dendrimer, and poly (ethylenimine) (PEI) have been widely studied for effective gene delivery (Gurzov et al. 2016; Guo et al. 2018). However, nonbiodegradability and cationic toxicity limited the in vivo application of these traditional cationic polymers. In recent decade, many efforts have been made to develop the biodegradable cationic polymers such as the poly(amino acid) conjugates (Li et al. 2014; Wang et al. 2015). Furthermore, the cationic carriers were usually modified with ligand molecule for targeting gene delivery (Zhou et al. 2016). Many studies have shown that the specific ligand-conjugated nanocarrier targeting HSCs improved therapeutic effect and reduced side effects of various drugs. These targeting ligands include vitamin A (VA), cRGD, 6-phosphate mannose-binding peptide, and platelet-derived growth factor receptor $\beta$-binding peptide (Bartneck et al. 2014). As an indirect targeting ligand, the VA first binds to the retinol binding protein (RBP) in the blood to form a complex of VA/RBP which is then uptaked by the HSCs via the overexpressed RBP receptor (RBPR) (Zhang et al. 2015). Through this mechaism, approximately 80% of VA is stored in HSCs in the human body (Sato et al. 2008). Sato et al. prepared a VA-coupled liposome for HSCs-targeting delivery of small interfering RNA (siRNA) against gp46, resulting in a effective treatemnt of liver fibrosis induced by $CCl_4$ or bile duct ligation in rat (Sato et al. 2008).

The gene-complexed nanocarrier would be internalized and entrapped into the acidic lysosome via endocytosis. In recent years, pH-responsive strategy shows feasibility in gene/drug delivery, as the "proton sponge" effect of pH-sensitive cationic nanocarriers facilitates the lysosomal escape (Zhou et al. 2017; Xiao et al. 2020). Moreover, the acidity-induced dissociation of nanoparticle causes the release of drug or gene (Lynn and Langer 2000; Huang et al. 2019; Huang et al. 2021). For instance, Huang et al. developed a cationic micelle based on a pH-sensitive copolymer monomethoxy-**poly(ethylene glycol)–poly(ethyleneimine)–poly(*N*-(*N*′,*N*′-diisopropylaminoethyl)-*co*-benzylamino) aspartamide** (mPEG-bPEI-PAsp (DIP-BzA) (PBP) (Huang et al. 2018). The complete protonation of DIP group led to a hydrophobic-to-hydrophilic transition of micellar core composed of PAsp (DIP-BzA) block, which induced the dissociation of nanoparticle and the release of both small molecule drug simvastatin and siRNA.

On the other hand, dynamic monitoring of miRNA delivery events and miRNA therapetic effect in vivo is essential for precision treatment of liver fibrosis. The superparamagnetic iron oxide (SPIO) nanoparticles have been demonstrated to significantly enhance the magnetic resonance imaging (MRI) signal via reducing the t2 relaxation time of adjacent proton of water (Wang et al. 2015; Yu et al. 2020). Therefore, Huang et al. further synthesized a VA-conjugated copolymer **poly(ethylene glycol)–poly(ethyleneimine)–poly(*N*-(*N*′,*N*′-diisopropylaminoethyl)-*co*-benzylamino) aspartamide (**mPEG-bPEI-PAsp(DIP-BzA) (Wu et al. 2019). The copolymer was then assembled into an SPIO-encapsulated micelle for the MRI-visible and HSC-targeted delivery of miRNAs (abbreviated as T-PBP/miRNAS/SPIO). The miRNA-29b and miRNA-122 were complexed into the cationic micelle via a electrostatic interaction and specifically codelivered into HSC in fibrotic liver of rat. In vitro and in vivo results demonstrated that a combination of miRNA-29b and miRNA-122 resulted in a synergistic amelioration of liver fibrosis and significantly improved the liver function (Fig. 1).

## 2 Protocol

***Materials***: Monomethoxy-poly(ethylene glycol) (mPEG-OH, *M*n: 2 kDa), vitamin A (VA), hyper-branched poly(ethylenemine) (PEI, *M*n: 1.8 kDa), N,N′-carbonyldiimidazole (CDI), n-butylamine (nBu-$NH_2$), succinic anhydride (SA), N, N-diisopropylamino ethylamine (DIP), dicyclohexylcarbodiimide (DCC), benzylamine (BzA), 3-(4,5-dimethyl-thiazol-2-yl)-2,5-diphenyltetrazo-lium bromide (MTT), 4′,6-diamidion-2-phenylindole (DAPI), and retinol binding protein (RBP) could be purchased from Sigma-Aldrich. The superparamagnetic iron oxide (SPIO) nanoparticle could be prepared using a solvothermal method according to a report (Sun et al. 2004). The HSC-T6 cell line could be purchased from the Institute of Biochemistry and Cell Biology, Chinese Academy of Sciences. Dulbecco's modified eagle medium (DMEM) and fetal bovine serum (FBS) were purchased from Gibco. Scrambled miRNA (SCR), miRNA-122 (sense, 5'-UGGAGUGUGACAAUGGUGUUUG; antisense, 5'-AACACCAUUGUCACACUCCAUU-3′), and miRNA-29b (sense, 5'-

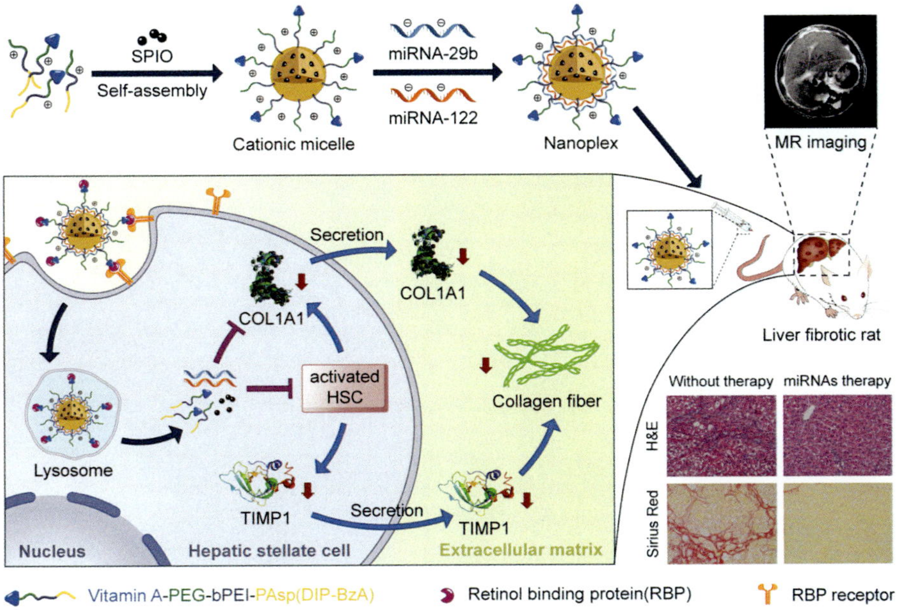


**Fig. 1** The synergistic anti-liver fibrotic performance of miRNA-29b and miRNA-122 using a vitamin A-tailed and SPIO-loaded nanocomplex T-PBP@miRNA/SPIO. The expression of COL1A1, TIMP1, and collagen fiber were downregulated synergistically as indicated by the red arrows. Reproduced with permission from the Wiley-VCH Verlag GmbH & Co. KGaA. (Wu et al. 2019)

UUUCAUAUGGUGGUUUAGAUUU-3′; antisense, 5’-AUCUAAACCACCAUAUGAAAUU-3′) could be purchased from GenePharma CO., Ltd. (Shanghai, China). PrimeScript™ RT Master Mix and FastStart Universal SYBR Green Master (ROX) for the RT-qPCR experiments could be purchased from Takara and Roche, respectively. The primary and second antibodies could be purchased from Abcam.

***Synthesis of VA-PEG-CDI***: Upon 0.25 g of vitamin A was dissolved in anhydrous THF (3 mL), 0.28 g of CDI was added dropwise (Sato et al. 2008). The above solution was stirred for 10 h at 25 °C. Then, 0.6 g of $NH_2$-PEG-OH (*M*n: 2.3 kDa) was added into the solution which was stirred for another 10 h at 25 °C. The mixture was precipitated into excess ether, frozen, filtrated, and vacuum-dried to obtain VA-PEG-OH (Yield: 85%). Next, 0.5 g of VA-PEG-OH and 97 mg of CDI were dissolved in anhydrous THF (5 mL) and stirred for 12 h at 25 °C. The mixture solution was precipitated into excess ether, frozen, filtrated, and vacuum-dried to obtain CDI-activated VA-PEG-CDI (Yield: 90%).

***Synthesis of bPEI-PAsp(DIP-BzA)-COOH***: As shown in Fig. 2, the n-butylamine-terminated poly(*β*-benzyl L-aspartate) (nBu-PBLA) was first synthesized via a ring-opening polymerization of BLA-NCA using n-butylamine as an initiator (Wang et al. 2012). Under $N_2$ atmosphere, 2.49 g of BLA-NCA and 25 μL of n-butylamine were dissolved in a mixture of 4 mL of DMF and 40 mL of anhydrous $CH_2Cl_2$. The mixture was stirred under $N_2$ atmosphere for 3 days at

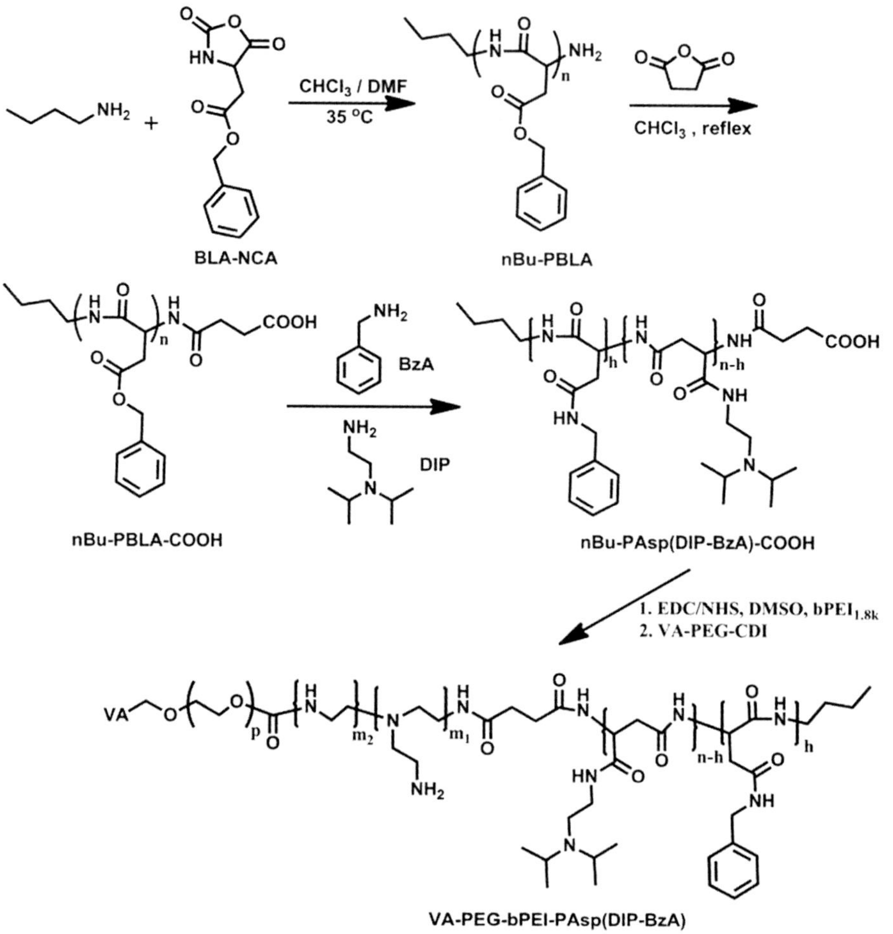


**Fig. 2** Synthetic approach of the vitamin A–coupled copolymer VA-PEG-bPEI-PAsp(DIP-BzA) abbreviated as T-PBP. Reproduced with permission from the Wiley-VCH Verlag GmbH & Co. KGaA. (Wu et al. 2019)

35 °C, precipitated into excess cold diethyl ether, filtered, and vacuum-dried to obtain nBu-PBLA (Yield: 87.5%). Then, the carboxylation of PBLA was performed using succinic anhydride. An amount of 1.7 g of PBLA and 0.2 g of succinic anhydride was added into a flask pre-containing 25 mL of $CHCl_3$. The above solution was heated at 80 °C, stirred for 48 h, precipitated into excess cold methanol, filtrated, and vacuum-dried to obtain nBu-PBLA-COOH as a white powder (Yield: 81.0%). Third, the 2-(diisopropylamino)ethylamine (DIP) and benzylamine (BzA) were incorporated into the polymer side chain via a quantitative aminolysis reaction of PBLA (Nakanishi et al. 2007). After the 0.83 g of nBu-PBLA-COOH was dissolved in 8 mL of anhydrous DMSO, 0.11 g of BzA and 0.58 g of DIP were

added and stirred for 5 h 40 °C. The mixture was dialyzed in methanol for 2 days, concentrated by rotary evaporation, and vacuum-dried to obtain nBu-PAsp (DIP-BzA)-COOH (Yield:75%). Finally, a reaction between nBu-PAsp(DIP-BzA)-COOH and bPEI was performed to synthesize bPEI-PAsp(DIP-BzA) using DCC and NHS as coupling reagents (Dai et al. 2011).

***Synthesis of VA-PEG-bPEI-PAsp(DIP-BzA)***: After 0.56 g of bPEI-PAsp (DIP-BzA) (*Mn:* 11.2 k) was dissolved in anhydrous DMSO (3 mL), 0.26 g of VA-PEG-CDI was added and stirred for 0.5 h at 25 °C. The mixture was dialyzed in methanol for 2 days, concentrated by rotary evaporation, and vacuum-dried to obtain the VA-decorated triblock copolymer VA-PEG-bPEI-PAsp(DIP-BzA) (Yield: 81%). In addition, The VA-free copolymer poly(ethylene glycol)-poly(ethyleneimine)-poly (*N*-(*N*′,*N*′-diisopropylaminoethyl)-*co*-benzylamino)aspartamide, abbreviated as PEG-bPEI-PAsp(DIP-BzA) or PBP, was also synthesized through a reaction between nBu-PAsp(DIP-BzA)-COOH and PEG-bPEI using DCC and NHS as coupling reagents. After 0.47 g of nBu-PAsp(DIP-BzA)-COOH, 62 mg of DCC, and 35 mg of NHS were resolved in a mixture of DMSO and $CHCl_3$ (8 mL, 1/1, v/v) and stirred for 1 h. Then, 0.21 g of PEG-bPEI was added and was stirred for another 48 h at 25 °C. The solution was dialyzed (MWCO: 3.5 kDa) in methanol for 2 days, concentrated by rotary evaporation, and evaporated to obtain PEG-bPEI-PAsp (DIP-BzA) (Yield:72%).

***Preparation of nanocomplex***: The SPIO-loaded micelles were prepared by self-assembly. As shown in Figs. 1, 25 mg of copolymer and 2.5 mg of SPIO were dissolved in 10 mL of $CHCl_3$ and 2 mL of MeOH. The mixture was emulsified in water (25 mL) under ultrasonication, evaporated to remove $CHCl_3$, and dialyzed (MWCO: 14 kDa) in water for 1 day. The resulted micelle solution was filtered through a filter (220 nm), concentrated, and stored at 4 °C. The micelle solution was diluted with Tris-HCl buffer (pH 7.4), which was then mixed with a certain amount of miRNA under vortex and kept still at 25 °C for 5 ~ 30 min to fully complex miRNA. By this means, various nanocomplexes including N-SCR, T-SCR, N-SCR/S, and T-SCR/S at different N/P ratios were successfully prepared. The N/P ratio indicated a value of the molar number of nitrogen atoms in the PEI block over phosphate groups in the miRNA.

***Characterizations of copolymer and nanocomplex***: $^1H$ NMR spectrum was obtained on a Bruker spectrometer (400 MHz). Dynamic light scattering (DLS, Malvern NANO ZS) measurement was performed to detect the particle size and zeta potential of nanocomplexes at 25 °C. The morphologies of nanocomplexes were detected using a JEM 1400 Plus transmission electron microscopy (TEM). The nanocomplex dried on copper grid was stained with uranyl acetate if needed.

***Agarose gel electrophoresis***: The nanocomplexes at various N/P ratios in pH 7.4 solutions were loaded in 1% agarose gel containing 0.5 μg/mL ethidium bromide (EB) and electrophoresed for 15 ~ 20 min under 120 V in a TAE buffer solution. The TAE buffer was composed of 40 mM Tris-HCl, 1% v/v acetic acid, and 1 mM EDTA. The EB-stained miRNA was imaged on a DNR Bio-Imaging System.

***Cell culture:*** HSC-T6 was cultured in DMEM supplemented with 10% FBS at 37 °C under 5% $CO_2$, trypsinized, and subcultured if the cell density reached 80%.

***Cell viability:*** HSCs were seeded in a 96-well plate, incubated for 24 h at 37 °C, and co-incubated with various nanocomplexes (i.e., N-SCR, T-SCR, and T-SCR/S) for another 24 h. Then, the medium was replaced with 100 μL of fresh medium, and the cell viability was measured using MTT assay in triplicate. After the MTT solution was incubated with cells at 37 °C for 2 h, the absorbance at 562 nm was recorded on a microplate reader (Tecan). The influences of N/P ratios on the cytotoxicities were investigated as well. The dose of SCR was set as 100 nM.

**In vitro *miRNA transfection and intracellular distribution of nanocomplexes***: For CLSM assay, HSCs were co-incubated with Cy3-labeled nanocomplexes at a miRNA concentration of 100 nM to evaluate the RBP receptor-mediated cellular uptake in the presence of RBP (0.7 μg/mL). In addition, HSCs were pretreated with 0.5 μg/mL free vitamin A for 2 h before addition of Cy3-labeled nanocomplexes. Moreover, the lysosomes of HSCs were stained with LysoTracker Green DND-26 if required. Afterward, the cells were washed with PBS, fixed with 4% paraformaldehyde, washed with PBS, and stained with DAPI. The fluorescent intensity of Cy3-labeled miRNA and intracellular distribution of nanocomplexes were detected on a CLSM (Nickon C2). For flow cytometric assay, HSCs were co-incubated with Cy3-labeled nanocomplexes at different N/P ratios, collected, and analyzed on a flow cytometric meter (CytoFlex S, Beckman Coulter). Furthermore, after HSCs were incubated with the T-SCR, N-SCR, T-SCR + RBP (0.7 μg/mL), or T-SCR + free vitamin A (0.5 μg/mL) at N/P 10, cells were washed with PBS, trypsinized, collected, and analyzed on a flow cytometric meter. The dose of Cy3-labeled SCR was set as 100 nM.

***Prussian blue staining:*** When the cell density reached 90%, HSCs seeded on a six-well plate were incubated with SPIO-encapsulated nanocomplexes (i.e., N-SCR/S or T-SCR/S) at N/P = 10 for 2 h. Then, the cells were washed with PBS, treated with Prussian blue solution (2% potassium ferrocyanide (II) trihydrate in 2% hydrochloride aqueous) for 30 min at 37 °C, washed with PBS, and observed under microscopy.

**In vitro *and* in vivo *MRI scanning:*** HSCs were seeded in a six-well plate, incubated with SPIO-encapsulated nanocomplexes (i.e., N-SCR/S or T-SCR/S) at various Fe concentrations for 2 h, washed with PBS, trypsinized, and resuspended in a 1% gelatin solution. A 3.0-T MR scanner (GE Healthcare) was used to detect the MR signals. For MRI of animals, the liver fibrotic rats induced by $CCl_4$ were received different nanocomplexes via the tail vein injection. Then, a clinical 1.5-T system (Intera, Philips Medical Systems) was used for in vivo MRI using an animal coil. The $T_2$-weighted images were obtained using the following parameters: TR/TE, 1836/100 ms; FOV, 70 × 60 × 28 mm; matrix, 232 × 258; slice thickness, 1.5 mm; and relative signal-to-noise ratio. The mean T2 signal intensity of three transverse sections of liver tissue over those of the muscle in the same section was calculated as the normalized MR signal intensity.

***Real-time quantitative PCR and Western blot***: After the HSCs or rats were treated with different nanocomplexes, the levels of mRNA and protein including α-SMA, COL1A1, and TIMP1 were evaluated via real-time quantitative PCR (RT-qPCR) and Western blot assays according the instruction of test kits. In addition, the miRNA-29b and miRNA-122 in liver of rat were also detected by RT-qPCR. The primer sequences for RT-qPCR were shown in Table 1.

**Table 1** Primer sequences for real-time quantitative PCR

| Genes | Sequences |
|---|---|
| $\beta$-Actin | 5'-GGAGATTACTGCCCTGGCTCCTA-3′<br>5'-GACTCATCGTACTCCTGCTTGCTG-3' |
| COL1A1 | 5'-CTGACTGGAAGAGCGGAGAG-3′<br>5'-GAGTGGGGAACACACAGGTC-3' |
| $\alpha$-SMA | 5'-CAGGGAGTGATGGTTGGAAT-3′<br>5'-GGTGATGATGCCGTGTTCTA-3' |
| TIMP1 | 5'-TGCAACTCGGACCTGGTTAT-3′<br>5'-ACAGCGTCGAATCCTTTGAG-3' |
| miR-29b<br>miR-122 | 5'-CGCGCGTTTCATATGGTGGTTTAGATTT-3′<br>5′-ACGTGGAGTGTGACAATGGTGTTTG-3' |

***Rat model of liver fibrosis***: All animal experiments on male Sprague-Dawley rat were in accordance with the Guide for the Care and Use of Laboratory Animals. In detail, a mixture of $CCl_4$ and olive oil (1/1, V/V) was intraperitoneally injected into the rat by twice a week at 2 mL/kg body weight per injection for 6 weeks to induce liver fibrosis (Issa et al. 2004). After the animals were anesthetized, serum and liver tissue were collected for pathological and functional analysis.

***Colocalization of miRNA and HSCs in fibrotic liver* in vivo**: The HSC-targeting miRNA delivery was revealed by the measurement of colocalization of nanocomplex and HSCs. The Rhodamine B (Rho) as a red fluorescence dye was used to label the nanocarrier. The $\alpha$-SMA as a marked of activated HSCs on the liver section is stained with Alexa Fluor 488 (AF488)-conjugated antibody which emits green fluorescence under CLSM. In detail, the liver fibrotic rats were intravenously injected with Rho-labeled nanocomplexes. The liver tissue was collected at 2 h after injection of nanocomplexes, and fixed in 4% formalin for 24 h, exposed to 10% and 30% sucrose for 12 h in sequence, embedded in Tissue Tek OTC compound (Sakura Finetek, CA), and frozen at −25 °C, and sliced. Then, approximately 5 μm thick sections were fixed with the acetone for 10 min, rinsed 4 times in PBS, blocked with 5% BSA for 1 h at 25 °C, incubated with a primary antibody (dilution 1:200) against $\alpha$-SMA at 4 °C overnight, washed with TBST, incubated with an AF488-conjugated secondary IgG (dilution 1:200) for 1.5 h at 25 °C, and imaged by a confocal microscopy.

**In vivo *synergistic treatment of miRNA-29b and miRNA-122***: The liver fibrotic rats were treated with different nanocomplexes via tail vein at 1 mL/kg body weight. The rat received with intraperitoneal injection of olive oil was set as the negative control (CTRL). The total miRNAs were administered at 1 mg/kg body weight with a 1:1 molar ratio of miRNA-29b and miRNA-122. The levels of serum liver functional markers including aspartate transaminase (AST), alanine transaminase (ALT), and total bilirubin (T-BIL) were detected according to the instructions of test kit.

***Immunohistochemistry:*** After various treatments, the liver tissue was collected, fixed in paraformaldehyde, embedded in paraffin, and sliced into approximately 5 μm thick sections. The Sirius red and H&E staining were performed on the sections according to instructions of staining kits, which were then detected on an Olympus BX51 microscopy (Olympus).

***Statistical analysis:*** The data was expressed as the mean ± standard deviation (SD). An analysis of variance was used for statistical analysis, and $^*P < 0.05$ meant statistical significance.

## 3 Discussion

***Preparation of nanocomplexes***: The as-synthesized copolymer VA-poly(ethylene glycol)-poly(ethyleneimine)-poly(*N*-(*N*′,*N*′-diisopropylaminoethyl) *co*-benzylamino) aspartamide, namely VA-PEG-bPEI-PAsp(DIP-BzA) or T-PBP (Figs. 2 and 3a), was characterized by $^1$H NMR. The characterized peaks of isopropyl group of DIP, vitamin A, –OC$\boldsymbol{H}_2$C$\boldsymbol{H}_2$O– of PEG, and benzyl group of BzA were at 0.9 ppm, 1.05-1.35 ppm, 3.6 ppm, and 7.25 ppm, respectively (Fig. 3b), indicating a successful synthesis of T-PBP copolymer. The nontargeting copolymer PEG-bPEI-PAsp(DIP-BzA) also named as PBP was synthesized as well according to the method of T-PBP. Then, the copolymers were prepared into SPIO-loaded cationic micelles by self-assembly under ultrasound. Furthermore, miRNA or scramble miRNA (SCR) was complexed with the above micelle to prepare the nanocomplex at predetermined N/P ratios. The names of miRNA and SCR-complexed nanocomplexes were shown in Table 2.

***Characterization of nanocomplex:*** Dynamic light scattering (DLS) measurement showed that the particle size of T-SCR/S nanocomplex was N/P ratio dependent, showing a decrease along with an increase in N/P ratio and a plateau at +149.8 ± 5.6 nm above N/P ≥ 20 (Fig. 3c). Due to the more amino groups at higher N/P ratios, an increase in zeta potential of T-SCR/S nanocomplex was observed along with the increase in N/P ratio. A weak positive charge and relatively small size of nanocomplex was reported to be favorable for gene transfection (Cheng et al. 2012; Li et al. 2014). Thus, the N/P 10 was chosen to prepare the nanocomplex having a particle size (168.8 ± 9.2 nm) with small particle distribution index (PDI = 0.11) and a weak positive charge of +12.2 ± 3.6 mV (Table 3).

Moreover, transmission electron microscopy (TEM) was used to analyze the morphology of nanocomplex. As shown in Fig. 3d, a roughly spherical shape with uniform size of 155.0 ± 10.8 nm in diameter at pH 7.4 was observed when the nanocomplex was prepared at N/P 10. The particle size measured by DLS measurement was slightly larger than that detected by TEM. In contrast, at pH 5.0, random polymeric aggregate was observed under TEM (Fig. 3e), which was in line with the result as detected by the DLS measurement (a particle size of 1088 ± 108.5 nm, Table 3). The complete protonation of DIP in PAsp(DIP-BzA) hydrophobic block led to a disassembly of nanocomplex. Therefore, the lysosomal escape and cytoplasm release of miRNA would be facilitated by the proton sponge effect of PEI and the pH-sensitive DIP group–induced disassembly.

***Optimization of miRNA complexation:*** The miRNA complexation ability was assessed by agarose gel electrophoresis. The negatively charged free miRNA would migrate to the anode if an electric filed was applied and marked as a fluorescent band with the staining of ethidium bromide (EB). However, above N/P 10, the miRNA migration was retarded because it was completely complexed by cationic micelles

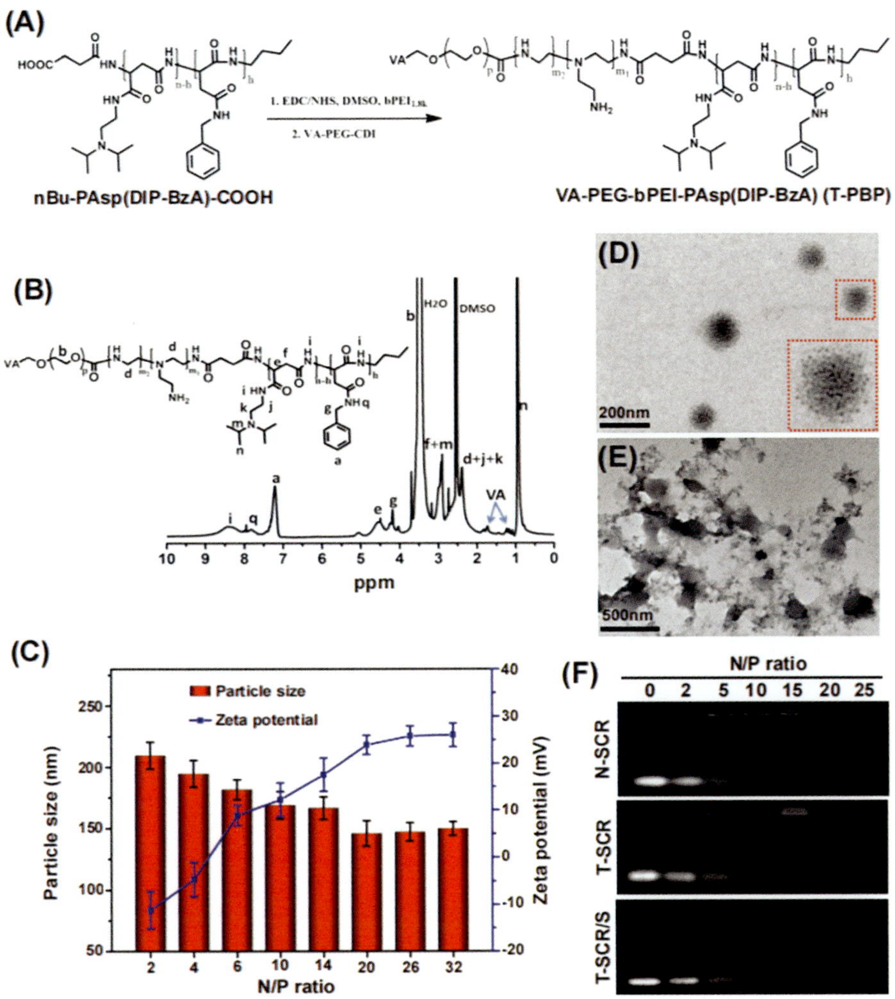


**Fig. 3** Synthetic route of copolymer and characterization of nanocomplex. (**a**) Synthesis of the VA-decorated copolymer VA-PEG-bPEI-PAsp(DIP-BzA), namely T-PBP. (**b**) $^1$H-NMR spectrum of T-PBP copolymer. (**c**) N/P ratio-dependent particle size and zeta potential of T-SCR/S nanocomplex in pH 7.4 solution (n = 3). (**d** and **e**) Transmission electron microscopic (TEM) imaging of T-SCR/S nanocomplex prepared at N/P 10 in pH 7.4 (**d**) and pH 5.0 (**e**) solution. (**f**) N/P ratio-dependent complexation of scrambled miRNA (SCR) using N-SCR, T-SCR, and T-SCR/S, measured by agarose gel. Reproduced with permission from the Wiley-VCH Verlag GmbH & Co. KGaA. (Wu et al. 2019)

(Fig. 3f). Notably, below N/P 10, the miRNA band was lengthened, which was likely because the incomplete complexation led to the differently charged miRNA. Moreover, T-SCR, T-SCR/S, and N-SCR showed very similar miRNA bands at the same N/P ratio, indicating both the decoration of vitamin A and the encapsulation of SPIO had negligible effect on the complexation of miRNA.

**Table 2** The abbreviations as used in this chapter

| Abbreviation | Full name | Abbreviation | Full name |
|---|---|---|---|
| SPIO | Superparamagnetic iron oxide | Rho | Rhodamine B |
| VA | Vitamin A | SCR | Scramble miRNA |
| N-SCR | Nontargeting PBP micelle complexing SCR | N-SCR/S | Nontargeting PBP micelle complexing scramble miRNA and encapsulating SPIO |
| T-SCR | Targeting T-PBP micelle complexing SCR | T-SCR/S | T-PBP micelle complexing SCR and encapsulating SPIO |
| N-mix | PBP micelle complexing miRNA-29b and miRNA-122 | T-mix | T-PBP micelle complexing miRNA-29b and miRNA-122 |
| T-29b | T-PBP micelle complexing miRNA-29b | T-122 | T-PBP micelle complexing miRNA-122 |
| CTRL | Cells without treatment or normal rat treated with equal quantity of olive oil | CTRL/T-SCR | Normal rats receiving T-SCR |
| CTRL/T-SCR/S | Normal rats receiving T-SCR/S | $CCl_4$/T-SCR/S | $CCl_4$-induced liver fibrotic rats receiving T-SCR/S |
| $CCl_4$/N-SCR | $CCl_4$-induced liver fibrotic rats receiving N-SCR | $CCl_4$/T-SCR | $CCl_4$-induced liver fibrotic rats receiving rho-labeled T-SCR |
| $CCl_4$/N-SCR/S | $CCl_4$-induced liver fibrotic rats receiving N-SCR/S | HSCs | Hepatic stellate cells |

**Table 3** Averaged particle size and zeta potential of nanocomplex prepared at N/P = 10 in PBS solution at different pH (n = 3)[a]

| Nanocomplex | pH | Size / nm | PDI[b] | ζ potential / mV |
|---|---|---|---|---|
| T-SCR/S | 7.4 | 168.8 ± 9.2 nm | 0.11 | +12.12 ± 3.59 |
| | 5.0 | 1088 ± 108.5 | 0.77 | +9.50 ± 0.75 |
| N-SCR/S | 7.4 | 166.2 ± 6.4 | 0.10 | +11.90 ± 3.32 |
| | 5.0 | 1306 ± 82.0 | 0.46 | +9.27 ± 1.29 |

[a]Measured by DLS
[b]PDI, particle distribution index

Then, the cytotoxicities of cationic nanocomplexes on HSCs were detected using MTT assay. Above 88.5% of cell viabilities in all groups were observed at a carrier concentration up to 400 μg/mL (Fig. 4a), suggesting little cytotoxicity of nanocomplex prepared at N/P 10. In addition, the N/P ratio-dependent cytotoxicities were also revealed. As shown in Fig. 4b, below N/P 10, negligible cytotoxicities were shown in cells incubated with both the N-SCR and T-SCR. Above N/P 10, due to the higher transfection efficiency mediated by the VA, the cytotoxicity of T-SCR (targeting nanocomplex) was higher than that of N-SCR. The transfection efficiency

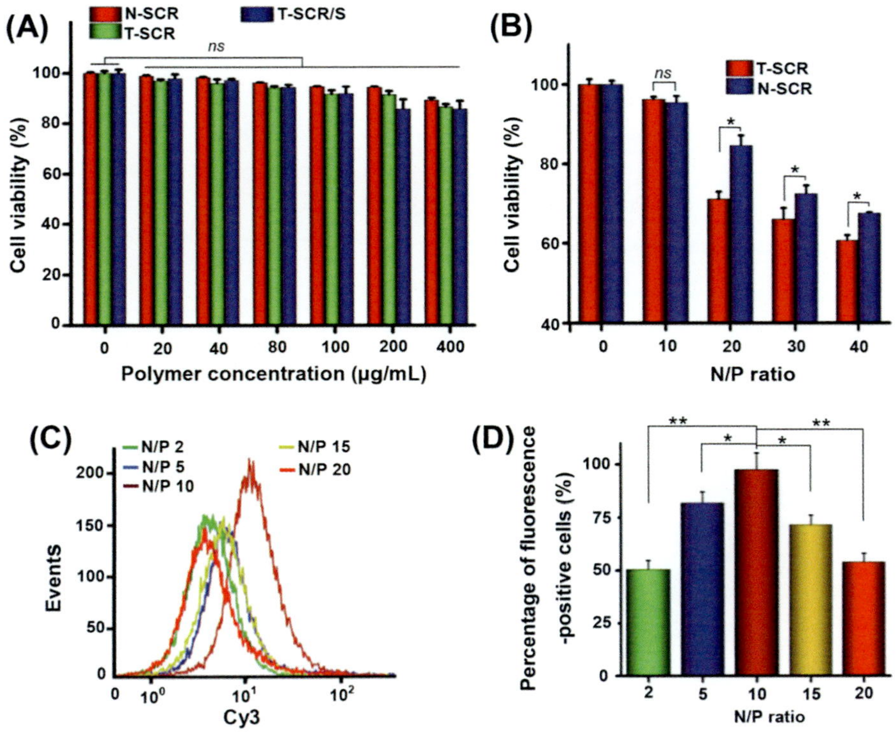


**Fig. 4** Cytotoxicity of nanocomplex and N/P ratio-dependent miRNA transfection efficiency. (**a**) Viabilities of HSCs incubated with different concentrations of N-SCR, T-SCR, and T-SCR/S for 24 h (n = 3). N/P ratio was 10. (**b**) Viabilities of HSCs incubated with 100 μg/mL T-SCR and 100 μg/mL N-SCR at different N/P ratios for 24 h. (**c–d**) Flow cytometric analysis of the effect of N/P ratios on the transfection efficiency of T-SCR. HSCs were incubated with nanocomplex for 2 h. $*P < 0.05$, $**P < 0.01$, and ns: no significant difference

at different N/P ratios was quantified by flow cytometric assay (Fig. 4c, d). The highest miRNA transfection efficiency was shown when the cells were incubated with T-SCR (N/P 10), in which 97.5% of HSCs was Cy3-SCR positive. Although the higher surface charge would enhance the internalization of nanoparticle, the highly positive charge-mediated cationic cytotoxicity may reduce the miRNA transfection efficiency (Roy et al. 1999; Li et al. 2015;Wang et al. 2015 ; Yu et al. 2020). Thus, the nanocomplex prepared at N/P 10 was ideal and chosen for miRNA delivery.

***MRI-visible targeting miRNA delivery:*** As shown in Fig. 5a, VA first binds to the RBP to form a VA/RBP complex which is uptaked by the HSCs via the over-expressed RBP receptor (RBPR) (Zhang et al. 2015). Thus, the VA on the surface of nanocomplex was expected to mediate a HSC-targeted miRNA delivery. The Cy3-labeled SCR was complexed with the cationic micelle, which was then incubated with HSCs for observation of cell uptake. Due to the presence of RBP in the serum, the Cy3 fluorescent intensity in HSCs incubated with T-SCR-Cy3 nano-complex was higher than that incubated with N-SCR-Cy3 (Fig. 5b). The Cy3

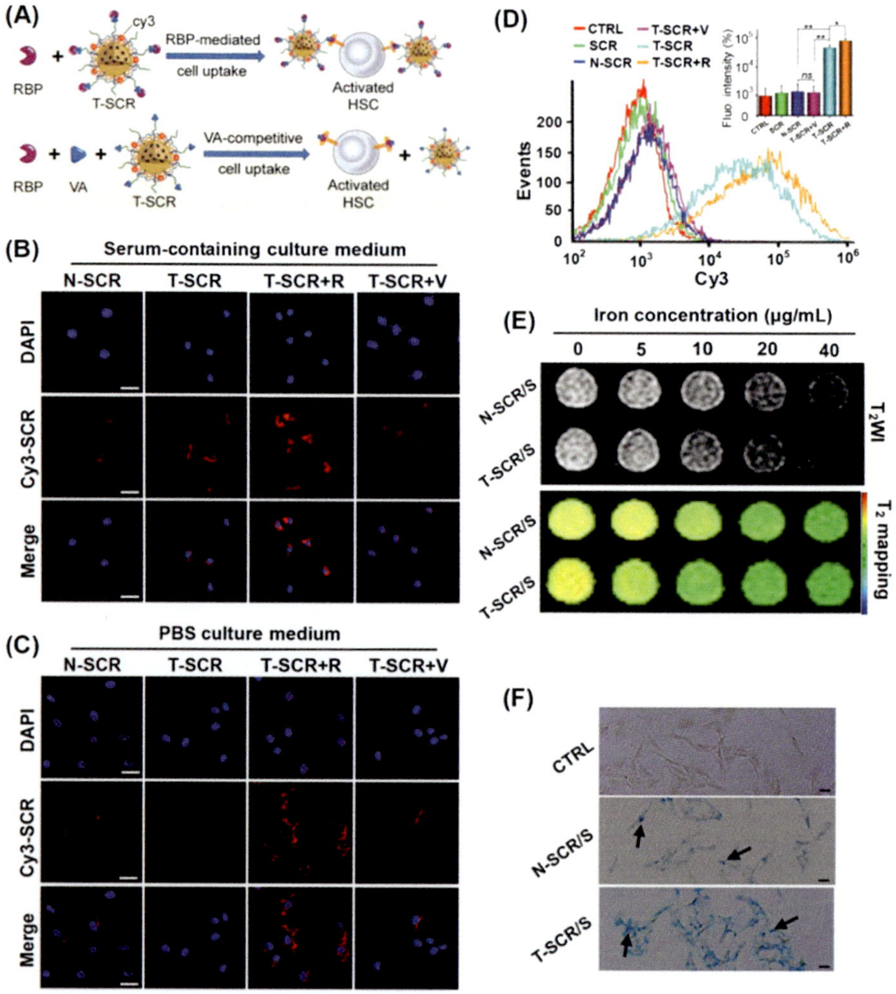


**Fig. 5** MRI-visible and HSCs-targeted miRNA delivery using T-SCR/S nanocomplex. (**a**) Illustration of the HSCs-targeted miRNA delivery via the RBP-mediated cell uptake of T-SCR/S nanocomplex. (**b** and **c**) CLSM imaging of HSCs-specific uptake of T-SCR/S nanocomplex. HSCs were incubated with various nanocomplexes (i.e., N-SCR, T-SCR, T-SCR + R, and T-SCR + V) in serum-containing medium for 2 h (**b**) or PBS medium for 0.5 h (**c**). DAPI-labeled nuclei and Cy3-labeled SCR (SCR-Cy3) emit blue and red fluorescence, respectively, under CLSM. (**d**) Flow cytometric analysis of miRNA transfection efficiency (n = 3). The SCR-Cy3-complexed nanocomplexes were incubated with HSCs in serum-containing medium for 2 h. $*P < 0.05$, $**P < 0.01$, and ns: no significant difference. (**e**) MRI-visible miRNA delivery in vitro. The $T_2$WI and $T_2$-mapping imaging of HSCs were conducted after the cells were incubated with nanocomplex (i.e., N-SCR/S or T-SCR/S) at various concentrations of Fe element. (**f**) Prussian blue staining of nanocomplex-incubated HSCs after the cells were incubated with nanocomplex (N/P 10) for 2 h. RBP concentration was 0.7 μg/mL if added. Reproduced with permission from the Wiley-VCH Verlag GmbH & Co. KGaA. (Wu et al. 2019)

fluorescent intensity further enhanced after adding extra RBP, i.e., T-SCR + R group. On the contrary, due to the competitive effect of excessive VA, the Cy3 fluorescent intensity in HSCs incubated with free VA plus T-SCR-Cy3 was significantly lower than that incubated with T-SCR-Cy3. The PBS solution was used to replace the serum-containing culture medium for clearly revealing the RBPR-mediated uptake of VA-decorated nanocomplex. As shown in Fig. 5c, due to the absence of RBP, the Cy3 fluorescent intensity in HSCs incubated with T-SCR-Cy3 in PBS was very similar to that incubated with N-SCR. In contrast, the Cy3 fluorescent intensity in HSCs incubated with T-SCR-Cy3 plus RBP was significantly enhanced, indicating that a HSC-targeting miRNA delivery was mediated by the VA-decorated nanocomplex in the presence of RBP.

Moreover, the flow cytometric assay was used to quantificationally detect the miRNA transfection efficiency using targeting nanocomplex in RBP-containing medium. As shown in Fig. 5d, the Cy3 fluorescent intensity in HSCs incubated with T-SCR-Cy3 was much higher than that incubated with N-SCR-Cy3 ($4.6 \times 10^4$ vs $1.4 \times 10^3$ a.u.). The Cy3 fluorescent intensity in HSCs incubated with T-SCR-Cy3 plus extra RBP (T-SCR + R group) was 1.7 times higher than that incubated with only T-SCR-Cy3. In contrast, the Cy3 fluorescent intensity in HSCs incubated with excessive vitamin A plus T-SCR-Cy3 was significantly lower than that incubated with T-SCR-Cy3 ($1.4 \times 10^3$ vs $4.6 \times 10^4$ a.u.). These data clearly revealed that the interaction between RBP and RBP receptor mediated a HSCs-targeting internalization of VA-decorated nanocomplex.

SPIO nanoparticles have been demonstrated to significantly enhance the magnetic MRI signal via reducing the $t_2$ relaxation time of adjacent proton of water, (Wang et al. 2015; Yu et al. 2020) which enabled MRI-monitoring miRNA delivery once incorporating the SPIO into the nanocomplex. After the HSCs were incubated with N-SCR/S or T-SCR/S nanocomplex, an obvious decrease in the $T_2$WI and $T_2$ mapping signal was recorded along with the increase in iron concentration (Fig. 5e). Moreover, HSCs incubated with T-SCR/S showed a more obvious decrease than that incubated with N-SCR/S. In addition, compared to the N-SCR/S nanocomplex, more Prussian blue stains in HSCs incubated with T-SCR/S nanocomplex were observed (Fig. 5f), which clearly suggested that the targeting nanocomplex was more efficiently internalized into the HSCs.

Then, the in vivo MRI scanning was conducted in rat received with N-SCR/S, T-SCR/S, or T-SCR/S. As shown in Fig. 6a, b, on day 2 after tail vein injection, the $T_2$WI signal intensity in fibrotic liver of rat received with T-SCR/S showed 60.0% and 33.3% of reduction than that in the normal liver of rat received with T-SCR/S and that in fibrotic liver of rat received with N-SCR/S, respectively. The data suggested a more effective accumulation of T-SCR/S nanocomplex in fibrotic liver which was due to the activated HSCs-targeting delivery (Sato et al. 2008; Hernandez-Gea and Friedman 2011). In addition, the $T_2$WI signal intensity of fibrotic liver of rat received with N-SCR/S is lower than that of normal liver of rat received with T-SCR (CTRL/T-SCR group), which was most likely due to the enhanced phagocytosis of activated Kupffer cells in fibrotic liver (Liu et al. 2010).

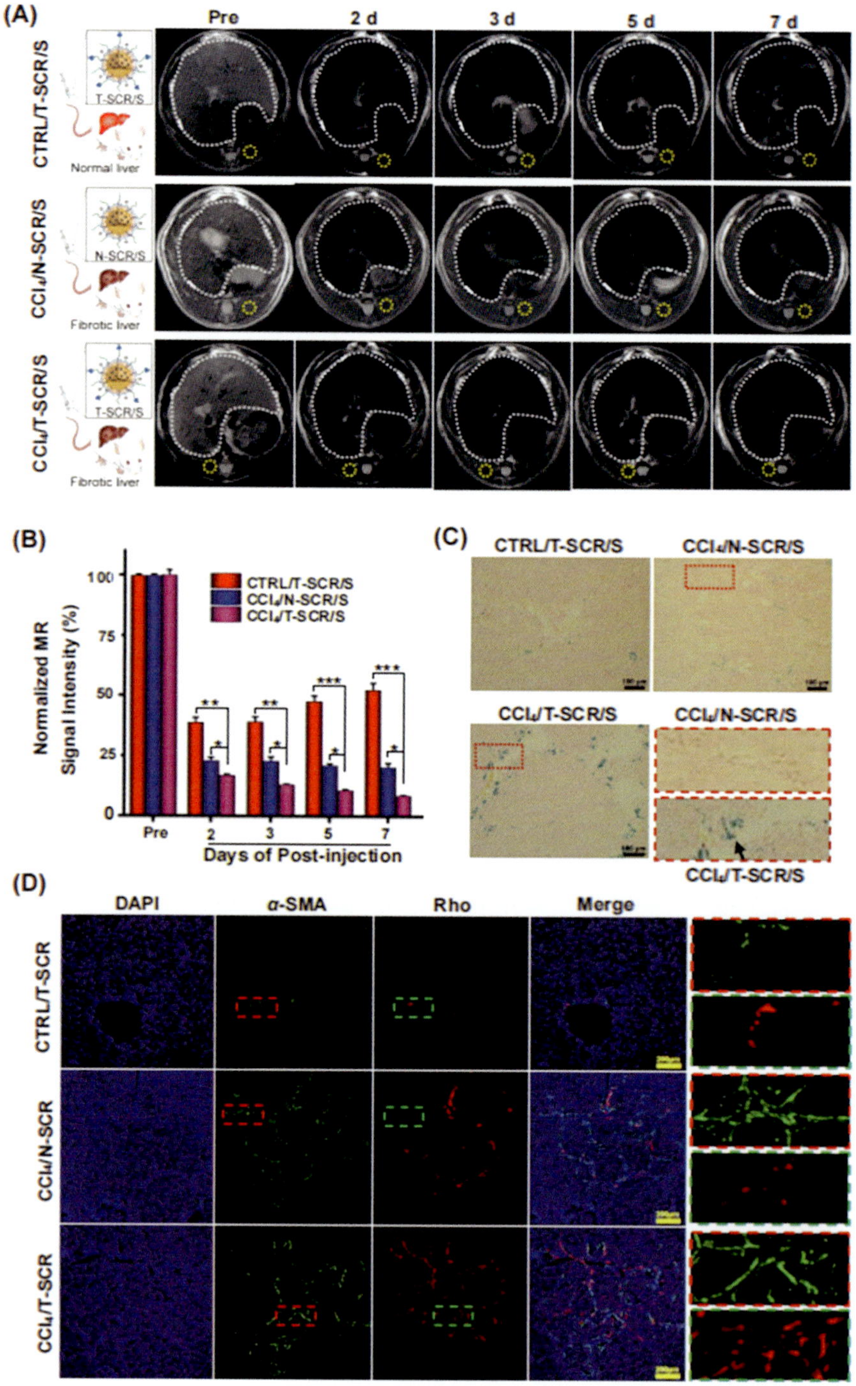


**Fig. 6** (continued)

Furthermore, Prussian blue staining was performed to verify the liver accumulation of SPIO. The blue stains in liver tissue from rat received with T-SCR/S were much more than that received with N-SCR/S (Fig. 6c). These results demonstrated the T-SCR/S nanocomplex showed a great potential in MRI-visible and HSC-targeted miRNA delivery.

The HSC-targeting miRNA delivery was further revealed by an immunofluorescent colocalization measurement of nanocomplex and HSCs. The nanocomplex and HSCs were stained with a red fluorescence dye Rho and AF488-labeled anti-$\alpha$-SMA-antibody (green fluorescence), respectively. As shown in Fig. 6d, the green fluorescent intensity in fibrotic liver tissue was much stronger than that that in normal liver tissue, indicating the high expression of $\alpha$-SMA as a marker of aHSCs in $CCl_4$-induced fibrotic liver. The highest red fluorescent intensity in fibrotic liver tissue from rat received with T-SCR/Rho was recorded, which was in line with the result of MRI and Prussian blue staining. Furthermore, most green fluorescence and red fluorescence were colocalizated, evidencing that the Rho-labeled nanocomplex was uptaked by the $\alpha$-SMA-expressing aHSCs in fibrotic liver.

***Accumulation of miRNA in fibrotic liver:*** The miRNA-29b and miRNA-122 have been demonstrated to inhibit several liver fibrosis–promoting signaling pathways (Roderburg et al. 2011; Li et al. 2013; Zhang et al. 2014; Zeng et al. 2015; Murakami and Kawada 2017). Because the HSCs may develop compensatory signaling pathways to secret collagen, a combination of miRNA-29b and miRNA-122 may achieve a synergistic treatment of liver fibrosis by acting different targets involving in HSCs activation and collagen metabolism. Therefore, the accumulation including the level and retention time of miRNA-29b and miRNA-122 in fibrotic liver mediated by the VA-decorated nanocomplex was investigated. Compared to the normal liver in rat (CTRL group), both the miRNA-29b and miRNA-122 levels in $CCl_4$-induced fibrotic liver tissue at 6 weeks were significantly decreased (Fig. 7a, b), suggesting the potential therapy of co-delivering miRNA-29b and miRNA-122. Compared to the T-SCR treatment, the levels of miRNA-29b and miRNA-122 in fibrotic liver increased after tail vein injection of targeting nanocomplex including T-29b, T-122, and T-Mix (those full names are shown in Table 2).

Then, the liver retention time of miRNA-29b and miRNA-122 were detected on day 1, 2, and 3 after tail vein injection of miRNA-carrying nanocomplexes (Fig. 7c, d). The levels of miRNA-29b and miRNA-122 in rat liver received with T-Mix increased on day 1 and decreased to the similar levels in rat liver received with T-SCR on day

**Fig. 6** MRI of normal liver and fibrotic liver after tail vein injection of nanocomplex, and detection of HSC-targeted miRNA delivery using fluorescence imaging of colocalization. (**a**) $T_2$W MR imaging and (**b**) normalized $T_2$W MR signal intensity of liver after tail vein injection of N-SCR/S and T-SCR/S with 10 mg Fe/kg body weight (n = 3). The liver tissue and muscle tissue were indicated by a white dotted closed curve and a yellow dotted closed curve, respectively. $^*P < 0.05$, $^{**}P < 0.01$, and $^{***}P < 0.001$. (**c**) The SPIO in liver sections revealed by Prussian blue staining. The dotted red rectangle-marked areas were amplified for clear view. (**d**) Detection of HSC-targeted miRNA delivery using fluorescence imaging of colocalization. Reproduced with permission from the Wiley-VCH Verlag GmbH & Co. KGaA. (Wu et al. 2019)

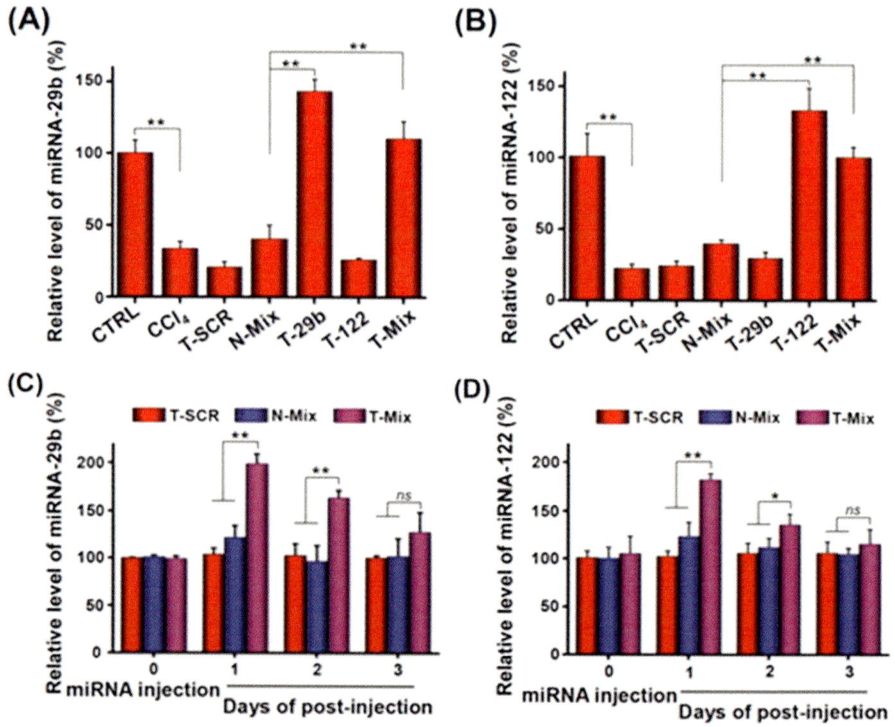


**Fig. 7** The miRNA content in normal liver and fibrotic liver of rat received with different nanocomplexes determined by RT-qPCR. (**a**) miRNA-29b and (**b**) miRNA-122 levels in liver on day 1 after tail vein injection of different nanocomplexes (n = 3). (**c and d**) Relative content of (**c**) miRNA-29b and (**d**) miRNA-122 on day 1, 2, and 3 after tail vein injection of different nanocomplexes (n = 3). One milligram of miRNA-29b, miRNA-122, or miRNA-29b plus miRNA-122 (molar ratio of 1:1) per kg body weight was administrated. $^*P < 0.05$ and $^{**}P < 0.01$. Reproduced with permission from the Wiley-VCH Verlag GmbH & Co. KGaA. (Wu et al. 2019)

3 after tail vein injection, suggesting that twice-a-week administration of nanocomplex was suitable for the treatment of liver fibrosis. However, compared to the injection of T-SCR, injection of N-Mix did not elevate the levels of miRNA-29b and miRNA-122. These data demonstrated the potential of HSC-targeted codelivery of miRNA-122 and miRNA-29b in the therapy of liver fibrosis.

***Synergistically downregulating the expression of fibrosis-related gene and protein:*** COL1A1, $\alpha$-SMA, and TIMP1 are the three typical pro-fibrotic genes that regulated by multiple signaling pathways. Given that the miRNA-29b and miRNA-122 act on different targets,(Roderburg et al. 2011; Li et al. 2013; Zhang et al. 2014; Zeng et al. 2015; Murakami and Kawada 2017) a synergistical inhibition of these three pro-fibrotic genes and collagen accumulation may be achieved (Fig. 8a). As shown in Fig. 8b, c, the COL1A1, $\alpha$-SMA, and TIMP1 were remarkably inhibited at 100 nM miRNA-29b and miRNA-122. Then, a mixture of miRNA-29b and miRNA-122 at a molar ratio of 1:1 was complexed with targeting and nontargeting cationic

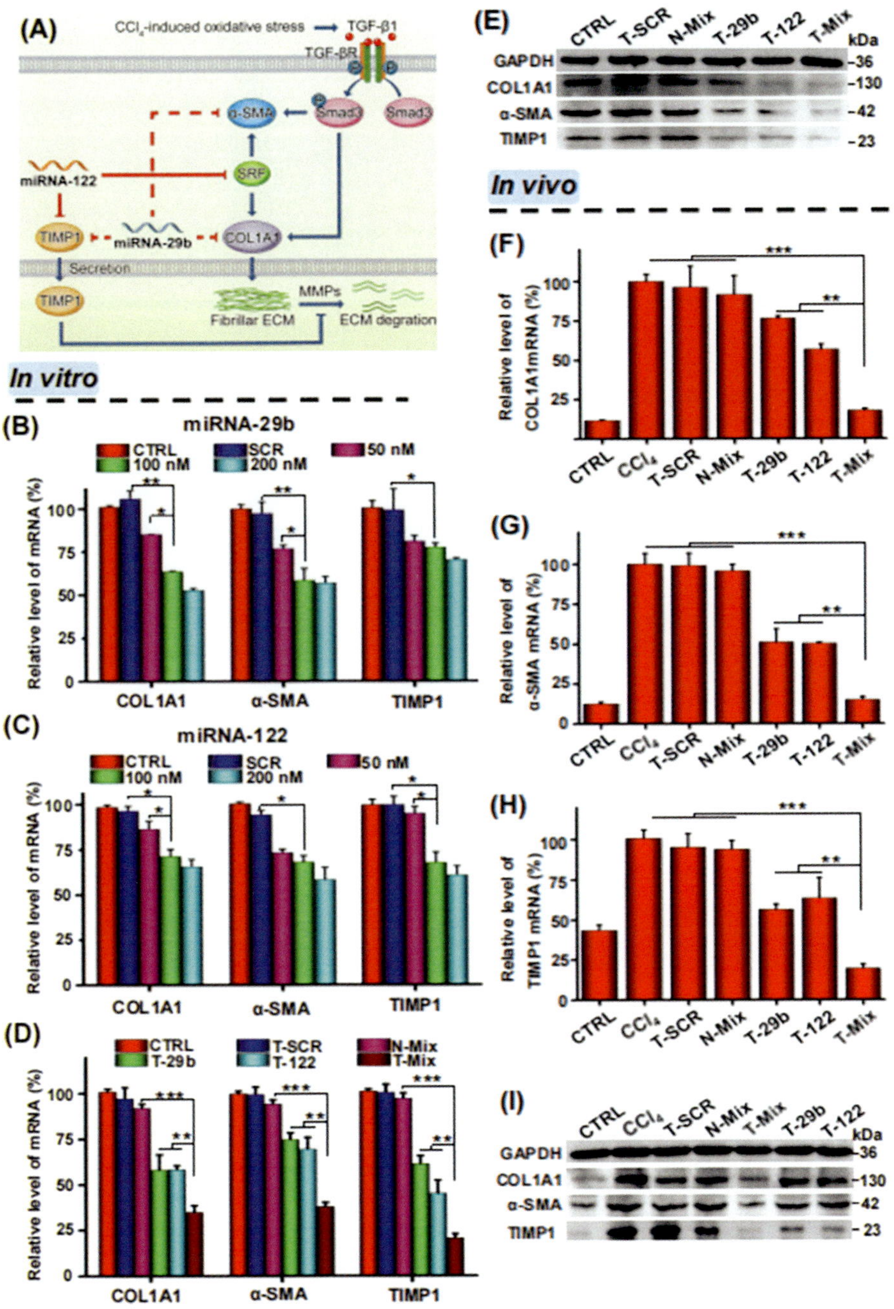


**Fig. 8** A combination of miRNA-29b and miRNA-122 synergistically inhibited the expressions of pro-fibrotic gene and protein in vitro and in vivo. (**a**) The synergistic mechanism of miRNA-29b and miRNA-122 in inhibition of pro-fibrotic gene. (**b** and **c**) Inhibition of COL1A1, $\alpha$-SMA, and

micelles, and used at a concentration of 100 nM. The combination therapy of miRNA-29b and miRNA-122 using the targeting micelle (T-Mix) showed a remarkably higher inhibition effect on the pro-fibrotic genes than the targeting micelle (N-Mix) did. Furthermore, the T-Mix treatment (a combination therapy of miRNA-29b and miRNA-122) showed an obviously higher inhibition effect on the pro-fibrotic genes than single miRNA treatment (i.e., T-29b and T-122). The result of pro-fibrotic protein level was in line with that of mRNA level (Fig. 8e). These data demonstrated the combined treatment of miRNA-29b and miRNA-122 using the targeting micelle (T-Mix) synergistically downregulating the expression of fibrosis-related gene and protein in vitro.

The two-in-one codelivery strategy has been demonstrated to enhance the synergistic therapeutic outcome of two drugs, because of the same pharmacokinetics of two drugs in one nanoparticle, targeting the same cell at a predetermined ratio, and drug release in a spatiotemporally controlled manner (Huang et al. 2019; Deng et al. 2020; Huang et al. 2021). Thus, the expression of pro-fibrotic genes (i.e., mRNA levels of COL1A1, α-SMA, and TIMP1) in liver were evaluated to investigate the synergistic treatment effect of codelivery of miRNA-29b and miRNA-22 in vivo. Compared to the normal rat (CTRL), the fibrotic liver of rat induced by $CCl_4$ ($CCl_4$ group) had an obvious upregulation of COL1A1, TIMP1, and $\alpha$-SMA (Fig. 8f–h), and was used as the liver fibrotic rat model. The expressions of pro-fibrotic genes were only slightly inhibited by the N-Mix treatment as compared to the T-SCR treatment and $CCl_4$ group. However, an obvious inhibition effect of pro-fibrotic genes was shown in fibrotic liver of rat received with T-29b or T-122 treatment. Notably, a highest inhibition effect of pro-fibrotic genes was shown in fibrotic liver of rat received with T-Mix treatment. Furthermore, the treatment results at protein levels were consistent with that at mRNA levels (Fig. 8i). These data demonstrated that a codelivery of miRNA-29b and miRNA-122 synergistically inhibited multiple targets regulating collagen synthesis and degradation, which may synergistically relieve liver fibrosis.

***Treatment of liver fibrosis by miRNA-29b and miRNA-122* in vivo*:*** The alleviation of liver fibrosis and recovery of liver function were investigated to evaluate the synergistic therapeutic effect of HSC-targeted codelivery of miRNA-29b and miRNA-122 by histopathological staining and analysis of blood biochemical function indicators. As shown in Fig. 9a, b, the $CCl_4$-induced liver fibrotic rat showed a significant increase in the levels of serum aspartate transaminase (AST), alanine

**Fig. 8** (continued) TIMP1 mRNA by miRNA-29b (**b**) and miRNA-122 (**c**) in a dose-dependent manner. (**d** and **e**) A combination of miRNA-29b and miRNA-122 synergistically inhibited the expressions of COL1A1, $\alpha$-SMA, and TIMP1 mRNA (**d**) and protein (**e**) revealed by real-time PCR and Western blot. 100 nM miRNA (a 1:1 molar ratio of miRNA-29b to miRNA-122 if combination applied) complexed with nanocarrier at N/P 10 was used. (**f–i**) Relative expressions of fibrosis-promoting mRNA (**f–h**) and protein (**i**) in liver after different treatments (n = 3). $^*P < 0.05$, $^{**}P < 0.01$, and $^{***}P < 0.001$. Reproduced with permission from the Wiley-VCH Verlag GmbH & Co. KGaA. (Wu et al. 2019). The abbreviations are shown in Table 2

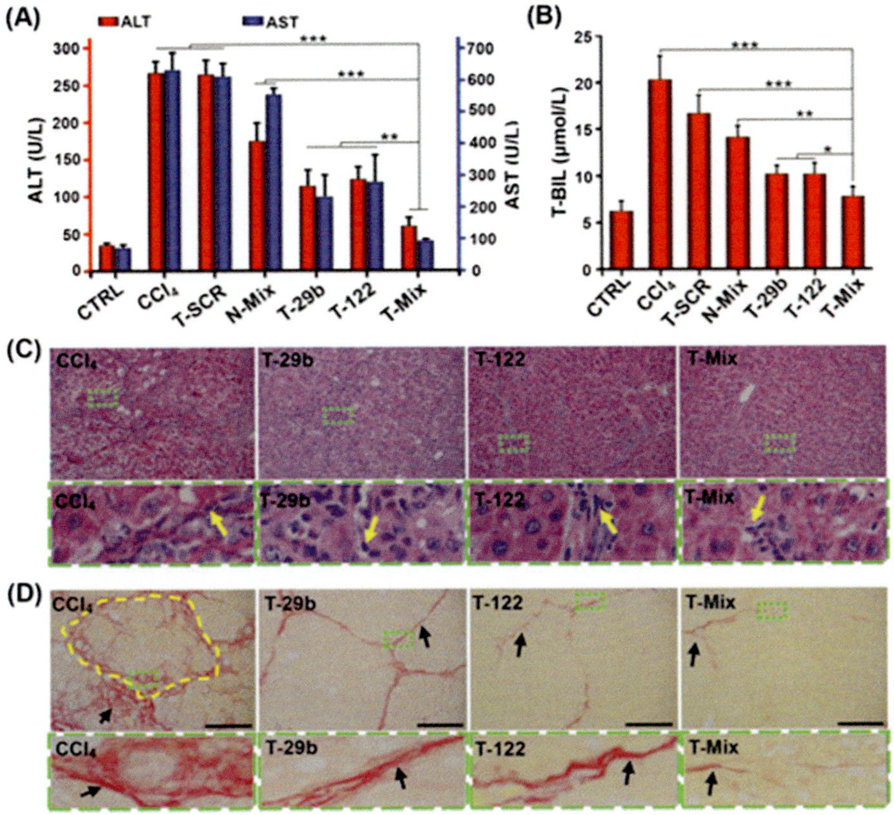


**Fig. 9** A combination of miRNA-29b and miRNA-122 synergistically alleviated liver fibrosis in vivo. (**a**) Levels of ALT and AST (**b**) levels of T-BIL in serum from rat after different treatments (n = 3) $^{*}P < 0.05$, $^{**}P < 0.01$, and $^{***}P < 0.001$. (**c**) H&E and (**d**) Sirius red staining of liver tissue from rat after different treatments. The dotted green rectangle-marked areas were enlarged for clear view. The inflammatory cells, collagen fiber, and pseudolobule were indicated by yellow arrows, black arrows, and yellow dotted portion, respectively. Scale bars indicate 100 μm. Reproduced with permission from the Wiley-VCH Verlag GmbH & Co. KGaA. (Wu et al. 2019). The abbreviations are shown in Table 2

transaminase (ALT), and total bilirubin (T-BIL) as the critical indicators for assessment of liver function damage (Ozer et al. 2008). The T-SCR treatment did not lower the ALT, AST, and T-BIL levels. On the contrary, the ALT, AST, and T-BIL levels were obviously decreased after the treatment of T-29b, T-122, or T-Mix. Furthermore, the ALT, AST, and T-BIL levels were most significantly decreased after the treatment of T-Mix, indicating a synergistic anti-liver fibrosis effect of HSC-targeted codelivery of miRNA-29b and miRNA-122. H&E and Sirius red staining of liver tissue sections were further conducted to reveal the histopathological damage and recovery. There was no inflammation and fibrosis in the liver of normal rat (Fig. 9c, d). However, large amount of inflammatory cell infiltration and fibrosis were shown in the fibrotic liver induced by $CCl_4$. Although the inflammatory cell infiltration and fibrosis were lower after the treatment of T-29b and T-122, they were maximally lowered after the treatment of T-Mix.

Although the PEG-modified PEI of 25 kDa has shown potential in gene delivery, there are still many challenges for miRNA delivery. First, the high molecular weight PEI often leads to high cationic toxicity. Second, the decomplexation of nucleic acids from nanocomplex is difficult but plays a key role in gene therapy. Third, the nonspecific cell uptake of cationic nanocomplex results in a low transfection efficacy. However, Huang et al. have demonstrated that the low molecular weight PEI of 1.8 kDa could effectively complex miRNA like high molecular weight PEI via micellization (Wu et al. 2019). In addition, intracellular miRNA release was shown via introducing a pH-sensitive DIP group responsible for the acidity of lysosomal microenvironment. Furthermore, VA decoration facilitated the HSC-targeted miRNAs codelivery, which was first reported.

## 4 Conclusion

Development of potent therapeutic strategy for anti-liver fibrosis is an urgent need. Huang et al. have developed an MRI-visible polymeric nanomedicine for the treatment of $CCl_4$-liver fibrosis via HSC-targeted codelivery of miRNA-29b and miRNA-122. In detail, a VA-conjugated copolymer VA-PEG-bPEI-PAsp(DIP-BzA) **has been synthesized and assembled into an SPIO nanoparticles-encapsulated micelle (T-PBP/SPIO). Then, the** miRNA-29b and miRNA-122 were complexed with **T-PBP/SPIO to form** T-PBP@miRNA/SPIO **which** specifically delivered the miRNA-29b and miRNA-122 into the HSCs in an MRI-monitorable manner. A synergistic anti-fibrosis outcome was shown in liver fibrotic rat model via acting on different regulation sites and downregulating the pro-fibrotic genes including COL1A1, $\alpha$-SMA, and TIMP1. The strategy of synergistic microRNA therapy using HSC-targeting and pH-sensitive polymeric nanocarrier greatly improved liver function and relieved hepatic fibrosis, showing great potential in the treatment of liver fibrosis.

## References

Abba ML, Patil N, Leupold JH, Moniuszko M, Utikal J, Niklinski J, Allgayer H (2017) Cancer Lett 387:84–94
Bartneck M, Warzecha KT, Tacke F (2014) Hepatobil Surg Nutr 3:364–376
Cheng D, Cao N, Chen J, Yu X, Shuai X (2012) Biomaterials 33:1170–1179
Dai J, Lin S, Cheng D, Zou S, Shuai X (2011) Angew Chem Int Ed 50:9404–9408
Deng SH, Li XX, Liu S, Chen JF, Li MQ, Chew SYA, Leong K, Cheng D (2020) Sci Adv 6:14
Esposito CL, Nuzzo S, Kumar SA, Rienzo A, Lawrence CL, Pallini R, Shaw L, Alder JE, Ricci-Vitiani L, Catuogno S, de Franciscis V (2016) J Control Release 238:43–57
Guo Y, Wu Z, Shen S, Guo R, Wang J, Wang W, Zhao K, Kuang M, Shuai X (2018) Nat Commun 9

Gurzov EN, Wang B, Pilkington EH, Chen P, Kakinen A, Stanley WJ, Litwak SA, Hanssen EG, Davis TP, Ding F, Ke PC (2016) Small 12:1615–1626
Hashimoto Y, Akiyama Y, Yuasa Y (2013) PLoS One 8:e42589
Hauff P, Gottwald U, Ocker M (2015) Expert Opin Investig Drugs 24:309–327
Hernandez-Gea V, Friedman SL (2011) Annu Rev Pathol-Mech Dis 6:425–456
Huang J, Lin C, Fang J, Li X, Wang J, Deng S, Zhang S, Su W, Feng X, Chen B, Cheng D, Shuai X (2018) ACS Appl Mater Interfaces 10:28471–28482
Huang J, Xiao Z, An Y, Han S, Wu W, Wang Y, Guo Y, Shuai X (2021) Biomaterials 269:120636
Huang J, Xu Y, Xiao H, Xiao Z, Guo Y, Cheng D, Shuai X (2019) ACS Nano 13:7036–7049
Issa R, Zhou X, Constandinou CM, Fallowfield J, Millward-Sadler H, Gaca MDA, Sands E, Suliman I, Trim N, Knorr A (2004) Gastroenterology 126:1795–1808
Koyama Y, Brenner DA (2017) J Clin Invest 127:55–64
Li J, Ghazwani M, Zhang Y, Lu J, Li J, Fan J, Gandhi CR, Li S (2013) J Hepatol 58:522–528
Li Z, Li J, Huang J, Zhang J, Cheng D, Shuai X (2015) Macromol Biosci 15:1497–1506
Li J, Yu X, Wang Y, Yuan Y, Xiao H, Cheng D, Shuai X (2014) Adv Mater 26:8217–8224
Liu C, Tao Q, Sun M, Wu JZ, Yang W, Jian P, Peng J, Hu Y, Liu C, Liu P (2010) Lab Investig 90: 1805–1816
Lynn DM, Langer R (2000) J Am Chem Soc 122:10761–10768
Murakami Y, Kawada N (2017) Hepatol Res 47:60–69
Nakanishi M, Park JS, Jang WD, Oba M, Kataoka K (2007) React Funct Polym 67:1361–1372
Ozer J, Ratner M, Shaw M, Bailey W, Schomaker S (2008) Toxicology 245:194–205
Roderburg C, Urban GW, Bettermann K, Vucur M, Zimmermann H, Schmidt S, Janssen J, Koppe C, Knolle P, Castoldi M, Tacke F, Trautwein C, Luedde T (2011) Hepatology 53:209–218
Roy K, Mao HQ, Huang SK, Leong KW (1999) Nat Med 5:387–391
Sato Y, Murase K, Kato J, Kobune M, Sato T, Kawano Y, Takimoto R, Takada K, Miyanishi K, Matsunaga T, Takayama T, Niitsu Y (2008) Nat Biotechnol 26:431–442
Schuppan D, Kim YO (2013) J Clin Invest 123:1887–1901
Seki E, Schwabe RF (2015) Hepatology 61:1066–1079
Sun S, Zeng H, Robinson DB, Raoux S, Rice PM, Wang SX, Li G (2004) J Am Chem Soc 126:273–279
Szabo G, Bala S (2013) Nat Rev Gastroenterol Hepatol 10:542–552
Trautwein C, Friedman SL, Schuppan D, Pinzani M (2015) J Hepatol 62:S15–S24
Wang W, Cheng D, Gong F, Miao X, Shuai X (2012) Adv Mater 24:115–120
Wang P, Koyama Y, Liu X, Xu J, Ma HY, Liang S, Kim IH, Brenner DA, Kisseleva T (2016) Front Physiol 7:47
Wang J, Ren L, Li J, Huang J, Cheng D, Shuai X (2015) RSC Adv 5:21103–21111
Wu J, Huang J, Kuang S, Chen J, Li X, Chen B, Wang J, Cheng D, Shuai X (2019) Adv Sci 6: 1801809
Xiao H, Li XX, Zheng CJ, Liu QM, Sun CY, Huang JS, Wang Y, Yuan YY (2020) J Nanopart Res 22:15
Yu B, Dong B, He J, Huang H, Huang J, Wang Y, Liang J, Zhang J, Qiu Y, Shen J, Shuai X, Tao J, Xia W (2020) Adv Sci n/a:2001657
Zeng C, Wang YL, Xie C, Sang Y, Li TJ, Zhang M, Wang R, Zhang Q, Zheng L, Zhuang SM (2015) Oncotarget 6:12224–12233
Zhang Y, Ghazwani M, Li J, Sun M, Stolz DB, He F, Fan J, Xie W, Li S (2014) Biochem Biophys Res Commun 446:940–944
Zhang ZP, Wang CM, Zha YH, Hu W, Gao ZF, Zang YH, Chen JN, Zhang JF, Dong L (2015) ACS Nano 9:2405–2419
Zhou ZX, Liu XR, Zhu DC, Wang Y, Zhang Z, Zhou XF, Qiu NS, Chen XS, Shen YQ (2017) Adv Drug Deliv Rev 115:115–154
Zhou GY, Xu YM, Chen MW, Cheng D, Shuai XT (2016) Polym Chem 7:3857–3863
Zhu WL, Zhao YL, Xu YQ, Sun Y, Wang Z, Yuan W, Du ZM (2013) PLoS One 8:e63342

# High DNA-Binding Affinity and Gene-Transfection Efficacy of Bioreducible Cationic Nanomicelles

15

Long-Hai Wang and Ye-Zi You

## Contents



**Abstract**

Cationic polymers have become one of the most promising nonviral vectors for gene delivery. However, complex formation of anionic nucleic acid molecules and cationic polymers are unstable because of their weak electrostatic interactions, resulting in polymer/nucleic acid polyplexes with poor serum resistance and a short circulation time in vivo. Furthermore, most polymer/nucleic acid polyplexes mixture exhibit high toxicity because an excess of high molecular weight cationic polymers that are typically required for complete gene condensation. This chapter introduces the preparation and characterizations of a class of bioreducible cationic nanomicelles endowed with high DNA-binding affinity, allowing for efficient DNA condensation and high transfection efficiency at a low nitrogen to phosphorus (N/P) ratio. These cationic nanomicelles hold promising potential as a high efficiency nonviral gene delivery vector for clinical use.

L.-H. Wang · Y.-Z. You (✉)
CAS Key Laboratory of Soft Matter Chemistry, Department of Polymer Science and Engineering, University of Science and Technology of China, Hefei, Anhui, China
e-mail: yzyou@ustc.edu.cn



H. Tian and X. Chen (eds.), *Gene Delivery*, Biomaterial Engineering,
https://doi.org/10.1007/978-981-16-5419-0_15

**Keywords**

Gene delivery · Nonviral vector · DNA-binding affinity · Cationic polymer · Nanomicelle · Stimulus-response

## 1 Overview

Efficient cellular delivery of nucleic acid molecules is critical to the success of many medical therapies, such as gene therapy (Mulligan 1993; Mastrobattista and Hennink 2012) and vaccine development (Pardi et al. 2018; Belete 2021). Although viral gene delivery vectors may be desirable in clinical applications because of their high gene transfection efficacy, overcoming safety issues remains a significant challenge (Bouard et al. 2009; Jackson et al. 2020). Moreover, other limitations are associated with viral vectors, including carcinogenesis, immunogenicity, limited gene packaging capacity, and difficulty of vector production (Thomas et al. 2003). Nonviral vectors have the potential to address many of these limitations, most notably, the safety concerns (Pack et al. 2005; Tan and Sun 2018). A powerful example demonstrating the potential of nonviral gene delivery is the successful COVID-19 vaccines developed by Moderna (Corbett et al. 2020) and Pfizer/BioNTech (Benenson et al. 2021), the first two Food and Drug Administration (FDA) authorized (emergency use) mRNA vaccines in history (Tanne 2020a, b), both of which employ lipid-based nonviral vectors. Several other lipid-based nonviral vectors for nucleic acid vaccines are promisingly undergoing clinical trials (Tan and Sun 2018; Belete 2021). In other efforts, another type of nonviral gene vectors, cationic polymers, could promisingly be employed as a safe, nonviral gene delivery vector for clinical applications (Pack et al. 2005; Lostalé-Seijo and Montenegro 2018; Wang et al. 2019).

Cationic polymers have become one of the most promising nonviral vectors for gene transfection in biotechnology over the past two decades because of their advantageous ease of synthesis and versatility of the chemical modification, which facilitates the development of vectors highly tailored for their specific biomedical applications. However, they have failed to enter clinical trials due to their low gene transfection efficacy (Tan and Sun 2018; Wang et al. 2019). Cationic polymers deliver anionic nucleic acid molecules by forming polyplexes through electrostatic interactions. The resulting polyplexes protect nucleic acids from degradation and facilitate their cellular uptake and intracellular gene transfection. Advantageously, strong interactions between anionic nucleic acids and cationic polymers can provide protection to the gene, better promoting effective gene delivery into cells. However, most cationic polymers exhibit weak interactions with anionic nucleic acids, and therefore the resulting polyplexes are generally unstable in physiological fluids containing serum components and salts, leading to the partial disassociation of these polyplexes (Zhou et al. 2012; Antila et al. 2015). Furthermore, most cationic polymers usually require a high molecular weight and a high

N/P ratio for a complete gene condensation, which results in a highly net-positive charge on the surface of polyplexes and redundant free cationic polymers within the polyplex mixture (Yue et al. 2011). Highly positive charges on the surface of the polyplexes can interact with cellular components (e.g., cell membranes) and inhibit normal cellular processes and the activity of ion channels, membrane receptors, and enzymes (Gao et al. 2011). Although the presence of redundant free cationic polymers can lead to higher gene-transfection efficiency, it is also associated with higher toxicity (Lv et al. 2006). In light of these undesirable effects, it is urgent to develop cationic polymer vectors with a high binding affinity towards nucleic acid molecules.

Some studies have reported several macromolecules with high DNA-binding affinities. For example, Smith et al. prepared a series of dendrons containing multiple spermine units exhibiting high DNA-binding affinity (Kostiainen et al. 2005). Schmuck et al. optimized a short sequence of amino acids within a tweezer-like molecule capped with a tailor-made anion-binding group which also showed high DNA-binding affinity (Li et al. 2015). Despite these macromolecules achieving high affinity for DNA and enabling the efficient shuttling of DNA into cells, their final gene transfection efficiency remained very low, most likely because their tight binding affinity prevented the efficient release of the entrapped DNA. Thus, an optimal gene delivery vector must not only have a high nucleic acid binding affinity, but likewise precisely release entrapped DNA after it enters the cell.

This chapter introduces a micellization method to construct a class of polymer-based bioreducible cationic nanomicelles as nonviral gene delivery vectors, representing a nonviral gene delivery vector which simultaneously achieves efficient gene condensation, good serum-resistance, facile endocytosis, stimulus-response intracellular gene release, and high gene transfection (Wang et al. 2016). Fluorocarbon chains are introduced into poly(ethylenimine) (PEI, Mw 25 kDa) structure via disulfide bonds. Taking the advantage of the hydrophobicity of fluorine materials (Wang et al. 2014; An et al. 2019; Fuchs et al. 2021), the fluorinated PEI can self-assembled into nanomicelles with extremely high zeta potential (+ 64 mV) and high DNA-binding affinity ($CE_{50} = 0.23$), supporting an efficient gene condensation. The lipophobicity of fluorocarbon chains lead to an improvement in the ability of the resulting complexes to traverse the lipid bilayers of cells, as well as the endosome/lysosome membrane, thereby facilitating endosomal escape (Kasuya et al. 2011; Wang et al. 2014). Moreover, the disulfide linkages can be reduced by intracellular glutathione, facilitating intracellular gene release and transfection (ca. 95% in 293 T cells). This micellization method has been expanded to various polymer systems to develop multiresponsive nanomicelles featuring high gene transfection efficiency accompanied by extremely low cytotoxicity (Cheng et al. 2016; Ding et al. 2016; Wang et al. 2016, 2017; Wu et al. 2017; Xu et al. 2017). On the basis of these advantages, it is envisaged that this bioreducible cationic nanomicelle system would be an excellent gene delivery vector.

# 2 Protocol

## 2.1 Materials

Pyridine disulfide (>98%, TCI), 2-mercaptoethylamine hydrochloride (98%, Sigma), pentadecafluorooctanoyl chloride (97%, Sigma), 2-iminothiolane hydrochloride (>98%, Sigma), triethylamine (>99.5%, Sigma), branched polyethylenimine PEI (Mn 10 kDa, Mw 25 kDa, Sigma), and Pyrene (98%, Sigma) can be used as received. Methanol, diethyl ether, isopropanol, dichloromethane, anhydrous sodium sulfate, silica gel, hexane, anhydrous dimethylformamide, acetone, chloroform, sodium acetate, glutaraldehyde, and ethanol can be purchased from Sinopharm Chemical Reagent *Co.* and used as received.

## 2.2 Methods

### 2.2.1 Synthesis of 2-(2-pyridyldithio)ethylamine Hydrochloride (Fig. 1)

1. Dissolve 6.6 g (30.0 mmol) pyridine disulfide in 50 mL methanol.
2. Prepare 1.05 g (10 mmol) 2-mercaptoethylamine hydrochloride in 20 mL methanol and slowly add it into the above solution using a dropping funnel.
3. Incubate the solution overnight at room temperature.
4. Concentrate the reaction mixture by vacuum rotary evaporation and precipitate the crude product in cold diethyl ether.
5. Purify the crude product by recrystallization in mixed solvent of isopropanol/water (8/2, v/v) to get the white crystalline product.

### 2.2.2 Synthesis of N-(2-(2-pyridyldithio)ethyl)perfluorooctanamide (Fig. 2)

1. Disperse 534.6 mg (2.4 mmol) 2-(2-pyridyldithio)ethylamine hydrochloride in 30 mL dichloromethane ($CH_2Cl_2$) and cool the system down to −10 °C.
2. Add 485.0 mg (2.4 mmol) triethylamine into the above suspension and stir it for 30 min.

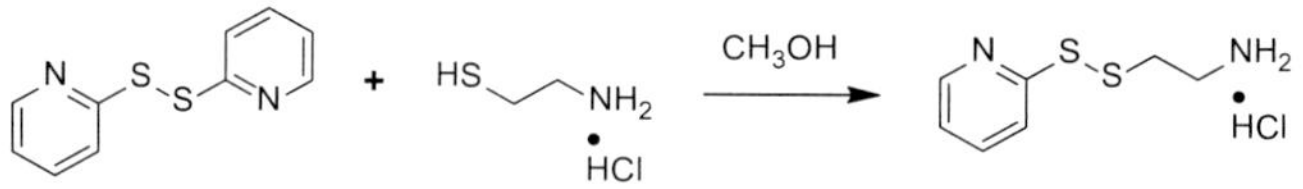


**Fig. 1** Synthesis of 2-(2-pyridyldithio)ethylamine hydrochloride

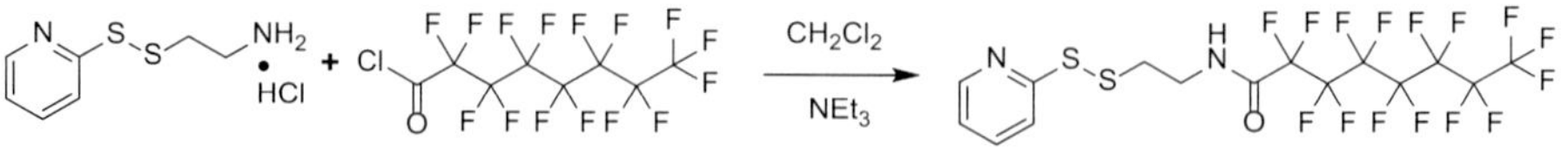


**Fig. 2** Synthesis of *N*-(2-(2-pyridyldithio)ethyl)perfluorooctanamide

3. Dissolve 865.0 mg (2.0 mmol) pentadecafluorooctanoyl chloride in 10 mL $CH_2Cl_2$ and slowly add it into the above solution using a dropping funnel.
4. Incubate the solution for 3 h at room temperature, then wash the organic solution with water for three times using a separatory funnel.
5. Collect the organic layer and treat it with anhydrous sodium sulfate.
6. Concentrate the solution by vacuum rotary evaporation to get a crude product.
7. Purify the crude product by column chromatography (silica gel, hexane/dichloromethane = 3/1, v/v) to get the final product as a colorless powder.

### 2.2.3 Synthesis of Fluorinated PEI (Fig. 3)

The fluorinated PEI (Mn, 10 kDa) was synthesized by the one-pot reaction using Traut's reagent (2-iminothiolane hydrochloride).

1. Dissolve PEI in anhydrous dimethylformamide.
2. Add *N*-(2-(2-pyridyldithio)ethyl) perfluorooctanamide at a molar ratio of 5 to PEI into the above solution.
3. Bubble the solution with argon to deoxygenate the system.
4. Add 2-iminothiolane hydrochloride at a same molar ratio of *N*-(2-(2-pyridyldithio) ethyl) perfluorooctanamide into the above solution.
5. Incubate the mixtures at room temperature for 4 h under argon atmosphere and then precipitate the product of PEI-SS-$5C_7F_{15}$ in diethyl ether.

### 2.2.4 Preparation of Nanomicelles (Fig. 4)

The nanomicelles are prepared via film dispersion method, and the sizes of the formed nanomicelles are related to the concentration of the polymer.

1. Dissolve fluorinated PEI (PEI-SS-$5C_7F_{15}$) in chloroform at a concentration of 2 mg/mL.
2. Add 1 mL PEI-SS-$5C_7F_{15}$ solution into 20 mL glass vials.

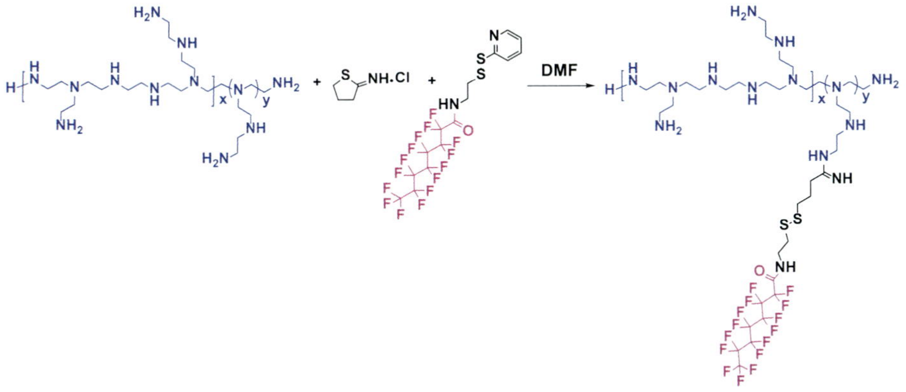


**Fig. 3** Synthesis of fluorinated PEI

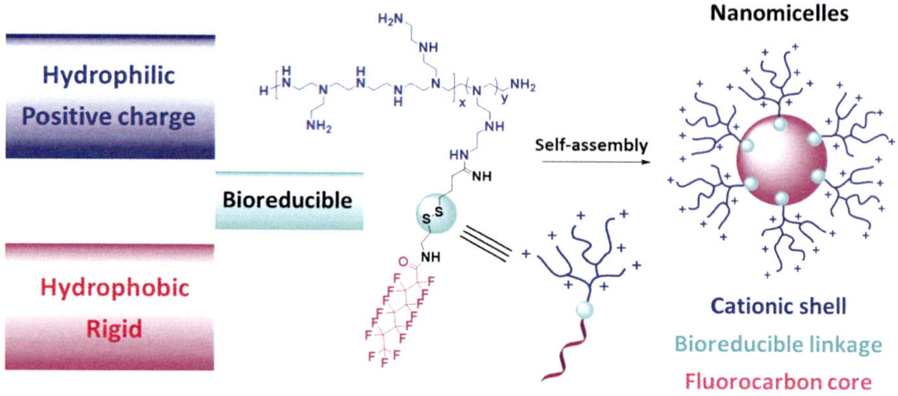


**Fig. 4** Self-assembly of fluorinated PEI into nanomicelles

3. Remove the chloroform solvent using vacuum rotary evaporation to form a dry polymer film on the wall of each glass vial.
4. Add different amounts of water (20 mL, 2 mL, and 1 mL) into the above vials with PEI-SS-5$C_7F_{15}$ film to target a final polymer concentration at 0.1 mg/mL, 1.0 mg/mL, and 2.0 mg/mL, respectively.
5. Sonicate the solutions for 30 min and then keep at rest for another 2 h to finalize the formation of the micelles.
6. The diameters of the forming micelles are about 10 nm, 30 nm, and 50 nm at the polymer concentration of 0.1 mg/mL, 1.0 mg/mL, and 2.0 mg/mL, respectively.
7. Use transmission electron microscopy (TEM) to verify the diameters of the formed nanomicelles.
8. Use NanoBrook 90Plus PALS Zeta Potential Analyzer to measure the zeta potential of the nanomicelles.

### 2.2.5 Critical Micelle Concentration of PEI25k-SS-5C7F15 (Fig. 5)

The critical micelle concentration of PEI25k-SS-5C7F15 is assessed using pyrene as the fluorescent probe. This method makes use of the environment-specific fluorescence of pyrene probe as a detection of organized hydrophobic environment.

1. Prepare pyrene stock solution in acetone at concentration of 0.6 mM.
2. Prepare PEI-SS-5$C_7F_{15}$ stock solution in chloroform at a concentration of 2 mg/mL.
3. Add a predetermined amount of pyrene acetone solution into vials and remove the acetone solvent using vacuum rotary evaporation, then add a predetermined amount of PEI-SS-5$C_7F_{15}$ chloroform solution into vials and remove the chloroform solvent using vacuum rotary evaporation.
4. Add water into above vials to get a set of PEI-SS-5$C_7F_{15}$ solution ranging from $1.0 \times 10^{-3}$ to 1.0 mg/mL with the concentration of pyrene fixed at $6.0 \times 10^{-7}$ M.

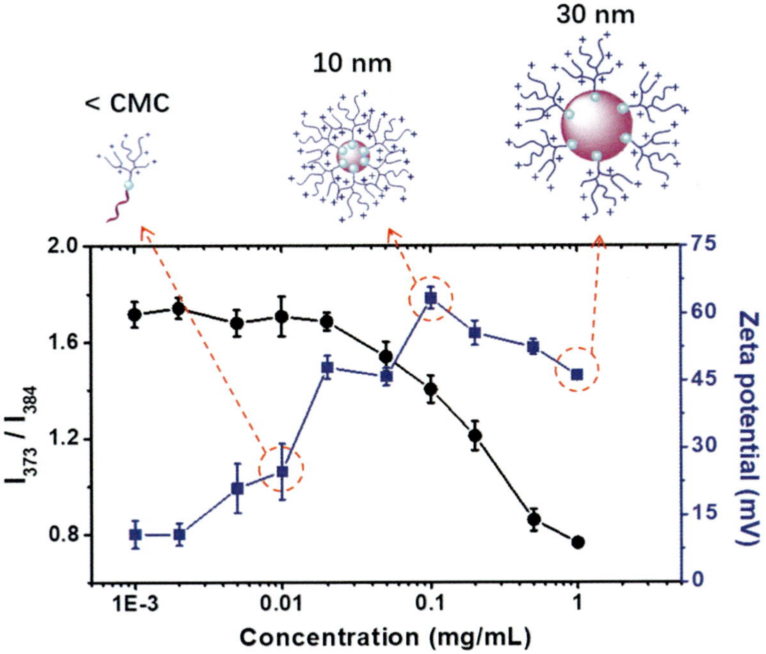


**Fig. 5** Plots of the ratio of intensities (I373/I384) of the vibrational bands in the pyrene fluorescence spectra as a function of polymer concentration in CMC test, and the zeta potential of solution at the corresponding concentration of CMC test. Figure reproduced with permission from reference Wang et al. 2016. Copyright 2016 Wiley

5. Sonicate the solutions for 30 min and then keep at rest for another 2 h to finalize the formation of the micelles.
6. Collect the fluorescent spectra of the above sonicated solutions at the excitation wavelength of 335 nm on a fluorescence spectrophotometer with the excitation and emission bandwidths set as 2 nm.
7. Measure the relative intensities at 373 nm and 384 nm of all collected spectra to get a plot of the fluorescent intensity ratio of I373/I384 as a function of PEI-SS-$5C_7F_{15}$ concentration.
8. CMC is deduced from the inflexion point in the obtained plot graph.

### 2.2.6 Isothermal Titration Microcalorimetry (ITC) Measurement (Fig. 6)

ITC200 (MicroCal) is used to evaluate the binding interactions between gene vectors and DNA.

1. Prepare 25 mM sodium acetate solution as buffer solution (pH = 5.0) for the ITC titrations.
2. Dilute polymer, nanomicelle, and DNA solutions using the above buffer.

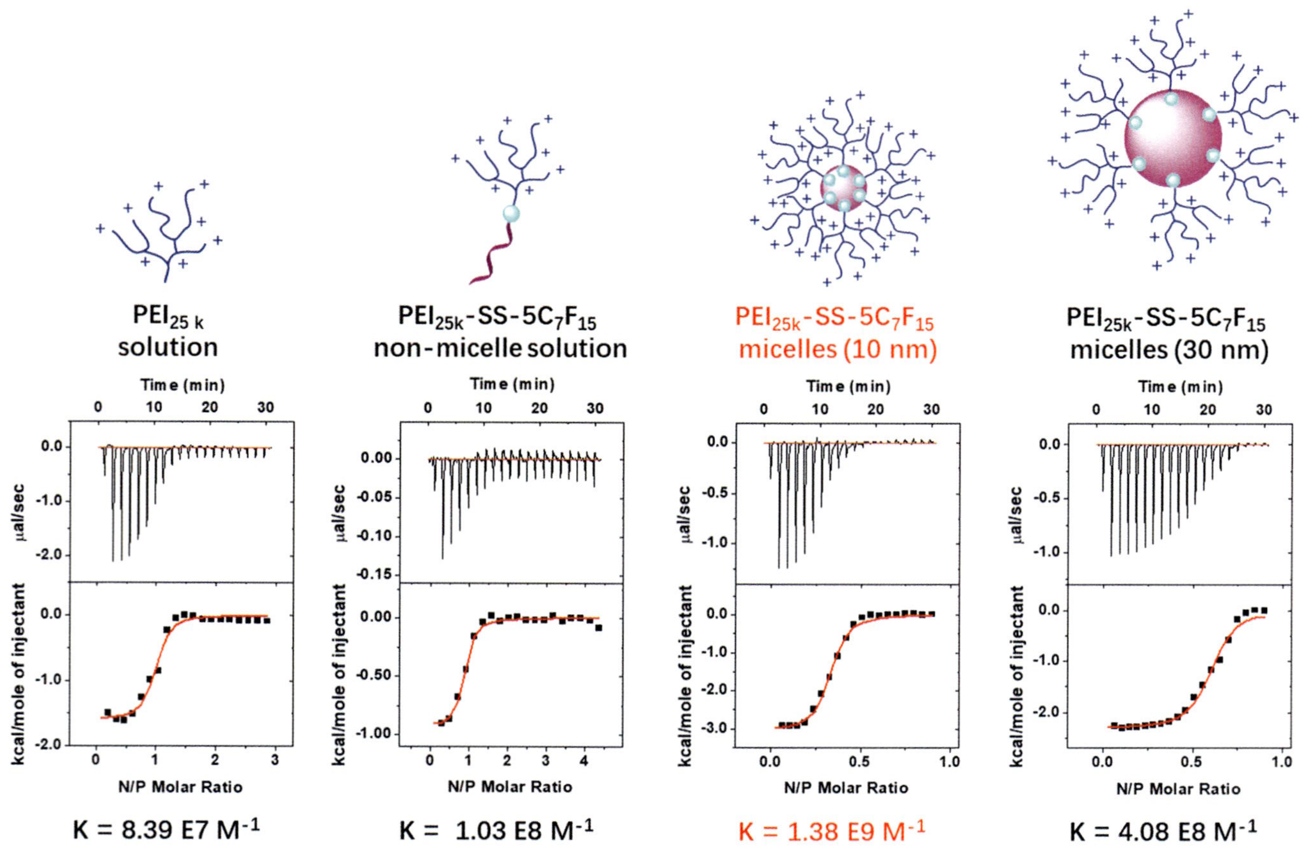


**Fig. 6** ITC curves obtained by titrating vectors into DNA showing their DNA-binding affinities. Figure reproduced with permission from reference Wang et al. 2016. Copyright 2016 Wiley

3. Degas all solutions under vacuum before ITC titrations.
4. Perform two ITC titrations for each group of vectors: first titration of polymer or nanomicelle solution into DNA buffer and second titration of polymer or nanomicelle solution into empty buffer. The settings during the titrations are given according to the following: the system temperature is set at 20 °C; solution in top syringe is injected into the solution in bottom cell by 20 steps with first injection of 1 μL and 19 following injections of 2 μL each; the duration of each injection is set as 4 s; the interval between each injection is set as 90s; the injector stirring speed is set at 1000 rpm to ensure fast mixing during the titrations.
5. Analyze calorimetric data using Origin 7.0 software (MicroCal) to get the binding affinities of the polymers and nanomicelles towards DNA.

### 2.2.7 Gene Transfection (Figs. 7 and 8)

Test transfection efficiency of nanomicelles in cells with gWiz-Luc plasmid DNA (Aldevron).

1. One day before transfection, seed 293 T cells (8000 cells/well) or HeLa cells (6000 cells/well) with 200 μL complete growth medium per well in 96-well cell culture plates. Incubate at 37 °C and 5% $CO_2$ for 24 h.

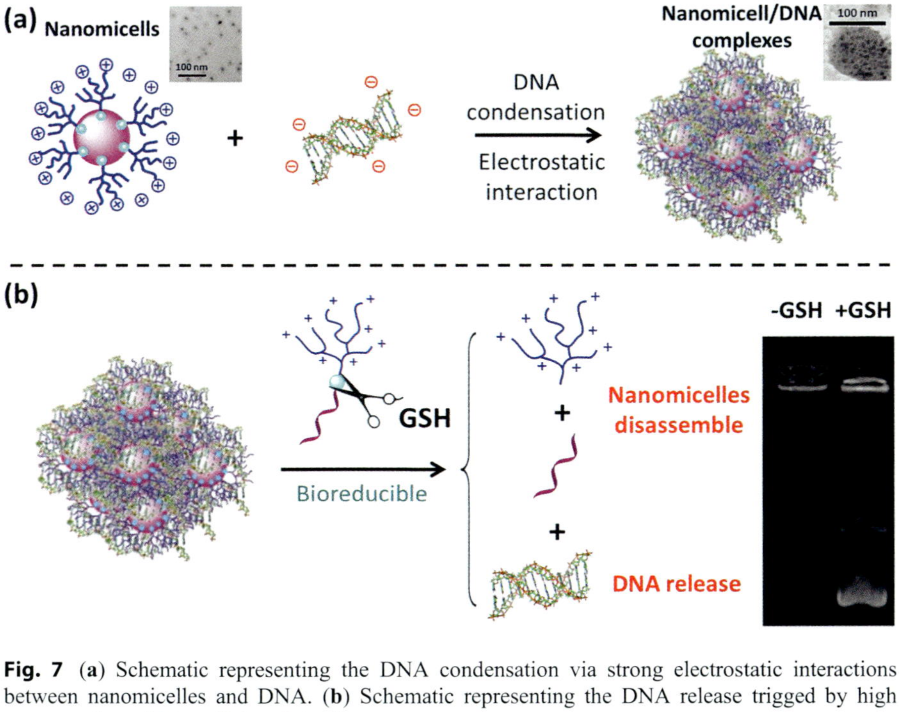


**Fig. 7** (**a**) Schematic representing the DNA condensation via strong electrostatic interactions between nanomicelles and DNA. (**b**) Schematic representing the DNA release trigged by high concentration of intracellular glutathione

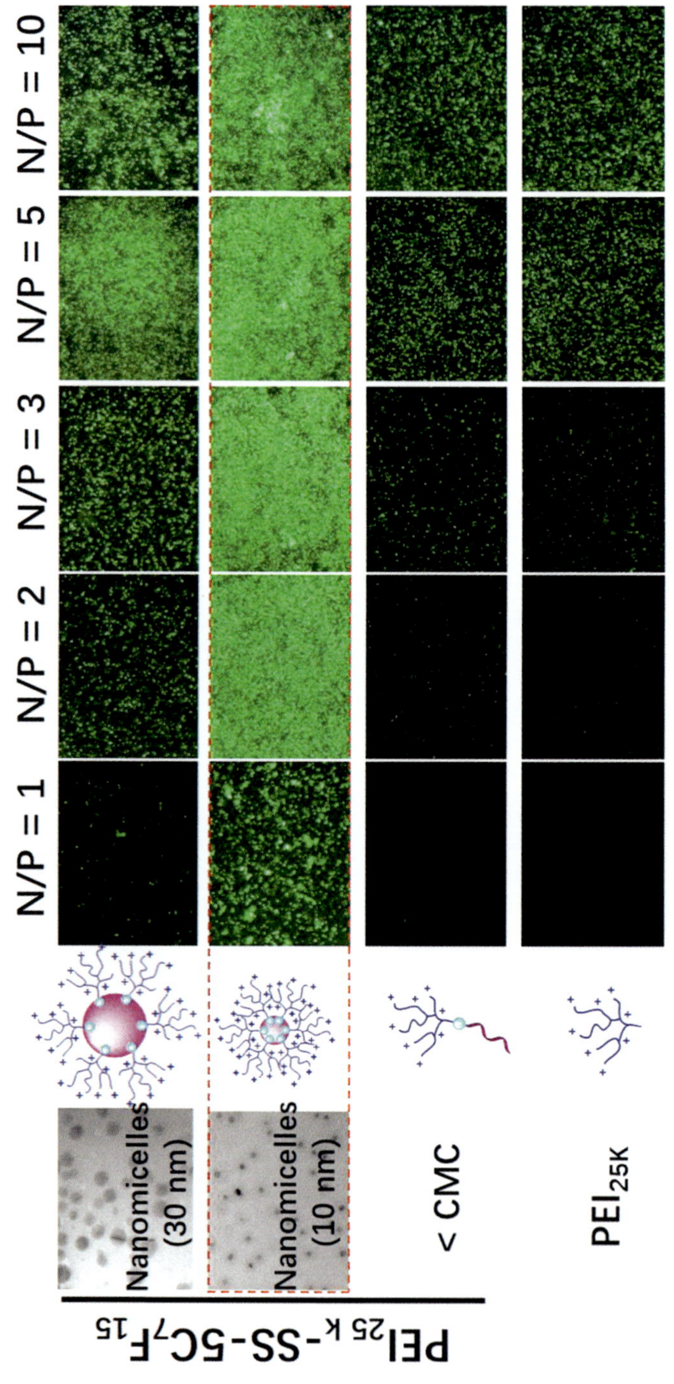


**Fig. 8** GFP expression results in 293 T cells transfected by nanomicelles (10 mm and 30 mm), non-micelle fluorinated PEI solution, and PEI solution at different N/P ratios. Figure reproduced with permission from reference Wang et al. 2016. Copyright 2016 Wiley

2. Prepare the nanomicelle/DNA complex at different N/P ratios by adding nanomicelle solutions into DNA solutions, vortexing for 5 s, and subsequently incubating at room temperature for 30 min. For a triplicate, prepare the nanomicelle/DNA complex with 1.5 μg DNA (0.5 μg DNA per well) for each N/P ratio set and dilute the complex into 300 μL with serum-free DMEM medium.
3. Remove the old 200 uL growth medium in wells and add 100 μL of the diluted complex solution from Step 2 into each well. Incubate at 37 °C and 5% $CO_2$ for 4 h.
4. After 4 h of incubation, refresh the medium in each well with 200 uL complete medium containing 10% FBS. Put the plates back to incubator and culture for an additional 48 h.
5. After 48 h of transfection, analyze luciferase expression and protein content according to the manufacturer's protocols (Promega). The luciferase transfection results are expressed as relative light units (RLU) per milligram of cellular protein.
6. To investigate the serum resistance of the nanomicelle/DNA complexes, the diluent of serum-free DMEM medium in Step 2 is replaced with DMEM medium containing 10%, 30%, or 50% FBS. Then repeat the following Steps 3–5.

Test transfection efficiency of nanomicelles in cells with gWiz-GFP plasmid DNA (Aldevron).

1. One day before transfection, seed 293 T cells (30,000 cells/well) or HeLa cells (20,000 cells/well) with 400 μL complete growth medium per well in 48-well cell culture plates. Incubate at 37 °C and a 5% $CO_2$ for 24 h.
2. Prepare nanomicelle/DNA complex at different N/P ratios by adding nanomicelle solutions into DNA solutions, vortexing for 5 s, and subsequently incubating at room temperature for 30 min. For a triplicate, prepare the nanomicelle/DNA complex with 3 μg DNA (1 μg DNA per well) for each N/P ratio set and dilute the complex into 600 μL with serum-free DMEM medium.
3. Remove the old 400 uL growth medium in wells and add 200 μL of the diluted complex solution from Step 2 into each well. Incubate at 37 °C and 5% $CO_2$ for 4 h.
4. After 4 h of incubation, refresh the medium in each well with 400 uL complete medium containing 10% FBS. Put the plates back to incubator and culture for an additional 48 h.
5. After 48 h of transfection, the expression of GFP in the cells is directly observed by a fluorescent microscopy (Olympus), and the transfection efficacy is quantitatively measured using flow cytometry.
6. To investigate the serum resistance of the nanomicelle/DNA complexes, the diluent of serum-free DMEM medium in Step 2 is replaced with DMEM medium containing 10%, 30%, or 50% FBS. Then repeat the following Steps 3–5.

### 2.2.8 Evaluation of Cytotoxicity of Fluorinated PEI Nanomicelles

1. Seed 293 T cells or HeLa cells in 96-well cell culture plates at a density of 10,000 cells per well with 200 μL complete growth medium. Incubate at 37 °C and 5% $CO_2$ for overnight.

2. Dilute the nanomicelle solution with complete cell culture medium to get final concentrations ranging from 5 μg/mL to 50 μg/mL.
3. Remove the old growth medium in wells and add 200 μL of the diluted nanomicelle solutions from Step 2 into each well. Incubate at 37 °C and 5% $CO_2$ for 48 h.
4. After 48 h of incubation, add 20 μL MTT stock solution (5.5 mg/mL, 11×) into each well. Incubate at 37 °C and 5% $CO_2$ for 4 h.
5. Remove all medium in wells and add 150 μL DMSO, mix thoroughly via pipette to dissolve the forming formazan crystals from MTT treatment.
6. Transfer 100 μL DMSO solution from each sample into a transparent 96-well plate and measure absorbance at 490 nm on a microplate reader.
7. Normalize the cell viability of cells treated with different concentration of nanomicelle solution using untreated cells serve as control (100% cell viability).

### 2.2.9 Erythrocyte Aggregation Test

1. Isolate erythrocytes from fresh heparinized mouse blood by centrifugation at 1500 rpm for 10 min at 4 °C, wash the erythrocytes with PBS buffer for three times.
2. Mix the nanomicelle/DNA complexes used in gene transfection experiments with erythrocyte suspension.
3. Add the above mixture in a 24-well plate, incubate at 37 °C and 5% $CO_2$ for 3 h.
4. Take erythrocyte aggregation phase contrast images under a microscopy.
5. Collect the above treated erythrocyte from the plate for further scanning electron microscopy imaging.
6. Fix the collected erythrocyte in 1% glutaraldehyde solution at 4 °C for 30 min.
7. After fixation, centrifuge and wash the erythrocytes with PBS for three times.
8. Dehydrate the erythrocytes with gradient ethanol/water solutions at volume fraction of 50%, 70%, 80%, 90%, and 100%. Each dehydration procedure lasts for 5 min and twice repeated.
9. Apply a drop of the dehydrated erythrocyte suspension on a slide for the scanning electron microscopy imaging.

## 3 Discussion

1. In synthesis of 2-(2-pyridyldithio)ethylamine hydrochloride, the pure product is a white crystalline. Repeat the recrystallization procedure if the produce is shown as light yellow.
2. In synthesis of *N*-(2-(2-pyridyldithio)ethyl)perfluorooctanamide, the molar ratio of 2-(2-pyridyldithio)ethylamine hydrochloride to pentadecafluorooctanoyl chloride is around 1.2. The excess 2-(2-pyridyldithio)ethylamine hydrochloride is easy to be washed out by water in separatory funnel and separated from the desired product because of the different retention time in column chromatography.
3. In synthesis of fluorinated PEI, the reaction is conducted under argon atmosphere which has a higher purity and higher density than normal nitrogen atmosphere, providing the system a better deoxygenated atmosphere. The Traut's reagent reacts with primary amines ($-NH_2$) on PEI to introduce

sulfhydryl (-SH) groups, then the sulfhydryl groups react with *N*-(2-(2-pyridyldithio)ethyl) perfluorooctanamide through a disulfide exchange reaction. The Traut's reagent should be added into reaction system last to prevent the recyclization or oxidization side reactions forming a nonreactive disulfide before its reaction with *N*-(2-(2-pyridyldithio)ethyl) perfluorooctanamide.

4. The obtained fluorinated PEI polymers containing disulfide bonds should be sealed under argon atmosphere and stored at −20 °C to avoid the crosslinking by disulfide exchange reactions among fluorinated PEI polymers.
5. In preparation of nanomicelles, the vacuum rotary evaporation procedure is recommended to get a thin polymer film on the wall of vials during spinning. (Note, an adapter is necessary to attach the vial onto the rotary evaporator.) Do not apply a hot water bath during the vacuum rotary evaporation to avoid a potential crosslinking reaction among fluorinated PEI polymers. Gently shake the vial during the sonication produce after introducing water. The obtained nanomicelle solutions after sonication should be clear and do not contain any polymer aggregates.
6. In CMC measurements, the acetone from pyrene solution should be removed before introducing of PEI-SS-5$C_7F_{15}$ solution. (Acetone is a poor solvent for PEI-SS-5$C_7F_{15}$, which may induce polymer aggregation and therefore affect the CMC result.)
7. Any non-micelle fluorinated PEI solution should be prepared at a low concentration under its CMC; it cannot be simply diluted from a micelle solution prepared at a higher concentration.
8. In ITC measurements, a buffer is necessary for the preparation of nanomicelle solution and DNA solution to avoid any artifactual heats produced by pH change during the titrations. Avoid introducing air bubbles into the system when loading solutions in top injector and bottom cell. Air bubbles may cause a noisy or stepping baseline. Delete the first data point before the curve fitting analysis.
9. The optimal cell density at the time of transfection and the following incubation time for transfection should be carefully determined for each cell line of interest. It is usually recommended to transfect cells at a confluence of 50–70% for 293 T cells and 70–90% confluency for Hela cells.
10. In erythrocyte aggregation test, to fix the erythrocytes, glutaraldehyde solution should be added into erythrocyte suspension dropwise to avoid osmotic shock. A sputter coating layer on erythrocytes is necessary before the SEM imaging because of the nonconductive nature of erythrocytes. And a sputter coating of platinum is recommended for the erythrocyte samples.

## 4 Conclusion

This chapter introduced the protocols and guidelines for the construction of bioreducible cationic nanomicelles which facilitate high gene transfection efficiency and low cytotoxicity. The nanomicelles exhibits excellent DNA-condensation ability, even at a low N/P ratio of 1. Moreover, the nanomicelle/DNA complexes are very stable under physiological conditions, but are disrupted by intracellular glutathione, which leads to the release of the entrapped DNA and high gene transfection efficacy at a level similar to that of the viral vector. These results therefore show that the construction of bioreducible cationic nanomicelles is an attractive strategy for producing effective gene vectors.

## References

An D, Wang LH, Ernst AU, Chiu A, Lu YC, Flanders JA, Datta AK, Ma M (2019) An atmosphere-breathing refillable biphasic device for cell replacement therapy. Adv Mater 31(52):e1905135. https://doi.org/10.1002/adma.201905135

Antila HS, Härkönen M, Sammalkorpi M (2015) Chemistry specificity of DNA–polycation complex salt response: a simulation study of DNA, polylysine and polyethyleneimine. Phys Chem Chem Phys 17(7):5279–5289

Belete TM (2021) Review on up-to-date status of candidate vaccines for COVID-19 disease. Infect Drug Resist 14:151–161. https://doi.org/10.2147/IDR.S288877

Benenson S, Oster Y, Cohen MJ, Nir-Paz R (2021) BNT162b2 mRNA Covid-19 vaccine effectiveness among health care workers. N Engl J Med 384:1775–1777

Bouard D, Alazard-Dany N, Cosset FL (2009) Viral vectors: from virology to transgene expression. Br J Pharmacol 157(2):153–165

Cheng B-F, Wang L-H, You Y-Z (2016) Photoinduced electron transfer-reversible addition-fragmentation chain transfer (PET-RAFT) polymerization using titanium dioxide. Macromol Res 24 (9):811–815

Corbett KS, Flynn B, Foulds KE, Francica JR, Boyoglu-Barnum S, Werner AP, Flach B, O'Connell S, Bock KW, Minai M (2020) Evaluation of the mRNA-1273 vaccine against SARS-CoV-2 in nonhuman primates. N Engl J Med 383(16):1544–1555

Ding S-G, Yu L, Wang L-H, Wang L-D, Yu Z-Q, You Y-Z (2016) Self-assembling Janus dendritic polymer for gene delivery with low cytotoxicity and high gene transfection efficiency. J Mater Chem B 4(39):6462–6467

Fuchs S, Ernst AU, Wang L-H, Shariati K, Wang X, Liu Q, Ma TC (2021) Hydrogels in emerging technologies for type 1 diabetes. Chem Rev 121(18):11458–11526

Gao X, Yao L, Song Q, Zhu L, Xia Z, Xia H, Jiang X, Chen J, Chen H (2011) The association of autophagy with polyethylenimine-induced cytotoxity in nephritic and hepatic cell lines. Biomaterials 32(33):8613–8625

Jackson NAC, Kester KE, Casimiro D, Gurunathan S, DeRosa F (2020) The promise of mRNA vaccines: a biotech and industrial perspective. npj Vaccines 5(1). https://doi.org/10.1038/s41541-020-0159-8

Kasuya MCZ, Nakano S, Katayama R, Hatanaka K (2011) Evaluation of the hydrophobicity of perfluoroalkyl chains in amphiphilic compounds that are incorporated into cell membrane. J Fluor Chem 132(3):202–206

Kostiainen MA, Hardy JG, Smith DK (2005) High-affinity multivalent DNA binding by using low-molecular-weight dendrons. Angew Chem 117(17):2612–2615

Li M, Schlesiger S, Knauer SK, Schmuck C (2015) A tailor-made specific anion-binding motif in the side chain transforms a tetrapeptide into an efficient vector for gene delivery. Angew Chem 127(10):2984–2987

Lostalé-Seijo I, Montenegro J (2018) Synthetic materials at the forefront of gene delivery. Nat Rev Chem 2(10):258–277. https://doi.org/10.1038/s41570-018-0039-1

Lv H, Zhang S, Wang B, Cui S, Yan J (2006) Toxicity of cationic lipids and cationic polymers in gene delivery. J Control Release 114(1):100–109

Mastrobattista E, Hennink WE (2012) Charged for success. Nat Mater 11(1):10–12

Mulligan RC (1993) The basic science of gene therapy. Science 260(5110):926–932
Pack DW, Hoffman AS, Pun S, Stayton PS (2005) Design and development of polymers for gene delivery. Nat Rev Drug Discov 4(7):581–593
Pardi N, Hogan MJ, Porter FW, Weissman D (2018) mRNA vaccines – a new era in vaccinology. Nat Rev Drug Discov 17(4):261–279. https://doi.org/10.1038/nrd.2017.243
Tan L, Sun X (2018) Recent advances in mRNA vaccine delivery. Nano Res 11(10):5338–5354. https://doi.org/10.1007/s12274-018-2091-z
Tanne JH (2020a) Covid-19: FDA approves moderna vaccine as US starts vaccinating health workers BMJ 2020;371:m4924. https://www.bmj.com/content/371/bmj.m4924
Tanne JH (2020b) Covid-19: FDA panel votes to authorise Pfizer BioNTech vaccine. British Medical Journal Publishing Group BMJ 2020;371:m4799. https://www.bmj.com/content/371/bmj.m4799
Thomas CE, Ehrhardt A, Kay MA (2003) Progress and problems with the use of viral vectors for gene therapy. Nat Rev Genet 4(5):346–358
Wang H, Ding S, Zhang Z, Wang L, You Y (2019) Cationic micelle: a promising nanocarrier for gene delivery with high transfection efficiency. J Gene Med 21(7). https://doi.org/10.1002/jgm.3101
Wang M, Liu H, Li L, Cheng Y (2014) A fluorinated dendrimer achieves excellent gene transfection efficacy at extremely low nitrogen to phosphorus ratios. Nat Commun 5(1):1–8
Wang L-H, Wu T, Wu D-C, You Y-Z (2016) Bioreducible gene delivery vector capable of self-scavenging the intracellular-generated ROS exhibiting high gene transfection. ACS Appl Mater Interfaces 8(30):19238–19244
Wang LH, Wu DC, Xu HX, You YZ (2016) High DNA-binding affinity and gene-transfection efficacy of bioreducible cationic nanomicelles with a fluorinated core. Angew Chem Int Ed Engl 55(2):755–759. https://doi.org/10.1002/anie.201508695
Wang L, Zhang Z, Zeng T, Xia L, Nie X, Chen G, Y-z Y (2017) Responsive cationic polymer and cationic nanomicelle vectors for gene delivery. Acta Polym Sin 12:1883–1904
Wu T, Wang L, Ding S, You Y (2017) Fluorinated PEG-polypeptide polyplex micelles have good serum-resistance and low cytotoxicity for gene delivery. Macromol Biosci 17(8):1700114
Xu C-T, Chen G, Nie X, Wang L-H, Ding S-G, You Y-Z (2017) Low generation PAMAM-based nanomicelles as ROS-responsive gene vectors with enhanced transfection efficacy and reduced cytotoxicity in vitro. New J Chem 41(9):3273–3279
Yue Y, Jin F, Deng R, Cai J, Chen Y, Lin MC, Kung H-F, Wu C (2011) Revisit complexation between DNA and polyethylenimine – effect of uncomplexed chains free in the solution mixture on gene transfection. J Control Release 155(1):67–76
Zhou J, Liu J, Cheng CJ, Patel TR, Weller CE, Piepmeier JM, Jiang Z, Saltzman WM (2012) Biodegradable poly (amine-co-ester) terpolymers for targeted gene delivery. Nat Mater 11(1): 82–90

# Preparation of Chimeric Polymersomes for Gene Delivery

16

Jun Shi, Liang Cheng, and Zhiyuan Zhong

## Contents



**Abstract**

RNA interference (RNAi) has become a powerful tool for the treatment of different diseases including virus infections and cancers. The clinical applications of RNAi are, however, limited by absence of safe, stable, and efficient delivery vehicles. Nonviral vectors such as lipid nanoparticles, liposomes, and cationic polymers with better safety compared with viral counterparts show only moderate transfection efficacy in vivo, due to poor stability, low target cell entry, and inefficient intracellular release of small interfering RNA (siRNA). This protocol describes preparation of chimeric polymersomes from poly(ethylene glycol)-b-poly(trimethylene carbonate-co-dithiolane trimethylene carbonate)-b-poly-ethylenimine/spermine (PEG-P(TMC-co-DTC)-PEI/spermine) as a versatile

J. Shi · L. Cheng · Z. Zhong (✉)
Biomedical Polymers Laboratory, College of Chemistry, Chemical Engineering and Materials Science, and State Key Laboratory of Radiation Medicine and Protection, Soochow University, Suzhou, People's Republic of China
e-mail: zyzhong@suda.edu.cn


H. Tian and X. Chen (eds.), *Gene Delivery*, Biomaterial Engineering,
https://doi.org/10.1007/978-981-16-5419-0_16

type of vehicle for efficient siRNA delivery. PEG-P(TMC-co-DTC)-PEI/spermine was synthesized by ring-opening copolymerization of trimethylene carbonate and dithiolane trimethylene carbonate using methoxy poly(ethylene glycol) as an initiator and diphenyl phosphate as a catalyst followed by activating the terminal hydroxyl group with N, N′-carbonyldiimidazole and conjugation with PEI or spermine. siRNA-loaded chimeric polymersomes were prepared with a size of 40–120 nm depending on the type of polycation, PEI molecular weights, and copolymer compositions through co-self-assembly of PEG-P(TMC-co-DTC)-PEI/spermine and siRNA in aqueous conditions. Targeted siRNA formulations could be easily prepared by either pre- or post-modification with peptides and antibodies. The in vivo studies showed that polymersomal siRNA was nontoxic and stable, and mediated efficient RNAi therapy of different tumor models. These self-regulating biodegradable polymersomes offer a robust, multifunctional, and viable nanoplatform for targeted gene therapy.

**Keywords**

Polymersomes · siRNA delivery · Gene therapy · Targeted delivery · RNA interference · Reduction sensitive

# 1 Overview

## 1.1 Introduction

RNA interference (RNAi) capable of targeting and silencing virtually any gene of interest has become a powerful tool for biomedical research and drug discovery. Small interfering RNA (siRNA) is double-stranded oligonucleotides consisting of 21–23 base pairs that guide RNAi via binding to RNA-induced silencing complex (RISC) in the cytoplasm and subsequently cleaving mRNA sequence to suppress the expression of specific genes (Elbashir et al. 2001). The past decades have seen the development of different therapeutic siRNAs that are able to effectively treat both genetic and acquired diseases. Notably, at present, four siRNA drugs have been approved by the FDA or EMA for treating hereditary transthyretin-mediated amyloidosis (hATTR), acute hepatic porphyria (AHP), primary hyperoxaluria type 1 (PH1), and hypercholesterolemia (Hu et al. 2020). A number of siRNA drugs are under phase I–III clinical trials for treating advanced solid tumors, acute kidney injury, hepatitis B, liver fibrosis, hypertrophic scars, cardiovascular diseases, and so on (Saw and Song 2020; Zhang et al. 2021).

siRNA with negative charge, easy degradation, and poor cell penetration has a low gene silencing efficacy in vivo. The clinical applications of siRNA therapeutics critically rely on the development of safe and efficient vehicles that are able to overcome the extracellular and intracellular barriers in the process of siRNA transportation (Dowdy 2017). Liposomes, lipid nanoparticles, and polymers that are mainly cationic and form nanocomplexes with siRNA are among the most used nonviral vectors for siRNA transfection. The first clinically approved siRNA drug, Patisiran, has utilized cationic lipid nanoparticles as a vehicle (Adams et al. 2018). The cationic polymers such as polyethylenimine and polylysine are less advanced than lipid nanoparticles and are primarily limited to preclinical studies. The positive charge of liposomes, lipid nanoparticles, and polymers, while playing an important role in condensing siRNA, protecting siRNA from degradation, and facilitating cellular uptake, will cause nonspecific interactions, poor cell selectivity, and potential toxic effects in vivo. Low stability and cell selectivity are further problems associated with cationic vehicles. Trivalent N-acetylgalactosamine (GalNAc)-siRNA conjugates provide a unique, safe, and liver-targeted platform for siRNA transfection (Springer and Dowdy 2018). However, GalNAc strategy is only limited to liver transfection and requires extensive chemical modification of siRNA to increase its in vivo stability and reduce immunogenicity.

Polymersomes with a similar structure to liposomes are of particular interest in drug and gene delivery. The watery core of polymersomes can be used to load different hydrophilic drugs including protein and siRNA. The loading content and efficacy of polymersomes toward siRNA is, however, typically marginal. We found that chimeric polymersomes formed from amphiphilic ABC triblock copolymers with poly(ethylene glycol) (PEG) as A block and a charged polymer as C block and A longer than C can efficiently load large biomacromolecules like proteins (Liu et al. 2010).

Recently, we developed disulfide-crosslinked biodegradable chimeric polymersomes based on PEG-b-poly(trimethylene carbonate-co-dithiolane trimethylene carbonate)-b-PEI/spermine (PEG-P(TMC-co-DTC)-PEI/spermine)) for efficient loading and targeted intracellular delivery of gene and protein (Fig. 1) (Jiang et al.

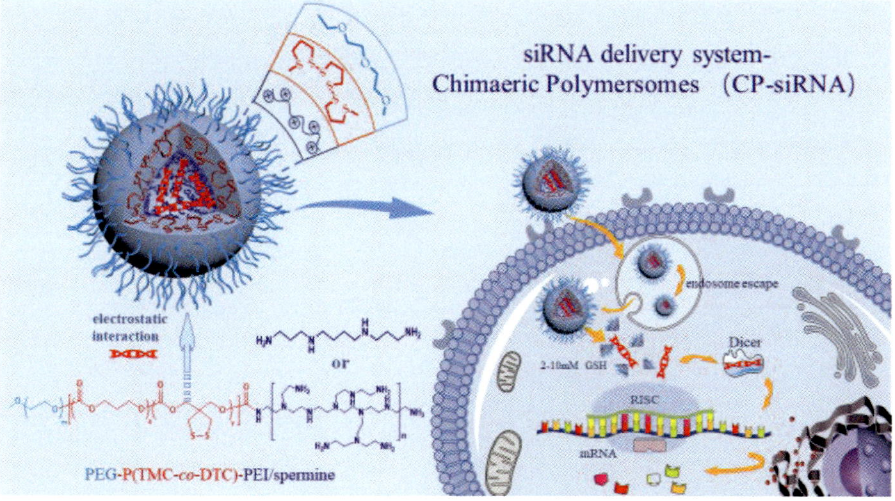


**Fig. 1** Schematic illustration of chimeric biodegradable polymersomes based on PEG-P(TMC-co-DTC)-PEI/spermine for siRNA delivery

2018; Yang et al. 2018). Dithiolane trimethylene carbonate (DTC) is our proprietary monomer (Zou et al. 2016). The polymersomes based on P(TMC-co-DTC) were found self-crosslinkable under aqueous condition to afford high stability and responsive to intracellular reductive conditions to enable fast release of payloads. The short PEI or spermine preferentially located inside the vesicles facilitates loading of siRNA via charge and hydrogen bonding interactions. The longer PEG is oriented at the outer surface of vesicles to equip them with good water dispersity, biocompatibility, and nonfouling properties. Moreover, polymersome surface can be functionalized with different ligands such as peptides and antibodies, via either premodification or post-modification method, to achieve high cell specificity and/or to overcome delivery barriers. For instance, cNGQ peptide-modified chimeric polymersomes loading siRNA against polo-like kinase 1 (siPLK1) effectively inhibited orthotopic lung tumor growth and prolonged mice survival time (Zou et al. 2017). Angeopep-2 peptide modified chimeric polymersomes were shown to penetrate blood-brain barrier and mediate effective gene silencing and tumor growth inhibition in an orthotopic glioblastoma model (Shi et al. 2018). These chimeric polymersomes have emerged as a simple, robust, multifunctional, and versatile platform for siRNA delivery. In this chapter, we give a comprehensive description about preparation of chimeric polymersomes for siRNA delivery, which can also extend to other genes such as micro-RNA, antisense oligonucleotide (ASO), etc.

## 2 Protocol

### 2.1 Materials

#### 2.1.1 Preparation and Characterization of PEG-P(TMC-co-DTC)

1. Methoxy poly(ethylene glycol) (mPEG-OH, $M_n = 5000$ g/mol, Sigma-Aldrich)
2. Trimethylene carbonate (TMC, Jinan Daigang Biomaterial Co., Ltd., China)
3. Dithiolane trimethylene carbonate (DTC)
4. Diphenyl phosphate (DPP, TCI Development Co., Ltd., Japan)
5. Dichloromethane (DCM)
6. Tetrahydrofuran (THF)
7. Toluene (Tol)
8. Phosphorus pentoxide
9. Ethanol
10. Vacuum desicator
11. Vacuum oil pump
12. Vacuum drying oven
13. Oil bath
14. Hot plate stirrer
15. Glove box
16. 100 ml Schlenk bottle
17. Solvent purification system (Innovative Technology, USA)

18. Bruker AVANCE NEO 400 MHz NMR spectrometer (Bruker Corporation, Germany)
19. Waters 1515 gel permeation chromatograph (GPC, USA)

#### 2.1.2 Preparation and Characterization of PEG-P(TMC-co-DTC)-PEI/Spermine

1. N,N′-Carbonyldiimidazole (CDI, J&K Chemical)
2. Dichloromethane (DCM)
3. Polyethylenimine (PEI, $M_w = 600/1200/1800$, Sigma-Aldrich)
4. Spermine (Sigma-Aldrich)
5. Constant pressure dropping funnel
6. Rotary evaporator (BUCHI Labortechnik AG, Switzerland)
7. Ethanol
8. Diethyl ether

#### 2.1.3 Preparation and Characterization of Peptide-Decorated Polymers

1. N-hydroxysuccinimide functionalized poly(ethylene glycol) (NHS-PEG-OH, $M_n = 6500$ g/mol)
2. Maleimide functionalized poly(ethylene glycol) (Mal-PEG-OH, $M_n = 7500$ g/mol)
3. Azide functionalized poly(ethylene glycol) ($N_3$-PEG-OH, $M_n = 7900$ g/mol)
4. Trimethylene carbonate (TMC)
5. Dithiolane trimethylene carbonate (DTC)
6. Diphenyl hydrogen phosphate (DPP, TCI Development Co., Ltd., Japan)
7. cRGD peptide (Sequence: cyclo (RGDfK), China Peptides Co., Ltd., China)
8. Angiopep-2 peptide (Sequence: TFFYGGSRGKRNNFKTEEYC, China Peptides Co., Ltd., China)
9. Dichloromethane (DCM)
10. N,N-Dimethylformamide (DMF)
11. Dimethyl sulfoxide (DMSO)
12. 25 ml Schlenk bottle
13. Oil bath
14. Hot plate stirrer
15. BCA protein quantitative analysis kit (Sangon Biotech Co., Ltd., China)
16. Microplate reader (Model 680, Bio-RAD, USA)
17. 7 kDa cutoff dialysis bag (XiAn Uber Biotechnology Co., China)
18. DD2–600 liquid superconducting NMR spectrometer (Agilent, USA)

#### 2.1.4 Preparation of Polymersomes

1. Phosphate buffer (PB, 2 mM, pH 6.0)
2. Phosphate buffer (PB, 10 mM, pH 7.4)
3. Phosphate buffer (PB, 10 mM, pH 8.5)
4. Hepes buffer (10 mM, pH 6.8)
5. Hepes buffer (10 mM, pH 7.4)

6. DEPC-treated water
7. Dimethyl sulfoxide (DMSO)
8. N, N-Dimethylformamide (DMF)
9. 7 and 14 kDa cutoff dialysis bag (XiAn Uber Biotechnology Co., China)
10. NanoDrop One/Onec spectrophotometer (Thermo Fisher Scientific, USA)
11. Ultrafiltration centrifuge tube (MWCO = 10 kDa)
12. Vortex mixer
13. NHS-$PEG_4$-DBCO
14. Daratumumab (Dar)
15. Dynamic light scattering analyzer (DLS, Malvern Instruments, UK)
16. E2695-Waters high-performance liquid chromatograph (HPLC)
17. Matrix-assisted laser desorption ionization time of flight mass spectrometry (MALDI-TOF-MS)

#### 2.1.5 Determination of siRNA Loading Content, Stability, and Reduction Responsivity of Chimeric Polymersomes (CP)

1. Agarose
2. TAE buffer (1×, pH 8.3)
3. Gel-Red (10,000×, Beyotime)
4. DNA loading buffer (6×, including bromophenol blue and xylene cyanol FF)
5. Electrophoresis apparatus
6. Fetal bovine serum (FBS)
7. Glutathione (GSH)
8. Dynamic light scattering analyzer (DLS, Malvem Instruments, UK)
9. Phosphate buffer (PB, 10 mM, pH 7.4)

#### 2.1.6 Characterization of CP by Transmission Electron Microscopy (TEM)

1. Copper mesh
2. Filter paper
3. Phosphotungstic acid solution (2%, pH 7.0)
4. Infrared lamp
5. Hitachi HT7700 TEM (Hitachi Limited, Japan)

#### 2.1.7 MTT Assays of Blank CP

1. Trypsin
2. Dulbecco's modified eagle medium (DMEM) and RPMI 1640 medium
3. solution (MTT, 5 mg/mL)
4. Dimethyl sulfoxide (DMSO)
5. Microplate reader (Thermo Scientific Varioskan LUX, USA)
6. 96-well tissue culture plates
7. $CO_2$ incubator
8. Optical microscope (Nikon, Japan)

#### 2.1.8 Flow Cytometry Assays and Confocal Microscopy of siRNA-Loaded CP

1. BD FACS calibur flow cytometer (Becton Dickinson, USA)
2. Dulbecco's modified eagle medium (DMEM) and RPMI 1640 medium
3. Phosphate buffered saline (PBS, 10 mM)
4. siRNA-Cy3 (siScramble, sense strand sequence: 5'-UUC UCC GAA CGU GUC ACG UDTDT-3′, and antisense strand sequence: 5'-ACG UGA CAC GUU CGG AGA ADTDT-3'-Cy3)
5. siRNA-Cy5 (siScramble, sense strand sequence: 5'-UUC UCC GAA CGU GUC ACG UDTDT-3′, and antisense strand sequence: 5'-ACG UGA CAC GUU CGG AGA ADTDT-3'-Cy5)
6. Lyso-Tracker red
7. 4′,6-Diamidino-2-phenylindole solution (DAPI)
8. Paraformaldehyde (4% (v/v))
9. Glycerol
10. Confocal laser scanning microscope (CLSM, Lecia TCS SP8 X, German)
11. Centrifuge
12. Six-well tissue culture plates
13. Twenty-four-well tissue culture plates
14. Glass slide
15. $CO_2$ incubator
16. Optical microscope (Nikon, Japan)

#### 2.1.9 In Vitro Gene Silencing Efficacy of CP-siRNA

1. siPLK-1 (sense strand sequence: 5′-AGA UCA CCC UCC UUA AAU AUU-3′ and antisense strand sequence: 5'-UAU UUA AGG AGG GUG AUC UUU-3′)
2. Phosphate buffered saline (PBS)
3. Six-well tissue culture plates
4. Isopropanol
5. DEPC-treated water
6. 75% ethanol
7. RNA isolation reagent (Biosharp, China)
8. Centrifuge
9. Oligo (dT)
10. Reverse transcription reagent
11. TB Green fast qPCR mix
12. Taq DNA polymerase
13. Oligo-deoxynucleotide primers (PLK1-fw: 5'-CGA CTT CGT GTT CGT GGT G-3′, PLK1-rev: 5'-CCC GTC ATA TTC GAC TTT GGT-3′, GAPDH-fw: 5'-CAT GAG AAG TAT GAC AAC AGC CT-3′, GAPDH-rev: 5′-AGT CCT TCC ACG ATA CCA AAG T-3′)
14. Reverse transcription instrument (Bio-Rad, USA)
15. PCR amplifier (Bio-Rad, USA)

### 2.1.10 Pharmacokinetic of CP-siRNA

1. Dithiothreitol (DTT)
2. BALB/c nude mice
3. Dimethyl sulfoxide (DMSO)
4. Capillary
5. siPLK1 (Cy5)
6. Cary eclipse fluorospectrophotometer (Agilent Technology, USA)

### 2.1.11 In Vivo Gene Silencing Efficacy of CP-siRNA

1. BALB/c nude mice
2. Electronic balance
3. Microinjector
4. Near-infrared fluorescence imaging system (Caliper IVIS Lumina II, Ex = 640 nm, Em = 668 nm, Perkin elmer, USA).

## 2.2 Methods

### 2.2.1 Preparation and Characterization of PEG-P(TMC-co-DTC) (Fig. 2, Notes 1, 2, 3, 4, 5, and 6)

1. Poly(ethylene glycol) (mPEG-OH) was dried by azeotropic distillation from dry toluene. mPEG-OH (20 g, $M_n$ = 5000 g/mol,) and dry toluene (20 ml) were heated to 120 °C and toluene was distilled off over 2 h. PEG was then dried under vacuum for 3 days.
2. An amount of 25 g of diphenyl phosphate organocatalyst was placed in a vacuum desicator containing 6–7 g of phosphorus pentoxide for 2 days.
3. DTC monomer was purified by recrystallization from dry THF. An amount of 15 g of DTC was added to 180 ml of dry THF and heated slowly to 60 °C with an oil bath to completely dissolve DTC. DTC crystalized upon slowly cooling down to room temperature. After completion, the supernatant was poured off, and the DTC crystals were dried under vacuum for 1 day.
4. TMC monomer was purified by recrystallization from dry toluene. A mass of 100 g of TMC was added to 180 ml of dry toluene, and heated slowly to completely dissolve TMC. TMC crystalized upon slowly cooling down to 4 °C

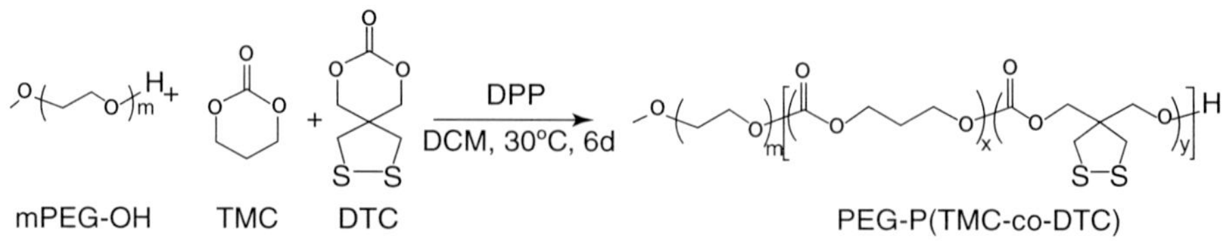


**Fig. 2** Synthesis of PEG-P(TMC-co-DTC)

in a refrigerator. After completion, the supernatant was poured off, and the TMC crystals were dried under vacuum for 2 days.

5. Under a $N_2$ atmosphere in a glove box, mPEG-OH (2.5 g, 0.5 mmol), TMC (7.5 g, 73.5 mmol), DTC (1 g, 5.2 mmol), anhydrous DCM (22.4 ml), and DPP (625 mg, 2.5 mmol) were added into a 100 ml Schlenk bottle containing a magnetic stirrer. The bottle was sealed and placed in an oil bath thermostated at 30 °C for 6 days.
6. After the reaction, PEG-P(TMC-co-DTC) copolymer was precipitated in cold ethanol, the supernatant was poured off, and the product was redissolved in DCM and precipitated in cold ethanol. The final product was dried under vacuum. Yield: 90%.
7. The structure of PEG-P(TMC-co-DTC) was characterized by $^1H$ NMR ($CDCl_3$, 400 MHz) and GPC.

### 2.2.2 Preparation of PEG-P(TMC-co-DTC)-PEI/Spermine (Fig. 3, Notes, 7, 8, and 9)

1. Typically, under a nitrogen atmosphere, PEG-P(TMC-co-DTC) (1.5 g, 0.0682 mmol) was dissolved in anhydrous DCM (3.75 mL). A mass of 33.1 mg of N, N′-carbonyldiimidazole (CDI, 0.205 mmol) was quickly added. The reaction vessel was sealed and placed in an oil bath thermostated at 30 °C.
2. After 4 h, 3.8 ml of DCM was added to dilute the reaction mixture. PEG-P (TMC-co-DTC)-CDI copolymer was isolated by precipitation in cold diethyl

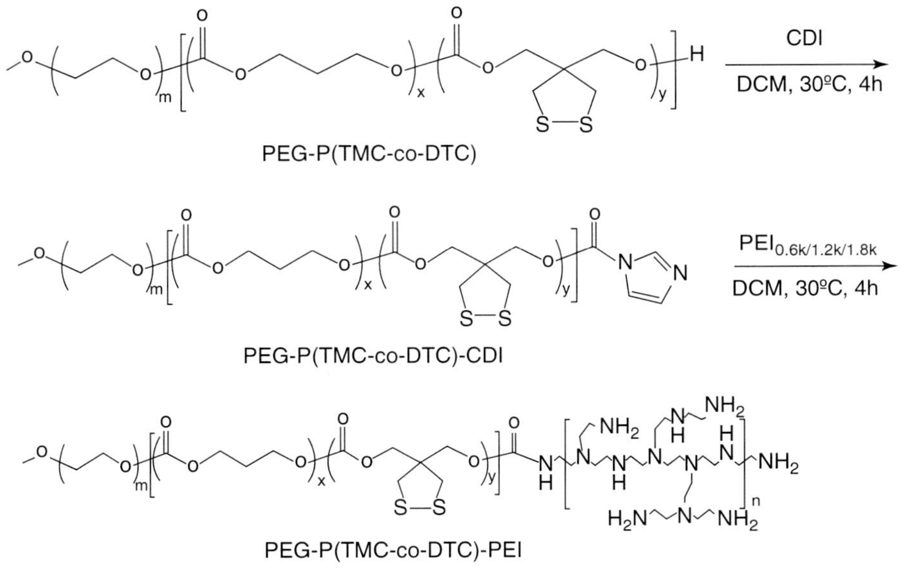


**Fig. 3** Synthesis of PEG-P(TMC-co-DTC)-PEI

ether. The copolymer was redissolved in DCM, and precipitated in cold diethyl ether for three times, to completely remove unconjugated CDI molecules. PEG-P(TMC-co-DTC)-CDI copolymer was dried under vacuum for 24 h. Yield: 88%.

3. The polymer of PEG-P(TMC-co-DTC)-CDI (1.1 g, 0.05 mmol) was dissolved in DCM to a concentration of 150 mg/ml, and then added dropwise to solution of polyethylenimine with different molecular weights ($M_w$ = 600/1200/1800 g/mol, 0.5 mmol, 50 mg/ml in DCM) at 0 °C under rapid stirring. After completion of addition, the reaction vessel was placed in 30 °C oil bath for 4 h.
4. After the reaction was completed, the reaction mixture was concentrated to 150 mg/ml by rotary evaporator; PEG-P(TMC-co-DTC)-PEI copolymer was isolated by precipitation in cold diethyl ether and ethanol (volume ratio = 4:1), filtered and washed again with cold diethyl ether. After drying for 10 min, the copolymer was redissolved in DCM, precipitated in cold diethyl ether and ethanol for three times, to completely remove unconjugated PEI molecules. PEG-P(TMC-co-DTC)-PEI copolymer was dried under vacuum for 24 h. Yield: 71%.
5. The structure of PEG-P(TMC-co-DTC)-PEI was characterized by $^1$H NMR ($CDCl_3$:$CD_4O$ = 4:1, 400 MHz).
6. PEG-P(TMC-co-DTC)-spermine was synthesized similarly.

### 2.2.3 Preparation of Peptide or $N_3$-Functionalized PEG-P(TMC-co-DTC)

**Synthesis of cRGD-Functionalized PEG-P(TMC-co-DTC) (Fig. 4, Notes 10, 11)**

1. Under a $N_2$ atmosphere in a glove box, NHS-PEG-OH ($M_n$ = 6500 g/mol, 325 mg, 0.05 mmol), TMC (750 mg, 7.4 mmol), DTC (100 mg, 0.52 mmol), anhydrous DCM (4 ml), and DPP (125 mg, 0.5 mmol) were added into 25 ml Schlenk bottle containing a magnetic stirrer. The bottle was sealed and placed in an oil bath at 30 °C for 4 days.
2. After the polymerization reaction, 2 ml of DCM was added to dilute the reaction mixture. NHS-PEG-P(TMC-co-DTC) copolymer was isolated by precipitation in cold diethyl ether. The polymer was dried under vacuum for 10 min, redissolved in 5 ml of DCM, precipitated in cold diethyl ether, and dried under vacuum. Yield: 85.7%.
3. Under a $N_2$ atmosphere, NHS-PEG-P(TMC-co-DTC) (0.5 g, 0.021 mmol) was dissolved in 4 ml of anhydrous DMF. cRGDfK peptide (20 mg, 0.033 mmol) dissolved in 1 ml of anhydrous DMF was dropwise added. After completion of addition, the reaction vessel was placed in an oil bath thermostated at 30 °C for 2 days.
4. The product of cRGD-PEG-P(TMC-co-DTC) was dialyzed (MWCO = 7 kDa) against DMF for 14 h, to remove unreacted cRGD peptide. cRGD-PEG-P (TMC-co-DTC) was obtained by precipitating in cold diethyl ether, filtration, and vacuum drying. Yield: 85.8%.

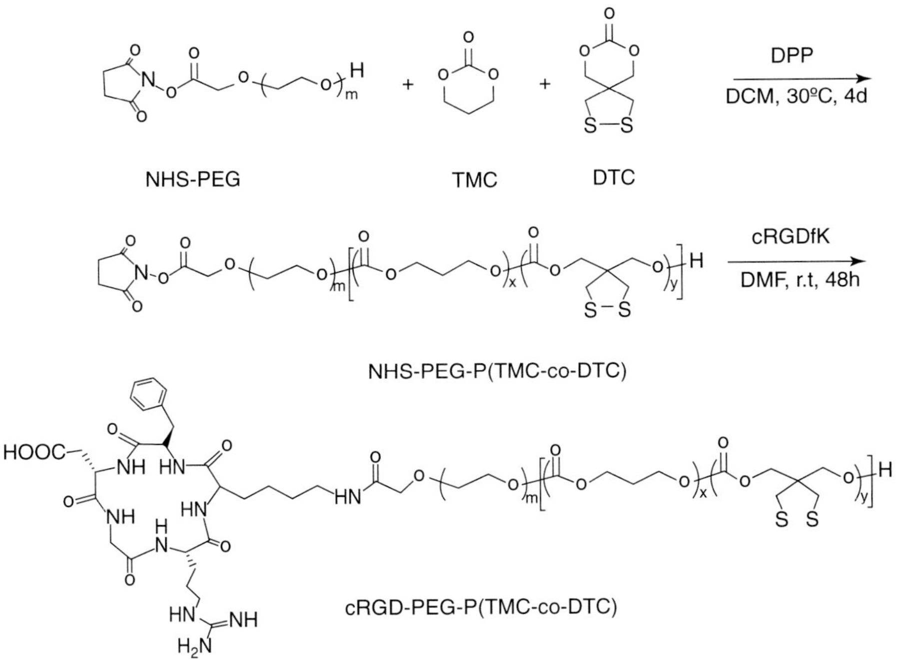


**Fig. 4** Synthesis of cRGD-PEG-P(TMC-co-DTC)

5. The structure of cRGD-PEG-P(TMC-co-DTC) was characterized by $^1$H NMR (DMSO-$d_6$, 600 Hz), the graft ratio of cRGD was 94% as determined by BCA protein quantitative analysis kit.

### Synthesis of ANG-Functionalized PEG-P(TMC-co-DTC) (Fig. 5, Notes 12, 13)

1. Under a $N_2$ atmosphere in a glove box, Mal-PEG-OH ($M_n = 7500$ g/mol, 750 mg, 0.1 mmol), TMC (1.5 g, 14.7 mmol), DTC (200 mg, 1.04 mmol), anhydrous DCM (8 ml), and DPP (250 mg, 1 mmol) were added into 25 ml Schlenk bottle containing a magnetic stirrer. The bottle was sealed and placed in an oil bath at 30 °C for 4 days.
2. After the polymerization reaction, 4.5 ml of DCM was added to dilute the reaction mixture. Mal-PEG-P(TMC-co-DTC) copolymer was isolated by precipitation in cold diethyl ether. The polymer was dried under vacuum for 10 min, redissolved in 12 ml of DCM, precipitated in cold diethyl ether, and dried under vacuum. Yield: 91.8%.
3. Under a $N_2$ atmosphere, Mal-PEG-P(TMC-co-DTC) (50 mg, 0.002 mmol) was dissolved in 2 ml of anhydrous DMSO. Angiopep-2 peptide (10 mg, 0.0042 mmol) dissolved in 0.5 ml of anhydrous DMSO was dropwise added.

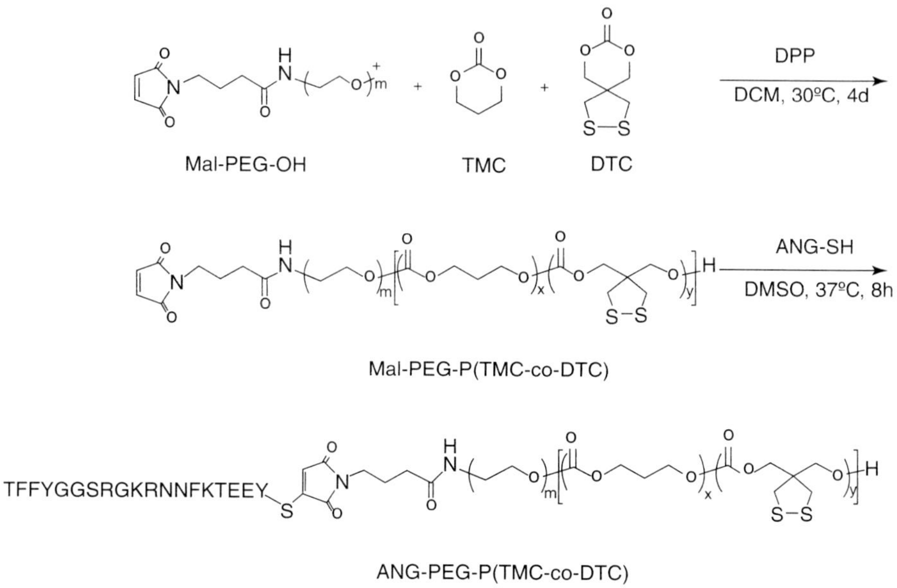


**Fig. 5** Synthesis of ANG-PEG-P(TMC-co-DTC)

After completion of addition, the reaction vessel placed in an oil bath thermostated at 37 °C for 8 h.

4. At room temperature, the product ANG-PEG-P(TMC-co-DTC) was dialyzed (MWCO = 7 kDa) against DMSO for 24 h (change dialysate four times), and then dialyzed against DCM for 4 h (change dialysate two times). After the dialysis was completed, the solution of ANG-PEG-P(TMC-co-DTC) was concentrated by rotary evaporator, precipitated in cold diethyl ether, filtration, and vacuum drying. Yield: 90.6%.
5. The structure of ANG-PEG-P(TMC-co-DTC) was characterized by $^{1}$H NMR (DMSO-$d_6$, 600 Hz), the graft ratio of ANG was 94% as determined by BCA protein quantitative analysis kit.

### Synthesis of $N_3$-PEG-P(TMC-co-DTC) (Fig. 6)

1. Under a $N_2$ atmosphere in a glove box, $N_3$-PEG-OH ($M_n$ = 7900 g/mol, 790 mg, 0.1 mmol), TMC (1.5 g, 14.7 mmol), DTC (200 mg, 1.04 mmol), anhydrous DCM (8.5 ml), and DPP (250 mg, 1 mmol) were added into 25 ml Schlenk bottle containing a magnetic stirrer. The bottle was sealed and placed in an oil bath at 30 °C for 4 days.
2. After the polymerization reaction, 4 ml of DCM was added to dilute the reaction mixture.

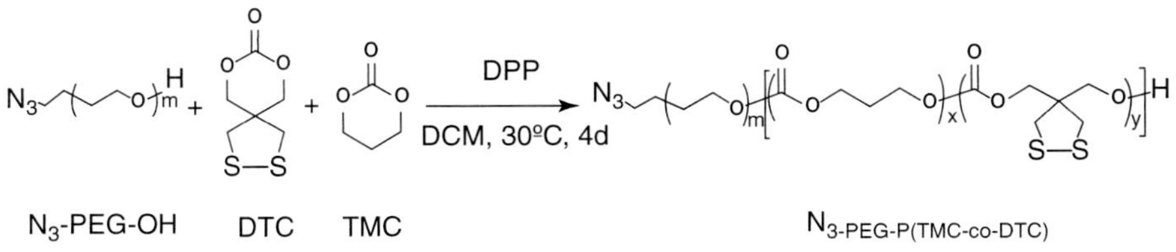


**Fig. 6** Synthesis of $N_3$-PEG-P(TMC-co-DTC)

3. $N_3$-PEG-P(TMC-co-DTC) copolymer was isolated by precipitation in cold diethyl ether. The polymer was dried under vacuum for 10 min, redissolved in 11 ml of DCM, precipitated in cold diethyl ether, and dried under vacuum. Yield: 87.9%.
4. The structure of $N_3$-PEG-P(TMC-co-DTC) was characterized by $^1$H NMR ($CDCl_3$, 400 MHz) and GPC.

### 2.2.4 Preparation of CP

**Preparation Method 1 (DMSO as a Solvent) (Notes 14,15)**

1. PEG-P(TMC-co-DTC)-PEI or PEG-P(TMC-co-DTC)-spermine was dissolved in DMSO to 5 mg/ml. siRNA was dissolved in Hepes buffer (10 mM, pH 7.4) to 1 μg/μl. siRNA content was measured with NanoDrop One/Onec spectrophotometer.
2. The polymer solution was mixed with the siRNA solution at a certain mass ratio, and 100 μl of the mixed solution was added dropwise to 900 μl of Hepes buffer (10 mM, pH 6.8) at room temperature with stirring, stirring speed: 300 r/min, stirring time: 10 min.
3. The vesicle dispersion was dialyzed against pH 6.8 Hepes buffer (MWCO = 7 kDa) at room temperature for 12 h with 5 times refreshing of Hepes buffer.
4. The CP-siRNA dispersion was concentrated in an ultrafiltration centrifuge tube (MWCO = 10 kDa) with a centrifugal force of 4000 g.
5. The CP-siRNA dispersion was diluted to the required concentration with pH 6.8 Hepes buffer.
6. The particle size and PDI of CP were determined by DLS.

**Preparation Method 2 (DMF as a Solvent) (Notes 16)**

1. PEG-P(TMC-co-DTC)-PEI or PEG-P(TMC-co-DTC)-spermine was dissolved in DMF to obtain 40 mg/ml polymer solution as organic phase.
2. A certain amount of siRNA was dissolved in DEPC water (1 μg/μl), and NanoDrop One/Onec spectrophotometer was used to determine the concentration.
3. The siRNA solution was diluted with pH 6.0 PB to desired concentration, as the water phase. The organic phase was added to the bottom of the water phase (the volume ratio of organic phase/water phase = 9:1) within 5–10 s at 25 °C water bath.

4. After adding the organic phase, the mixture was stirred at 300 rpm for 10 min.
5. The resultant polymersomes were initially dialyzed against pH 6.0 PB buffer (MWCO = 7 kDa), and then change the dialysate to pH 7.4 PB. The whole dialysis process lasts for 5 h, and the medium was changed every hour.
6. The CP-siRNA dispersion was concentrated in an ultrafiltration centrifuge tube (MWCO = 10 kDa) with a centrifugal force of 4000 g.
7. The CP-siRNA dispersion was diluted to the required concentration with pH 7.4 PB.
8. The size and PDI of CP-siRNA were determined by DLS.

**Preparation of Polypeptide Functionalized CP (Notes 17)**

1. cRGD-PEG-P(TMC-co-DTC) or ANG-PEG-P(TMC-co-DTC) was mixed with PEG-P(TMC-co-DTC)-PEI/spermine at a predetermined mass ratio (mass of peptide-PEG-P(TMC-co-DTC) = 5%, 10%, 20%) and dissolved in DMF to a concentration of 40 mg/ml.
2. siRNA was dissolved in DEPC water (1 μg/μl) and then added to pH 6.0 PB.
3. The polymer solution was slowly injected into the bottom of PB containing siRNA. The mixture was stirred at 300 r/min for 10 min.
4. The polymersome dispersion was dialyzed against pH 6.0 PB buffer and then pH 7.4 PB (MWCO = 7 kDa).
5. The vesicle dispersion was measured by DLS.

**Preparation of Monoclonal Antibody Functionalized CP (Fig. 7, Notes 18)**

1. $N_3$-PEG-P(TMC-co-DTC) and PEG-P(TMC-co-DTC)-PEI were weighed and mixed at a certain ratio, and dissolved in DMSO (40 mg/ml).

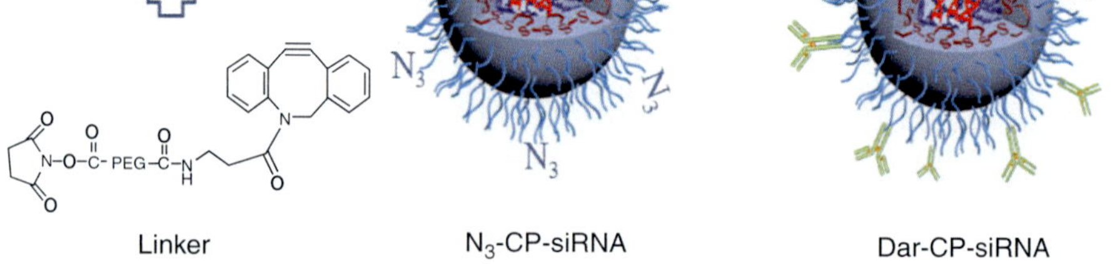


**Fig. 7** Preparation of antibody functionalized CP-siRNA by post-modification

2. An amount of 0.5 ml of polymer solution was injected into 4.5 ml of Hepes buffer (pH 6.8, 10 mM) containing siRNA.
3. After magnetic stirring at 300 rpm for 10 min, $N_3$-CP-siRNA dispersion was dialyzed (MWCO = 14 kDa) against Hepes buffer (pH 7.4, 10 mM) for 6 h.
4. Dar-DBCO was prepared by reacting NHS-$PEG_4$-DBCO with the amino group of Dar. Briefly, the PBS solution of Daratumumab (Dar, 21.7 mg/ml) was diluted to 10 mg/ml with PB buffer (pH 8.5, 10 mM). An amount of 5.26 or 8.78 μl DMSO solution (5 mg/ml) of NHS-$PEG_4$-DBCO was added to 200 μl PBS solution of Dar under oscillation. The mixture was placed in a shaker at 27 °C and 120 rpm for overnight. The unreacted NHS-$PEG_4$-DBCO was removed by ultrafiltration (MWCO = 10 kDa, 3000 rpm) and the final product Dar-DBCO was washed twice with PBS (pH 7.4, 10 mM).
5. Dar-CP-siRNA was prepared by click reaction between Dar-DBCO and $N_3$ on the surface of $N_3$-CP-siRNA. The surface density of Dar can be adjusted by changing the feeding ratios of Dar-DBCO to $N_3$ (e.g., 0.25:1, 0.5:1, or 1:1). In a typical example, 10.4 μl of Dar-DBCO solution (5.6 mg/ml) was added to 107.5 μl of $N_3$-CP-siRNA (18.6 mg/ml), and the reaction was carried out overnight in a shaker at 25 °C and 100 rpm/min.
6. The unbound Dar-DBCO was removed by ultracentrifugation (58 krpm, 4 °C) and the product was washed twice with Hepes buffer (pH 7.4, 10 mM).
7. Dar-CP-siRNA was collected, and the efficacy of Dar conjugation was determined by quantification of free Dar-DBCO in the supernatant with HPLC.

### 2.2.5 Characterization of CP

#### siRNA Loading Efficiency of CP Was Characterized by Gel Electrophoresis (Fig. 8, Notes 19)

1. CP-siRNA was prepared with varying siRNA loading contents.
2. One percent (w/v) agarose gel was prepared with TAE buffer and 5 μl Gel-Red was added into the gel solution.
3. After the gel coagulated, samples were mixed with DNA loading buffer and added to gel wells, and the electrophoresis was performed for 10 min under 80 V.

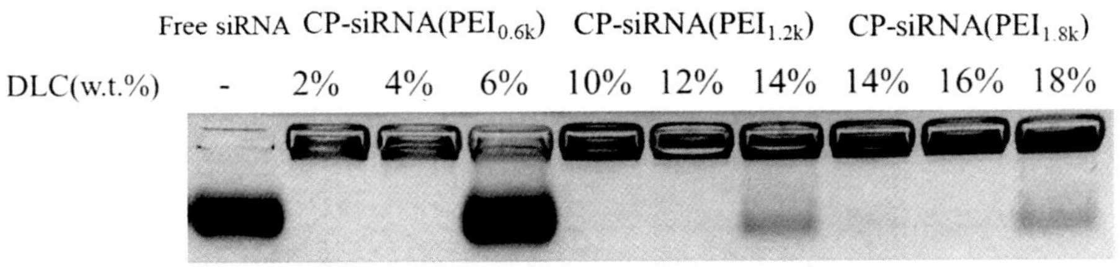


**Fig. 8** Gel electrophoresis of CP-siRNA formed with PEI of different molecular weights

4. Five percent free siRNA solution (relative to the concentration of CP-siRNA sample) was used as an external standard, and the entrapment efficiency of CP-siRNA samples was roughly evaluated by comparison.
5. After electrophoresis, the gel image was photographed by Chem Studio multi-function imaging system (lambda Ex/Em = 532/605 nm).
6. The drug loading capacity of CP with different molecular weight PEI was evaluated.

### Evaluate Stability and Reduction Responsivity of CP-siRNA (Notes 20)

1. Prepare polymersomes using the step 1–7 of section "Preparation Method 2 (DMF as a Solvent)" S18.
2. For stability evaluation, CP was incubated in PB (10 mM, pH 7.4) containing 10% FBS for 24 h or diluted with 50 times PB (10 mM, pH 7.4). The size and PDI of CP-siRNA were measured by DLS.
3. The polymer vesicle dispersion was diluted to 1 mg/ml and added to GSH solution (10 mM) for 6 h, 12 h, or 24 h. The size and PDI of vesicles were measured by DLS.

### Characterization of CP by TEM (Fig. 9, Notes 21)

1. Prepare cNGQ-CP using the step 1–5 of section "Preparation of Polypeptide Functionalized CP."
2. An amount of 20 μl of the prepared vesicle dispersion was dropped onto a copper mesh, held for 30 s, and then blotted with filter paper.

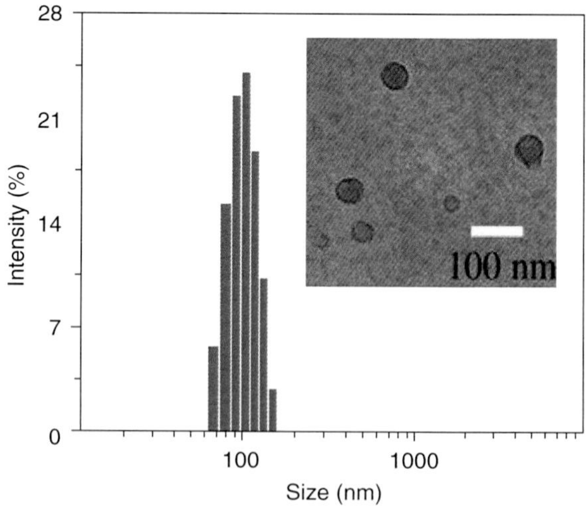


**Fig. 9** Size distribution of cNGQ-CP (10 wt% siRNA) determined by DLS and TEM. (Adapted from reference Zou et al. 2017, with permission)

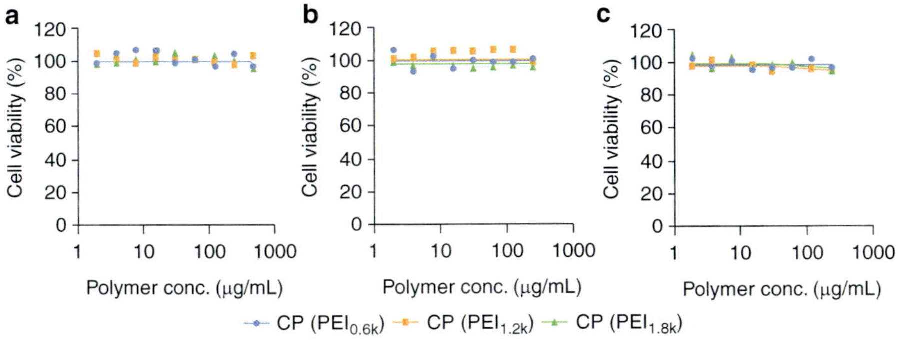


**Fig. 10** Cytotoxicity of CP with different molecular weight PEI after 48 h incubation (Polymer concentration: 1.95, 3.9, 7.8, 15.6, 31.25, 62.5, 125, 250, 500 μg/ml). (**a**) L929 cells, (**b**) A549 cells, and (**c**) U87 cells

3. An amount of 20 μl of 2% phosphotungstic acid solution was slowly added to the prepared copper mesh, held for 30 s, blotted with filter paper, and dried at room temperature overnight.
4. The copper mesh was then baked under an infra-red lamp for about 60 s to remove residual water, and installed into a Hitachi HT7700 TEM device (120 kV) to observe the vesicle structure.

### 2.2.6 MTT Assay of CP (Fig. 10)

1. Murine fibroblasts (L929), human alveolar basal epithelial adenocarcinoma cells (A549), or human glioma cells (U87) were plated in a 96-well plates ($3 \times 10^3$ cells/well) containing 80 μL of DMEM or RPMI 1640 medium for 24 h.
2. An amount of 20 μL of CP-siRNA in PB (10 mM, pH 7.4) was added to yield final concentrations ranging from 1.95–500 μg/mL.
3. The cells were cultured for 48 h.
4. An amount of 10 μL of 3-(4,5-dimethylthiazol-2-yl)-2,5-diphenyltetrazolium-bromide solution (MTT, 5 mg/mL) was added.
5. The cells were cultured for another 4 h, the medium was aspirated, the MTT-formazan generated by live cells was dissolved in 150 μL of DMSO, and the absorbance at 570 nm of each well was measured by using a microplate reader.
6. The relative cell viability (%) was determined by comparing the absorbance at 570 nm with control wells only containing culture medium.

### 2.2.7 Flow Cytometry and Confocal Laser Scanning Microscopy Assays of CP-siRNA

#### Flow Cytometry Assays of CP-siRNA-Cy3 (Fig. 11)

1. A549/U87 cells seeded in a six-well plates ($4 \times 10^5$ cells/well) were incubated with CP-siRNA-Cy3 at 37 °C for 4 h.

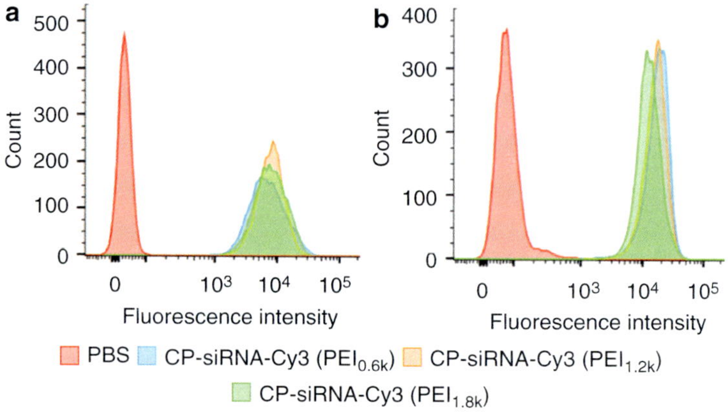


**Fig. 11** Endocytosis of CP-siRNA-Cy3 with different molecular weight PEI. (A) A549 cells and (B) U87 cells

2. The suspensions were centrifuged at 1000 × g for 3 min, and the cells were digested by 300 μl trypsin, washed twice with PBS, and then resuspended in 500 μL of PBS.
3. Fluorescence histograms were immediately recorded with a BD FACS Calibur flow cytometer and analyzed using Cell Quest software based on 10,000 gated events.
4. The gate was arbitrarily set for the detection of Cy3 fluorescence.

**Confocal Laser Scanning Microscopy of CP-siRNA (Fig. 12)**

1. U87 cells were cultured on microscope slides in a 24-well plates ($5 \times 10^4$ cells/well) using DMEM for 24 h.
2. The cells were incubated with CP-siScramble(Cy5) for 1, 2, and 4 h before DMEM was removed.
3. The cell endo/lysosomes were stained with Lyso-Tracker red in culture medium.
4. The culture medium was removed and the cells on microscope plates were washed three times with PBS before fixation with 4% paraformaldehyde solution for 15 min, then washed three times with PBS.
5. The cell nuclei was stained with 4′,6-diamidino-2-phenylindole (DAPI) for 5 min.
6. The cells on microscope plates were washed five times with PBS.

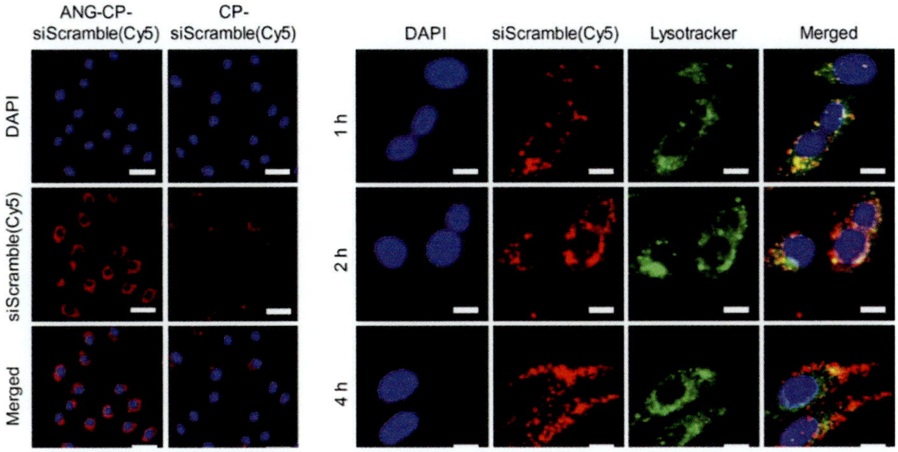


**Fig. 12** Confocal laser scanning microscopy images of U87 cells following transfection with ANG-CP-siScramble(Cy5) or CP-siScramble(Cy5) (siRNA dosage: 200 nM); CLSM images of U-87 MG cells following transfection with ANG-CP-siScramble(Cy5) (siRNA dosage: 200 nM). For each panel, the images from left to the right were cell nuclei stained by DAPI (blue), lysosomes stained by lysotracker red (green), siScramble(Cy5) (red), and overlays of the three images. Bar: 20 μm. (Adapted from reference Shi et al. 2018, with permission)

7. The fluorescence images were recorded using Confocal laser scanning microscopy.

## 2.3 In Vitro Gene Silencing Determined by RT-PCR (Fig. 13)

1. U87 cells were seeded into a six-well plates ($3 \times 10^5$ cells/well) for 24 h.
2. ANG-CP-siPLK1 was added at a final siPLK1 concentration of 200 nM or 400 nM (n = 4) and the cells were further cultured for 4 h.
3. The medium was removed and replaced with an equal volume of fresh medium, and the cells were further cultured for 44 h.
4. The transfected U87 cells were collected and total RNA was isolated using total RNA isolation reagent according to the protocol of manufacturer and tested by qPCR.
5. Gene silencing efficiency was denoted as the fold changes in PLK1 expression relative to the untreated control cells and normalized with the house keeping gene, glyceraldehyde phosphate dehydrogenase (GAPDH) as the endogenous reference.
6. The mRNA expression levels were calculated by the $2^{-\Delta\Delta CT}$ method, and data were presented as mean value ± standard deviation.

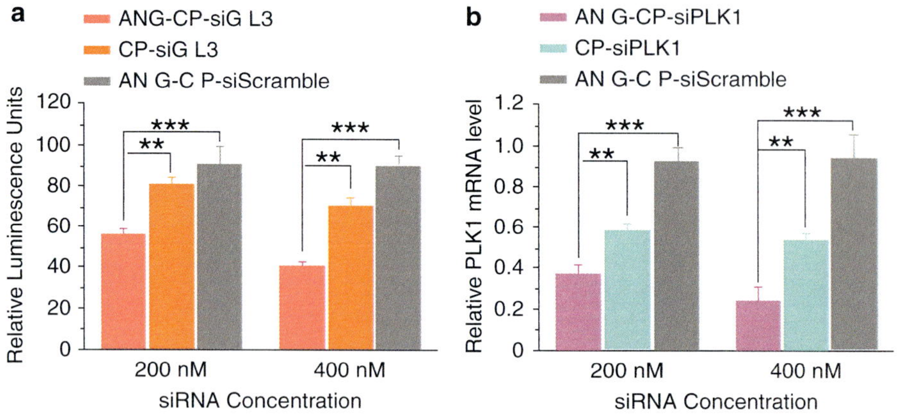


**Fig. 13** Gene silencing ability of ANG-CP-siGL3 (A) and ANG-CP-siPLK1 (B) in U87-Luc cells after 48 h transfection (dosage: 200 or 400 nM siRNA). (Adapted from reference Shi et al. 2018, with permission)

**Fig. 14** In vivo pharmacokinetics of ANG-CP-siPLK1(Cy5), CP-siPLK1(Cy5), and free siPLK1(Cy5); siPLK1(Cy5) was quantified by fluorescence spectroscopy (n = 3). (Adapted from reference Shi et al. 2018, with permission)

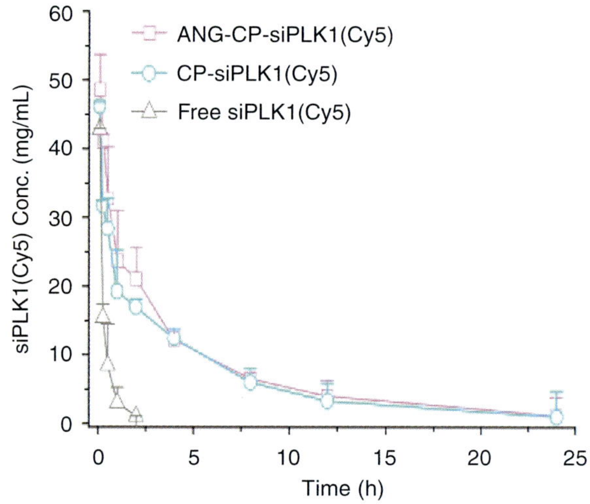


## 2.4 Pharmacokinetics of CP-siRNA (Fig. 14)

1. siPLK1(Cy5) was used for studying the pharmacokinetics at a siPLK1(Cy5) dosage of 1 mg/kg.
2. Free siPLK1(Cy5), CP-siPLK1(Cy5), and ANG-CP-siPLK1(Cy5) were administered to BALB/c athymic nude mice via the tail vein, respectively.

3. At pre-set time points post-administration, 50 μL of blood sample was withdrawn from the orbital of animal and centrifuged at 3000 rpm for 5 min immediately.
4. The supernatant was then added to 700 μL of DMSO (containing 40 mM dithiothreitol [DTT] for reduction-triggered CP destabilization) and extracted at 37 °C overnight, followed by another centrifugation of $1.5 \times 10^4$ rpm for 30 min.
5. The Cy5 content in the supernatant was quantified by fluorometry using Cary Eclipse fluorospectrophotometer.

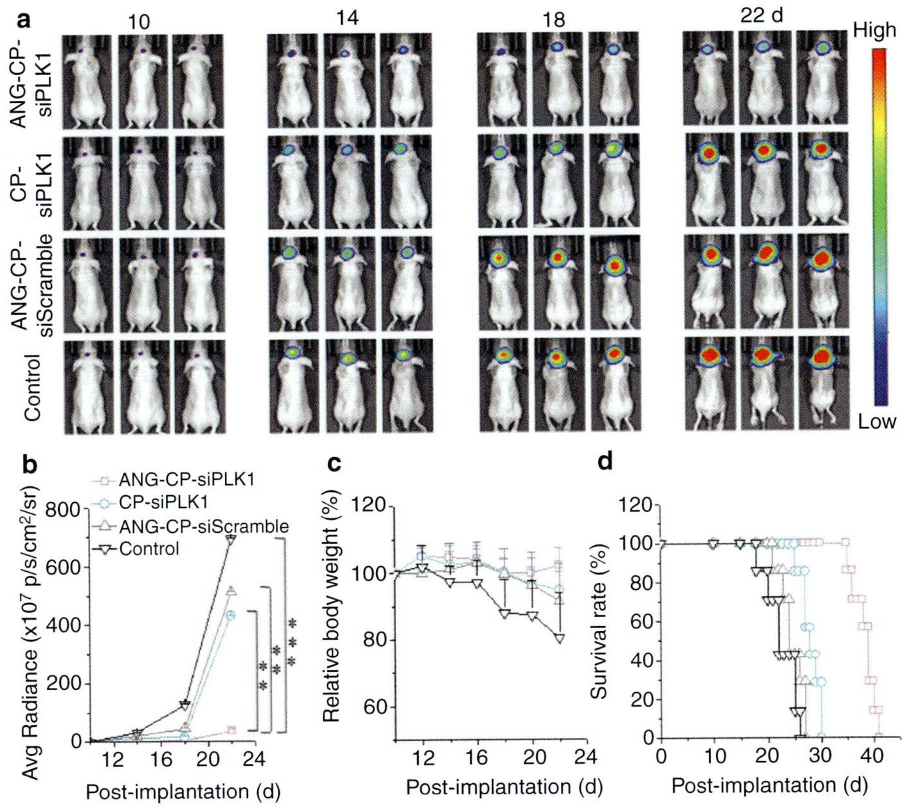


**Fig. 15** (**a**) Luminescence optical images of orthotopic U-87-Luc brain tumor–bearing nude mice following treatment with ANG-CP-siPLK1, CP-siPLK1, ANG-CP-siScramble, and PBS. (**b**) Quantified luminescence levels after different treatments. (**c**) Relative body weight changes of mice. (**d**) Kaplan-Meier survival curve of mice. (Adapted from reference Shi et al. 2018, with permission)

## 2.5 The Gene Silencing Efficiency *In Vivo* (Fig. 15)

1. On day 10 post-tumor implantation, BALB/c nude mice bearing orthotopic U87-Luc glima were imaged via bioluminescence.
2. Mice with similar tumor burden were randomly divided into four groups ($n = 8$) and intravenously injected with ANG-CP-siPLK1, CP-siPLK1, ANG-CP-siScrambe, or PBS (as control) at siRNA dose of 60 μg/mouse on day 10, 12, 14, 16, and 18 post-implantation.
3. The tumor progression was monitored by bioluminescence imaging on day 14, 18, and 22 using near-infrared fluorescence imaging system.
4. Mice were weighed and normalized to their initial weights on day 10.
5. The survival of animals was recorded throughout the treatment.

## 2.6 Statistical Analysis

1. All data are presented as the mean ± standard deviation (SD).
2. One way analysis of variance (ANOVA) was used to determine significance among groups, after which post-hoc tests with the Bonferroni correction were used for comparison between individual groups. Statistical significance was established at $^{*}p < 0.05$, $^{**}p < 0.01$, and $^{***}p < 0.001$.

# 3 Discussion

There are common mistakes when following the above procedure. Here are some notes which can be used to solve possible problems.

# 4 Notes

1. Dithiolane trimethylene carbonate (DTC) monomer was synthesized according to the patent CN 104031248 A.
2. The copolymers can be synthesized with metal catalysts such as Zinc Bis[bis(trimethylsilyl)amide] or organic catalysts such as diphenyl phosphate (DPP) and triazabicyclo[4.4.0]dec-5-ene (TBD). Our studies found that DPP is a best catalyst in that it promotes controlled statistical copolymerization of TMC and DTC under very mild conditions to afford PEG-P(TMC-co-DTC) copolymers with prescribed molecular weight and narrow molecular weight distribution (Wei et al. 2018). Moreover, unlike metal catalysts, DPP can be easily removed by repeated precipitation.
3. By adjusting the feed ratio of PEG (initiator) and monomers, polymers of PEG-P(TMC-co-DTC) with different hydrophilic and hydrophobic blocks were obtained. In this protocol, two copolymers, $PEG_{5k}$-P($TMC_{24.2k}$-co-$DTC_{1.8k}$) and $PEG_{5k}$-P($TMC_{15k}$-co-$DTC_{2k}$), were used with a major focus on $PEG_{5k}$-P($TMC_{15k}$-co-$DTC_{2k}$).

4. The existence of traces of water will influence the polymerization and lead to formation of oligomers, so it is important to control the water residue in the polymerization system. All chemicals and solvents were dried prior to polymerization and the polymerization was carried out in the Schlenk bottle. The experiment was operated under a $N_2$ atmosphere in the glove box.
5. When PEG/DPP ratio was set at 1/10, polymerization would be completed in 4 d. When PEG/DPP ratio was set at 1/5, polymerization would be completed in 6 d.
6. For the determination of GPC, DMF was used as the mobile phase at a flow rate of 0.8 ml/min and the test temperature was 40 °C. A series of monodisperse linear poly(methyl methacrylate) were used as the molecular weight standard.
7. N, N′-carbonyldiimidazole (CDI) is widely used as enzyme and protein binders, antibiotic intermediates, especially as bonding agents for peptide compounds. There are several advantages of CDI, such as strong reaction activity, wide application, low toxicity, simple product purification, and especially high selectivity for different functional groups, which is of great significance in the field of organic synthesis and polymer. The small molecules of imidazole formed in the reaction process are directly removed by cold diethyl ether precipitation. The operation is simple and controllable.
8. PEG-P(TMC-co-DTC) following activation with CDI can easily react with spermine or PEI of different molecular weights to form PEG-P(TMC-co-DTC)-spermine or PEG-P(TMC-co-DTC)-PEI triblock copolymers. To ensure equivalent coupling, PEG-P(TMC-co-DTC)-CDI was slowly added into tenfold excess of spermine or PEI solution.
9. Spermine and PEI have good solubility in ethanol. To remove excess spermine or PEI, PEG-P(TMC-co-DTC)-spermine and PEG-P(TMC-co-DTC)-PEI were purified by precipitation in cold ethanol/diethyl ether (1/4, v/v) mixture for three times.
10. To synthesize peptide-functionalized PEG-P(TMC-co-DTC) copolymers, NHS-PEG-OH and MAL-PEG-OH were used as initiators. Notably, both NHS and MAL groups were intact during DPP-catalyzed polymerization and subsequent workup procedures.
11. The length of PEG chain in the peptide-functionalized PEG-P(TMC-co-DTC) copolymers is generally longer than that in PEG-P(TMC-co-DTC)-PEI/spermine. In the self-assembly process, hydrophilic PEG is exposed on the surface of vesicle, and the longer PEG chain with targeted molecules increases the probability of binding with receptor.
12. Michael addition reaction of sulfhydryl group with maleimide is a kind of click chemistry, which has many features such as fast reaction, high conversion under mild conditions, specific selectivity, and single product. In this synthesis scheme, the functional PEG with molecular weight of 6500, 7500, or 7900 Da is mainly used. After the reaction, the residue targeting molecules are removed by dialysis, and the grafting rate is very high (generally, >90%).
13. The peptides with strong polarity are difficult to dissolve in DCM, while DMSO is a good solvent to get clear peptide solution, which is preferred as a solvent in

the experiment. The same solvent should be chosen in the process of dialysis. The polymer of PEG-P(TMC-co-DTC) dissolved in DMSO is difficult to precipitate in cold diethyl ether or ethanol, so it needs to be replaced by DCM.

14. For small-scale preparation of polymersomes, when the preparation volume is 1–2 ml, the appropriate size of magnetic stirrer is directly added into the EP tubes, and the rotating speed is kept constant at 300–400 r/min.
15. In the first preparation method of CP, DMSO was used to dissolve the polymer and dropped into Hepes buffer to prepare polymersomes with larger particle size of 100–120 nm.
16. In the second preparation method of CP, the polymer was dissolved in DMF, and slowly added into the PB (pH 6.0, 2 mM), and CP was formed by stirring the mixture. The size of polymersomes is usually in the range of 40–80 nm.
17. Peptide-functionalized CP was obtained by premodification method, in which peptide-functionalized PEG-P(TMC-co-DTC) and PEG-P(TMC-co-DTC)-PEI/spermine at prescribed weight ratios were dissolved in DMF prior to assembly.
18. The concentration of Dar-DBCO was determined by HPLC (mobile phase: 150 mM PB/acetonitrile = 90/10, detection wavelength: 214 nm, and column temperature: 30 °C). Matrix-assisted laser desorption ionization time-of-flight mass spectrometry (MALDI-TOF-MS) was used to determine the number of grafted DBCO on each Dar. The concentrations of Dar and Dar-DBCO were fixed at 1.0 mg/ml.
19. The charge density of PEG-P(TMC-co-DTC)-PEI copolymers increased with increasing PEI molecular weights from 600 and 1200 to 1800, which in turn leads to increased siRNA loading efficiency of corresponding CP. High molecular weight PEI (e.g., $M_w$ = 25,000 g/mol), as one of the most used cationic polymers for gene delivery both in vitro and in vivo, suffers a high toxicity. Low molecular weight PEI has a low toxicity but also a low transfection activity. Here, PEG-P(TMC-co-DTC)-PEI copolymers were all based on low molecular weight PEI.
20. The stability and reduction-sensitivity of CP was studied in FBS and GSH conditions. CP while possessing a good stability against FBS showed fast response to 10 mM GSH.
21. TEM images of CP formed from PEG-P(TMC-co-DTC)-PEI with a molecular weight of 5.0-24.2-1.8 kg/mol showed a vesicular structure.

## 5 Conclusion

This protocol presents preparation of chimeric polymersomes based on PEG-P(TMC-co-DTC)-PEI triblock copolymers for nontoxic and efficient siRNA transfection. Notably, with these chimeric polymersomes, peptide or antibody-targeted siRNA delivery systems can be easily prepared by either premodification or post-modification strategy. The cell and animal experiments reveal that targeted chimeric polymersomes can effectively overcome the extracellular and intracellular barriers and mediate specific gene silencing, achieving high-efficacy RNAi therapy for orthotopic human glioblastoma xenograft and lung tumor xenograft in mice. These virus-mimicking chimeric polymersomes have emerged as a simple, robust, multifunctional, and versatile platform for targeted siRNA therapy.

## References


Adams D, Gonzalez-Duarte A, O'Riordan WD et al (2018) Patisiran, an RNAi therapeutic, for hereditary transthyretin amyloidosis. N Engl J Med 379(1):11–21

Dowdy SF (2017) Overcoming cellular barriers for RNA therapeutics. Nat Biotechnol 35(3):222–229

Elbashir SM, Harborth J, Lendeckel W et al (2001) Duplexes of 21-nucleotide RNAs mediate RNA interference in cultured mammalian cells. Nature 411(6836):494–498

Hu B, Zhong L, Weng Y et al (2020) Therapeutic siRNA: state of the art. Signal Transduct Target Ther 5(1):101

Jiang Y, Zhang J, Meng F et al (2018) Apolipoprotein E peptide-directed chimeric Polymersomes mediate an ultrahigh-efficiency targeted protein therapy for glioblastoma. ACS Nano 12(11): 11070–11079

Liu G, Ma S, Li S et al (2010) The highly efficient delivery of exogenous proteins into cells mediated by biodegradable chimaeric polymersomes. Biomaterials 31(29):7575–7585

Saw PE, Song EW (2020) siRNA therapeutics: a clinical reality. Sci China-Life Sci 63(4):485–500

Shi YN, Jiang Y, Cao JS et al (2018) Boosting RNAi therapy for orthotopic glioblastoma with nontoxic brain-targeting chimaeric polymersomes. J Control Release 292:163–171

Springer AD, Dowdy SF (2018) GalNAc-siRNA conjugates: leading the way for delivery of RNAi therapeutics. Nucl Acid Ther 28(3):109–118

Wei J, Meng H, Guo B et al (2018) Organocatalytic ring-opening copolymerization of Trimethylene carbonate and Dithiolane Trimethylene carbonate: impact of Organocatalysts on copolymerization kinetics and copolymer microstructures. Biomacromolecules 19(6):2294–2301

Yang W, Wei Y, Yang L et al (2018) Granzyme B-loaded, cell-selective penetrating and reduction-responsive polymersomes effectively inhibit progression of orthotopic human lung tumor in vivo. J Control Release 290:141–149

Zhang MM, Bahal R, Rasmussen TP et al (2021) The growth of siRNA-based therapeutics: updated clinical studies. Biochem Pharmacol 189(5):114432

Zou Y, Fang Y, Meng H et al (2016) Self-crosslinkable and intracellularly decrosslinkable biodegradable micellar nanoparticles: a robust, simple and multifunctional nanoplatform for high-efficiency targeted cancer chemotherapy. J Control Release 244:326–335

Zou Y, Zheng M, Yang WJ et al (2017) Virus-mimicking Chimaeric Polymersomes boost targeted cancer siRNA therapy in vivo. Adv Mater 29(42):1703285

# Preparation of Ultrasmall Gold Nanoparticles for Nuclear-Based Gene Delivery

# 17

Zhihuan Liao, Shuaidong Huo, and Xing-Jie Liang

## Contents



**Abstract**

The construction of safe and efficient gene delivery vectors is still facing challenges during effective gene therapy. We previously reported a nuclear-based gene delivery strategy in which the surface of ultrasmall gold nanoparticles (Au NPs) is further conjugated with oncogene silencing sequence. Here, we summarize the preparation method of ultrasmall Au NPs for direct nucleus targeting, the followed test method can be used to demonstrate the excellent stability and high efficiency of the nuclear-targeting ultrasmall Au NPs which provides a promising gene delivery vector for gene therapy.

**Keywords**

Gene delivery · Ultrasmall gold nanoparticles · Cancer cell nucleus · Nuclear targeting · Oncogene

Z. Liao · S. Huo (✉)
Fujian Provincial Key Laboratory of Innovative Drug Target Research, School of Pharmaceutical Sciences, Xiamen University, Xiamen, Fujian, China
e-mail: huosd@xmu.edu.cn

X.-J. Liang (✉)
Chinese Academy of Sciences (CAS) Key Laboratory for Biomedical Effects of Nanomaterials and Nanosafety, CAS Center for Excellence in Nanoscience, National Center for Nanoscience and Technology of China, Beijing, China
e-mail: liangxj@nanoctr.cn



H. Tian and X. Chen (eds.), *Gene Delivery*, Biomaterial Engineering,
https://doi.org/10.1007/978-981-16-5419-0_17

# 1 Overview

Gene therapy, a concept that was once dismissed as an unsafety operation to introduce alien genes to human cells, is becoming a potential approach to treat genetic diseases nowadays (Roemer and Friedmann 1992). It is used to treat inherited or acquired diseases by correcting gene defects or regulating disease-related protein expressions at the molecule level (Rideout et al. 2002; Perrin et al. 2019). However, there are still several hurdles exist before realizing effective gene delivery. On one hand, nucleic acids are unstable negatively charged biomacromolecules that are easily degraded by nucleases in cells (Fujiwara et al. 2016; Qian et al. 2017). On the other, they cannot cross cell membranes and other biological barriers in vivo (Sajid et al. 2020). Therefore, more efficient delivery vectors are needed for gene transferring which should meet the requirements with excellent stability protecting genes from nuclease degradation and effective targeting capability penetrating barriers (Naso et al. 2017; Shi et al. 2017).

Generally, gene delivery vectors were divided into two categories, one is virus-based vectors such as adenovirus (ADV) (Fernandez-Frias et al. 2020), adeno-associated virus (AAV) (Gao et al. 2020), and herpes simplex virus (HSV), etc. (Zhang et al. 2020). The other is nonviral vehicles, including cationic polymers (Van Bruggen et al. 2019), liposomes (Barba et al. 2019), inorganic nanoparticles (Wu et al. 2019), and so on. Although the former has entered clinical trials, they have some undesired drawbacks such as potential cytotoxicity, low packaging capacity, cellular immunogenicity, etc. (Guo and Huang 2012). Fortunately, a large number of nonviral vehicles have been developed for gene delivery in recent years. Compared with the virus-based vectors, safety is one of the most superior characteristics of the nonviral ones (Fernandes et al. 2020, Mashel et al. 2020). Moreover, the feasible preparation and controllable physicochemical properties make the non-viral vehicles more reliable candidates for gene delivery. For example, an oligopeptide for nucleus targeting was used to enhance the anti-osteosarcoma effect significantly (Sahin et al. 2018). Similarly, a multifunctional polymer with actively cellular penetration and nuclear targeting capabilities has been constructed to inhibit liver tumor growth (Hua et al. 2019). Besides, a higher gene transfection efficiency has been demonstrated by using magnetic nanoparticles via high-gradient magnets (Salvatore et al. 2016). In addition, other stimulus-responsive strategies have been utilized to deliver target genes to specific tumor microenvironments (e.g., pH (Homayun et al. 2018), redox potential (Radtke et al. 2019), enzymes (Santos et al. 2020), and temperature (Cheng et al. 2011) to overcome intracellular barriers and improve gene transfection efficiency. However, in these studies, gene delivery was achieved indirectly through nuclear localization sequence (NLS) or triggered under specific stimuli. To this end, we previously reported a typical inorganic vehicle to directly target the nucleus by using ultrasmall Au NPs (Huo et al. 2014, 2019). In our study, for the first time, the ultrasmall 2 nm Au NPs were used as carriers to deliver triplex-forming oligonucleotides (TFO) into the nucleus, selectively regulating the expression of oncogenes.

Herein, we summarize the preparation method of ultrasmall Au NPs for gene delivery. The synthesis steps of Au NPs were firstly described, then followed by the conjugation method with the oligo sequence. To test the nanoparticle-mediated gene regulation, MTT assay, real-time PCR, and Western blot analyses were introduced. The conjugation with ultrasmall carriers not only enhanced the entry of TFOs to the nucleus but also achieved protection of oligonucleotides from nuclease degradation, thus provide a stable and effective carrier to realize nuclear targeting for biomedical application.

# 2 Protocol

## 2.1 Materials

### 2.1.1 Preparation of 2 nm Au-TIOP NPs and Au-POY2T NPs

1. Gold (III) chloride trihydrate (≥99.9%, $HAuCl_4 \cdot 3H_2O$)
2. *N*-(2-mercap-topropionyl)-glycine (tiopronin)
3. Methanol
4. Acetic acid
5. Sodium borohydride (≥98.0%, $NaBH_4$)
6. Hydrochloric acid (HCl)
7. Nitric acid ($HNO_3$, MOS grade)
8. *N*-(3-dimethylaminopropyl)-*N*′-ethylcarbodiimide hydrochloride (EDC, $C_8H_{17}N_3 \cdot HCl$)
9. *N*-Hydroxy succinimide (98%, NHS, $C_4H_5NO_3$)
10. $NH_2$–5′ TGGGTGGGTGGTTTGTTTTTGGG 3′ ($NH_2$-POY2T)
11. Dialysis membrane (MWCO = 8000–14,000)
12. Milli-Q water

### 2.1.2 Characterization of 2 nm Au-TIOP NPs and Au-POY2T NPs

1. Transmission Electron Microscope (TEM, Philips, Netherlands)
2. Lambda 950 UV/vis/NIR spectrophotometer (25 °C, Perkin-Elmer, USA)
3. X′Pert PRO MPD X-ray diffractometer (PANalytical B. V., Netherlands)
4. Nano ZS Zetasizer (25 °C, Malvern, England)
5. Plasma Optical Emission Spectrometer (ICP-OES, Perkin-Elmer, USA)

### 2.1.3 Cell Viability Study

1. MCF-7 cells (human breast cancer cell line)
2. Dulbecco 's modified Eagle's medium (DMEM)
3. Glucose
4. Fetal bovine serum (FBS)
5. Water-jacketed $CO_2$ incubator (Thermo Fisher Scientific Inc., USA)
6. Phosphate buffer saline (PBS)
7. Au-POY2T (at 1 μM in POY2T), $NH_2$-POY2T (at 1 μM in POY2T), POY2T sequence (0.1, 1, 2.5, 5, and 10 μM) and 2 nm Au NPs (1 μM)

8. 3-(4,5-Dimethyl-2-Thiazolyl)-2,5-Diphenyl Tetrazolium Bromide (MTT)
9. Dimethyl sulfoxide (DMSO)
10. Microplate reader (Infinite M200, Tecan, Durham, USA)

#### 2.1.4 Determination of the Gene Conjugation Efficiency

1. Agarose
2. Electrophoresis buffer (TBE)
3. Roti dye
4. Glycerin
5. Unpurified solution of 2 nm Au-TIOP NPs
6. Electrophoresis apparatus
7. VILBER E-Box gel imaging system

#### 2.1.5 Determination of the mRNA Level and Protein Expression

1. cDNA synthesis kit (Takara, Shiga, Japan)
2. c-myc fwd, 5' TGAGGAGACACCGCCCAC 3′
   c-myc rev, 5' CAACATCGATTTCTCTCATCTTC 3'
   GAPDH fwd, 5' GACTTCAACAGCAACTCCCAC 3'
   GAPDH rev, 5' TCCACCACCCTGTTGCTGTA 3′
3. TNE lysis buffer (0.5% NP-40, 10 mM Tris, 150 mM NaCl, 1 mM EDTA and protease inhibitors)
4. 10% SDS-PAGE gel
5. PVDF membrane
6. Rabbit monoclonal c-myc (diluted 1:1000, BS 246; Bioworld Technology, Inc., Minnesota, USA)
7. Peroxidase-conjugated secondary antibody (1:5000, zsBio, Beijing, China)

### 2.2 Methods

#### 2.2.1 Preparation Before the Experiment

##### Preparation of Aqua Regia

Aqua regia was prepared by mixing concentrated $HCl/HNO_3$ 3:1 (v/v) in a large beaker in a fume hood. Extreme caution should be exercised during this process, and protective measures (wear goggles and gloves, etc.) should be taken. Aqua regia should never be stored in a closed vessel.

##### Clean the Glassware, Etc.

Soak all glassware, magnetic stirring bars, and stoppers in aqua regia for no less than 15 min, and then rinse them with Milli-Q water. Make sure there is no contamination of all the starting materials which is important for the synthesis of Au NPs.

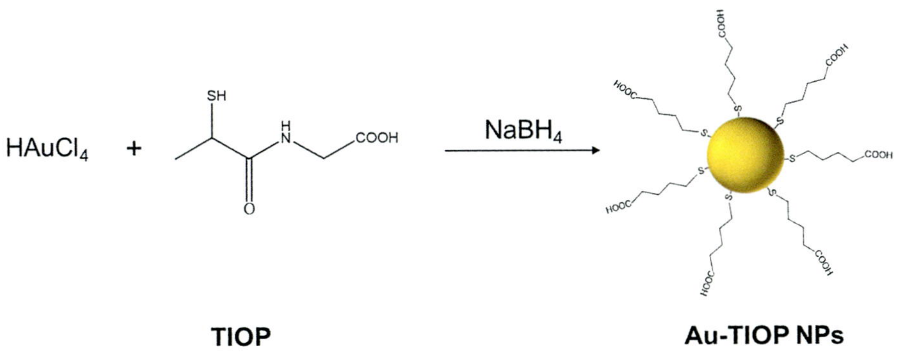


**Fig. 1** Synthetic routes of the Au-TIOP NPs with 2 nm

### 2.2.2 Preparation of 2 nm Au-TIOP NPs (Fig. 1)

1. 0.4 mM $HAuCl_4 \cdot 3H_2O$ and 1.2 mM tiopronin were mixed and stirring in a 20 mL solution containing methanol and acetic acid (6:1, v/v), then producing a ruby red mixture.
2. 8.0 mM $NaBH_4$ dissolved in 7.5 mL cold Milli-Q water was added dropwise into the above mixture with rapid stirring, producing a black solution gradually. Stop the reaction after 2 h, and the solvent was removed by a rotary evaporator.
3. Redissolve the residue with 20 mL Milli-Q water and then add hydrochloric acid continuously to adjust pH to 1.
4. Dialyze (dialysis membrane, MWCO = 8000–14,000) the solution against Milli-Q water for 72 h and change the water every 8 h. The obtained 2 nm Au-TIOP NP was ready for further characterization and study.

### 2.2.3 Preparation of Au-POY2T NPs (Fig. 2)

1. $NH_2$-POY2T sequence was conjugated with 2 nm Au-TIOP NP through an amide reaction which was catalyzed by EDC/NHC at room temperature. The reaction molar ratio of –COOH/-$NH_2$/EDC/NHS was 1:1.2:5:5, and the reaction time is 24 h.
2. Dialyze the obtained solution against Milli-Q water for 48 h and change the water every 8 h.
3. The purified Au-POY2T NP was collected and ready for further characterization and study.

### 2.2.4 Determination of the Gene Conjugation Efficiency

1. Prepare a 3% agarose gel (containing Roti dye).
2. Load 20 μL unpurified Au-POY2T NP and glycerol (1/4 in volume) mixture into an agarose gel.
3. The electrophoresis was carried out at 130 V for 30 min in TBE (1 ×) running buffer.
4. Use a VILBER E-Box gel imaging system to photograph and analyze the fluorescence intensity to determine the sequence conjugation efficiency.

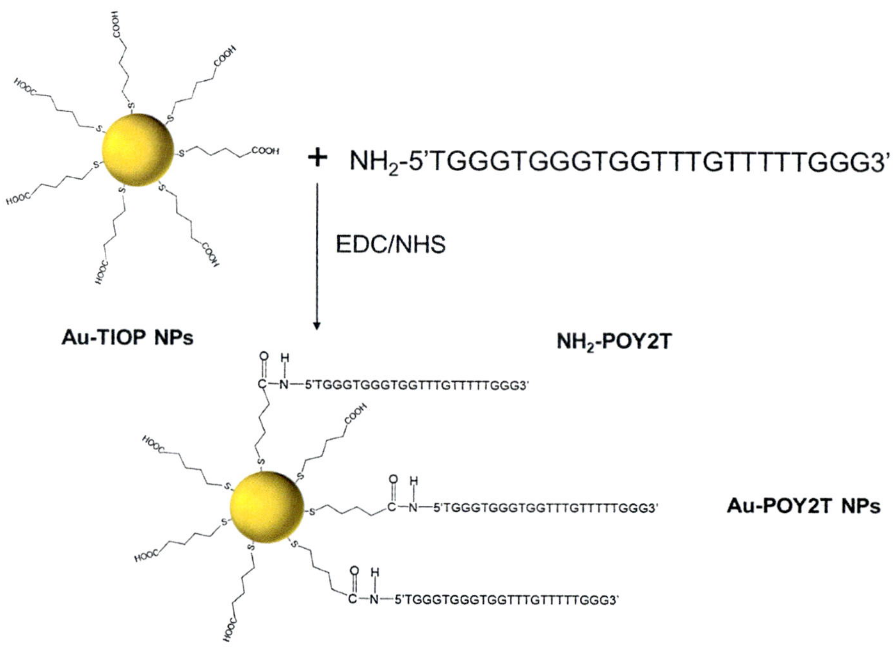


**Fig. 2** Synthetic routes of 2 nm Au-POY2T NPs

### 2.2.5 Cell Viability Study

1. Culture MCF-7 cells in DMEM containing 10% FBS and 4.5 g/L glucose in a water-jacketed $CO_2$ incubator.
2. MCF-7 cells were seeded in a 96-well plate ($5 \times 10^3$ cells per well) and preincubated for 24 h.
3. Samples with Au-POY2T (at 1 μM in POY2T), $NH_2$-POY2T (at 1 μM in POY2T), POY2T sequence (0.1, 1, 2.5, 5, and 10 μM), and 2 nm Au NPs (1 μM) were added into the 96-well plates, respectively, and incubated for another 24 h.
4. Replace the medium with 100 μL 0.5 mg/mL MTT and then replace the MTT solution with 150 μL DMSO solution after 3 h incubation.
5. Measure the absorbance at 570 nm and 630 nm (as a reference) in each well by a microplate reader.
6. Use untreated cells as controls, and calculate all standard deviations from three replicates.

### 2.2.6 Determination of the mRNA Level and Protein Expression

1. Culture MCF-7 cells with a DMEM containing 10% FBS and 4.5 g/L glucose in a water-jacketed $CO_2$ incubator.
2. MCF-7 cells were seeded in a 6-well plate ($10^6$ cells per well) and preincubated for 80% confluences.

3. 5 μM Au-POY2T NPs was added to a 6-well plate, then incubated for 24 h.
4. Wash the cells with PBS buffer solution and digest with trypsin for 3 min. After centrifuging, the supernatant was removed and cell precipitation was obtained.
5. Mix the above cells with a certain amount of PBS buffer and divide into two groups evenly.
6. Extract mRNA from MCF-7 cells and using a PrimeScript first-strand cDNA synthesis kit synthesize the first-strand cDNA in one group. Real-time PCR was used to detect the transcription level of c-myc and the reduction of the transcription level of c-myc was quantitatively analyzed. GAPDH was used as a reference gene.

   PCR parameters were as follows:

   One cycle of 2 min at 95 °C, followed by 20 s at 95 °C, 20 s at 55.6 °C, and 40 s at 72 °C for 45 cycles.

   Specific forward and reverse primer sequences were as follows:

   c-myc fwd, 5' TGAGGAGACACCGCCCAC 3′
   c-myc rev, 5' CAACATCGATTTCTCTCATCTTC 3'
   GAPDH fwd, 5' GACTTCAACAGCAACTCCCAC 3'
   GAPDH rev, 5' TCCACCACCCTGTTGCTGTA 3′
7. Extract protein lysates by using TNE lysis buffer in another group. Total protein was separated by 10% SDS-PAGE gel, transferred to a PVDF membrane, treated with primary rabbit monoclonal c-myc (diluted 1:1000), and then immunoblotted with peroxidase-conjugated secondary antibody (1:5000).

## 3 Discussion

As the regulatory center of cell growth and metabolism, the disordered gene expression of the nucleus is closely related to the occurrence of diseases. By interfering with the transcription process, some so-called incurable diseases could be cured. As mentioned above, TFO is an antisense oligonucleotide that has the potential for gene therapy. Moreover, due to the high salt concentration around the Au NPs and the steric hindrance between nucleic acid strands, the antisense nucleotides are protected from being degraded by endogenous DNase enzymes. Besides, the TFOs can be stably transported into the nucleus by the ultrasmall nanocarriers. The results show that the conjugation between Au NPs and TFOs is highly selective and cooperative for gene delivery application.

## 4 Conclusion

In summary, taking advantage of the feasible surface modification techniques, this protocol presents the synthesis and conjugation method of 2 nm Au NP with oligo sequence for gene silencing. The excellent nuclear targeting ability and antitumor effect can be proved by test cell viability (MTT assays), gene and protein expression level (real-time PCR and Western blot analyses). Moreover, Au NPs can protect nucleic acids from degradation and further greatly increases the concentration of TFO in the nucleus. This typical preparation protocol of ultrasmall Au NPs provides an effective strategy for gene delivery and other biomedical application.

**Acknowledgments** This work was supported by the National Natural Science Foundation of China (NSFC) (grant No. 82001959 and 31630027) and NSFC-German Research Foundation (DFG) project (grant No. 31761133013). The authors also appreciate the support by the "Ten Thousand Elite Plan" (grant No. Y9E21Z11), CAS international collaboration plan (grant No. E0632911ZX), the National Key Research & Development Program of China (grant No. 2018YFE0117800), as well as the Key Laboratory of Biomedical Effects of Nanomaterials and Nanosafety, CAS (No: NSKF202003) and Fujian Provincial Key Laboratory of Innovative Drug Target Research (No. FJ-YW-2021KF04). S.H. is grateful for the financial support of the Nanqiang Outstanding Young Talents Program from Xiamen University.

**Conflict of Interest** The authors declare no conflict of interest.

## References

Barba AA, Bochicchio S, Dalmoro A, Lamberti G (2019) Lipid delivery Systems for Nucleic-Acid-Based-Drugs: from production to clinical applications. Pharmaceutics 11(8):360–385

Cheng R, Feng F, Meng FH, Deng C, Feijen J, Zhong ZY (2011) Glutathione-responsive nano-vehicles as a promising platform for targeted intracellular drug and gene delivery. J Control Release 152(1):2–12

Fernandes F, Kotharkar P, Chakravorty A, Kowshik M, Talukdar I (2020) Nanocarrier mediated siRNA delivery targeting stem cell differentiation. Curr Stem Cell Res Ther 15(2):155–172

Fernandez-Frias I, Perez-Luz S, Diaz-Nido J (2020) Enhanced production of herpes simplex virus 1 amplicon vectors by gene modification and optimization of packaging cell growth medium. Mol Ther Methods Clin Dev 17:491–496

Fujiwara Y, Wada K, Kabuta T (2016) Lysosomal degradation of intracellular nucleic acids—multiple autophagic pathways. J Biochem 161(2):145–154

Gao J, Zhang WL, Ehrhardt A (2020) Expanding the Spectrum of adenoviral vectors for cancer therapy. Cancer 12(5):1139–1163

Guo X, Huang L (2012) Recent advances in nonviral vectors for gene delivery. Acc Chem Res 45(7):971–979

Homayun B, Sun CM, Kumar A, Montemagno C, Choi HJ (2018) Facile fabrication of microparticles with pH-responsive macropores for small intestine targeted drug formulation. Eur J Pharm Biopharm 128:316–326

Hua Q, Qiang Z, Chu M, Shi D, Ren J (2019) Polymeric drug delivery system with actively targeted cell penetration and nuclear targeting for cancer therapy. ACS Appl Bio Mater 2(4):1724–1731

Huo SD, Gong NQ, Jiang Y, Chen F, Guo HB, Gan YL, Wang ZS, Herrmann A, Liang XJ (2019) Gold-DNA nanosunflowers for efficient gene silencing with controllable transformation. Sci Adv 5(10):eaaw6264

Huo SD, Jin SB, Ma XW, Xue XD, Yang KN, Kumar A, Wang PC, Zhang JC, Hu ZB, Liang XJ (2014) Ultrasmall gold nanoparticles as carriers for nucleus-based gene therapy due to size-dependent nuclear entry. ACS Nano 8(6):5852–5862

Mashel TV, Tarakanchikova YV, Muslimov AR, Zyuzin MV, Timin AS, Lepik KV, Fehse B (2020) Overcoming the delivery problem for therapeutic genome editing: current status and perspective of non-viral methods. Biomaterials 258:120282

Naso MF, Tomkowicz B, Perry WL, Strohl WR (2017) Adeno-associated virus (AAV) as a vector for gene therapy. BioDrugs 31(4):317–334

Perrin GQ, Herzog RW, Markusic DM (2019) Update on clinical gene therapy for hemophilia. Blood 133(5):407–414

Qian H, Tay CY, Setyawati MI, Chia SL, Lee DS, Leong DT (2017) Protecting microRNAs from RNase degradation with steric DNA nanostructures. Chem Sci 8(2):1062–1067

Radtke A, Ehlert M, Jedrzejewski T, Bartmanski M (2019) The morphology, structure, mechanical properties and biocompatibility of Nanotubular Titania coatings before and after autoclaving process. J Clin Med 8(2):272–293

Rideout WM, Hochedlinger K, Kyba M, Daley GQ, Jaenisch R (2002) Correction of a genetic defect by nuclear transplantation and combined cell and gene therapy. Cell 109(1):17–27

Roemer K, Friedmann T (1992) Concepts and strategies for human gene-therapy. Eur J Biochem 208(2):211–225

Sahin A, Eke G, Buyuksungur A, Hasirci N, Hasirci V (2018) Nuclear targeting peptide-modified, DOX-loaded, PHBV nanoparticles enhance drug efficacy by targeting to Saos-2 cell nuclear membranes. J Biomater Sci Polym Ed 29(5):507–519

Sajid MI, Moazzam M, Kato S, Cho KY, Tiwari RK (2020) Overcoming barriers for siRNA therapeutics: from bench to bedside. Pharmaceuticals 13(10):294–318

Salvatore A, Montis C, Berti D, Baglioni P (2016) Multifunctional Magnetoliposomes for sequential controlled release. ACS Nano 10(8):7749–7760

Santos A, Veiga F, Figueiras A (2020) Dendrimers as pharmaceutical excipients: synthesis, properties, toxicity and biomedical applications. Materials 13(1):65–95

Shi BY, Zheng M, Tao W, Chung R, Jin DY, Ghaffari D, Farokhzad OC (2017) Challenges in DNA delivery and recent advances in multifunctional polymeric DNA delivery systems. Biomacromolecules 18(8):2231–2246

Van Bruggen C, Hexum JK, Tan Z, Dalai RJ, Reineke TM (2019) Nonviral gene delivery with cationic Glycopolymers. Acc Chem Res 52(5):1347–1358

Wu YH, Gu WY, Li L, Chen C, Xu ZP (2019) Enhancing PD-1 gene silence in T lymphocytes by comparing the delivery performance of two inorganic nanoparticle platforms. Nano 9(2): 159–170

Zhang XT, Chai Z, Samulski RJ, Li CW (2020) Bound protein- and peptide-based strategies for adeno-associated virus vector-mediated gene therapy: where do we stand now? Hum Gene Ther 31:1146–1154

# Polypeptide Cationic Micelles–Mediated Co-delivery of Docetaxel and siRNA for Synergistic Tumor Therapy

# 18

Hong Pan, Lanlan Liu, and Lintao Cai

## Contents



**Abstract**

The combination chemotherapy with other anticancer techniques is of great clinical importance to reduce side effects and enhance the effectiveness of cancer treatment. Co-delivery of chemotherapy drugs and small interfering RNA (siRNA) through advanced nanotechnology provides a reliable and effective strategy for combination therapy with synergistic effect. In this regard, this protocol focuses on the fabrication of polypeptide cationic micelles and delivery of chemical drug and siRNA for synergistic antitumor therapy. Here, the preparation and characterization techniques of polypeptide cationic micelles are described. A triblock copolymer poly (ethylene glycol)-b-poly (L-lysine)-b-poly (L-leucine) (PEG-PLL-PLLeu) was prepared through ring-opening polymerization reaction. These cationic copolymers could effectively encapsulate the hydrophobic drug and negatively charged siRNA in a single nanomicelle for co-delivery of drug/gene. The co-delivery system of chemotherapy drugs (docetaxel, DTX) and siRNA (siRNA-Bcl-2) obviously reduced the expression of antiapoptotic Bcl-2 gene and synergistically promoted antitumor activity of

H. Pan · L. Liu · L. Cai (✉)
Guangdong Key Laboratory of Nanomedicine, CAS-HK Joint Lab for Biomaterials, Shenzhen Engineering Laboratory of Nanomedicine and Nanoformulations, Shenzhen Institute of Advanced Technology (SIAT), Chinese Academy of Sciences, Shenzhen, China
e-mail: lt.cai@siat.ac.cn


H. Tian and X. Chen (eds.), *Gene Delivery*, Biomaterial Engineering,
https://doi.org/10.1007/978-981-16-5419-0_18

DTX. The present results demonstrate that the polypeptide cationic micelle is an effective chemotherapeutic drug/siRNA co-delivery system, thereby further improving the combined therapeutic efficacy for tumor in vivo.

**Keywords**

Polypeptide cationic micelles · siRNA · Co-delivery system · Synergistic effect · Tumor therapy

## 1 Overview

Combination of multiple therapeutic strategies with diverse mechanisms is currently an effective way to eliminate tumors. Recent studies have demonstrated small interference RNA (siRNA) as a potential therapeutic choice in various diseases for silencing target genes (Dykxhoorn et al. 2003). However, due to the short half-life of siRNA in serum and its poor ability to penetrate cells, effective delivery vehicles are required for siRNA to overcome the multiple cellular barriers and achieve successful clinical application (Kim and Rossi 2007). In addition, chemotherapy, a traditional and primary treatment strategy for anticancer therapy, has been also hold back because of potential off target side effect, acute toxicity on normal tissues, and drug resistance. Therefore, there is an urgent need of chemotherapeutic drug/gene co-delivery systems to improve the efficacy of tumor-targeted drug/gene delivery and antitumor treatment.

More and more evidences have indicated that the uptake of positively charged nanoparticles by cells is more effective than that of neutral/negatively charged nanoparticles due to the electrostatic interaction between nanoparticles and cell membranes. In the past decades, drug delivery systems for such co-delivery purpose have been developed based on polymeric (Zhu et al. 2010), liposomal (Xu et al. 2010), and silica-based cationic NPs (Meng et al. 2010). By comparison, polymer-based micelles show better performance than cationic lipids in term of safety, convenience for mass production, and physiological stability.

So far, multiple synthetic and natural cationic polymers have been reported as gene or drug vehicles, including poly(ethylene imine) (PEI) (Merdan et al. 2002), poly(L-lysine) (Miyata et al. 2005), and chitosan (Cheng et al. 2012). Synthetic polypeptides are unique supramolecular nanostructured polymers formed through self-assembly. They not only have sophisticated biological functions but also have biocompatible and biodegradable properties. Numerous studies have also shown that polymer micelles based on amphiphilic block copolymers play a significant role in synergistic chemotherapy and siRNA antitumor therapy. Encouragingly, the current polymeric micelles based on amphiphilic block copolymers widely explored in drug delivery and have been entering clinical trials (Yap et al. 2009) or obtaining clinical approval (for example, Genexol in Korea).

In this protocol, a polypeptide micelle system based on triblock copolymers poly (ethylene glycol)-b-poly-L-lysine-b-poly-L-leucine for a highly effective drug/gene co-delivery was described (Deng et al. 2012; Luo et al. 2013). The triblock polypeptide copolymers are amphiphilic and can self-assemble into micelle nanoparticles. PLLeu severed as the hydrophobic core, PLL is the cationic shell, and PEG is the hydrophilic corona. These polypeptide cationic micelles are enable to encapsulate negatively charged siRNA (siRNA-Bcl-2) and hydrophobic drug (docetaxel, DTX) in a single nanoparticle as a reliable drug/gene co-delivery system. The capability of polypeptide cationic micelles to simultaneously deliver siRNA and DTX into the same tumor cells, as well as the antitumor therapeutic efficacy are evaluated in vitro and the tumor xenograft mice (Zheng et al. 2013).

## 2 Protocol

### 2.1 Materials

#### 2.1.1 Preparation of Polypeptide $PEG_1$-$PLL_{10}$-$PLLeu_{40}$

1. N-carboxyanhydride (NCA) (GL Biochem, Shanghai, China)
2. ε-benzyloxycarbonyl-L-lysine (LLZe-NCA) (GL Biochem, Shanghai, China)
3. O-(2-Aminoethyl)-O′-(2-methyl) polyethylene glycol ($PEG$-$NH_2$, Mw = 2000) (Sigma-Aldrich, Natick, MA)
4. Ethyl acetate (J&K Scientific, Shanghai, China)
5. Diethyl ether (J&K Scientific, Shanghai, China)
6. N, N′-Dimethylformamide (DMF) (J&K Scientific, Shanghai, China)
7. Trifluoroacetic acid (J&K Scientific, Shanghai, China)
8. Hydrobromic acid (Sinopharm Chemical Reagent, Shanghai, China)
9. Acetic acid (Sinopharm Chemical Reagent, Shanghai, China)
10. Dialysis membrane (MWCO 3500 Da)

#### 2.1.2 Characterization of Polypeptide $PEG_1$-$PLL_{10}$-$PLLeu_{40}$

1. Proton nuclear magnetic resonance (1H NMR) (Bruker)
2. $CF_3COOD$ (J&K Scientific, Shanghai, China)
3. $PEG_1$-$PLL_{10}$-$PLLeu_{40}$ copolymers

#### 2.1.3 Preparation of Drug Loaded Micelle Nanoparticles (NPs)

1. Docetaxel (DTX) (Advanced Technology & Industrial Co. Ltd., Hong Kong, China)
2. Dimethyl sulfoxide (DMSO) (J&K Scientific, Shanghai, China)
3. Deionized water
4. $PEG_1$-$PLL_{10}$-$PLLeu_{40}$ copolymers
5. Dialysis membrane (MWCO 3500 Da)

#### 2.1.4 Characterization of Drug Loaded Micelle NPs

1. Micelle NPs
2. DTX loaded micelle NPs (DTX-NPs)
3. Zetasizer Nano ZS (Malvern Instrument)

4. Transmission electron microscope (TEM)
5. Deionized water

### 2.1.5 Preparation of Micelleplex

1. DEPC water (Sinopharm Chemical Reagent, Shanghai, China)
2. Micelle NPs
3. DTX-NPs
4. Targeting human Bcl-2 siRNA (siRNA-Bcl-2) (sense: 5-′-CCGGGAGAUAGUGAUGAAGdTdT-3′, anti-sense: 5'-CUUCAUCACUAU-CUCCCGGdTdT-3′) (Shanghai GenePharma Co. Ltd., Shanghai, China)
5. Negative control siRNA (NC siRNA) (sense: 50-UUCUCCGAACGUGU-CACGUdTdT-3′, anti-sense: 5′-ACGUGACACGUUCGGAGAAdTdT-3′) (Shanghai GenePharma Co. Ltd., Shanghai, China)
6. Deionized water

### 2.1.6 Gel Retardation Assay

1. UV illuminator with gel red staining
2. 2% (w/v) agarose gel
3. TAE buffer containing Tris-HCl (40 mM), acetic acid (1% v/v), and EDTA (1 mM)
4. DTX-siRNA-NPs

### 2.1.7 Stability Analysis of DTX-NPs and Characterization of Micelleplex

1. DTX-NPs
2. Phosphate buffer saline (PBS)
3. Fetal bovine serum (FBS)
4. Dulbecco's Modified Eagle Medium (DMEM)
5. DTX-siRNA-NPs
6. Zetasizer Nano ZS instrument

### 2.1.8 Cell Culture

1. Human breast cancer cells (MCF-7)
2. DMEM medium supplemented with 10% FBS
3. Cell incubator

### 2.1.9 Animals and Antitumor Model

1. 6–8-week-old female BALB/c nude mice (18–22 g)
2. MCF-7 cells ($2 \times 10^6$)

### 2.1.10 In Vitro Study on Co-delivery of Drug and siRNA

1. FAM-labeled siRNA NPs (siRNA-NPs). Fluorescein-labeled siRNA (FAM-siRNA) was produced by fluorescence modification of the 3′ end of the sense strand of the scrambled siRNA and was purchased from GenePharma Co. Ltd. (Shanghai, China).

2. Rhoda mine-labeled micelle NPs (DTX-NPs).
3. MCF-7 cells
4. 8-well cover glass plate.
5. PBS.
6. 4% paraformaldehyde solution.
7. Hoechst 33258 (Sigma-Aldrich, St. Louis, MO).
8. Confocal laser scanning microscope (CLSM, Leica TCS SP5, Germany).

#### 2.1.11 In Vitro siRNA-Bcl-2 Transfection

1. MCF-7 cells
2. 6-well plates
3. PBS
4. Blank NPs
5. NC-NPs
6. siRNA-NPs (50, 100, 150 nM of siRNA)
7. siRNA-Lipofectamine (100 nM of siRNA)

#### 2.1.12 Analysis of Bcl-2 Expression by PCR

1. AxyPrep Multisource total RNA Miniprep Kit (Axygen, USA)
2. Prime Script first Strand cDNA Synthesis Kit (Takara, Japan)
3. SYBR Green qPCR Mix (Maygene Biotech, China)
4. Applied Biosystems StepOne Real-Time PCR Systems
5. Step One Software v 2.1 (Applied Biosystems)

#### 2.1.13 Western Blot Analysis of Bcl-2 Expression

1. Transfected cells
2. Cold PBS
3. Lysis buffer (pH 7.5, 50 mM Hepes, 150 mM NaCl, 1% Triton X-100, 10% glycerol, 1.5 mM $MgCl_2$, 1 mM EGTA) freshly supplemented with ROCHE cOmplete™ Protease Inhibitor Cocktail
4. Ice
5. Centrifuge
6. BCA Protein Assay Kit (Tiangen, China)
7. 12% Bis-Tris-poly-acrylamide gels
8. PVDF membranes (Millipore, Bedford, MA)
9. 5% nonfat milk powder (Merck, Germany)
10. Phosphate-buffered saline supplemented with Tween-20 (pH 7.2)
11. Antibody against human antiapoptotic protein (Bcl-2) (Cell Signaling Technology, USA)
12. Goat anti rabbit IgG-HRP antibody (Sigma-Aldrich, St. Louis, MO)
13. ECL system (Pierce)

#### 2.1.14 Analysis of Cell Proliferation

1. Micelle NPs
2. DTX-siRNA-NPs

3. MCF-7 cells
4. 96-well plates
5. MTT solution
6. DMSO
7. Microplate reader (Synergy 4, Bio Tec, USA)

#### 2.1.15 Micelle NPs Distribution in Nude Mice

1. Rhodamine-labeled micelle nanoparticles (DTX-NPs)
2. Maestro in vivo imaging system (CRi, Inc., USA)
3. PBS
4. Balb/c nude mice-bearing MCF-7 tumors

#### 2.1.16 Tumor Suppression Study

1. Nude mice-bearing MCF-7 tumor cells
2. PBS
3. Blank NPs
4. NC-NPs
5. siRNA-NPs
6. Taxotere
7. DTX-NPs
8. DTX-siRNA-NPs

#### 2.1.17 Detection of Bcl-2 Gene Expression in Tumor

1. Tumor tissues
2. RIPA tissue lysis buffer (include 1% 100 mM PMSF) freshly supplemented with the lysates
3. Centrifuge
4. BCA Protein Assay Kit

## 2.2 Methods

### 2.2.1 Preparation of $PEG_1$-$PLL_{10}$-$PLLeu_{40}$ Copolymer (Note 1, 2)

1. Synthesize the PEG-PLLZ copolymers by ring-opening polymerization of LLZ-NCA initiated with $PEG$-$NH_2$. Concisely, given amounts of $PEG$-$NH_2$ and LLZ-NCA were dissolved in dried DMF (10 wt %) and stirred at 40 °C under nitrogen atmosphere for 48 h. Next, the obtained product was precipitated using an excess diethyl ether under vigorous stirring to produce a white solid (PEG-PLLZ).
2. Synthesize $PEG_1$-$PLLZ_{10}$-$PLLeu_{40}$ via further ring-opening polymerization of LLeu-NCA using PEG-PLLZ as initiator. A certain amounts of PEG-PLLZ and LLeu-NCA were dissolved in dried DMF (10 wt %) and stirred at 40 °C under a nitrogen atmosphere for 48 h.
3. Precipitate the PEG-PLLZ-PLLeu copolymer in diethyl ether and purified by repeated precipitation by diethyl ether.

4. PEG-PLL-PLLeu copolymers were obtained by the deprotection of PEG-PLLZ-PLLeu (Fig. 1).

### 2.2.2 Characterization of $PEG_1$-$PLL_{10}$-$PLLeu_{40}$ Copolymer (Note 3)

1. Proton nuclear magnetic resonance ($^1H$ NMR) spectra were recorded on Bruker NMR spectrometers (400 MHz) with CF3COOD/CDC13 as the solvent (Fig. 2).

### 2.2.3 Preparation of DTX-Loaded Micelle NPs

1. DTX-loaded micelle nanoparticles (DTX-NPs) were produced by directly dissolving 2 mg $PEG_1$-$PLL_{10}$-$PLLeu_{40}$ copolymers with DTX in DMSO of 2 mg/mL with sonication for 10 min.
2. The mixture solution above was titrated with water to reach copolymers' final concentration to 1 mg/mL.
3. At last, the solution was dialyzed for another 24 h under magnetic stirring.

### 2.2.4 Characterization of DTX-Loaded Micelle NPs (Note 4, 5, 6)

1. The sizes and zeta potentials of the self-assembled micelles were determined at 25 °C by Zetasizer Nano ZS (Malvern Instrument).

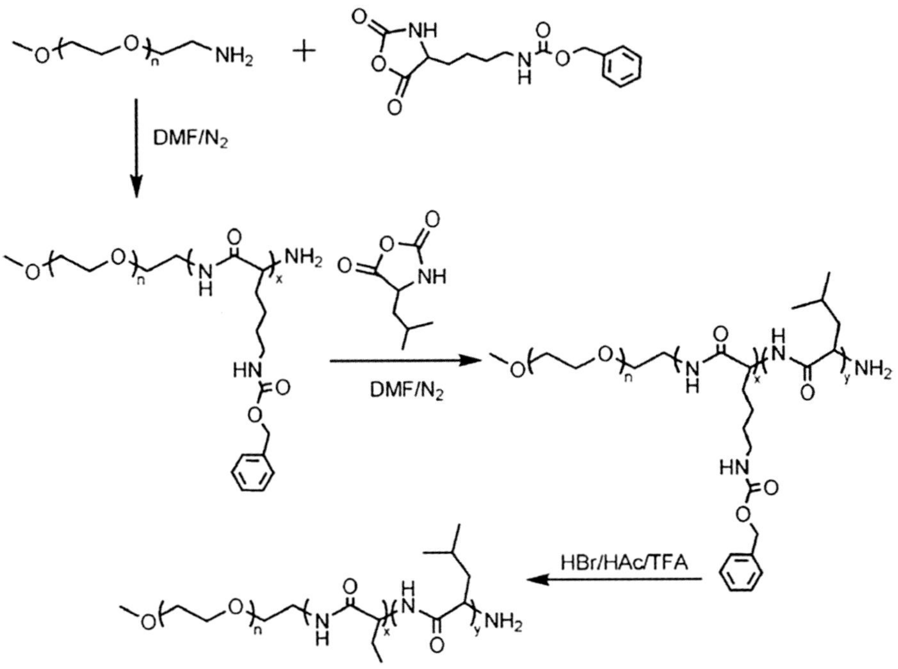


**Fig. 1** Synthesis of PEG-PLL-PLLeu copolymers. First, the diblock copolymer PEG-PLLZ was prepared. Next, the copolymer PEG-PLLZ-PLLeu was prepared by further ring opening polymerization of LLeu-NCA. Finally, the amphiphilic PEG-PLL-PLLeu products were gained after copolymer deprotection. (Adapted from Deng et al. (2012), with permission)

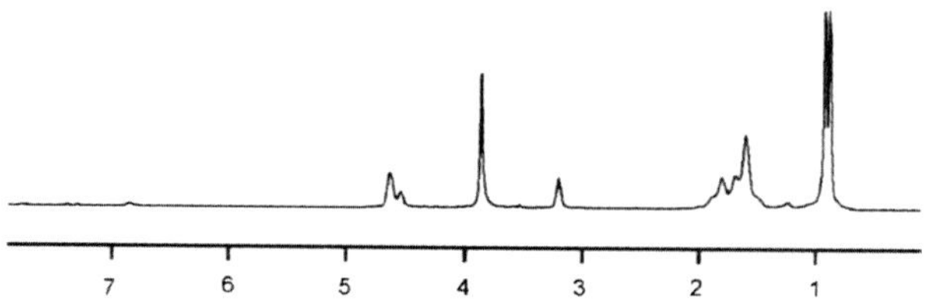


**Fig. 2** $^1$H NMR spectra of PEG-PLL-PLLeu triblock copolymers. The peaks mainly from 0.8 to 0.9 ppm are attributable to the protons ($-CH_3$) in PLLeu. (Adapted from Deng et al. (2012), with permission)

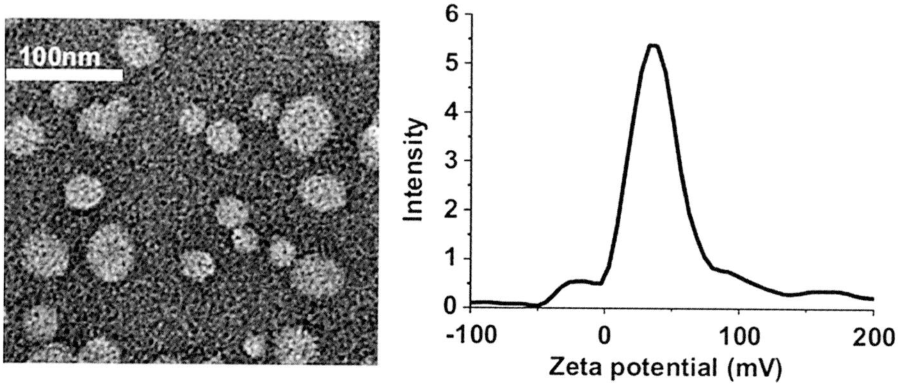


**Fig. 3** TEM image and zeta potential characterization of docetaxel micelle NPs. (Adapted from Zheng et al. (2013), with permission)

2. The morphology and sizes of the self-assembled micelles were determined by transmission electronic microscopic (TEM) at 2 °C (Fig. 3).

### 2.2.5 Preparation of Micelleplex (Note 7, 8, 9)

1. Dilute micelle NPs or DTX-NPs with DEPC water at a serious of concentrations.
2. Various concentration of siRNA (siRNA-Bcl-2 or NC siRNA) in DEPC water was then mixed with equal volume of NPs above by gentle pipetting.
3. The formed micelleplex was incubated at room temperature for 20 min before further treatments.
4. The morphology and zeta potential of micelleplex were separately determined using TEM imaging and dynamic light scattering (DLS) (Fig. 4).

### 2.2.6 Gel Retardation Assay of siRNA-Loading Micelleplex

1. The electrophoretic mobility of micelleplex was visualized on a UV illuminator with gelred staining after electrophoresis on a 2% (w/v) agarose gel in TAE buffer (40 mM Tris-HCl, 1% v/v acetic acid, 1 mM EDTA) for 15 min at 100 V.

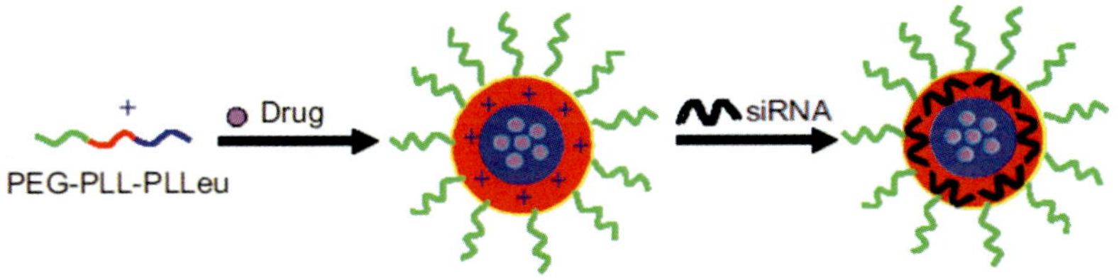


**Fig. 4** Schematic illustration of self-assembled cationic micelle and loading of siRNA and drug. The polypeptide self-assembled a micelle structure in aqueous solution and exhibited the ability of simultaneous loading of siRNA and DTX. (Adapted from Zheng et al. (2013), with permission)

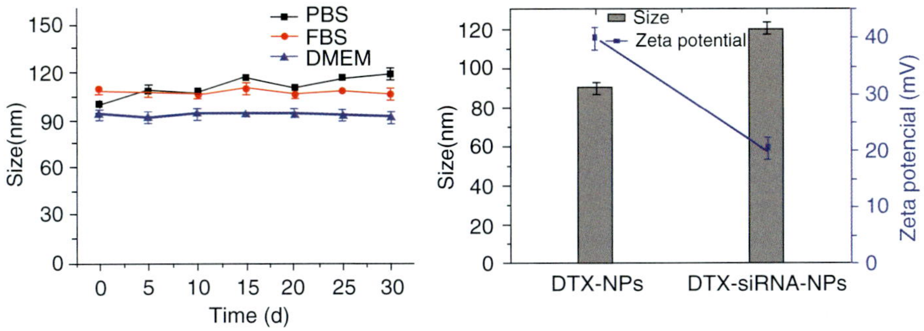


**Fig. 5** Long time colloid stability test of DTX-NPs in three different solvents (left panel), and the size and zeta potential variation of DTX-NPs after loading siRNA. (Adapted from Zheng et al. (2013), with permission)

### 2.2.7 Stability of DTX-NPs and Characterization of Micelleplex (Note 10, 11)

1. Dilute DTX-NPs with phosphate buffer saline (PBS), fetal bovine serum (FBS), or Dulbecco's Modified Eagle Medium (DMEM).
2. The size of NPs were recorded every week in 1 month.
3. The size and zeta potential of DTX-NPs and DTX-siRNA-NPs were recorded by Zetasizer Nano ZS instrument (Fig. 5).

### 2.2.8 Cell Culture

1. MCF-7 human breast cancer cells over-expressing Bcl-2 protein were cultured for following experiments.
2. The cell culture medium were prepared by DMEM medium supplemented with 10% FBS and 1% penicillin/streptomycin.
3. MCF-7 cells were cultured in an incubator at 37 °C with 5% $CO_2$.
4. MCF-7 cells were pre-cultured until cell confluence reached to 75% before experiments.

### 2.2.9 Animals and Tumor Model Study

1. Six to eight weeks female BALB/c nude mice (18–22 g) were obtained from Vital River Laboratory Animal Technology Co. Ltd. (Beijing, China).
2. All animals received care in compliance with the Guidelines outlined in the Guide for the Care and Use of Laboratory Animals.
3. All experiment procedures were approved by the University of Science and Technology of China Animal Care and Use Committee.
4. The tumor xenograft model was built by subcutaneous injection of MCF-7 cells ($2 \times 10^6$) into the armpit of the mice.
5. Tumor-bearing mice were used for following experiments after 2 weeks tumor-inoculation.

### 2.2.10 Co-delivery Analysis of Drug and siRNA into Tumor Cells

1. FAM-labeled siRNA NPs (siRNA-NPs) or rhodamine-labeled micelle NPs (DTX-NPs) were produced as the same procedure described above.
2. MCF-7 cells ($5 \times 10^4$ cells/well) were seeded into an 8-well chambered cover-slips (Corning Ltd) and followed culturing for 24 h at 37 °C in 5% $CO_2$.
3. The DTX-NPs, siRNA-NPs, and DTX-siRNA-NPs solutions were added into the above cells.
4. After 2 h incubation, remove the cell culture medium.
5. Cells were rinsed twice with the same temperature PBS.
6. The cells were fixed by 4% paraformaldehyde solution for 15 min.
7. Stain the nuclei with Hoechst 33258 (10 mg/mL) for 5 min and wash three times with PBS.
8. Observe cell uptake for different nanoparticles by confocal laser scanning micro-scope (CLSM, Leica TCS SP5, Germany).

### 2.2.11 siRNA-Bcl-2 Transfection in Cells

1. Seed MCF-7 cells ($5 \times 10^4$) in 6-well plates and incubate for 24 h at 37 °C in 5% $CO_2$ until 70% cell confluence.
2. Various formulations, including PBS, Blank NPs, NC-NPs, siRNA-NPs (50, 100, 150 of nM siRNA), and siRNA-Lipofectamine (100 nM siRNA) were added into the above cells and co-incubated for another 24 h (for mRNA isolation) or 72 h (for protein extraction).

### 2.2.12 Analysis of Bcl-2 mRNA Expression by PCR Test

1. The expression level of Bcl-2 mRNA and protein were assessed by quantitative real-time PCR (qRT-PCR) and Western blot assay, respectively.
2. During qRT-PCR analysis, total RNA from administered cells was extracted by the AxyPrep Multisource total RNA Miniprep Kit (Axygen, USA) followed as the manufacture's protocols.
3. 1 μg total RNA were reverse transcribed into cDNA using the Prime Script first Strand cDNA Synthesis Kit (Takara, Japan).
4. Next, cDNA (1 mL) was subjected to qRT-PCR analysis of target gene Bcl-2 and β-actin using the SYBR Green 1 qPCR Mix (Maygene Biotech, China).

5. Data analysis was conducted under the Applied Biosystems StepOne$^{TM}$ Real-Time PCR Systems.
6. PCR parameters consisted of 30 s of Taq enzyme activation at 95 °C.
7. Forty cycles of PCR at 95 °C, 5 s, 60 °C, 30 s, and 1 cycle of 95 °C, 15 s, 60 °C, 60 s, and 95 °C, 15 s.
8. Standard curves were figured by the relative amount of target gene mRNA to β-actin mRNA as the standard protocols. Reaction specificity was further confirmed by melt curve analysis.
9. The relative gene expression values were analyzed by the ΔΔCT method by using of Step One Software v 2.1 (Applied Biosystems).
10. Data are presented as the fold difference in Bcl-2 mRNA expression related to reference gene β-actin, and relative to the untreated control cells.
11. Primer sequences used in qRT-PCR analysis for Bcl-2 and β-actin are:
    Bcl-2-forward 5′-AACATCGCCCTGTGGATGAC-3′, Bcl-2-reverse 5′-AGA GTCTTCAGAGACAGCCAGGAG-3′ and β-actin-forward 5′-CGCGAGAAGAT GACCCAGATC-3′, β-actin-reverse 5′-CATGAGGTAGTCAGTCAGGTCCC-3′.

### 2.2.13 Analysis of Bcl-2 Protein Expression by Western Blot

1. Wash transfected cells twice with precooled PBS.
2. Resuspended cells in 50 mL of pH 7.7 lysis buffer, which containing 50 mM HEPES, 150 mM NaCl, 1% Triton X-100, 10% glycerol, 1.5 mM $MgCl_2$, 1 mM EGTA), and freshly supplemented with Roche's Complete Protease Inhibitor Cocktail Tablets.
3. Incubate the cell lysates on ice for 30 min and vortexed it every 5 min.
4. The lysates were then centrifuged for 10 min at 12,000 × g, 4 °C.
5. The total protein concentration in lysate was further determined by using of BCA Protein Assay Kit (Tiangen, China).
6. Sixty milligram of total protein in each sample was separated by electrophoresis on 12% Bis-Tris-poly-acrylamide gels and then transferred to PVDF membranes at 150 mA for 2 h (Millipore, Bedford, MA).
7. Incubate PVDF membranes in phosphate-buffered saline containing 5% nonfat milk powder (Merck, Germany) and Tween-20 (PBST, pH 7.2) for 1 h at room temperature.
8. Incubate the membranes in 5% nonfat milk powder in PBST with Bcl-2 primary antibodies (1:500) overnight at 4 °C.
9. Incubate the membranes in 5% nonfat milk powder in PBST with goat anti rabbit IgG-HRP antibody (1:3500) for 2 h at room temperature.
10. Protein bands were observed using a standard ECL system (Pierce).

### 2.2.14 Analysis of Cell Proliferation

1. The cytotoxicity of micelle NPs and DTX-siRNA-NPs over a wide range of concentrations were evaluated by MTT assay in MCF-7 cells.
2. MCF-7 cells ($5 \times 10^3$ cells/well) were seeded into 96-well plates and cultured in an incubator at 37 °C, 5% $CO_2$ for 12 h.

3. Replace cell culture supernatant with the fresh medium containing the different NPs samples with a range of concentrations from 0.5 to 80 mg/mL NPs and other controls (contain 0.05 mg/mL DTX).
4. Cells in culture media without treatment were performed as the blank control.
5. Incubate the above MCF-7 cells at 37 °C, 5% $CO_2$ for another 24 h.
6. 20 mL/well MTT solution (5 mg/mL) was added and incubated for 4–6 h.
7. Carefully removed supernatant and add 150 mL DMSO to dissolve the MTT formazan crystal.
8. The solution's absorbance at a wavelength of 490 nm was determined by a microplate reader (Synergy 4, Bio Tec, USA).
9. The cell viability (%) was defined as the percentage of $OD_{490}$ value of the cells administrated with the NPs suspension over the blank control.
10. Repeat this experiments for 3–5 times.

### 2.2.15 Micelle NPs Distribution In Vivo

1. Rhodamine-labeled micelle NPs (DTX-NPs) solution and PBS control were intravenously injected into MCF-7 tumor-bearing Balb/c nude mice.
2. At 24 h post-administration, the mice were sacrificed and the organs including heart, liver, spleen, lung, kidneys, and tumor were harvested and determined the fluorescence signal by the Maestro in vivo imaging system (CRi, Inc., USA).
3. Analyze the distributions of rhodamine-tagged micelle nanoparticles (DTX-NPs) in Balb/c nude mice by using of a Maestro in vivo imaging system.

### 2.2.16 Tumor Suppression Assay (Note 12)

1. Randomly divided experimental mice into different groups ($n = 5$), when the tumor volume was approximately 100 $mm^3$.
2. Balb/c mice were i.v. injected with various formulations (100 μl/mouse)
3. Groups are set as follows: Group 1: PBS, Group 2: Blank NPs, Group 3: NC-NPs, Group 4: siRNA-NPs, Group 5: Taxotere, Group 6: DTX-NPs, Group 7: siRNA-NPs + DTX-NPs, and Group 8: DTX-siRNA-NPs.
4. The i.v. injection administration was performed every 3 days. The dosage of siRNA-Bcl-2 (or NC siRNA) and DTX of each experiment mouse were qualified at 0.2 mg/kg and 0.5 mg/kg, respectively.
5. The antitumor efficiency was evaluated according to the tumor size during different treatment. The tumor size was estimated by the following formulas: $V = 6 \times \text{larger diameter} \times (\text{smaller diameter})^2/\pi$.
6. Both tumor size and mice weights were regularly monitored at post-administration every time (Fig. 6).

### 2.2.17 Analysis of Tumorous Bcl-2 Expression In Vivo

1. Collect tumor tissues at 24 h post last administration.
2. Lyse tumor tissues by 500 mL RIPA tissue lysis buffer (with 1% 100 mM PMSF) and supplemented with fresh lysates.
3. Vortex the tumor lysate by the Tissue-Tearor for 10 min
4. Centrifuge the lysates at 12,000 × g for 10 min.
5. Total protein concentration was quantified by using of BCA Protein Assay Kit.

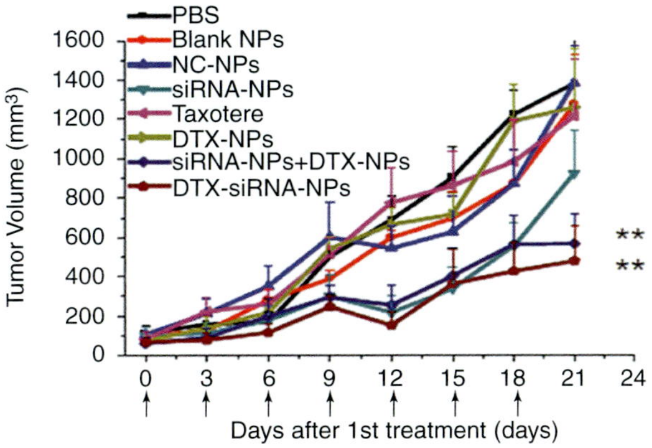


**Fig. 6** The antitumor effects of DTX-siRNA-NPs and other controls (including PBS, Blank NPs, NC-NPs, siRNA-NPs, Taxotere, DTX-NPs, DTX-NPs + siRNA-NPs, DTX-siRNA-NPs) were evaluated in MCF-7 xenografts tumor-bearing nude mice. $^{**}p < 0.001$ ($n = 5$). (Adapted from Zheng et al. (2013), with permission)

6. Protein semiquantitative analysis was performed to determine Bcl-2 expression by the Western blot assay as described in Sect. 2.1.13.

#### 2.2.18 Statistical Analysis

1. All of the experimental data are reported as mean ± SE of three independent measurements.
2. The difference among groups were determined using a Student's t-test (two-tailed).
3. Statistical significance was assigned at $^{*}p < 0.05$, $^{**}p < 0.001$ (95% confidence level).

## 3 Notes

1. During the preparing procedure of PEG-PLLZ copolymers, the feed molar ratio of $PEG\text{-}NH_2$ to LLZ-NCA was 1:10, and the PEG-PLLZ copolymers precursor ($PEG_1\text{-}PLLZ_{10}$) were obtained. The $PEG_1\text{-}PLL_{10}\text{-}PLLeu_{40}$ polypeptide was synthesized according to the molar ratio of PEG-PLLZ to LLeu-NCA at 1:40.
2. After completing the reaction, PEG-PLLZ or PEG-PLLZ-PLLeu was dissolved in a given volume of trifluoroacetic acid (5 wt %) and 4 equiv. of a 33 wt % solution of HBr in HAc with respect to the benzyloxycarbonyl (Z) groups, and then followed by stirring in ice for 2 h under a nitrogen atmosphere. The reaction mixture was further precipitated slowly in excessive ice diethyl ether to obtain the crude product.
3. For further identification of the structure of copolymers, $^1H$ NMR spectra of the polypeptide were analyzed at 25 °C using a Bruker 400 MHz instrument with the use of $CF_3COOD$ solvents. The fluorescence spectra were further measured using a Perkin-Elmer LS55 luminescence spectrometer.
4. DTX-loaded micelle nanoparticles were synthesized by the direct mixture of 2 mg $PEG_1\text{-}PLL_{10}\text{-}PLLeu_{40}$ copolymers with DTX in DMSO at a concentration

of 2 mg/mL with another sonication for 10 min. Next, dd$H_2O$ was added into the above mixture to dilute the copolymers concentration to 1 mg/mL.

5. Particle size and zeta potential of polypeptide cationic micelle were measured at 25 °C using transmission electron microscopy (TEM) and Zetasizer Nano ZS (Malvern Instrument Ltd), respectively.
6. To remove DMSO and free drug, NPs should dialysis against deionized water for 24 h with replace fresh deionized water every 4 h.
7. RNA is easily degraded by RNA enzymes, so the raw materials without RNA enzymes should be selected and the introduction of RNA enzymes should be avoided in the process of polypeptide cationic micelles synthesis.
8. For efficient siRNA binding by NPs or DTX-NPs, nitrogen/phosphate (N/P ratio) in the vector and siRNA should be greater than 10.
9. Nanoparticles with positive surface charge are more likely to cross the cell membrane and enter cytoplasm. Based on above reasons, the maximum encapsulation rate of siRNA/drug was not chosen for the polypeptide cationic micelles. Polypeptide cationic micelles loaded with siRNA/drug should maintain the zeta potential about +20 mV ~ +40 mV.
10. DTX-NPs micelles with the size of 100 nm were quite stable in 30 days in the experimental condition, such as PBS, FBS, and DMEM solution.
11. Polypeptide cationic micelles, if not used in a short period of time, should be prepared as lyophilized powders and stored at −20 °C or −80 °C.
12. Since endotoxin in the body can cause some uncertain immune stimulation, the reagents and water used in the synthesis of polypeptide cationic micelles is supposed to remove endotoxins in advance.

## 4 Discussion

This protocol presents a kind of polypeptide cationic micelle based on triblock copolymers poly(ethylene glycol)-*b*-poly-L-lysine-*b*-poly-L-leucine (PEG-PLL-PLLeu) for a highly effective drug/gene carrier, which are designed to co-deliver anticancer drugs and siRNA for enhancing the tumor targeting and combined therapy. A kind of amphiphilic PEG-PLL-PLLeu hybrid polypeptide micelle was synthesized through electrostatic interaction between PLL polypeptide and siRNA. The nanoparticles were characterized for particle size, surface morphology, stability, and encapsulation efficiency. Results clearly demonstrate that the micelleplex carrier system exhibits great potential in simultaneously delivering the antitumor agent and gene into the tumor in vivo, which could significantly block tumor progression in a synergistic manner.

## References

Cheng D, Cao N, Chen J, Yu X, Shuai X (2012) Multifunctional nanocarrier mediated co-delivery of doxorubicin and siRNA for synergistic enhancement of glioma apoptosis in rat. Biomaterials 33(4):1170–1179

Deng J, Gao N, Wang Y, Yi H, Fang S, Ma Y, Cai L (2012) Self-assembled cationic micelles based on PEG-PLL-PLLeu hybrid polypeptides as highly effective gene vectors. Biomacromolecules 13(11):3795–3804

Dykxhoorn DM, Novina CD, Sharp PA (2003) Killing the messenger: short RNAs that silence gene expression. Nat Rev Mol Cell Biol 4(6):457–467

Kim DH, Rossi JJ (2007) Strategies for silencing human disease using RNA interference. Nat Rev Genet 8:173–184

Luo Z, Li P, Deng J, Gao N, Zhang Y, Pan H, Liu L, Wang C, Cai L, Ma Y (2013) Cationic polypeptide micelle-based antigen delivery system: a simple and robust adjuvant to improve vaccine efficacy. J Control Release 170(2):259–267

Meng H, Liong M, Xia T, Li Z, Ji Z, Zink JI, Nel AE (2010) Engineered design of mesoporous silica nanoparticles to deliver doxorubicin and P-glycoprotein siRNA to overcome drug resistance in a cancer cell line. ACS Nano 4(8):4539–4550

Merdan T, Kopeček J, Kissel T (2002) Prospects for cationic polymers in gene and oligonucleotide therapy against cancer. Adv Drug Deliv Rev 54(5):715–758

Miyata K, Kakizawa Y, Nishiyama N, Yamasaki Y, Watanabe T, Kohara M, Kataoka K (2005) Freeze-dried formulations for in vivo gene delivery of PEGylated polyplex micelles with disulfide crosslinked cores to the liver. J Control Release 109(1–3):15–23

Xu Z, Zhang Z, Chen Y, Chen L, Lin L, Li Y (2010) The characteristics and performance of a multifunctional nanoassembly system for the co-delivery of docetaxel and iSur-pDNA in a mouse hepatocellular carcinoma model. Biomaterials 31(5):916–922

Yap TA, Carden CP, Kaye SB (2009) Beyond chemotherapy: targeted therapies in ovarian cancer. Nat Rev Cancer 9(3):167–181

Zheng C, Zheng M, Gong P, Deng J, Yi H, Zhang P, Zhang Y, Liu P, Ma Y, Cai L (2013) Polypeptide cationic micelles mediated co-delivery of docetaxel and siRNA for synergistic tumor therapy. Biomaterials 34(13):3431–3438

Zhu C, Jung S, Luo S, Meng F, Zhu X, Park TG, Zhong Z (2010) Co-delivery of siRNA and paclitaxel into cancer cells by biodegradable cationic micelles based on PDMAEMA-PCL-PDMAEMA triblock copolymers. Biomaterials 31(8):2408–2416

# Preparation and Evaluation of Reduction-Controlled Hierarchical Unpacking Terplexes for Gene Delivery

# 19

Yiyan He and Zhongwei Gu

## Contents



Y. He
Research Institute for Biomaterials, Tech Institute for Advanced Materials, College of Materials Science and Engineering, Suqian Advanced Materials Industry Technology Innovation Center, Jiangsu Collaborative Innovation Center for Advanced Inorganic Function Composites, Nanjing Tech University, Nanjing, People's Republic of China

Z. Gu (✉)
Research Institute for Biomaterials, Tech Institute for Advanced Materials, College of Materials Science and Engineering, Suqian Advanced Materials Industry Technology Innovation Center, Jiangsu Collaborative Innovation Center for Advanced Inorganic Function Composites, Nanjing Tech University, Nanjing, People's Republic of China

Huaxi MR Research Center (HMRRC), Department of Radiology, Functional and Molecular Imaging Key Laboratory of Sichuan Province, West China Hospital, Sichuan University, Chengdu, People's Republic of China
e-mail: zwgu@scu.edu.cn


H. Tian and X. Chen (eds.), *Gene Delivery*, Biomaterial Engineering,
https://doi.org/10.1007/978-981-16-5419-0_19

**Abstract**

Much effort has been devoted to developing virus-inspired gene delivery systems that are able to invade target cells and release cargos in a controlled and programmed manner inside cells. In this regard, a new concept of reduction-controlled hierarchical unpacking is proposed for developing a virus-mimicking gene delivery system. This protocol describes the fabrications of the reduction-controlled hierarchical unpacking terplexes based on the disulfide bonds functionalized hyaluronic acid and diselenide-crosslinked oligoethylenimine, which is designed to be stepwise triggered by gradient reduced reagent both at the tumor site and intracellular compartment. Here, the synthesis techniques of disulfide bonds functionalized hyaluronic acid and diselenide-crosslinked oligoethylenimine are described. A GSH level-dependent responsive behavior of the disulfide and diselenide deposited core-shell shaped terplexes is introduced. The sequential disassembly of cationic core and release of gene payload is confirmed by size, morphology, and FRET signals. Finally, the hierarchical unpacking terplexes achieve highly accelerated gene transfection *in vitro* and *in vivo*. The outstanding outcome of the GSH-controlled hierarchical unpacking gene delivery systems provides a powerful approach to achieve efficient gene delivery.

**Keywords**

Diselenide linkage · Disulfide linkage · Reduction-stimuli · Hierarchical unpacking · Gene delivery

# 1 Introduction

Gene therapy has attracted much attention as a promising treatment for genetic diseases and cancer through correcting genetic defects. The outcome of gene therapy relies on the secure delivery of nucleic acids through the extracellular barriers to the desired tissue and a capacity to reach the intracellular targets. It has proved to be a challenge to design gene delivery systems capable of overcoming extracellular and intracellular obstacles to maximize nucleic acids cargo at desired sites while minimizing the undesired side effects. As the most powerful natural gene vectors, viruses infect host cells with the "Trojan Horse" tactic and undergo dynamic transformation to unpack and dissociate the genome according to the signals from extracellular or intracellular (Smith and Helenius 2004). However, the potential dangers of immunogenicity and mutagenesis hinder its large-scale clinical applications (Brun et al. 2017). A growing number of studies indicate that designed gene delivery systems in a stimuli-sensitive fashion can be used as a useful approach for facilitating the delivery efficiency and specificity of gene payload, which is desired for highly efficient gene transfection (Ahmadi et al. 2020; Zhang et al. 2020). Virus-inspired mimics have been gaining strong momentum as the next generation of gene delivery systems (Luo et al. 2019), especially the profiles alter in response to stimuli including reduced reagents (Wang et al. 2021; Wang et al. 2020; Liang et al. 2020), reactive oxygen species (ROS) (Zhang et al. 2019; Zhou et al. 2021), pH gradients (Guan et al. 2016), and so on.

The different signals generated from extracellular and intracellular microenvironments, or biological sites and disease tissues, can be explored as biological triggers when designing stimuli-responsive gene carriers. This might be one of the highly promising methods for conquering the series of extracellular and intracellular hurdles. The main hurdles toward successful gene delivery (Whitehead et al. 2009) include (1) packaging of the nucleic acids by the carrier, (2) keeping stability during the circulation, and (3) specific cellular binding, (4) endosomal escape, (5) intracellular trafficking, (6) nucleic acids release, and (7) nuclear transportation. One approach to constructing stimulus-responsive gene vectors is to design them triggered by one specific stimulus, such as temperature, protease, and redox potential. In the case of redox-sensitive cationic polymers (Yue et al. 2014; Cheng et al. 2012), the reducing intracellular condition can facilitate disassembly of polyplexes and release the gene payload, which is beneficial for the delivery of nucleic acid in the intracellular target site. An alternative approach utilizes the pH gradient in the tumor microenvironment and intracellular region to trigger the dissociation of dual-pH sensitive carrier (Du et al. 2011; Mo et al. 2012), this design endowed the carrier improved physical stability, facilitated cellular uptake at the tumor site, and enhanced the release of the cargo inside cells.

Polyplexes formed by electrostatic interactions between cationic polymers and nucleic acids have gained increasing interest as gene delivery systems. The composition of the polyplexes can be manipulated to possess desired stimuli-sensitive features. Inspired by the dynamic transformations of viruses when sensing and responding to signals from the microenvironment, a new concept of reduction-controlled hierarchical unpacking is proposed for developing a virus-mimicking gene delivery system, which is designed to be stepwise triggered by gradient reduced reagent both at the tumor site and inside the cells. In this protocol, instructions to synthesize the disulfide bonds functionalized hyaluronic acid (HA-SS-COOH) (He et al. 2013a, b; He et al. 2014; He et al. 2016) and the diselenide-crosslinked oligoethylenimine (OEI-SeSex) (Yue et al. 2014) are described, and most important items are introduced. The fabrication and characterization of reduction-controlled hierarchical unpacking terplexes (DNA/OEI-SeSex/HA-SS-COOH) are mentioned. A GSH concentration-dependent responsive behavior of the disulfide-and diselenide-crosslinked polymers was investigated by the degradability of polymers and the dissociation of polyplexes. The sequential disassembly of the inner core and release of gene cargos of the hierarchical unpacking terplexes were confirmed by size, morphology, and FRET signals (He et al. 2013a, b). The hierarchical unpacking designed terplexes can achieve significantly improved and negligible cytotoxicity.

## 2 Materials

### 2.1 Preparation of 3, 3′-Diselanediyldipropanoic Acid

1. Selenium powder
2. Nitrogen
3. Sodium borohydride ($NaBH_4$)
4. MilliQ ultrapure water
5. 3-Chloropropanoic acid
6. Sodium carbonate ($Na_2CO_3$)
7. Hydrochloric acid (HCl), 1 mol/L
8. Ethyl acetate
9. Anhydrous magnesium sulfate ($MgSO_4$)

### 2.2 Preparation of Diselenide-Crosslinked Oligoethylenimine (OEI-SeSex)

1. 3, 3′-disulfanediyldipropanoic acid
2. 3, 3′-diselanediyldipropanoic acid
3. N-hydroxysuccinimide (NHS)
4. Anhydrous tetrahydrofuran (THF)
5. Oligoethylenimine (OEI 800 Da)
6. Anhydrous dimethyl sulfoxide (DMSO)
7. Ethyl-3-[3-(dimethylamino)-propyl] carbodiimide (EDC)
8. Hydrochloric acid (HCl)
9. Dialysis membrane (MWCO 7 kDa)

### 2.3 Preparation of Disulfide Bonds Functionalized HA (HA-SS-COOH)

1. Ethyl-3-[3-(dimethylamino)-propyl] carbodiimide (EDC)
2. Cystamine dihydrochloride
3. PBS pH 6.8
4. Sodium hyaluronate (HA, 1.6 MDa)
5. Ethanol
6. Hydroxybenzotriazole (HOBt)
7. Dithiothreitol (DTT)
8. 3-mercaptopropionic acid
9. Hydrochloric acid (HCl)
10. Sodium chloride (NaCl)

### 2.4 Preparation of Reduction-Controlled Hierarchical Unpacking Terplexes

1. Diselenide-crosslinked oligoethylenimine (OEI-SeSex)
2. Disulfide bonds functionalized HA (HA-SS-COOH)
3. HBG buffer (20 mM HEPES in 5 % aqueous glucose solution, pH 7.4)
4. Plasmid DNA

### 2.5 Determination of Particle Size and Zeta Potential

1. KCl (1 mM)
2. DNA/PEI biplexes, PEI:DNA = 1.3 (w/w)
3. DNA/OEI-SeSex/HA-SS-COOH terplexes, HA-SS-COOH:DNA = 0 ~ 5 (w/w), OEI-SeSex:DNA = 10 (w/w)

### 2.6 Reduction-Responsive Degradability of OEI-SeSex and OEI-SSx

1. DNA/OEI-SeSex binary polyplexes (biplexes), OEI-SeSex:DNA = 1 (w/w)
2. DNA/OEI-SSx biplexes, OEI-SSx:DNA = 1 (w/w)
3. DNA/PEI biplexes, PEI:DNA = 1.3 (w/w)
4. DNA/OEI biplexes, OEI:DNA =1 (w/w)
5. Naked DNA
6. Reduced glutathione (GSH)
7. Sodium chloride (NaCl)
8. Agarose gel
9. Ethidium bromide
10. Tris-acetate-EDTA

### 2.7 Reduction-Controlled Hierarchical Unpacking Behavior of Terplexes

1. Reduced glutathione (GSH)
2. DNA/OEI-SeSex/HA-SS-COOH terplexes, OEI-SeSex:DNA = 10 (w/w), HA-SS-COOH/DNA = 2 (w/w)
3. Label IT™ Nucleic Acid Labeling Kit, Cy5
4. Label IT™ Nucleic Acid Labeling Kit, Cy3
5. pGL3 (5.2 kb) plasmid
6. Lacy carbon-coated copper grid

### 2.8 Cell Culture and *In Vitro* Viability Assay

1. DNA/OEI-SeSex/HA-SS-COOH terplexes, OEI-SeSex:DNA = 10 (w/w), HA-SS-COOH:DNA = 0 ~ 5 (w/w)
2. DNA/PEI biplexes, PEI:DNA = 1.3 (w/w)
3. HepG2 cells
4. B16F10 cells
5. Heat-inactivated fetal bovine serum
6. DMEM-HG
7. Streptomycin
8. Penicillin
9. 3-(4,5-dimethylthiazol-2-yl)-2,5-diphenyltetrazolium bromide (MTT)
10. PBS, pH 7.4
11. DMSO
12. 96-well plate

### 2.9 *In Vitro* Gene Transfection of Reduction-Controlled Hierarchical Unpacking Terplexes

1. DNA/OEI-SeSex/HA-SS-COOH terplexes, OEI-SeSex:DNA = 10 (w/w), HA-SS-COOH:DNA = 0 ~ 5 (w/w)
2. DNA/PEI biplexes, PEI:DNA = 1.3 (w/w)
3. pEGFP (4.7 kb)
4. pGL3 (5.2 kb)
5. HepG2 cells
6. B16F10 cells
7. Heat-inactivated fetal bovine serum
8. DMEM-HG
9. Streptomycin
10. Penicillin

11. Luciferase reporter assay substrate kit
12. Bicinchoninic acid (BCA) protein assay kit
13. 96-well plate
14. 24-well plate

## 2.10 *In Vivo* Gene Transfection of Reduction-Controlled Hierarchical Unpacking Terplexes

1. BALB/c nude mice
2. Human hepatoma cell line HepG2
3. PBS, pH 7.4
4. Vernier calliper
5. DNA/OEI-SeSex/HA-SS-COOH terplexes, OEI-SeSex:DNA = 10 (w/w), HA-SS-COOH/DNA = 2 (w/w)
6. DNA/PEI biplexes, PEI:DNA = 1.3 (w/w)
7. pEGFP (4.7 kb)

## 2.11 Analytical Instruments

1. Use Zetasizer Nano ZS (Malvern, UK) to record the size and zeta potential of the terplexes.
2. Determine the degradability of OEI-SSx and OEI-SeSex polymers by a Waters 2690D HPLC and a 2410 refractive index detector, equipped with ultrahydrogel 120 and 1000 columns.
3. Record the resulted DNA migration patterns of DNA/OEI-SeSex biplexes and DNA/OEI-SSx biplexes by using the Molecular Imager ChemiDoc XRS+ system (Bio-Rad, USA).
4. Utilize Transmission Electron Microscopy (TEM, FEI Company, USA) to observe the changes in the structure of the terplexes after GSH treatment.
5. Perform fluorescence resonance energy transfer (FRET) by a Spectrophotometer (Hitachi) to evaluate the condensation and reduction-controlled hierarchical unpacking of the terplexes in a reduced environment.
6. Monitor the cell cytotoxicity by the use of a microplate reader (Bio-Rad, USA) to detect the UV absorbance at 490 nm.
7. Utilize an inverted fluorescence microscope to evaluate the in vitro green fluorescent protein expression.
8. Measure the luciferase transfection efficiency through a microplate reader (Bio-Rad, USA).
9. Utilize confocal laser-scanning microscope (Leica TCS SP5) to analyze in vivo GFP expression.

# 3 Methods

## 3.1 Preparation of 3, 3′-Diselanediyldipropanoic Acid (Koch et al. 1990)

1. Add 60 mmol (4.74 g) of selenium powder in $H_2O$ (20 mL) to a three-necked flask under a $N_2$ condition.
2. Dissolve 120 mmol (4.54 g) of $NaBH_4$ in 50 mL of cold water then inject to the above mixture.
3. Stir the reaction solution in an ice-bath, react until the selenium dust was dissolved completely and the reaction system became colorless.
4. Add another 60 mmol of selenium dust and heat to 105 °C for 20 min.
5. Dissolve 120 mmol (13.0 g) of 3-chloropropanoic acid in $H_2O$ (30 mL) and adjust the pH to 8.0 with $Na_2CO_3$.
6. Add the above 3-chloropropanoic acid solution to the reddish-brown reaction mixture and react overnight at r.t. at a $N_2$ condition.
7. Filter the reaction solution after another 4 h of stirring under a nitrogen atmosphere.
8. Adjust the yellow supernatant to pH 3 ~ 4 by adding 1 mol/L HCl solution, and extract two times with ethyl acetate.
9. Wash the ethyl acetate layers with water, dry with anhydrous $MgSO_4$, filter, and recrystallize from ethyl acetate to afford the final product.
10. Confirm the structure of the product with $^1$H-NMR (Fig. 1).

## 3.2 Preparation of Diselenide or Disulfide-Crosslinked Oligoethylenimine

1. Dissolve 2.4 mmol (0.73 g) of 3, 3′-diselanediyldipropanoic acid, or 2.4 mmol (0.50 g) of 3, 3′-disulfanediyldipropanoic acid and 5.8 mmol of NHS (0.66 g) in anhydrous THF (10 mL). Then add it to a three-necked flask at a $N_2$ condition.
2. Dissolve 5.8 mmol (0.89 g) of EDC in 10 mL of anhydrous THF then add to the mixture at 0 °C.
3. Stir the reaction solution overnight at r.t.

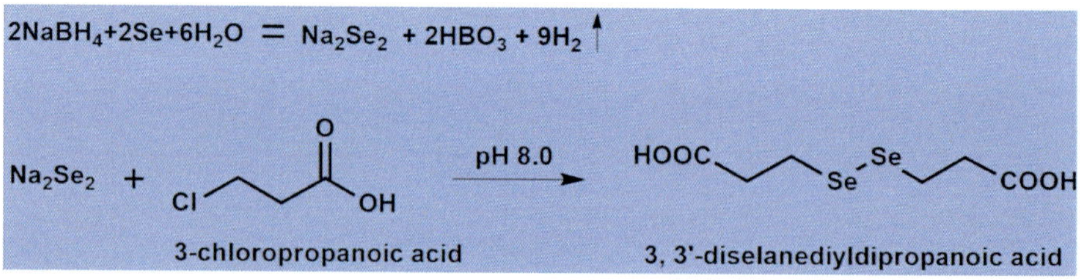


**Fig. 1** Synthesis diagram of 3, 3′-diselanediyldipropanoic acid

4. Filter, evaporate, and re-dissolve in 1.0 mL of anhydrous DMSO.
5. Dissolve 2.0 mmol of oligoethylenimine (1.60 g) in $H_2O$ maintaining the pH 7.4 and then lyophilized.
6. Re-dissolve the above oligoethylenimine in DMSO (4 mL), and mix with the obtained NHS ester under nitrogen.
7. Stir the solution for 48 h at 35 °C, and dialyze with $H_2O$ using dialysis membrane (MWCO 7 kDa).
8. Freeze-dry and obtain the final products of $OEI_{800}$-SeSex or $OEI_{800}$-SSx (Figs. 2 and 3).

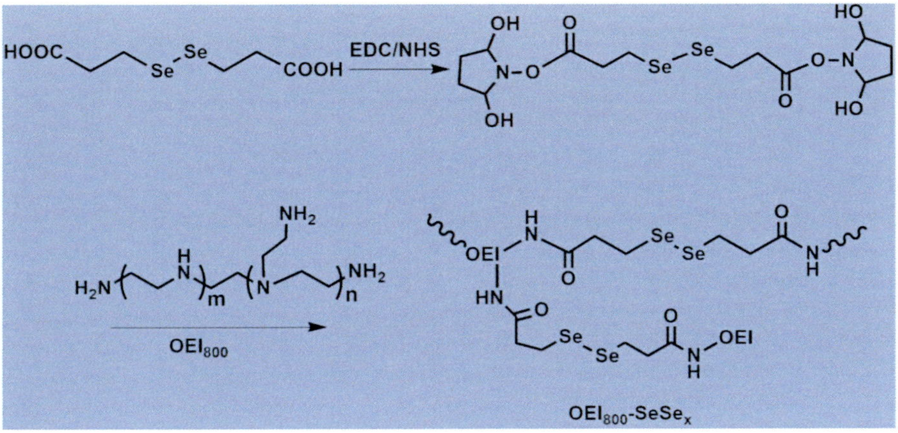


**Fig. 2** Synthesis diagram of diselenide-conjugated oligoethylenimine (OEI-$SeSe_x$)

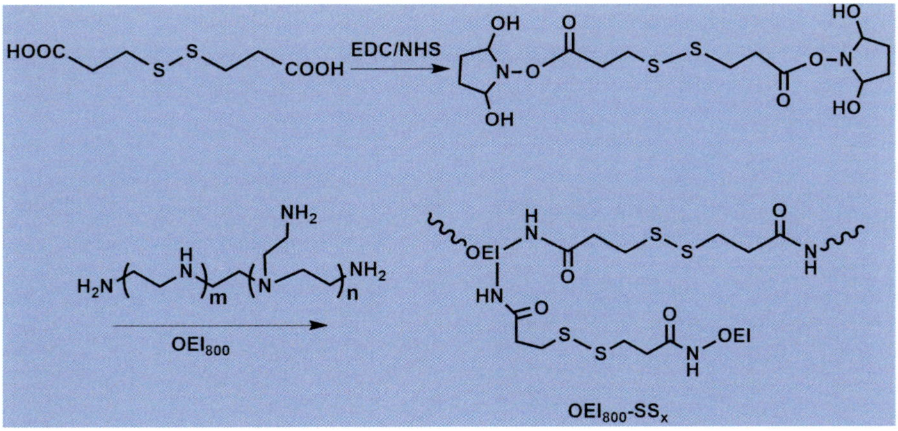


**Fig. 3** Synthesis diagram of disulfide-conjugated oligoethylenimine (OEI-$SS_x$)

### 3.3 Preparation of HA-SS-COOH (Note 1)

1. Add 3.0 mmol (575.2 mg) of EDC and 3.0 mmol (405.4 mg) of HOBt to 1.0 mmol of HA (400 mg) in 80 mL of PBS pH 6.8 for 2 h to activate the carboxyl groups.
2. Add 3.0 mmol (675.6 mg) of cystamine dihydrochloride to the solution at r.t. for 1 day to obtain cystamine modified HA.
3. Dialyze exhaustively the reaction solution against deionized water with a dialysis membrane (MWCO 3.5 kDa).
4. Treat HA-cys with a five-fold excess of DTT to reduce disulfide linkage in PBS pH 8.5 at r.t. for 4 h.
5. Maintain the solution at pH 3.5.
6. Add sodium chloride to achieve a concentration of 5 % (w/v).
7. Precipitate the thiol groups modified HA with ethanol, re-dissolve it in water, centrifuge, and freeze-dry to obtain thiolated HA.
8. React 1.0 mmol of the obtained thiolated HA in 50 mL of PBS with 100 equiv. of 3-mercaptopropionic acid overnight at room temperature.
9. Dialyze and freeze-dry to obtain HA-SS-COOH.
10. Prepare the HA-SS-COOH with different disulfide contents by optimizing the EDC: HOBt: cystamine: HA ratios.
11. Confirm the HA-SS-COOH product by $^1$H-NMR (Fig. 4).

### 3.4 Preparation of Reduction-Controlled Hierarchical Unpacking Terplexes (Note 2)

1. First, mix DNA and OEI-SeSex solution at an appropriate ratio in HBG buffer and incubate at r.t. for 20 min to form DNA/OEI-SeSex binary polyplexes.
2. Subsequently, add the DNA/OEI-SeSex biplexes to a solution of HA-SS-COOH at HA-SS-COOH/DNA ratio of 0–5 (w/w) and incubate for another 20 min to form DNA/OEI-SeSex/HA-SS-COOH terplexes.
3. Prepare DNA/OEI-SeSex/HA-SS-COOH terplexes used in the following experiments with OEI-SeSex/DNA = 10 (W/W) and HA-SS-COOH/DNA = 2 (W/W), respectively, unless otherwise specified (Fig. 5).

### 3.5 Determination of Particle Size and Zeta Potential

1. Prepare DNA/OEI-SeSex/HA-SS-COOH terplexes at a concentration of 3 μg/mL DNA (total volume 1 mL) for size measurement.
2. Dilute five-fold in 1 mM KCl solution and determine the zeta potential of the terplexes.
3. Use DNA/PEI biplexes, PEI/DNA = 1.3 (w/w) as a control (Fig. 6).

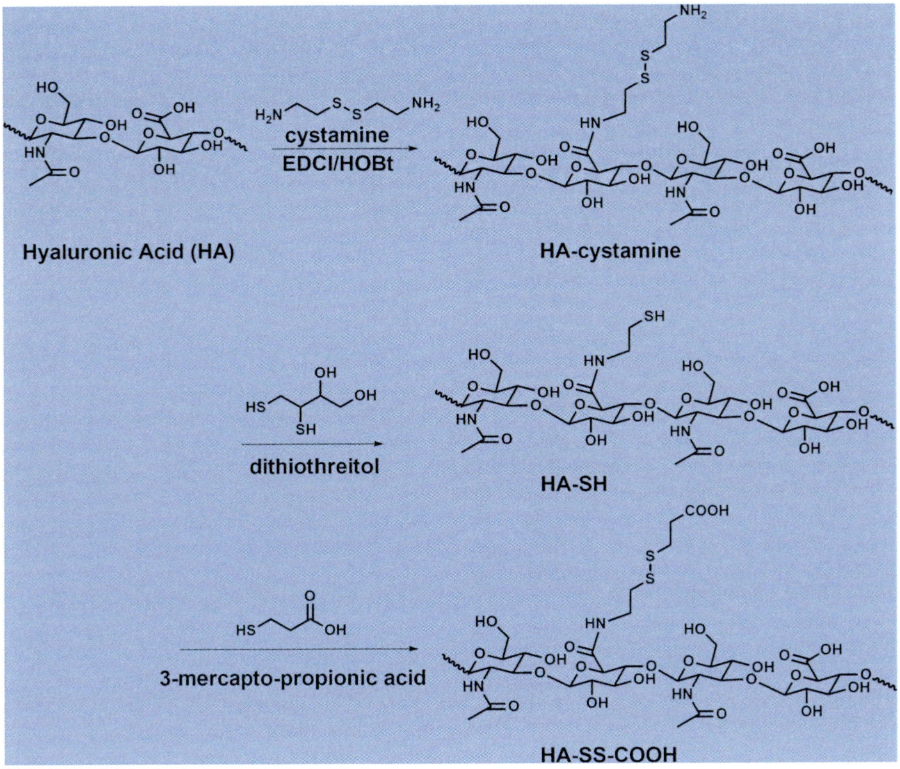


**Fig. 4** Preparation diagram of the HA-SS-COOH

### 3.6 Reduction-Responsive Degradability of OEI-SeSex and OEI-SSx (Note 3 and 4)

1. Incubate OEI-SSx and OEI-SeSex in redox stimuli (10 μM for 8 h and 100 μM GSH for 4 h) at 37 °C, respectively, to evaluate the reduction-responsive degradability of diselenide-crosslinked oligoethylenimine (OEI-SeSex) with its disulfide-crosslinked analogue (OEI-SSx).
2. Before and after the treatment, determine the molecular weight of the OEI-SSx and OEI-SeSex polymers by using gel permeation chromatography.
3. Use oligoethylenimine 800 Da and polyethylenimine 25 kDa as controls.
4. In addition, compare the reduction-responsiveness of OEI-SeSex with OEI-SSx by using gel retardation assay in the form of DNA/OEI-SeSex and DNA/OEI-SSx polyplexes.
5. Select the weight ratio of 1 (OEI-SeSex/DNA or OEI-SSx/DNA) for DNA/OEI-SeSex or DNA/OEI-SSx polyplexes.
6. Use naked DNA, DNA/OEI polyplexes and DNA/PEI polyplexes as controls.

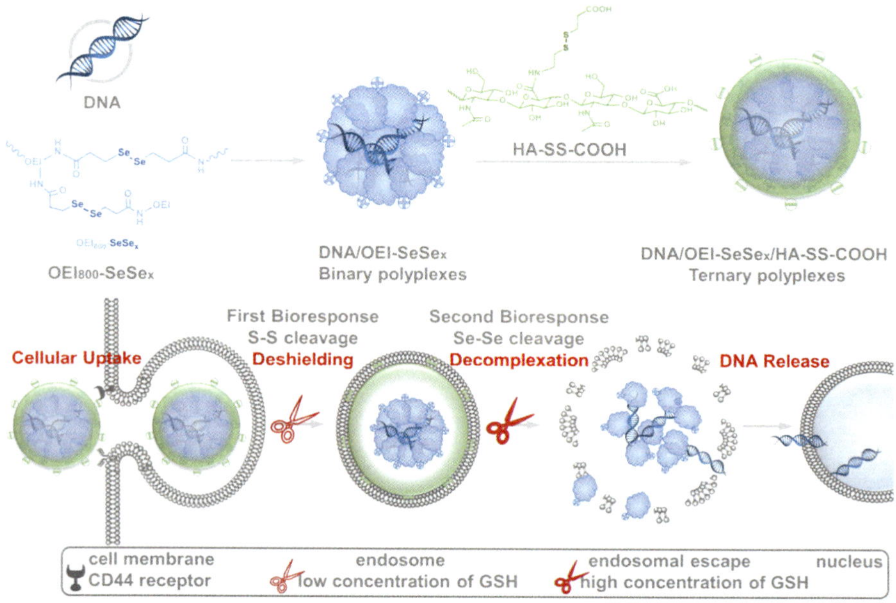


**Fig. 5** Schematic illustration for the preparation of reduction-controlled hierarchical unpacking terplexes for gene delivery: CD44 receptor-mediated endocytosis, low concentration of GSH regulated deshielding of HA-SS-COOH, high concentration of GSH triggered decomplexation of polyplexes, the release of DNA and delivery to nuclei

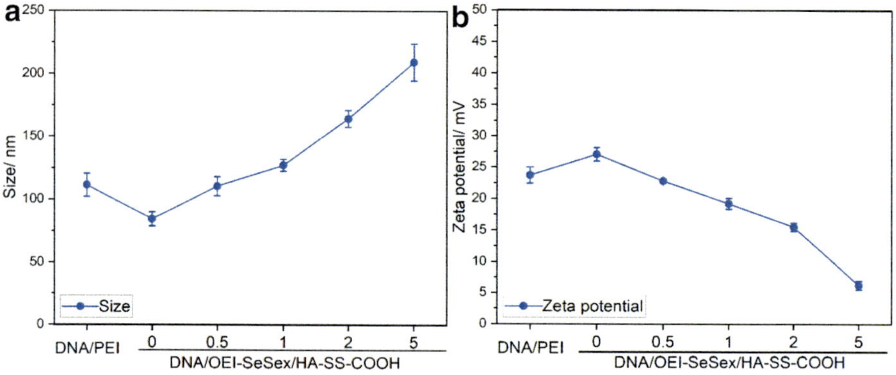


**Fig. 6** Particle size and zeta potential measurements. DNA/OEI-SeSex/HA-SS-COOH terplexes: OEI-SeSex/DNA = 10 (w/w) and HA-SS-COOH/DNA = 0 ~ 5 (w/w). DNA/PEI biplexes, PEI/DNA = 1.3 (w/w)

7. Select the weight ratio of 1 (OEI/DNA) for DNA/OEI polyplexes.
8. Select the weight ratio of 1.3 (PEI/DNA) for DNA/PEI polyplexes.
9. Incubate polyplexes at indicated GSH concentrations (0, 10 μM, 20 μM, 100 μM and 5 mM) in the absence of 0.3 M NaCl for 2 h at 37 °C.

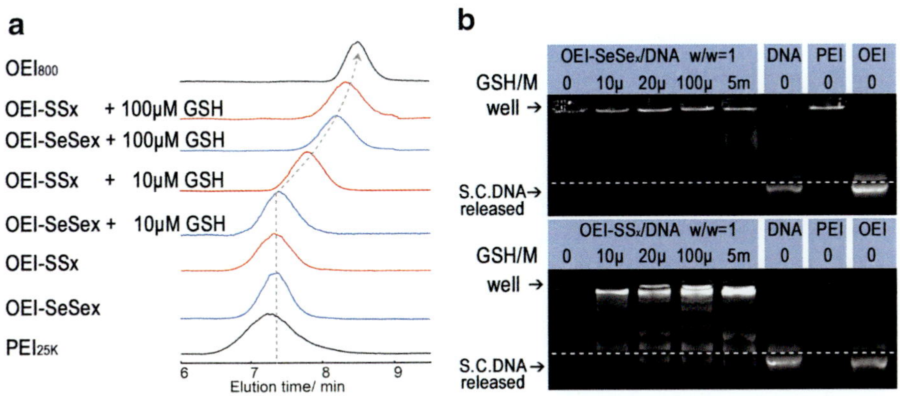


**Fig. 7** (**a**) Gel-permeation chromatography diagrams of OEI-SSx and OEI-SeSe$_x$ after treatment with GSH. (**b**) Gel retardation assay of supercoiled (S.C.) DNA released from OEI-SSx/DNA and OEI-SeSe$_x$/DNA biplexes after treatment with different concentrations of GSH

10. Record expansion kinetics of the OEI-SeSex/DNA and OEI-SSx/DNA polyplexes (weight ratio = 10) at 37 °C with the treatment of 10 μM or 20 μM GSH every 5 min for 6 h.
11. Electrophorese ten microliters of polyplexes solution containing 0.2 μg DNA on the 0.8 % (w/v) agarose gel with Tris-acetate-EDTA running buffer at 80 V for 60 min.
12. Stain the agarose gels with ethidium bromide after electrophoresis.
13. Use the Molecular Imager ChemiDoc XRS+ system to observe the DNA migration patterns (Fig. 7).

### 3.7 Reduction-Controlled Hierarchical Unpacking Behavior of Terplexes (Note 5 and 6)

1. Add gradient GSH concentrations into DNA/OEI-SeSex/HA-SS-COOH terplexes solution to simulate the physiological condition in circulation (no GSH), weak reducing milieu (10 μM GSH) around the tumor (Kuppusamy et al. 2002) and intracellular reduction environments (5 mM GSH) (Saito et al. 2003).
2. Incubate the DNA/OEI-SeSex/HA-SS-COOH polyplexes with various GSH levels (0, 10 μM and 5 mM) for 2 h at 37 °C.
3. Deposit a drop of polyplexes solution on a lacy carbon-coated copper grid and air-dried. Investigate the changes in the structure of the terplexes through transmission electron microscopy (TEM).
4. Study the kinetics of size changes of the terplexes through Malvern Instruments.
5. Perform fluorescence resonance energy transfer (FRET) spectrofluorometry to evaluate the complexation and reduction-controlled hierarchical unpacking of the terplexes in a reduced environment.
6. Label the pGL3 plasmid with Cy3 and Cy5 for monitoring FRET spectrofluorometry.

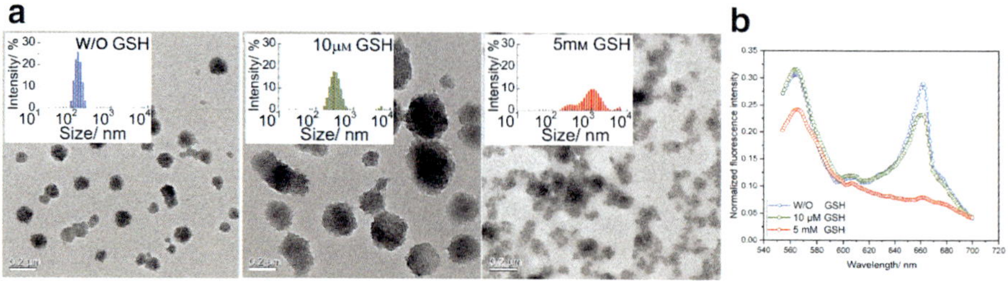


**Fig. 8** Redox responsive hierarchical unpacking behaviors of DNA/OEI-SeSex/HA-SS-COOH terplexes. (**a**) Morphology and size distributions. Scale bar: 0.2 μm. (**b**) FRET spectra of the terplexes after incubation with GSH for 2 h. DNA/OEI-SeSex/HA-SS-COOH terplexes: OEI-SeSex/DNA = 10 (w/w) and HA-SS-COOH/DNA = 2 (w/w)

7. Use the Cy3 and Cy5 dual-labeled DNA to prepare the terplexes.
8. Incubate the Cy3 and Cy5 dual-labeled terplexes with various GSH concentrations (0, 10 μM and 5 mM) for 2 h at 37 °C.
9. Use 200 microliters of Cy3 and Cy5 dual-labelled terplexes solution containing 3 μg DNA for the spectrofluorometry study.
10. Choose 543 nm as excitation wavelength, record the fluorescence emission spectrum from 550 to 700 nm, and the step length and bandwidth are both 5 nm (Fig. 8).

## 3.8 Cell Culture and *In Vitro* Viability Assay

1. Maintain HepG2 and B16F10 cells in DMEM-HG medium containing 10 % (v/v) fetal bovine serum, 100 μg/mL streptomycin and 100 IU/mL penicillin.
2. Perform all cell cultures at 37 °C in a humidified incubator with 5 % carbon dioxide.
3. Determine the metabolic activity of the cells treated with the terplexes by MTT assay.
4. Seed cells at a density of $1 \times 10^4$ cells per well in 96 wells culture plates.
5. Culture cells overnight to achieve 70 ~ 80 % cell confluence.
6. Replace the culture medium with a fresh medium containing 10 % (v/v) fetal bovine serum.
7. Add DNA/OEI-SeSex/HA-SS-COOH terplexes with OEI-SeSex/DNA = 10 and HA-SS-COOH/DNA = 0 ~ 5 (w/w), to achieve a final concentration of 0.4 μg/well DNA.
8. Culture the cells for 24 h.
9. Prepare 5 mg/mL MTT PBS solution, add 10 μL to each well, and incubate for another 4 h.
10. Replace the medium with DMSO (100 μL).
11. Detect the UV absorbance at 490 nm by using a microplate reader.
12. Use untreated cells as a positive control.
13. Use DNA/PEI biplexes, PEI/DNA = 1.3 (w/w) as a negative control.
14. Express the metabolic activity as a relative to the untreated control (Fig. 9).

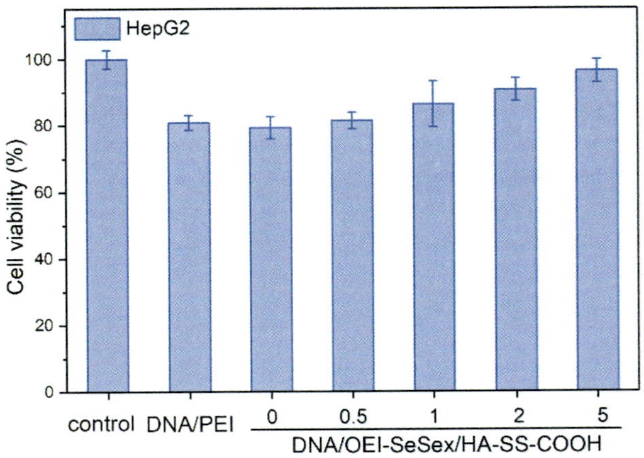


**Fig. 9** Cell viability exposed to different polyplexes against HepG2 cells. DNA/OEI-SeSex/HA-SS-COOH terplexes: OEI-SeSex/DNA = 10 (w/w) and HA-SS-COOH/DNA = 2 (w/w)

### 3.9 *In Vitro* Gene Transfection of Reduction-Controlled Hierarchical Unpacking Terplexes (Note 7)

1. Investigate gene transfection ability of the reduction-controlled hierarchical unpacking terplexes in HepG2 and B16F10 cells in the presence of 10 % fetal bovine serum.
2. Use binary polyplexes of PEI and DNA with the weight ratio of 1.3 (DNA/PEI polyplexes) as a golden standard control.
3. Use Plasmid pGL3 and pEGFP as reporter genes for the quantitative and qualitative studies, respectively.
4. For the quantitative study, seed HepG2 cells at a density of $1 \times 10^4$ cells per well in 96-well plates.
5. Culture cells to achieve 70 ~ 80 % cell confluence.
6. Replace the culture medium with a fresh medium containing 10 % (v/v) fetal bovine serum.
7. Add DNA/OEI-SeSex/HA-SS-COOH terplexes: OEI-SeSex/DNA = 10 (w/w) and HA-SS-COOH/DNA = 0 ~ 5 (w/w) to achieve a final concentration of DNA 0.2 μg per well.
8. Change the culture medium with 100 μL fresh complete medium after 4 h incubation.
9. Cultivate cells for an additional 20 h and then process them for the luciferase expression analysis.
10. Measure the luciferase activity by a microplate reader.
11. Determine the total protein content by BCA protein assay.
12. Express the luciferase transfection level as relative light units per mg protein (RLU/mg protein).
13. For the qualitative study, select DNA/OEI-SeSex/HA-SS-COOH terplexes: OEI-SeSex/DNA = 10 (w/w) and HA-SS-COOH/DNA = 2 (w/w).
14. Seed HepG2 or B16F10 cells at a density of $5 \times 10^4$ cells per well in 24-well plates.

15. Cultivate cells to achieve 70 ~ 80 % cell confluence.
16. Replace the culture medium with 0.5 mL of fresh medium containing 10 % (v/v) fetal bovine serum.
17. Add DNA/OEI-SeSex/HA-SS-COOH terplexes, DNA/OEI-SeSex biplexes, and DNA/PEI biplexes to give a final concentration of 1.0 μg/well DNA.
18. Change the culture medium with 0.5 mL fresh complete medium after 4 h incubation.
19. Cultivate cells for additional 44 h of incubation.
20. Evaluate enhanced green fluorescent protein (EGFP) expression level using an inverted fluorescence microscope (Fig. 10).

### 3.10 *In Vivo* Gene Transfection of Reduction-Controlled Hierarchical Unpacking Terplexes

1. Carry out all mice experiments following the ethics of our institutional and NIH guidelines.
2. Maintain BALB/c nude mice under specific pathogen-free (SPF) conditions at 24 ± 1 °C, 55 ± 10 % humidity with a 12-h day and night alternate, and allow free eating.
3. Inject subcutaneously 50 μL of $1 \times 10^6$ HepG2 cells suspension in sterile PBS in the right-back of five-week old mice.
4. Use a vernier calliper to measure the longest and shortest diameters of the tumor. Calculate its volume by the following equation: $\text{Volume} = 0.5 \times \text{longest} \times \text{shortest}^2$.
5. Randomly divide mice into four groups ($n = 6$) when the sizes of tumors reach 80–100 $mm^3$.
6. Inject intratumorally either PBS, naked DNA, DNA/PEI biplexes, or DNA/OEI-SeSex/HA-SS-COOH terplexes into tumors at a dosage of 15 μg pEGFP.
7. Two days after injection, sacrifice the mice and resect their tumors.
8. Wash tumors with ice-cold PBS, freeze and cut tumors into 5 μm thick cryosections.
9. Use a confocal laser-scanning microscope to analyze the GFP transfection (Fig. 11).

### 3.11 Statistical Analysis

1. Show results as the average ± standard deviation.
2. Record results from at least triplicated experiments.
3. Analyze differences between two groups by a two-tailed unpaired Student's t-test.
4. Consider a value of $P < 0.05$ to be significant.

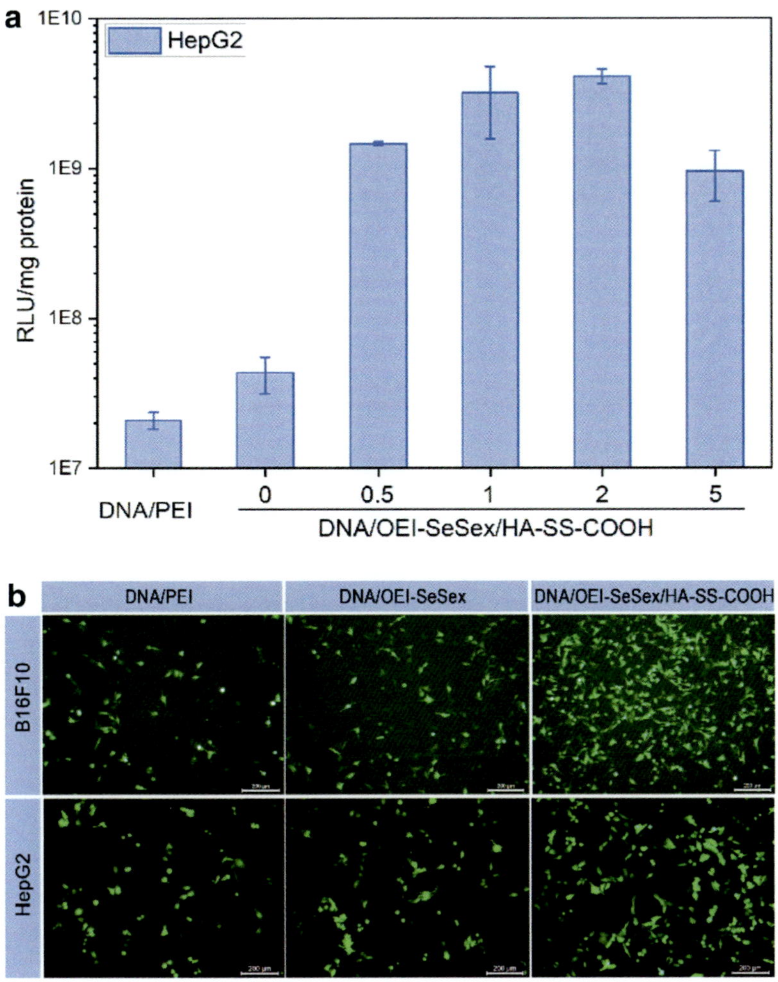


**Fig. 10** (**a**) Luciferase gene transfection of the terplexes with 10 % serum in HepG2 cells. DNA/OEI-SeSex/HA-SS-COOH terplexes: OEI-SeSex/DNA = 10 (w/w) and HA-SS-COOH/DNA = 0 ~ 5 (w/w). (**b**) EGFP gene transfection with 10 % serum in B16F10 and HepG2 cells. DNA/OEI-SeSex/HA-SS-COOH terplexes: OEI-SeSex/DNA = 10 (w/w) and HA-SS-COOH/DNA = 2 (w/w). DNA/OEI-SeSex biplexes: OEI-SeSex/DNA = 10 (w/w)

## 4 Notes

1. pH should be controlled accurately for the preparation of disulfide bonds functionalized hyaluronic acid (HA-SS-COOH) (He et al. 2013a, b; He et al. 2014), which contains condensation, reduction, and oxidation. For the

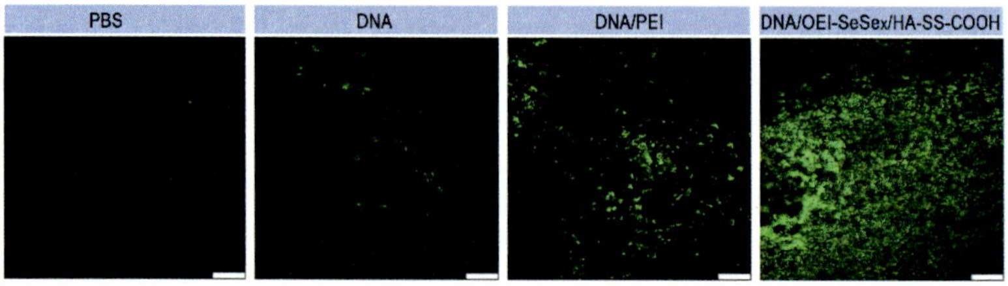


**Fig. 11** EGFP transfection in HepG2-tumor-bearing nude mice at 48 h post-intratumoral administration (15 μg DNA per mouse). DNA/OEI-SeSex/HA-SS-COOH terplexes: OEI-SeSex/DNA = 10 (w/w) and HA-SS-COOH/DNA = 2 (w/w). DNA/PEI biplexes, PEI:DNA = 1.3 (w/w). Scale bar:100 μm

condensation step, the neutral pH 6.8 was optimized for the viscous hyaluronic acid to conjugate with cystamine. For the reduction step, cystamine conjugated HA was treated with excess DTT in alkaline condition (pH 8.5) for the cleavage of disulfide linkages to afford thiolated HA. After cleavage, the pH was adjusted to 3.5 to avoid self-crosslinking of thiolated HA.

2. For the preparation of the terplexes, the mixing sequence of anionic nucleic acids, cationic OEI-SeSex polymer, and anionic HA-SS-COOH could affect the complexation including size and surface charge and thus correlate to the transfection efficiency and cytotoxicity (Cho et al. 2015; Cai et al. 2013). In this study, anionic nucleic acids solution was added to cationic OEI-SeSex polymer to form binary polyplexes. Then the DNA/OEI-SeSex binary polyplexes solution was transferred to the anionic HA-SS-COOH for shielding the binary polyplexes and forming the terplexes.
3. To study the differences between diselenide linkages and disulfide linkages, OEI-SeSex and OEI-SSx with similar molecular weight and its distribution were synthesized from oligoethylenimine 800 Da (Yue et al. 2014; Cheng et al. 2012). Particularly, the golden standard branched PEI 25 kDa and low molecular weight of oligoethylenimine were used as controls when investigating the reductive stimuli degradability, DNA binding, and release abilities. The results showed in Fig.7 indicate a GSH level-dependent sensitive behavior of the disulfide and diselenide linkages, indicating they could construct as a reduction-controlled hierarchical unpacking gene delivery system.
4. It is noteworthy that the stability of the DNA/OEI-SeSex polyplexes and DNA/OEI-SSx polyplexes highly depends on the reduced conditions. Moreover, the polyplexes stability is also affected by the ionic strength (Yu et al. 2009). A sufficient level of GSH could destabilize the DNA/OEI-SeSex polyplexes or DNA/OEI-SSx polyplexes. However, GSH in the absence of ionic buffer is not sufficient for DNA release from the destabilized polyplexes. Therefore, all samples were incubated with 0.3 M sodium chloride to ensure the release of DNA could be detected.
5. FRET was performed to monitor the reduction-controlled hierarchical unpacking behavior of the terplexes under reduced conditions. An ideal FRET donor-acceptor pair should possess separated emission spectra and a certain degree of overlap between donor emission and acceptor absorption (Xu et al. 2009). In addition, only when the distance between the donor and the receptor is less than

10 nm, the emit FRET signals can be detected. In this study, the Cy3-Cy5 pair is selected and labeled onto DNA molecules for FRET analysis.
6. To study the reduction-controlled hierarchical unpacking behavior of the terplexes, 10–20 μM GSH and 5 mM GSH were used to simulate weak reducing milieu around tumor (Kuppusamy et al. 2002) and intracellular reduction environments (Saito et al. 2003), respectively.
7. In general, the transfection capacity of cationic polymers is prominently inhibited in the serum-containing condition, which is a significant obstacle for the in vivo application (Li et al. 2018; Liu et al. 2021). Because of the shielding effect of HA-SS-COOH from negatively charged serum proteins, and CD44 receptor-mediated cellular uptake profile (He et al. 2013a, b), the terplexes achieved much stronger gene transfection than DNA/OEI-SeSex polyplexes or DNA/PEI biplexes in the presence of 10 % serum.

## 5 Summary

This protocol presents a virus-mimicking gene delivery system based on the disulfide bonds functionalized hyaluronic acid and diselenide-crosslinked oligoethylenimine. This reduction-controlled hierarchical unpacking terplexes could be triggered by gradient GSH level, thus disassembly of the inner core and release of DNA in a controlled and programmed manner. In vitro and in vivo studies demonstrated that the designed gene carriers achieve significantly improved gene transfection and negligible cytotoxicity.

## References

Ahmadi S, Rabiee N, Bagherzadeh M, Elmi F, Fatahi Y, Farjadian F, Baheiraei N, Nasseri B, Rabiee M, Dastjerd NT, Valibeik A, Karimi M, Hamblin MR (2020) Stimulus-responsive sequential release systems for drug and gene delivery. Nano Today 34:100914

Brun MJ, Gomez EJ, Suh J (2017) Stimulus-responsive viral vectors for controlled delivery of therapeutics. J Control Release 267:80–89

Cai X, Dong H, Ma J, Zhu H, Wu W, Chu M, Li Y, Shi D (2013) Effects of spatial distribution of the nuclear localization sequence on gene transfection in catiomer–gene polyplexes. J Mater Chem B 1:1712–1721

Cheng G, He Y, Xie L, Nie Y, He B, Zhang Z, Gu Z (2012) Development of a reduction-sensitive diselenide-conjugated oligoethylenimine nanoparticulate system as a gene carrier. Int J Nanomedicine 7:3991–4006

Cho SK, Dang C, Wang X, Ragan R, Kwon YJ (2015) Mixing-sequence-dependent nucleic acid complexation and gene transfer efficiency by polyethylenimine. Biomater Sci 3:1124–1133

Du J-Z, Du X-J, Mao C-Q, Wang J (2011) Tailor-made dual pH-sensitive polymer–doxorubicin nanoparticles for efficient anticancer drug delivery. J Am Chem Soc 133:17560–17563

Guan X, Guo Z, Lin L, Chen J, Tian H, Chen X (2016) Ultrasensitive pH triggered charge/size dual-rebound gene delivery system. Nano Lett 16:6823–6831

He Y, Cheng G, Xie L, Nie Y, He B, Gu Z (2013a) Polyethyleneimine/DNA polyplexes with reduction-sensitive hyaluronic acid derivatives shielding for targeted gene delivery. Biomaterials 34:1235–1245

He Y, Nie Y, Cheng G, Xie L, Shen Y, Gu Z (2013b) Viral mimicking ternary Polyplexes: a reduction-controlled hierarchical unpacking vector for gene delivery. Adv Mater 26: 1534–1540
He Y, Nie Y, Xie L, Song H, Gu Z (2014) p53 mediated apoptosis by reduction sensitive shielding ternary complexes based on disulfide linked PEI ternary complexes. Biomaterials 35:1657–1666
He Y, Zhou J, Ma S, Nie Y, Yue D, Jiang Q, Wali ARM, Tang JZ, Gu Z (2016) Multi-responsive "turn-on" Nanocarriers for efficient site-specific gene delivery in vitro and in vivo. Adv Healthc Mater 5:2799–2812
Koch T, Suenson E, Henriksen U, Buchardt O (1990) The oxidative cleavability of protein cross-linking reagents containing organoselenium bridges. Bioconjug Chem 1:296–304
Kuppusamy P, Li H, Ilangovan G, Cardounel AJ, Zweier JL, Yamada K, Krishna MC, Mitchell JB (2002) Noninvasive imaging of tumor redox status and its modification by tissue glutathione levels. Cancer Res 62:307–312
Li D, Sharili AS, Connelly J, Gautrot JE (2018) Highly stable RNA capture by dense cationic polymer brushes for the design of cytocompatible, Serum-stable SiRNA delivery vectors. Biomacromolecules 19:606–615
Liang H, Bi Q, Hu A, Chen X, Jin R, Song X, Ke B, Barz M, Nie Y (2020) A nitroreductase and glutathione responsive nanoplatform for integration of gene delivery and near-infrared fluorescence imaging. Chem Commun 56:6949–6952
Liu H, Liu C, Ye L, Ma D, He X, Tang Q, Zhao X, Zou H, Chen X, Liu P (2021) Nanoassemblies with effective serum tolerance capability achieving robust gene silencing efficacy for breast cancer gene therapy. Adv Mater 33:2003523
Luo T, Liang H, Jin R, Nie Y (2019) Virus-inspired and mimetic designs in non-viral gene delivery. J Gene Med 21:e3090
Mo R, Sun Q, Xue J, Li N, Li W, Zhang C, Ping Q (2012) Multistage pH-responsive liposomes for mitochondrial-targeted anticancer drug delivery. Adv Mater 24:3659–3665
Saito G, Swanson JA, Lee K-D (2003) Drug delivery strategy utilizing conjugation via reversible disulfide linkages: role and site of cellular reducing activities. Adv Drug Deliv Rev 55:199–215
Smith AE, Helenius A (2004) How viruses enter animal cells. Science 304:237–242
Wang G, Zhu D, Zhou Z, Piao Y, Tang J, Shen Y (2020) Glutathione-specific and intracellularly labile polymeric Nanocarrier for efficient and safe cancer gene delivery. ACS Appl Mater Interfaces 12:14825–14838
Wang Y, Shahi PK, Wang X, Xie R, Zhao Y, Wu M, Roge S, Pattnaik BR, Gong S (2021) In vivo targeted delivery of nucleic acids and CRISPR genome editors enabled by GSH-responsive silica nanoparticles. J Control Release 336:296–309
Whitehead KA, Langer R, Anderson DG (2009) Knocking down barriers: advances in siRNA delivery. Nat Rev Drug Discov 8:129–138
Xu PS, Quick GK, Yeo Y (2009) Gene delivery through the use of a hyaluronate-associated intracellularly degradable crosslinked polyethyleneimine. Biomaterials 30:5834–5843
Yu H, Russ V, Wagner E (2009) Influence of the molecular weight of bioreducible oligoethylenimine conjugates on the polyplex transfection properties. AAPS J 11:445–455
Yue D, Cheng G, He Y, Nie Y, Jiang Q, Cai X, Gu Z (2014) Influence of reduction-sensitive diselenide bonds and disulfide bonds on oligoethylenimine conjugates for gene delivery. J Mater Chem B 2:7210–7221
Zhang Y, Zhou J, Ma S, He Y, Yang J, Gu Z (2019) Reactive oxygen species (ROS)-degradable polymeric Nanoplatform for hypoxia-targeted gene delivery: unpacking DNA and reducing toxicity. Biomacromolecules 20:1899–1913
Zhang M, Guo X, Wang M, Liu K (2020) Tumor microenvironment-induced structure changing drug/gene delivery system for overcoming delivery-associated challenges. J Control Release 323:203–224
Zhou J, Ma S, Zhang Y, He Y, Mao H, Yang J, Zhang H, Luo K, Gong Q, Gu Z (2021) Bacterium-mimicking sequentially targeted therapeutic nanocomplexes based on O-carboxymethyl chitosan and their cooperative therapy by dual-modality light manipulation. Carbohydr Polym 264:118030

# Bioreducible Zinc (II)-Coordinative Polyethylenimine with Low Molecular Weight for Robust Gene Delivery of Primary and Stem Cells

# 20

Shuai Liu and Tianying Guo

## Contents



**Abstract**

Low molecular weight (LMW) cationic polymers show safety profile and biocompatibility, but are hindered of limited efficacy in gene delivery. This protocol describes a zinc(II) coordinative strategy to transform common LMW cationic polymers to highly efficient and safe gene vehicles. LMW cationic polymers exhibit lower efficacy compared to their high molecular weight counterparts, largely attributed to weaker nucleic acid binding. From this point of view, zinc dipicolylamine (Zn-DPA) analogs showing high phosphate binding affinity are used to functionalize LMW cationic polymers to obtain higher DNA encapsulation. In addition, for the purpose of DNA release, a bioreducible disulfide bond is introduced between cationic polymers and Zn-DPA analogues, which can be cleaved by abundant glutathione in cytoplasm. The Zn coordination strategy dramatically enhances transfection efficacy of LMW cationic polymers across diverse cell types, including primary and stem cells.

S. Liu · T. Guo (✉)
College of Chemistry, Nankai University, Tianjin, China
e-mail: tyguo@nankai.edu.cn



H. Tian and X. Chen (eds.), *Gene Delivery*, Biomaterial Engineering,
https://doi.org/10.1007/978-981-16-5419-0_20

**Keywords**

Low molecular weight · Cationic polymers · Zn coordination · Gene delivery

## 1 Introduction

Gene therapy has demonstrated tremendous potential for the treatment of various inherited and acquired human diseases (Cheng et al. 2020; Liu et al. 2019; Zhou et al. 2012). Viral gene vectors show high efficacy, however, are impeded by immunogenicity and sophisticated manufacture (Wang et al. 2016; Wei et al. 2013; Yen et al. 2016). Nonviral vectors provide an alternative option because of safety profiles and scalable production (Liu et al. 2017b; Yu et al. 2020; Zhou et al. 2016). Among them, cationic polymers, such as polyethylenimine (PEI) and poly(L-lysine) (PLL), have emerged as one of the major class for gene delivery; however, they fall short in in vivo and clinical applications (Chi et al. 2014; Liu et al. 2016; Seib et al. 2007). A paradox exists between efficacy and cytotoxicity in cationic polymers (Gao et al. 2016; Mastrobattista and Hennink 2012): high molecular weight (HMW) cationic polymers are capable of inducing high transfection efficacy but are associated with increased cytotoxicity, while well cell tolerated low molecular weight cationic polymers lack efficiency in gene delivery (Liu et al. 2018a). Therefore, transforming LMW cationic polymers to efficient gene vectors meanwhile retaining their low toxicity is of great significance.

LMW cationic polymers perform inferior efficacy to their HMW counterparts, largely due to the lack of multivalency for tight DNA binding (Liu et al. 2018a). To improve the performance of LMW cationic polymers, Breunig et al. (2007) and Liu et al. (2012b) used a cross-linking strategy to cross-link LMW polymers with disulfide bonds, which is followed by cleavage in cytosol via glutathione (GSH) reduction (Lin et al. 2006; Liu et al. 2017a; Lu et al. 2016). Nonetheless, these polymers have thus become HMW cationic polymers, and the polymer/DNA polyplexes might face instability in serum. To maintain the LMW, a specific functionalization strategy is in urgent demand. Based on this consideration, metal coordination, such as zinc dipicolylamine (Zn-DPA) analogs, may provide an option for tight DNA binding because of its high affinity toward phosphate groups (Liu et al. 2012a, 2017c, 2018b, c). Moreover, as phospholipids largely exist in biological membranes, the Zn-coordinative ligand modification on LMW cationic polymers not only can strengthen the DNA binding but also may enable the enhancement of the polyplex cellular uptake.

This protocol reports the synthesis a disulfide-containing Zn-coordinative DPA analog (Zn-DDAC), and subsequent functionalization on cationic polymers to give the efficient and safe nonviral gene vectors. In this section, LMW cationic polymers PEI ($M_w \sim 1.8$ k Da) and ε-polylysine (PLL, $M_w < 5$ k Da) were used. The disulfide bonds between Zn coordinative ligand and LMW cationic polymers are designed to induce DNA release upon entering into the cytosol by GSH-triggered reduction. Transfection is conducted across various cell types, including conventional cell lines, myeloma cells, primary cells, and stem cells. This strategy achieves the goal of transforming easily obtained LMW cationic polymers to highly effective and safe gene vehicles, even capable of transfecting primary and stem cells with high performance. It is worth noting that this method has universal applicability: there are plenty of metal coordination structures, numerous cationic polymers, and various stimuli-response linkages, and therefore, this system leads to inspiration to the development of massive nonviral gene vectors.

# 2 Protocol

## 2.1 Materials

### 2.1.1 Synthesis of Ligand DDAC

1. 2,2'-Dipicolylamine (DPA)
2. Alpha, alpha'-dichloro-p-xylene (Dx)
3. 5-Amino-1-pentanol (AP)
4. Cystamine bisacrylamide (CBA)
5. Dichloromethane ($CH_2Cl_2$, analytical reagent grade)
6. Methanol (analytical reagent grade)
7. Ethanol (analytical reagent grade)
8. Ethyl acetate (EA, analytical reagent grade)
9. Potassium carbonate ($K_2CO_3$)
10. Sodium sulfate ($Na_2SO_4$)

### 2.1.2 Synthesis of Zn-Coordinative Cationic Polymers

1. Polyethylenimine (PEI, Mw ~ 1.8 k Da)
2. ε-Polylysine (PLL, $M_w < 5$ k Da)
3. Methanol
4. Zinc nitrate hexahydrate ($Zn(NO_3)_2 \cdot 6H_2O$)
5. DDAC
6. Anhydrous diethyl ether (analytical reagent grade)
7. Triethylamine

### 2.1.3 Gel Retardation Assays

1. Sodium acetate (pH 5.2 ± 0.1, 50 mM)
2. Gaussia princeps secreted luciferase plasmid (pCMV-GLuc)
3. $PEI_{1.8k}$ polymer
4. Zn-PD2 polymer
5. PD2 polymer
6. 1.2% agarose gel
7. Tris-boric acid-EDTA, pH = 8.0
8. Ethidium bromide

#### 2.1.4 Polyplex Size and Zeta Potential Measurements

1. Sodium acetate buffer (pH 5.2 ± 0.1, 50 mM)
2. Gaussia princeps secreted luciferase plasmid (pCMV-GLuc)
3. $PEI_{1.8k}$ polymer
4. Zn-PD2 polymer
5. Zn-PD4 polymer
6. PD2 polymer
7. Phosphate-buffered saline (PBS, 10 mM, pH 7.2 ~ 7.4)

#### 2.1.5 In Vitro Gene Transfection

1. The human embryonic kidney cell line 293 T
2. The human cervical cancer cell line HeLa
3. The human colon cancer cell line HCT116
4. The mouse myeloma cell line SP2/0
5. Primary rat Schwann cells SC
6. Rat adipose-derived stem cells rADSC
7. Rat bone marrow stromal cells rBMSC
8. Human bone marrow stromal cells hBMSC
9. Fetal bovine serum (FBS)
10. Trypsin-EDTA
11. Dulbecco's modified Eagle Medium (DMEM)
12. RPMI-1640 medium
13. 50% DMEM/50% F12 Ham media
14. α-MEM medium
15. Gaussia princeps secreted luciferase plasmid (pCMV-GLuc)
16. $PEI_{1.8k}$ polymer
17. Zn-PD2 polymer
18. Zn-PD4 polymer
19. Commercial transfection reagents branched PEI (Mw ~ 25 kDa)
20. Commercial transfection reagents Xfect
21. BioLux™ Gaussia luciferase Assay Kit (New England Biolabs)

#### 2.1.6 Cytotoxicity Assays

1. 3-(4,5-dimethylthiazol-2-yl)-2,5-diphenyl-tetrazolium bromide (MTT)
2. Dimethyl sulfoxide (DMSO)
3. PBS

#### 2.1.7 Cellular Uptake of Polyplexes

1. Gaussia princeps secreted luciferase plasmid (pCMV-GLuc)
2. *Label* IT® Cy™3 Labeling Kit (Mirus)
3. The human colon cancer cell line HCT116
4. Fluorescein isothiocyanate (FITC)
5. 4′,6-diamidino-2-phenylindole (DAPI)
6. $PEI_{1.8k}$ polymer
7. methanol

8. DDAC
9. Zinc nitrate hexahydrate ($Zn(NO_3)_2{\cdot}6H_2O$)
10. Trypsin-EDTA
11. RPMI-1640 medium
12. PBS
13. 4% paraformaldehyde

## 2.2 Methods

### 2.2.1 Synthesis of Ligand DDAC

1. DPA (1.59 g, 8 mmol) and Dx (2.80 g, 16 mmol) were dissolved in 20 mL of dichloromethane.
2. Anhydrous $K_2CO_3$ (5.52 g, 40 mmol) was added to above mixture.
3. The mixture was stirred at room temperature for 48 h under $N_2$ atmosphere.
4. Silica gel column purification was conducted with dichloromethane:methanol (20:1, v/v) elution to give DxDA as yellowish oil (yield, 72%).
5. AP (1.04 g, 10 mmol) and $K_2CO_3$ (1.66 g, 12 mmol) were mixed with 8 mL of ethanol, then DxDA (0.84 g, 2.4 mmol) was dropwise added into the mixture.
6. Above reaction was occurred at 60 °C overnight.
7. The obtained mixture was precipitated with deionized water three times, and aqueous product suspension was extracted with 100 mL of $CH_2Cl_2$.
8. The organic phase was dried over anhydrous $Na_2SO_4$ and concentrated under vacuum to give DxDA-AP (yield, 71%).
9. DxDA-AP (0.3 g, 0.75 mmol) and CBA (0.39 g, 1.5 mmol) were dissolved in 5 mL of methanol, and the mixture was stirred at 40 °C for 48 h.
10. The product was purified using silica gel column with EA:methanol (4:1, v/v) elution. The final DDAC was obtained as yellowish solid (yield, 36%).

### 2.2.2 Synthesis of Zn Coordinative Cationic Polymers

1. To prepare Zn-PDm polymers, calculated DDAC, $Zn(NO_3)_2{\cdot}6H_2O$ and $PEI_{1.8k}$ were dissolved in methanol, then the reaction occurred at 60 °C for 48 h.
2. The solution was concentrated under vacuum to give Zn coordinative cationic polymers Zn-PDm (Fig. 1). "m" indicates the Zn-DDAC number modified on each $PEI_{1.8k}$ molecule.
3. DDAC (10.0 mg, 0.015 mmol), $Zn(NO_3)_2{\cdot}6H_2O$ (4.5 mg, 0.015 mmol), and $PEI_{1.8k}$ (13.5 mg, 0.0075 mmol) were used to prepare Zn-PD2.
4. DDAC (13.2 mg, 0.02 mmol), $Zn(NO_3)_2{\cdot}6H_2O$ (6.0 mg, 0.02 mmol), and $PEI_{1.8k}$ (9.0 mg, 0.005 mmol) were used to prepare Zn-PD4.
5. To synthesize PLL derived Zn-PLD, Zn-DDAC was first prepared (Note 1). Equimolar $Zn(NO_3)_2{\cdot}6H_2O$ and DDAC were dissolved in methanol, and stirred for 3 h to get Zn-DDAC.
6. Zn-DDAC (0.01 mmol), LMW PLL (16 mg), and triethylamine (30 μL) were dissolved in 1 mL of methanol, then the mixture was stirred at 60 °C for 48 h.

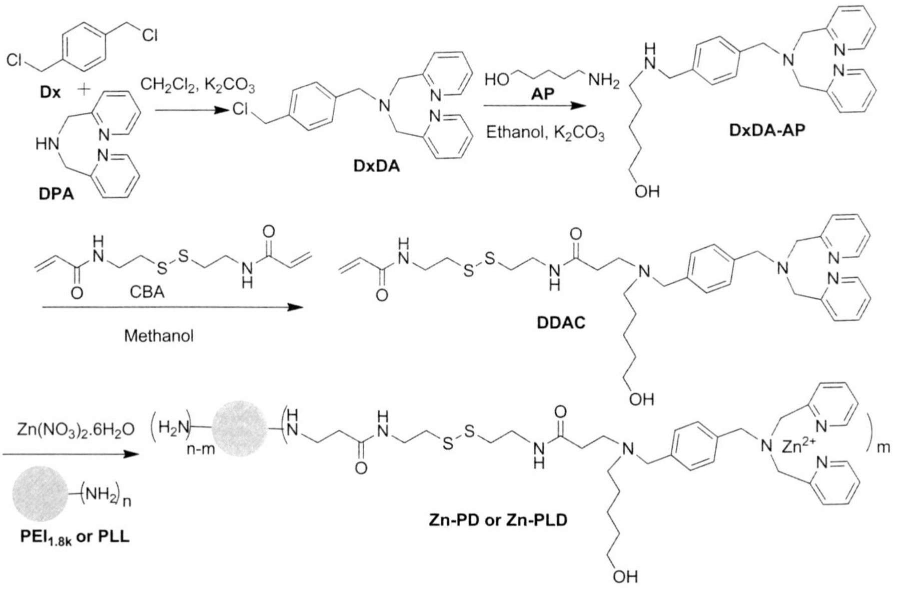


**Fig. 1** Design and synthesis of Zn coordinative cationic polymers

7. Above mixture was precipitated in cold diethyl ether three times and dried under vacuum for 24 h to give Zn-PLD.

### 2.2.3 Gel Retardation Assays

1. DNA was diluted with sodium acetate buffer (pH 5.2 ± 0.1).
2. Polymers were diluted with sodium acetate buffer (pH 5.2 ± 0.1) (Note 2).
3. DNA and polymer diluted solutions were mixed rapidly at a 1:1 volume ratio.
4. Above mixture was incubated for 20 min at room temperature to get polymer/DNA polyplexes. 1 μg DNA/sample was used. The polymer/DNA weight ratios of 0.01, 0.05, 0.1, 0.2, and 0.3 were used.
5. The polyplexes were transferred to 1.2% agarose gel wells (Tris-boric acid-EDTA, pH = 8.0).
6. Gels were run for 45 min at 100 V.
7. DNA bands were stained with ethidium bromide and visualized with an UV illuminator.

Figure 2 showed that Zn-PD2 could condense DNA at a lower polymer/DNA weight ratio compared to $PEI_{1.8k}$, because of high affinity between Zn coordinative ligand and phosphate groups in DNA. PD2 indicated the polymer without Zn coordination.

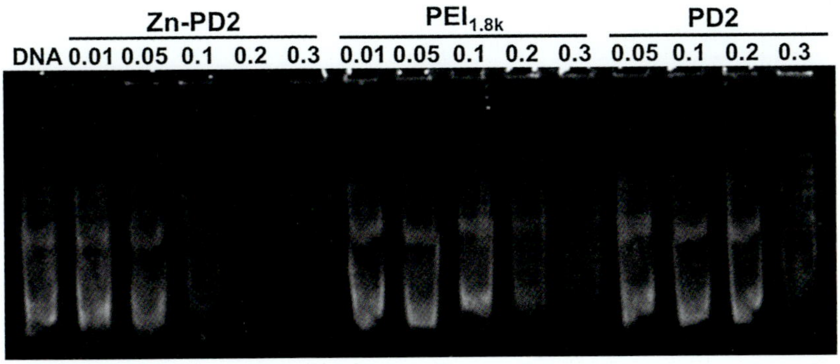


**Fig. 2** Gel retardation assays of polyplexes at different polymer/DNA weight ratios (0.01, 0.05, 0.1, 0.2, and 0.3). (Adapted with permission from Liu et al. (2017c), Copyright (2017) American Chemical Society)

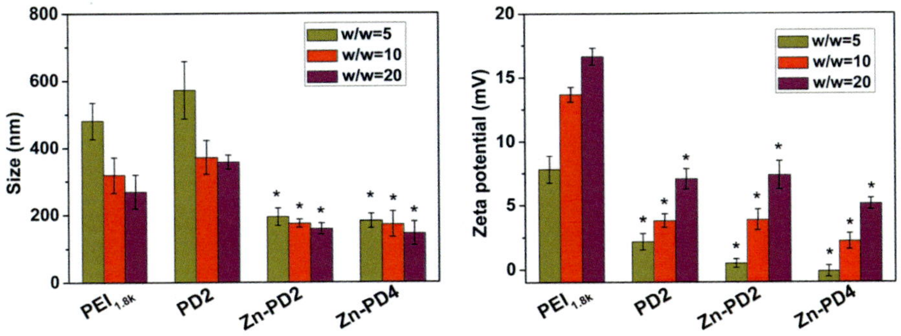


**Fig. 3** Size and zeta potentials of polyplexes at different polymer/DNA weight ratios (5, 10, and 20). (Adapted with permission from Liu et al. (2017c), Copyright (2017) American Chemical Society)

### 2.2.4 Polyplex Size and Zeta Potential Measurements

1. DNA was diluted with sodium acetate buffer (pH 5.2 ± 0.1).
2. Polymers were diluted with sodium acetate buffer (pH 5.2 ± 0.1).
3. DNA and polymer diluted solutions were mixed rapidly at a 1:1 volume ratio.
4. Above mixture was incubated for 20 min at room temperature to get polymer/DNA polyplexes. 2 μg DNA/sample was used. The polymer/DNA weight ratios of 5, 10, and 20 were used.
5. The polyplexes were diluted in 1 mL PBS (pH 7.2 ~ 7.4) for size and zeta potential measurement (Note 3).

Figure 3 showed that Zn-PD2 and Zn-PD4 mediated lower sizes and lower zeta potentials, attributed to Zn coordinative ligand modification. Lower nanoparticle sizes and zeta potentials could benefit polyplex cellular uptake and stability in serum, respectively.

### 2.2.5 In Vitro Gene Transfection

1. 293 T and HeLa cells were maintained DMEM medium with 10% FBS.
2. HCT116 and SP2/0 cells were cultured in RPMI-1640 medium containing 10% FBS.
3. SC, rADSC, and rBMSC cells were cultured in 50% DMEM/50% F12 Ham media with 10% FBS.
4. hBMSC cells were cultured in α-MEM with 10% FBS.
5. All these cells were digested with Trypsin-EDTA and seeded in 96-well plates at a density of $1 \sim 2 \times 10^4$ cells per well and cultured until 70–80% confluence.
6. The formulated polymer/pCMV-GLuc DNA polyplexes were mixed with 100 μL fresh cell culture media, replacing the old media in 96-well plates (Note 4). 0.25 μg DNA per well was used.
7. $PEI_{25k}$ was used at a polymer/DNA weight ratio of 3:1, and Xfect was utilized as per the protocol.
8. 48 h post transfection, cell supernatant were collected (Note 5).
9. BioLux™ Gaussia luciferase Assay Kit was used to determine the transfection efficiency (Gluciferase activity, plotted as relative light units (RLU)).

Figure 4 showed that Zn-PD4 not only exhibited higher transfection efficacy than commercial transfection reagents Xfect and $PEI_{25k}$, but only enabled transfection of diverse cell types, including primary and stem cells.

### 2.2.6 Cytotoxicity Assays

1. After transfection and cell supernatant were collected, fresh media were added to 96-well plates (Note 6).
2. μL MTT solution (5 mg/mL in PBS) was added to each well.
3. After 4 h incubation at 37 °C, above media were replaced by 100 μL DMSO to completely dissolve the generated formazan.
4. Absorbances were measured in a microplate reader at a wavelength of 570 nm.

Figure 5 showed that apart from PEI, Zn coordinative ligand functionalization strategy could be broadened to other cationic polymers (e.g., PLL, and the resultant polymer was Zn-PLD). High transfection efficacy and low cytotoxicity could be simultaneously achieved.

### 2.2.7 Cellular Uptake of Polyplexes

1. $PEI_{1.8k}$ and FITC were dissolved in methanol and stirred at room temperature for 24 h under dark. The solution was vacuum dried to give FITC-$PEI_{1.8k}$.
2. DDAC, $Zn(NO_3)_2 \cdot 6H_2O$, and FITC-$PEI_{1.8k}$ were dissolved in methanol, then the reaction occurred at 60 °C for 48 h under dark. The solution was concentrated under vacuum to give FITC-Zn-PD4 (Note 7).
3. pCMV-GLuc DNA was labeled using *Label* IT® Cy™3 Labeling Kit to get Cy3-DNA.
4. HCT116 cells were digested with Trypsin-EDTA and seeded in 96-well plates at a density of 3000 cells per well.

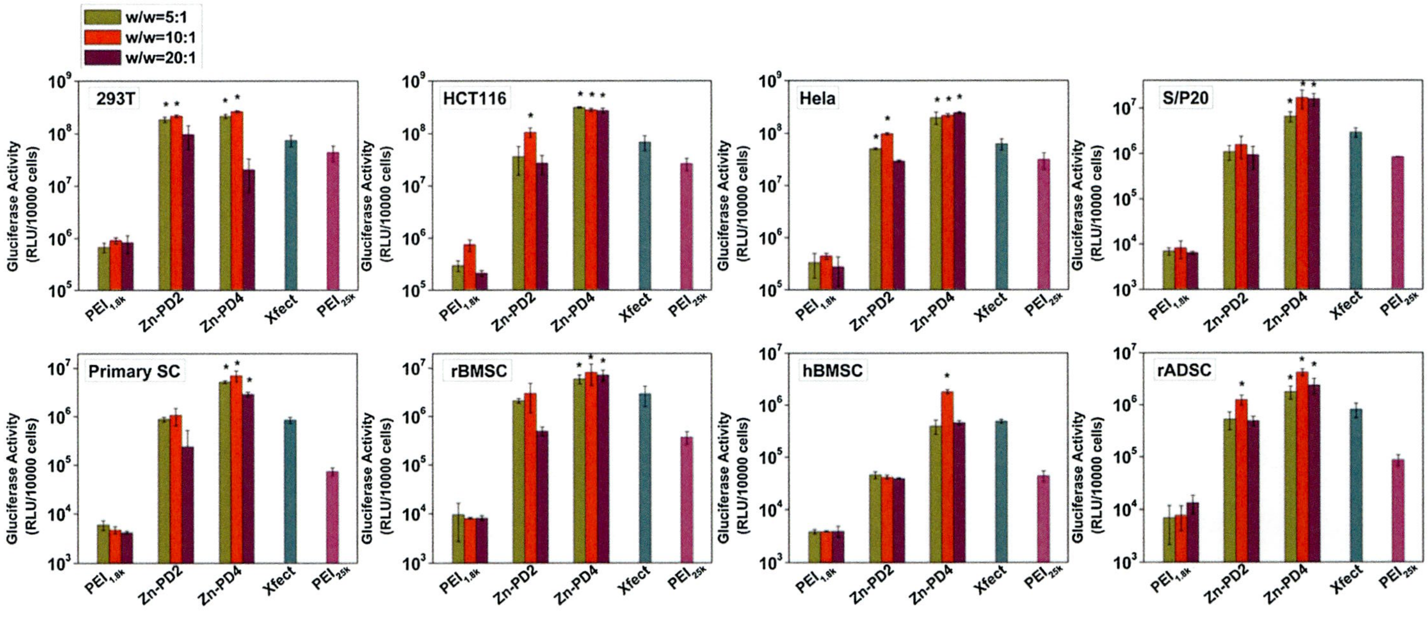


**Fig. 4** Zn-PD4 shows higher transfection efficacy than $PEI_{1.8k}$, Xfect, and $PEI_{25k}$ over diverse cell types. *$P < 0.05$ indicates superior Gluciferase activity compared to Xfect group. (Adapted with permission from Liu et al. (2017c), Copyright (2017) American Chemical Society)

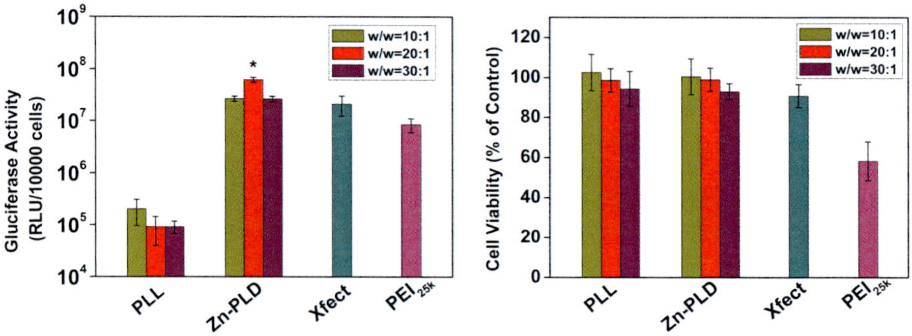


**Fig. 5** Zn-PLD mediates high transfection efficacy and low cytotoxicity in 293 T cells. *P < 0.05 superior Gluciferase activity compared to Xfect group. (Adapted with permission from Liu et al. (2017c), Copyright (2017) American Chemical Society)

5. 24 h later, polyplexes were formulated with FITC-polymer and Cy3-DNA at a weight ratio of 10:1. 6. The formulated polyplexes were mixed with 100 μL fresh cell culture media, which was then used to replace the old media in 96-well plates. 0.1 μg Cy3-DNA per well was used.
6. Post 4 h incubation, cells were washed with PBS three times, and fixed with 4% paraformaldehyde for 15 min.
7. DIPA was used to stain the cell nucleus for 5 min.
8. Cells were visualized with an inverted fluorescent microscopy.

Figure 6 showed that FITC-Zn-PD4/Cy3-DNA polyplexes mediated high cellular uptake, and then DNA could be released from polyplexes and accumulation around cell nuclei, attributed to disulfide linkage cleavage in Zn-PD4 backbone. Zn-PH4 indicated similar Zn coordinative polymer without disulfide bonds.

### 2.2.8 Statistical Analysis

All data were analyzed with GraphPad Prism version 5. A two-tailed unpaired t-test was used to determine the significance of the indicated comparisons. P-values <0.05 (*) were considered to be statistically significant. All transfection experiments were conducted in quadruplicate unless otherwise stated, with error bars indicating ± standard deviation (SD).

## 3 Notes

1. To prepare Zn-PLD polymers, $Zn(NO_3)_2{\cdot}6H_2O$ and DDAC should be firstly mixed to get Zn-DDAC. Then cationic polymer PLL and triethylamine are added to stir and heat.
2. Polymers are dissolved in dimethyl sulfoxide to get stock solutions at a high concentration. Before use, the polymers are diluted with sodium acetate buffer for polyplex preparation.

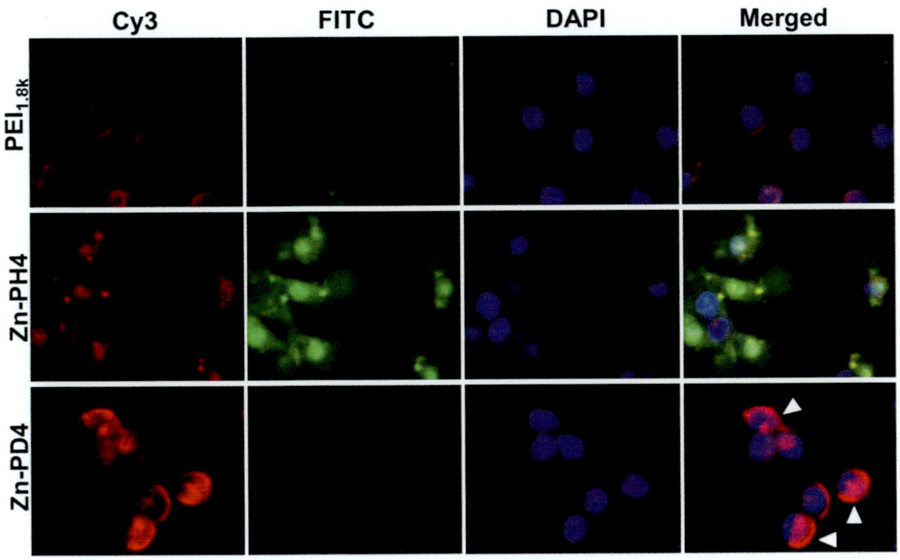


**Fig. 6** Cellular uptake evaluation of HCT116 cells treated with FITC-polymer/Cy3-DNA polyplexes. The cell nuclei are stained with DAPI. The arrows represent DNA release from polyplexes and accumulation around cell nuclei. (Adapted with permission from Liu et al. (2017c), Copyright (2017) American Chemical Society)

3. The polymer/DNA polyplexes are prepared in sodium acetate buffer (pH 5.2 ± 0.1). Before size and zeta potential measurement, the polyplexes should be diluted with PBS to adjust a neutral pH.
4. When transfection is conducted, polyplexes are mixed with fresh cell culture media with 10% FBS. Then, old media in 96-well plates were replaced by above mixtures.
5. For pCMV-GLuc DNA, the expressed luciferase protein was released to cell supernatant. Therefore, we do not need cell lysis to measure the transfection efficacy.
6. Using pCMV-GLuc DNA, cytotoxicity can be directly measured after luciferase containing cell supernatant was taken.
7. To prepare FITC-Zn-PD4, $PEI_{1.8k}$ was modified with FITC first, then DDAC and $Zn(NO_3)_2{\cdot}6H_2O$ were added to react.

## 4 Conclusion

This protocol achieved the goal of transforming LMW cationic polymers to highly efficient and safe nonviral vectors. Zn-DDAC ligand was used to functionalize $PEI_{1.8k}$ and PLL to dramatically improve their DNA binding affinity. Moreover, stimuli responses (disulfide bonds) provide controlled DNA release post nanoparticle internalization. This bioreducible Zn coordinative functionalization strategy breaks up the paradox between low molecular weight and high transfection efficacy. Overall, this strategy demonstrates great potential to be applicable in other nonviral gene delivery systems, altering cationic polymers, stimuli response linkages, and metal coordinative moieties as researchers need.

## References

Breunig M, Lungwitz U, Liebl R, Goepferich A (2007) Breaking up the correlation between efficacy and toxicity for nonviral gene delivery. Proc Natl Acad Sci U S A 104(36): 14454–14459

Cheng Q, Wei T, Farbiak L, Johnson LT, Dilliard SA, Siegwart DJ (2020) Selective organ targeting (SORT) nanoparticles for tissue-specific mRNA delivery and CRISPR–Cas gene editing. Nat Nanotechnol 15(4):313–320

Chi W, Liu S, Yang J, Wang R, Ren H, Zhou H, Chen J, Guo T (2014) Evaluation of the effects of amphiphilic oligomers in PEI based ternary complexes on the improvement of pDNA delivery. J Mater Chem B 2(33):5387–5396

Gao Y, Huang JY, O'Keeffe Ahern J, Cutlar L, Zhou D, Lin FH, Wang W (2016) Highly branched poly(beta-amino esters) for non-viral gene delivery: high transfection efficiency and low toxicity achieved by increasing molecular weight. Biomacromolecules 17(11):3640–3647

Lin C, Zhong Z, Lok MC, Jiang X, Hennink WE, Feijen J, Engbersen JF (2006) Linear poly(amido amine)s with secondary and tertiary amino groups and variable amounts of disulfide linkages: synthesis and in vitro gene transfer properties. J Control Release 116(2):130–137

Liu G, Choi KY, Bhirde A, Swierczewska M, Yin J, Lee SW, Park JH, Hong JI, Xie J, Niu G, Kiesewetter DO, Lee S, Chen X (2012a) Sticky nanoparticles: a platform for siRNA delivery by a bis(zinc(II) dipicolylamine)-functionalized, self-assembled nanoconjugate. Angew Chem Int Ed Engl 51(2):445–449

Liu H, Wang H, Yang W, Cheng Y (2012b) Disulfide cross-linked low generation dendrimers with high gene transfection efficacy, low cytotoxicity, and low cost. J Am Chem Soc 134(42): 17680–17687

Liu S, Yang J, Ren H, O'Keeffe-Ahern J, Zhou D, Zhou H, Chen J, Guo T (2016) Multifunctional oligomer incorporation: a potent strategy to enhance the transfection activity of poly(l-lysine). Biomater Sci 4(3):522–532

Liu S, Gao Y, Zhou D, Greiser U, Guo T, Guo R, Wang W (2017a) Biodegradable highly branched poly(β-amino Ester)s for targeted cancer cell gene transfection. ACS Biomater Sci Eng 3(7): 1283–1286

Liu S, Sun Z, Zhou D, Guo T (2017b) Alkylated branched poly(β-amino esters) demonstrate strong DNA encapsulation, high nanoparticle stability and robust gene transfection efficacy. J Mater Chem B 5(27):5307–5310

Liu S, Zhou D, Yang J, Zhou H, Chen J, Guo T (2017c) Bioreducible zinc(II)-coordinative polyethylenimine with low molecular weight for robust gene delivery of primary and stem cells. J Am Chem Soc 139(14):5102–5109

Liu S, Jia H, Yang J, Pan J, Liang H, Zeng L, Zhou H, Chen J, Guo T (2018a) Zinc coordinated cationic polymers break up the paradox between low molecular weight and high transfection efficacy. Biomacromolecules 19(11):4270–4276

Liu S, Jia H, Yang J, Pan J, Liang H, Zeng L, Zhou H, Chen J, Guo T (2018b) Zinc coordination substitute amine: a noncationic platform for efficient and safe gene delivery. ACS Macro Lett 7(7):868–874

Liu S, Yang J, Jia H, Zhou H, Chen J, Guo T (2018c) Virus spike and membrane-lytic mimicking nanoparticles for high cell binding and superior endosomal escape. ACS Appl Mater Interfaces 10(28):23630–23637

Liu S, Gao Y, Zhou D, Zeng M, Alshehri F, Newland B, Lyu J, O'Keeffe-Ahern J, Greiser U, Guo T, Zhang F, Wang W (2019) Highly branched poly(β-amino ester) delivery of minicircle DNA for transfection of neurodegenerative disease related cells. Nat Commun 10(1):3307

Lu Y, Aimetti AA, Langer R, Gu Z (2016) Bioresponsive materials. Nat Rev Mater 2:16075

Mastrobattista E, Hennink WE (2012) Polymers for gene delivery: charged for success. Nat Mater 11(1):10–12

Seib FP, Jones AT, Duncan R (2007) Comparison of the endocytic properties of linear and branched PEIs, and cationic PAMAM dendrimers in B16f10 melanoma cells. J Control Release 117(3): 291–300

Wang LH, Wu DC, Xu HX, You YZ (2016) High DNA-binding affinity and gene-transfection efficacy of bioreducible cationic nanomicelles with a fluorinated core. Angew Chem Int Ed 55(2):755–759

Wei H, Volpatti LR, Sellers DL, Maris DO, Andrews IW, Hemphill AS, Chan LW, Chu DSH, Horner PJ, Pun SH (2013) Dual responsive, stabilized nanoparticles for efficient in vivo plasmid delivery. Angew Chem Int Ed 52(20):5377–5381

Yen J, Ying H, Wang H, Yin L, Uckun F, Cheng J (2016) CD44 mediated nonviral gene delivery into human embryonic stem cells via hyaluronic-acid-coated nanoparticles. ACS Biomater Sci Eng 2(3):326–335

Yu X, Liu S, Cheng Q, Wei T, Lee S, Zhang D, Siegwart DJ (2020) Lipid-modified aminoglycosides for mRNA delivery to the liver. Adv Healthc Mater 9(7):1901487

Zhou J, Liu J, Cheng CJ, Patel TR, Weller CE, Piepmeier JM, Jiang Z, Saltzman WM (2012) Biodegradable poly(amine-co-ester) terpolymers for targeted gene delivery. Nat Mater 11(1): 82–90

Zhou D, Cutlar L, Gao Y, Wang W, O'Keeffe-Ahern J, McMahon S, Duarte B, Larcher F, Rodriguez BJ, Greiser U, Wang W (2016) The transition from linear to highly branched poly(beta-amino ester)s: branching matters for gene delivery. Sci Adv 2(6):e1600102

# Virus-Mimetic DNA-Ejecting Polyplexes for Cancer Gene Delivery

# 21

## Preparation and Evaluation

Guowei Wang, Siqin Chen, and Youqing Shen

## Contents



---

G. Wang · S. Chen · Y. Shen (✉)
Zhejiang Key Laboratory of Smart BioMaterials and Center for Bionanoengineering, and Key Laboratory of Biomass Chemical Engineering of the Ministry of Education, College of Chemical and Biological Engineering, Zhejiang University, Hangzhou, China
e-mail: shenyq@zju.edu.cn



H. Tian and X. Chen (eds.), *Gene Delivery*, Biomaterial Engineering,
https://doi.org/10.1007/978-981-16-5419-0_21

**Abstract**

Many viruses infect cells via anchoring on the cell membrane and ejecting their genetic materials into the cytosol to bypass the degradative pathways. This protocol presents such a virus-mimicking polymeric vector capable of sticking onto the cell membrane and ejecting DNA into the cytoplasm for efficient gene transfection. The said polymer is a linear quaternized polyethyleneimine with *N*-[(*p*-acyloxybenzyloxycarbonyl)-ethyl]-*N*-methyl ammonium units hydrolyzable by esterases to water-soluble zwitterions. The polymer packs DNA into the nano-sized polyplexes with pendant acyl chains. The polymers with different acyl chain lengths are synthesized. The luciferase reporter plasmid (pLuci) is used as a model DNA for optimizing polyplex preparations and characterizations, and a functional plasmid is used to test gene expression. Their polyplexes' cell-membrane anchoring abilities, esterase-catalyzed cation-to-anion charge-reversal rates, and intracellular pathways are investigated. The polymer with octanoyl groups, L4, condenses plasmids into DNA-ejecting polyplexes, whose long octanoyl chains can insert and tightly bind on the cell membrane and thus make the polyplexes partially exposed to the cytosol, where the esterases hydrolyze the phenol esters and turn the polymers negatively charged, freeing and driving the plasmids into the cytosol. This protocol provides the fabrication of highly efficient polyplexes with advantages in bypassing endo−/lysosomal DNA degradation and avoiding the safety concerns of the internalized carrier materials. Moreover, the polyplexes can be further coated with a poly(γ-glutamic acid) layer for in vivo gene transfection.

**Keywords**

Gene delivery · Nonviral vectors · Virus-mimicking · Esterase-responsive polymer · Charge-reversal · DNA ejection

## 1 Overview

Gene therapy has been demonstrated highly effective in curing many genetic diseases, (Wang et al. 2015, 2020; Mitchell et al. 2020) but its clinical applications are still bottlenecked by safe and efficient delivery of genetic materials.(Bulcha et al. 2021; Wang et al. 2019) Nonviral vectors such as cationic polymers(Malik et al. 2018; Fang et al. 2019) and lipids(Qiu et al. 2016, 2021; Liu et al. 2016) hold great promise for gene therapy attributed to their advantages such as multi-transgenic ability, non-immunotoxicity, biosafety, high cargo capacity, and low costs.(Van Bruggen et al. 2019; Wu et al. 2016; Chen et al. 2019; Hardee et al. 2017; Li et al. 2019)

However, nonviral vectors generally suffer inefficient transfection due to the delivery barriers,(Zhou et al. 2017; Sun et al. 2019; Liu et al. 2019) particularly lysosome-trapping caused degradation of nucleic acids,(Bus et al. 2018; Degors et al. 2019) and high cationic-charge density caused cytotoxicity.(Yan et al. 2018) Therefore, new carriers and strategies overcoming these problems, including tuning packaging, (Wu et al. 2020; Chen et al. 2018; Vermeulen et al. 2018) alternating endocytosis pathway by manipulating nanostructures,(Zhuang et al. 2019; Zhou et al. 2020; Qiu et al. 2019) facilitating lysosomal escape,(Liu et al. 2016; Zhou et al. 2020; Sun et al. 2018) promoting DNA release,(Curley et al. 2020; Tang et al. 2021) lowering cationic charge densities, and making polymers degradable into short chains or zwitterionic (Qiu et al. 2016; Li et al. 2014, 2019; Shen et al. 2020) have been widely explored.

In the nonviral gene delivery process, nearly all of the current gene vectors are engineered to enter cells via endocytosis, escape from endo/lysosomes, and then release the delivered genetic materials into the cytosol.(Hardee et al. 2017; Bus et al. 2018; Degors et al. 2019; Vermeulen et al. 2018) However, the endocytosed carrier materials and their degradation products in the cytoplasm may inevitably interfere with the transfection process and cause possible side effects,(Pollard et al. 1998; Zhu et al. 2017) further complicating the transfection efficiency and clinical translation. Inspired by some viruses like bacteriophages,(Molineux and Panja 2013) which can attach to the cell membrane, eject their genome into the cytoplasm via pore-mediated penetration, and leave their capsid proteins outside the cell, we hypothesize that a nonviral vector ejecting DNA into the cytoplasm without entering the cell would bypass the endo-/lysosomal trapping and avoid interference with the transcription and cytotoxicity of the carrier materials. Such a bacteriophage-mimicking vector should be able to (1) complex with DNA to form nanoparticles, (2) insert into the lipid bilayer of the cell membrane, and (3) unpack and squeeze the DNA through the cell membrane into the cytosol.

This protocol presents such a "DNA-ejecting vector" using esterase-labile cationic polymers with long acyl chains. The cationic polymer is a quaternized linear polyethyleneimine (QPEI) whose ammonium moieties have *N*-(*p*-acyloxy benzyloxycarbonyl)ethyl groups. The phenol ester hydrolysis can trigger the elimination reaction and turn the polymer from cation to zwitterion. The acyl chain length determines the QPEI's DNA condensation ability, cell-membrane binding ability, and esterase-triggered hydrolysis rate. The QPEI with the proper long acyl chain, L4 (acyl = octanoyl), can condense DNA plasmids into nano-sized L4/DNA polyplex nanoparticles. The L4's pendant long octanoyl chains can insert into the cell lipid bilayer and anchor the polyplex stably on the cell membrane. Subsequently, some of the phenol esters on the L4 chains facing the cytoplasm can be quickly hydrolyzed by cytosolic esterase, thereby turning some L4 neutral to liberalize the DNA. The phosphate anions' strong electrostatic repulsion of free DNA can squeeze the DNA into the cytoplasm for efficient gene transfection. Moreover, the L4/DNA polyplex coated with a poly($\gamma$-glutamic acid) layer maintains the DNA-injection ability and has high efficiency for in vivo gene transfection.

## 2 Materials

### 2.1 Synthesis of the Polymers

1. Acetyl chloride
2. Acryloyl chloride
3. Benzoyl chloride
4. Butyryl chloride
5. Bruker ARX 400 NMR spectrometer
6. Decanoyl chloride
7. Dialysis tubing (molecular weight cut-off 3.5 kDa)
8. Dichloromethane (DCM)
9. *N,N*-Dimethylformamide (DMF)
10. Ethyl acetate
11. Ethyl ether
12. Hexanoyl chloride
13. *n*-Hexane
14. *p*-Hydroxylmethylenephenol (HMP)
15. Iodomethane
16. Lauryl chloride
17. Linear polyethyleneimine (LPEI, 25 kDa)
18. Lyophilizer
19. Octanoyl chloride
20. *2*-Propylvaleroyl chloride
21. Silica gel column chromatography
22. Sodium chloride
23. Sodium sulfate
24. Triethylamine (TEA
25. Tertiary butylhydroquinone (TBHQ).
26. Thin layer chromatograph
27. Water bath kettle

### 2.2 Preparation of the Fluorescent Dye-Labeled Polymers and DNA

1. Cyanine5.5-hydroxysuccinimide active ester (Cy5.5-NHS)
2. Cy5$^{TM}$ Label IT$^{®}$ Nucleic Acid Labeling Kit (Mirus Bio Co., Ltd., USA)
3. Dialysis tubing (molecular weight cut-off 3.5 kDa)
4. DMF
5. Fluorescein isothiocyanate (FITC)
6. Linear polyethyleneimine (LPEI, 25 kDa)
7. Sephadex G15 column

## 2.3 Fabrication of Polymer/DNA Polyplexes

1. Dimethylsulfoxide (DMSO)
2. *N*-(2-Hydroxyethyl)piperazine-N′-(2-ethane sulfonic acid) (HEPES, pH 7.4, 10 mM)
3. Luciferase reporter plasmid (pLuci)
4. Poly(γ-glutamic acid) (γPGA, 20 kDa)
5. The polymers
6. Vortex generator

## 2.4 Size and Zeta Potential Measurements

1. Disposable capillary cell (DTS1070 from Malvern Panalytical)
2. HEPES (pH 7.4, 10 mM)
3. Low-volume disposable cuvette (ZEN0040 from Malvern Panalytical)
4. Zetasizer Nano (Malvern Instrument Ltd. Inc.)

## 2.5 Transmission Electron Microscope Measurements

1. Copper grid mesh (100-mesh type)
2. Filter paper
3. Saturated uranyl acetate solution
4. Transmission electron microscope (TEM) (JEOL, JEM-1010)

## 2.6 Agarose Gel Retardation Electrophoresis

1. Agarose gel
2. Chemiluminescence imaging system
3. DNA-loading buffer
4. Ethidium bromide
5. Electrophoresis apparatu
6. Tris-Acetate-EDTA buffer

## 2.7 Esterase-Responsive Activities of the Polymer

1. DMSO
2. High performance liquid chromatography (HPLC, Waters 1525, equipped with a 1525 binary Pump, 2475 multi-λ-Fluorescence Detector and 2998 Photodiode Array Detector, and a SunFireTM $C_{18}$ column (4.6 × 250 mm, 5 μm))

3. HPEPS (10 mM, pH 7.4)
4. Methanol
5. NaCl (100 mM)
6. Porcine liver esterase
7. Phosphorous acid (0.1 wt%)
8. Tris-HCl buffer (100 mM, pH 7.4)

## 2.8 Esterase-Responsive Activities of the Polyplexes

1. Chemiluminescence imaging system
2. Copper grid mesh (100-mesh type)
3. Electrophoresis apparatus
4. Filter paper
5. Porcine liver esterase solution (200 U/mL)
6. Saturated uranyl acetate solution
7. Transmission electron microscope (TEM) (JEOL, JEM-1010)
8. Zetasizer Nano (Malvern Instrument Ltd. Inc.)

## 2.9 Cell Line

1. Fetal bovine serum (FBS)
2. Human cervical carcinoma cell line (HeLa)
3. Penicillin
4. RPMI 1640 medium
5. Streptomycin
6. Trypsin

## 2.10 In Vitro Gene Transfection

1. BCA protein assay kit (Sangon Biotech Co., Ltd., Shanghai)
2. FB12 Tube Luminometer (Titertek-Berthold Co., Ltd., Germany)
3. Luciferase assay system (Luciferase assay substrate, Luciferase assay buffer, Cell culture lysis 5X reagent) (PromegaBiotech Co., Ltd., USA)
4. HeLa cells
5. The luciferase expression was normalized with the total protein concentration (the relative luciferase light units per milligram protein, RLU/mg)
6. 48-Well plates

### 2.11 Subcellular Distribution and Colocalization

1. Cy5™ Label IT® Nucleic Acid Labeling Kit (Mirus Bio Co., Ltd., USA)
2. Confocal laser scanning microscopy (CLSM, Nikon A1, Japan)
3. FITC-labeled wheat germ agglutin (Invitrogen™, USA)
4. HeLa cells
5. Hoechst 33342 (Invitrogen™, USA)
6. Lysotracker green (Invitrogen™, USA)
7. PBS buffer (10 mM, pH 7.4)
8. The glass-bottom petri dish

### 2.12 Effects of Inhibitors on Cellular Uptake

1. Chlorpromazine
2. Cytochalasin D
3. Filipin III
4. Flow cytometry (BD FACS Calibur™, USA)
5. HeLa cells
6. 24-Well plates
7. Wortmannin

## 3 Protocols

### 3.1 Synthesis of the Polymers

1. Taking the L1 polymer as an example (Fig.1a), a 250 mL round-bottomed flask equipped with a 2.0 cm Teflon-coated barbell-shaped stir bar is loaded with HMP (7.5 g, 60 mmol), TEA (10 mL, 72 mmol) and anhydrous DCM (100 mL). The resulting solution is magnetically stirred (500 rpm) and immersed in an ice bath.
2. A 25 mL predried dropping funnel is connected with the flask. In a fume hood with strong ventilation, acetyl chloride (4.7 mL, 60 mmol) is taken into a 5 mL syringe and charged into the funnel. Acetyl chloride is then added dropwise (within about 5 min) via the dropping funnel that is capped with a rubber septum.
3. The reaction mixture is further stirred in the ice bath for 1 h, and then the flask is taken out from the ice bath and stirred at 25 °C for 4 h.
4. The reaction mixture is filtered through a Buchner funnel. The filtrate is concentrated to 10 mL as thick, orange liquid using a rotary evaporator (200 mmHg to 50 mmHg, 35 °C).

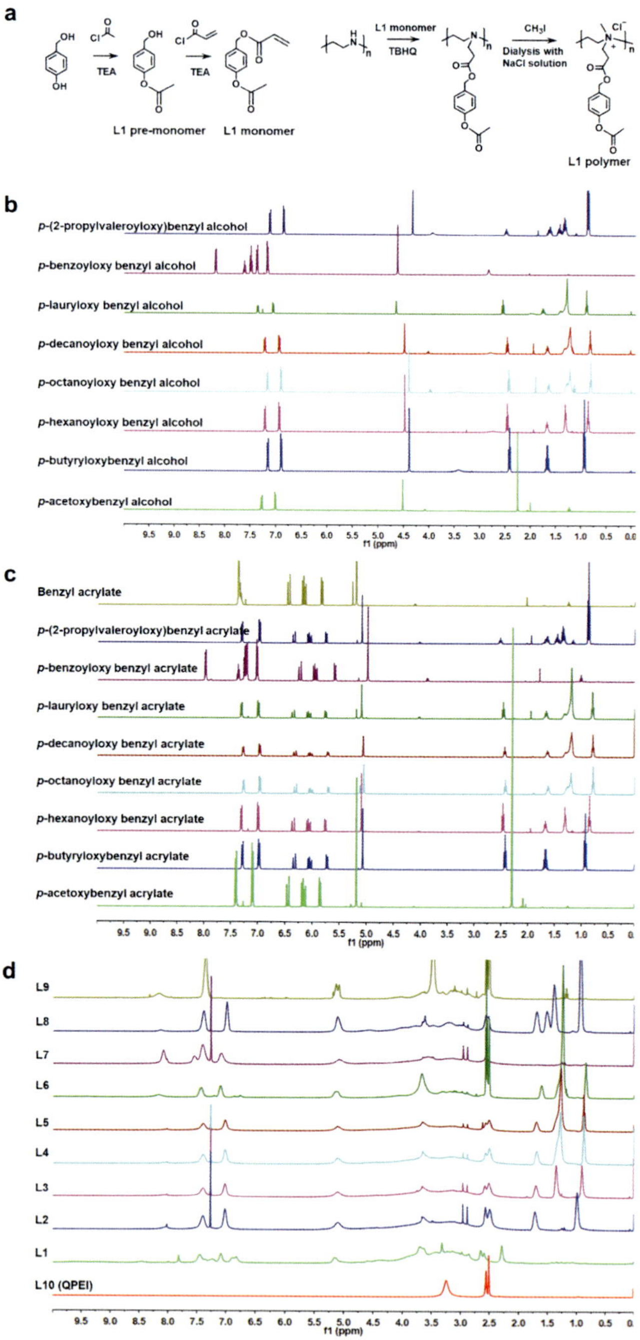


**Fig. 1** Synthesis and characterizations of the polymers. (**a**) The synthesis of *N*-[*p*-acetoxy benzyloxycarbonyl]ethyl-*N*-methyl LPEI (L1). (**b**) The $^{1}$H NMR spectra of *p*-acyloxybenzyl alcohols. (**c**) The $^{1}$H NMR spectra of *p*-acyloxybenzyl acrylates. (**d**) The (Wang et al. 2015) H NMR spectra of L1 ~ L9 and quaternized LPEI (L10)

5. In parallel, a column chromatography (50 mm in diameter and 400 mm long) is prepared using 250 ~ 300 g of reagent silica gel (200–300 mesh) and *n*-hexane (300 ~ 400 mL).
6. The concentrate is carefully added onto the top of the silica gel and then flushed using the eluent of *n*-hexane/ethyl acetate (volume ratio 5/2). An initial elution with 100% *n*-hexane (about 400 mL) does not contain product and is discarded. Per fraction of 50 mL is collected after this point, and eluting is successively collected for a total of 20 fractions.
7. The fractions are monitored using thin-layer chromatography (TLC). TLC is performed on aluminum-backed silica gel plates (GF254-plates) eluting with *n*-hexane/ethyl acetate (volume ratio 5/2), visualized first with UV light and then with iodine-staining. The desired product is observed at the staining spot with $R_f$ value of 0.31 on the TLC plate.
8. The desired product is obtained in the eluting of 8 ~ 18 fractions. Fractions containing the product are combined, the solvent is removed by rotary evaporation (200 mmHg to 50 mmHg, 35 °C) and then dried in a vacuum drying oven (0.1 mmHg, 25 °C). *p*-Acetoxy benzyl alcohol is obtained as colorless oil (7.0 g, yield 75%) (Fig.1b).
9. A 250 mL round-bottomed flask equipped with a 2.0 cm Teflon-coated barbell-shaped stir bar is added with *p*-acetoxybenzyl alcohol (1.66 g, 10 mmol), TEA (1.7 mL, 12 mmol) and anhydrous DCM (100 mL). The resulting solution is magnetically stirred (500 rpm) and immersed in an ice bath.
10. A 25 mL predried dropping funnel is connected with the flask. In a fume hood with strong ventilation, acryloyl chloride (0.95 mL, 12 mmol) is taken into a 1 mL syringe and charged into the dropping funnel, and 5 mL of anhydrous DCM is added to the funnel. The funnel is then capped with a rubber septum. Acryloyl chloride is then added dropwise (within about 2 min) into the flask.
11. The reaction mixture is further stirred in the ice bath for 1 h, and then the flask is taken out from the ice bath and stirred at 25 °C for 4 h. The reaction mixture is filtered through a Buchner funnel. The filtrate is poured into a 1 L separatory funnel containing a saturated solution of $NaHCO_3$ (300 mL) at 25 °C. The reaction flask is rinsed with DCM (2 x 10 mL) and the resulting solutions are added to the separatory funnel. After vigorously shaking (CAUTION: Gas may be produced, so the stopcock must be open from time to time to release the gas), the funnel is on standing for phase separation. The yellow-orange organic layer is obtained and further washed with water (2 × 300 mL) and a saturated aqueous NaCl solution (300 mL), dried on $Na_2SO_4$ (50 g), filtered, and concentrated to 10 mL using a rotary evaporator (200 mmHg to 50 mmHg, 35 °C).
12. In parallel, a column chromatography (50 mm in diameter and 400 mm long) is prepared using 250 ~ 300 g of reagent silica gel (200–300 mesh) and n-hexane (300 ~ 400 mL).
13. The concentrate is carefully added onto the top of the silica gel and then flushed using the eluent of n-hexane/ethyl acetate (volume ratio 10/1). An initial elution with 100% n-hexane (about 400 mL) does not contain product and is discarded. Per fraction of 50 mL is collected after this point, and eluting is successively collected for a total of 15 fractions.

14. TLC monitoring is performed on aluminum-backed silica gel plates (GF254-plates) eluting with n-hexane/ethyl acetate (volume ratio 10/1), visualized first with UV light and then with iodine-staining. The desired product is observed at the staining spot with $R_f$ value of 0.53 on the TLC plate.
15. The desired product is obtained in the eluting of 2 ~ 12 fractions. Fractions containing the product are combined, the solvent is removed by rotary evaporation (200 mmHg to 50 mmHg, 35 °C) and then dried using vacuum drying oven (0.1 mmHg, 25 °C). *p*-acetoxy benzyl acrylate is obtained as light yellow oil (1.5 g, yield 60%) (Fig.1c).
16. A 10 mL round-bottomed flask equipped with a 1.0 cm Teflon-coated barbell-shaped stir bar is charged with LPEI (88 mg, -NH- equivalent 2 mmol), TBHQ (1.7 mg, 0.01 mmol) and anhydrous DMF (2.0 mL). The resulting solution is magnetically stirred (500 rpm) at 25 °C. *p*-Acetoxybenzyl acrylate (660 mg, 3 mmol) is dissolved in DMF (2.0 mL) and added into the reaction mixture.
17. The reaction mixture is stirred at 25 °C for 48 h and then at 45 °C in a water bath for an additional 24 h (see Note 1).
18. The flask is wrapped with aluminum foil and stirred at 25 °C. Iodomethane (1.0 g, 7.0 mmol) is taken into a 1 mL syringe and added to the reaction mixture slowly. The reaction mixture is stirred at 25 °C for 12 h in the dark environment.
19. The reaction mixture is poured into 30 mL precooled ethyl ether with stirring (200 rpm) in a 50 mL centrifuge tube (see Note 2). The centrifuge tube is centrifuged at 5,000 rpm for 10 min at 4 °C. The supernate is discarded.
20. The precipitate is redissolved in 2.0 mL DMF, and loaded into a dialysis tube (molecular weight cut-off 3.5 kDa). The mixture is first dialyzed against saturated sodium chloride solution (2 × 500 mL, replace the dialyzate every 4 h) for 8 h and then against deionized water (2 × 500 mL, replace the dialyzate every 4 h) for 8 h in the dark environment.
21. The solution in the dialysis tube is collected into a 10 mL beaker, prefreezed at −80 °C for 2 h, and then lyophilized using a lyophilizer (0.05 mmHg, −50 °C) for 24 h to obtain the L1 polymer as pale-yellow powder (0.52 g, yield 67%) (see Note 3).
22. L1 polymer (20 mg) is taken and dissolved in 0.5 mL $CDCl_3$, and confirmed using the $^1$H-NMR spectrometer (Fig.1d).
23. In preparing the polymers with long acyl chains, L4, L5 and L6, the *p*-acyloxybenzyl acrylates are less reactive, so the acrylate to -NH- ratio is increased to two or more.

## 3.2 Preparation of the Fluorescent Dye-Labeled Polymers

1. Taking the Cy5.5-labeled L1 polymer ($L1^{Cy5.5}$) as an example, LPEI (100.0 mg) and Cy5.5-NHS ester (1.0 mg, 1.0 wt%) are dissolved in 2 mL anhydrous DMF in a 10 mL flask equipped with a 1.0 cm Teflon-coated barbell-shaped stir bar. The flask is wrapped with aluminum foil. The mixture is stirred for 12 h at room temperature in the dark.

2. The mixture is loaded into a dialysis tube (molecular weight cut-off 3.5 kDa). The mixture is dialyzed against deionized water ($3 \times 500$ mL, replace the dialyzate every 8 h) for 24 h.
3. The solution in the dialysis tube is collected into a 10 mL beaker, prefreezed in a $-80$ °C refrigerator for 2 h, and then lyophilized using a lyophilizer (0.05 mmHg, $-50$ °C) for 24 h to obtain the $LPEI^{Cy5.5}$ as navy-blue powder (92 mg, yield 91%).
4. $L1^{Cy5.5}$ is synthesized using $LPEI^{Cy5.5}$ and *p*-acetoxybenzyl acrylate as described protocol above in Sect. 3.1.

## 3.3 Preparation of the Fluorescent Dye-Labeled DNA

1. The Cy5-labeled pLuci ($pLuci^{Cy5}$) is prepared using Cy5™ Label IT® Nucleic Acid Labeling Kit (Mirus Bio., USA) according to the manufacturer's instructions. The protocol can be found on the link of https://www.mirusbio.com/.

## 3.4 Fabrication of Polymer/DNA Polyplexes

1. The HEPES buffer and centrifugal tubes are treated by autoclaved sterilization (121 °C, 30 min) before use.
2. Because the L4/DNA polyplex has preferable cell-membrane anchoring and DNA-ejecting abilities, the fabrication of the L4/pLuci polyplex is described as an example in detail. L4 (10 mg) is accurately weighed and dissolved in DMSO (0.2 mL) in a 5 mL centrifugal tube, and then diluted with HEPES buffer (10 mM at pH 7.4, 3.8 mL) to obtain the stock solution at 2.5 mg/mL of L4.
3. A frozen-reserved stock solution of pLuci (0.1 mL, 1.0 mg/ mL) is warmed to room temperature.
4. At the defined nitrogen (N, cation) to phosphate (P, anion) molar ratio (N/P ratio) of 24, The L4 stock solution (0.2 mL) is diluted with 0.71 mL HEPES buffer (10 mM, pH 7.4) to give a L4 solution at 550 μg/mL. The pLuci stock solution (0.05 mL) is also diluted with 1.2 mL HEPES buffer (10 mM, pH 7.4) to prepare a solution at 40 μg/mL pLuci.
5. L4 solution (0.5 mL, 550 μg/mL) is introduced into a 1.5 mL centrifugal tube at room temperature, and 0.5 mL of pLuci solution (40 μg/mL) is added to the polymer solution using a pipette. The mixture is gently vortexed for 10 s using a vortex vibrator, and incubated for 5 min at room temperature to obtain the L4/pLuci polyplex (see Note 4).

## 3.5 γPGA-Coating Polyplexes

1. For in vivo transfection, L4/pLuci polyplex needs coating with γPGA polymer. γPGA (20 kDa, 10 mg) is weighed and dissolved in HEPES (10 mM, pH 7.4) to give a solution at 20 nmol/mL γPGA.

2. The prepared L4/pLuci polyplex (0.2 mL, pLuci-equivalent dose of 20 μg/mL) is introduced into a 1.5 mL centrifugal tube at room temperature, and 0.2 mL of γPGA solution (20 nmol/mL) is added to the L4/pLuci polyplex solution using a pipette. The mixture is gently shaken for 10 min using a shaker (100 rmp), then sonicated for 1 min at room temperature using an ultrasonic bath to obtain the γPGA/L4/pLuci (N/P ratio is 24, and γPGA/pLuci ratio is 1 nmol/μg).

### 3.6 Size and Zeta Potential Measurements

1. The L4/pLuci polyplex is prepared at an N/P ratio of 24 at a DNA dose of 20 μg/mL as described protocol in Sect. 3.4.
2. The polyplex sample (100 μL) is transferred into a low-volume disposable cuvette (ZEN0040) for size measurement using a Zetasizer Nano (Nano ZS90, Malvern Instrument Ltd. Inc.). The Zetasizer Nano is equipped with a 4 mW He-Ne laser at a wavelength of 633 nm at 25 °C. Each sample is measured in triplicate (Fig.2a).
3. The polyplex sample (100 μL) is then diluted with 900 μL HEPES (pH 7.4, 10 mM) in a 1.5 mL centrifugal tube and transferred into a disposable capillary cell (DTS1070) for zeta potential measurement using a Zetasizer Nano. Each sample is measured in triplicate (Fig.2b).

### 3.7 Transmission Electron Microscope Imaging

1. The L4/pLuci polyplex is prepared at an N/P ratio of 24 at a DNA dose of 20 μg/mL as described protocol in Sect. 3.4.
2. The 100-mesh copper grid is immersed into the polyplex sample for 10 s using microforceps. Then, the copper grid is taken out, and the excess solution on the copper grid is removed using filter paper.
3. A drop of uranyl acetate solution (2 wt% in $H_2O$) is added to the copper grid to stain the sample for 10 s, and the excess solution on the copper grid is removed with filter paper.
4. The morphology of the polyplex is observed using TEM (JEOL, JEM-1010) at 100 kV voltage.

### 3.8 Agarose Gel Retardation Electrophoresis

1. Agarose gel is prepared at 1 wt% in Tris-Acetate-EDTA buffer containing 0.1% ethidium bromide.
2. The L4/pLuci polyplex is prepared with an N/P ratio of 24 at a DNA dose of 20 μg/mL as described protocol in Sect. 3.4.

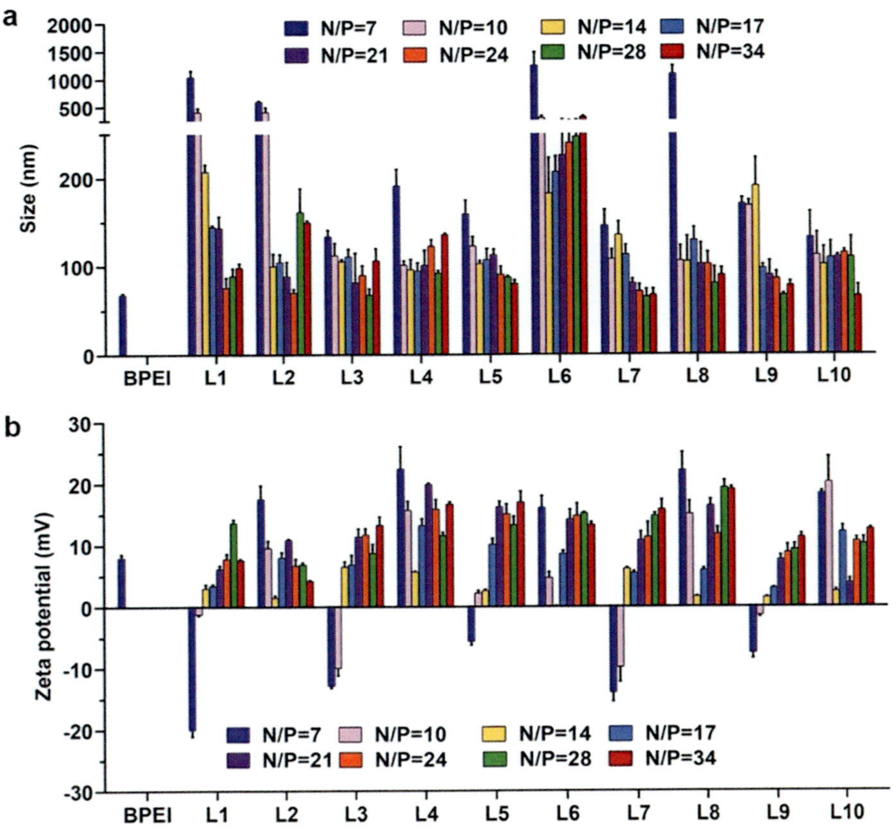


**Fig. 2** Fabrication and characterization of polymer/DNA polyplexes. (**a**) Hydrodynamic diameters and (**b**) zeta potentials of the polyplexes formed at different N/P ratios

3. The polyplex sample is mixed with DNA-loading buffer at the volume ratio of 1/5 in a 0.5 mL centrifugal tube. The mixture is gently vortexed for 10 s using a vortex vibrator.
4. The mixture (20 μL) is added to the agarose gel for electrophoresis at 120 V for 25 min.
5. The DNA bands are imaged via a chemiluminescence imaging system (Clinx Science Instruments Co., Ltd., China) (Fig. 3).

## 3.9 Esterase-Responsive Activities of the Polymer

1. Porcine liver esterase (200 U/mL) is dissolved in the Tris-HCl buffer (100 mM, pH 7.4) containing NaCl (100 mM).
2. L4 is dissolved in DMSO at 50 mg/mL, and then diluted with HPEPS (10 mM, pH 7.4) to 0.4 mg/mL L4.

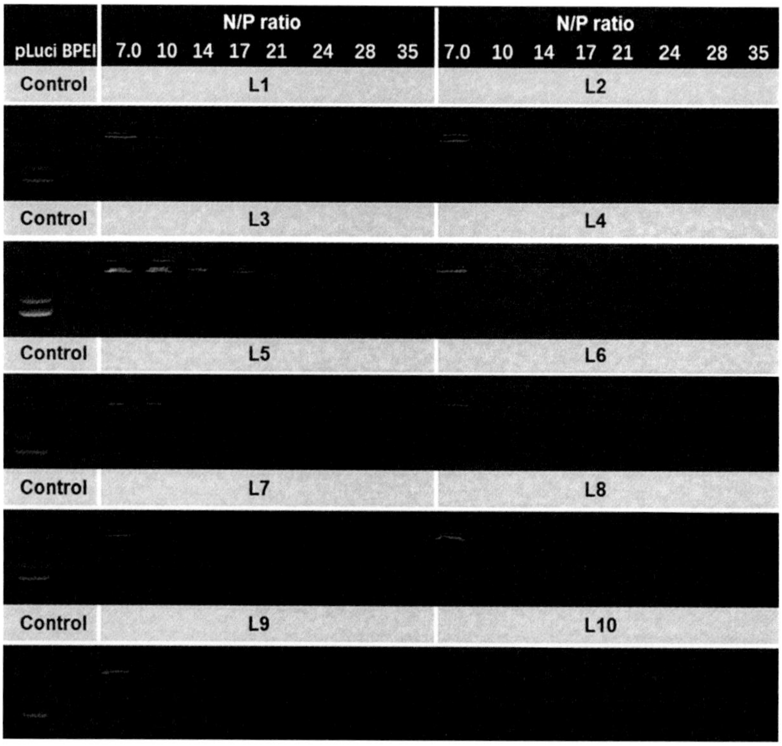


**Fig. 3** Agarose gel retardation electrophoresis of the polymer/pLuci polyplexes at different N/P ratios with the naked pLuci and BPEI/pLuci as controls; pLuci equivalent dose is 20 μg/mL

3. The polymer solution is mixed with an equal volume of the esterase solution in a 1.5 mL centrifugal tube and incubated at 37 °C in a water bath.
4. At timed intervals, 200 μL of the mixture is sampled and mixed with 400 μL methanol. Then, the mixed solution is vortexed and centrifuged (10,000 rpm for 10 min).
5. The supernate is analyzed by HPLC (The injecting volume is 20 μL, the mobile phase is methanol/phosphorous acid (0.1 wt%) solution (3/1, v/v) at a flow rate of 1.0 mL/min at 35 °C, UV-vis: $\lambda$max = 275 nm) (Fig. 4).

## 3.10 Esterase-Responsive Activities of the Polyplexes

1. Porcine liver esterase (200 U/mL) is dissolved in the Tris-HCl buffer (100 mM, pH 7.4) containing NaCl (100 mM).
2. The L4/pLuci polyplex is prepared with an N/P ratio of 24 at a DNA-equivalent dose of 20 μg/mL as described protocol in Sect. 3.4.

**Fig. 4** The esterase-responsiveness of the polymer incubated with porcine liver esterase at 37 °C in terms of the polymer hydrolysis rates

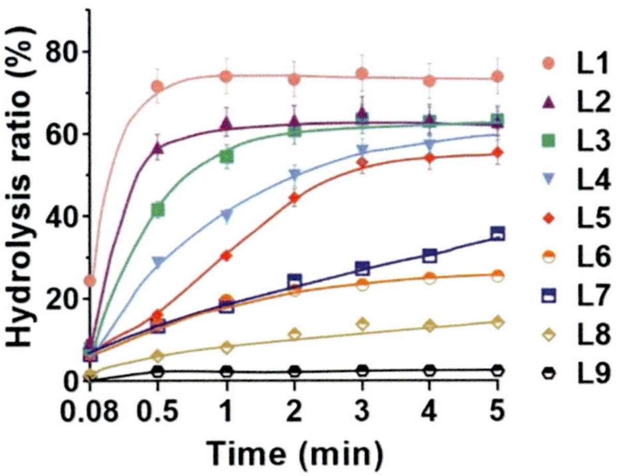


**Fig. 5** The esterase-responsiveness of the L4/pLuci polyplexes incubated with porcine liver esterase at 37 °C in terms of the changes in particle size and zeta potential at different times

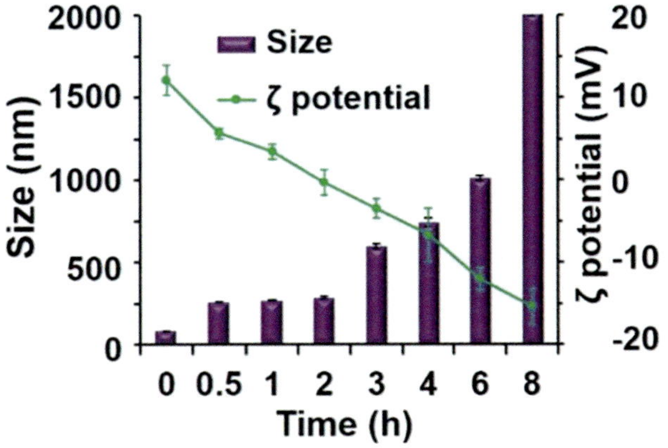


3. The polyplex solution is mixed with an equal volume of porcine liver esterase solution (200 U/mL) in a 1.5 mL centrifugal tube and incubated at 37 °C in a water bath.
4. At timed intervals, the size and zeta potential of polyplexes are measured using Zetasizer Nano as described protocol in Sect. 3.6 (Fig. 5).
5. The morphology changes of the polyplex are observed using TEM as described in Sect. 3.7 (Fig.6).
6. pLuci-releasing from the polyplex is detected by gel retardation electrophoresis as described protocol in Sect. 3.8 (Fig.7).

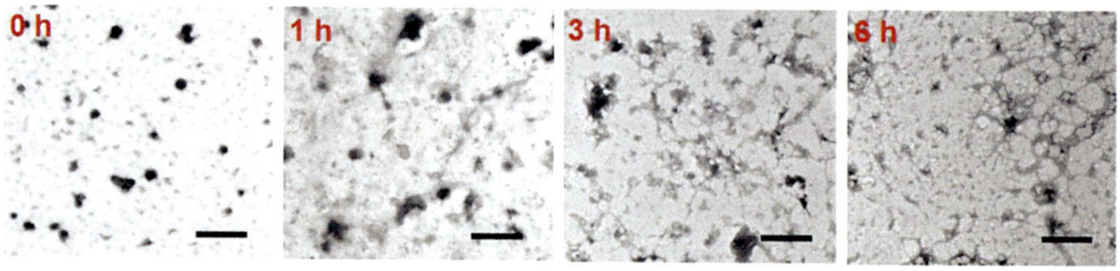


**Fig. 6** The morphological changes of L4/pLuci observed by TEM after incubation with porcine liver esterase at 37 °C (Scale bars = 100 nm)

**Fig. 7** The agarose gel retardation electrophoresis of the L4/pLuci polyplexes after incubated in esterase solution at different times

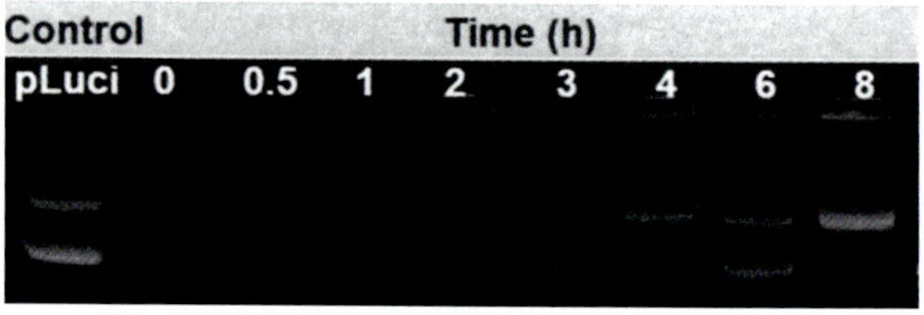


## 3.11 Gene Transfection

1. The L4/pLuci polyplex is prepared with an N/P ratio of 24 at a DNA dose of 20 μg/mL as described in Sect. 3.4.
2. HeLa cells are maintained in RPMI 1640 supplemented with 10% FBS, penicillin (100 units/mL), and streptomycin (100 μg/mL) in a humidified atmosphere of 5% $CO_2$ at 37 °C.
3. Cells are seeded in 48-well plates at a density of 25,000 cells per well and incubated in 10% FBS-containing medium (0.4 mL) for 12 h.
4. The cell medium in each well is replaced with fresh medium (0.4 mL) without FBS supplement and added with 10 μL of the L4/pLuci polyplex solution (pLuci in the medium is 0.5 μg/mL) using a pipettor. The plates are then placed back in the incubator.
5. After 4 h incubation, the culture medium in each well is replaced with fresh 10% FBS-containing medium (0.4 mL) and incubated for 44 h.
6. The cells are washed twice with PBS and lysed using a RIPA lysis buffer (100 μL per well) (PromegaBiotech Co., Ltd., USA). The plates are gently vortexed for 1 min to ensure complete coverage of the cells.
7. The cell lysate (20 μL) is mixed with luciferase substrate (5 μL, containing 1 mg/mL *D*-luciferin) in a polystyrene round bottom test tube and gently vortexed for 5 s. The chemiluminescence is immediately measured with an FB12 Tube Luminometer (Titertek-Berthold Co., Ltd., Germany).
8. The total protein content is measured by a BCA protein assay kit (Sangon Biotech Co., Ltd., Shanghai) according to the manufacturer's instructions.
9. The luciferase expression is normalized with the total protein concentration (the relative luciferase light units per milligram protein, RLU/mg) (Fig. 8).

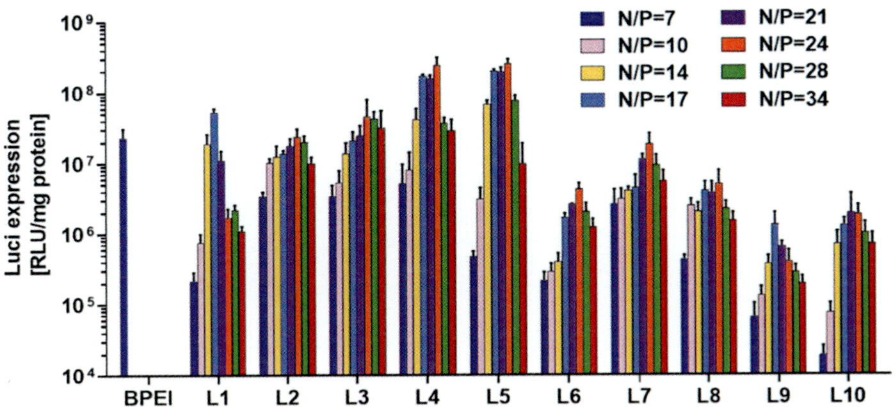


**Fig. 8** Luciferase expression in HeLa cells of the polymer/pLuci at different N/P ratios. Data are presented as mean ± SD of biological replicates

## 3.12 Subcellular Distribution and Colocalization

1. The fluorescent dye-labeled L4/pLuci polyplexes are prepared with an N/P ratio of 24 at a DNA dose of 20 μg/mL using the $L4^{FITC}$ or $pLuci^{Cy5}$ as described in Sect. 3.4.
2. HeLa cells are maintained in RPMI 1640 supplemented with 10% FBS, penicillin (100 units/mL) and streptomycin (100 μg/mL) in a humidified atmosphere of 5% $CO_2$ at 37 °C.
3. Cells are seeded in a glass-bottom petri dish at a density of 100,000 per dish and incubated in 10% FBS-containing culture medium (1.0 mL) for 24 h.
4. The cell medium is replaced with fresh serum-free medium (1.0 mL), and added with 50 μL fluorescent dye-labeled polyplexes (Taking the $L4^{FITC}/pLuci^{Cy5}$ as an example, N/P = 24, $pLuci^{Cy5}$ equivalent 1 μg/mL).
5. At the predesignated time, the nuclei are stained with Hoechst 33342 (2 μM) for 20 min, the lysosomes are stained with Lysotracker green (0.2 μM) for 20 min, or the cell membrane is stained with FITC-labeled wheat germ agglutin ($WGA^{FITC}$, 0.2 μM) for 10 min.
6. The cells are then washed three times with PBS and imaged using CLSM (Nikon A1) with excitation wavelengths at 405 nm for Hoechst 33342, 488 nm for LysoTracker green or FITC, and 640 nm for Cy5 or Cy5.5 (Fig.9).

## 3.13 Effects of Inhibitors on Cellular Uptake

1. HeLa cells are maintained in RPMI 1640 supplemented with 10% FBS, penicillin (100 units/mL) and streptomycin (100 μg/mL) in a humidified atmosphere of 5% $CO_2$ at 37 °C.

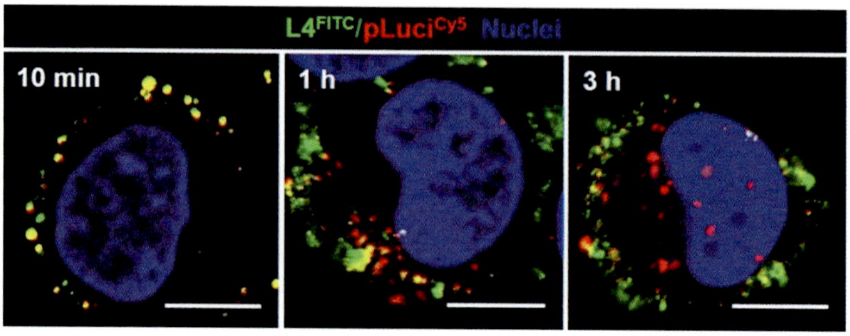


**Fig. 9** CLSM observation of the dissociation of the dually labeled L4$^{FITC}$/pLuci$^{Cy5}$ polyplexes in HeLa cells at different times (Scale bars = 25 μm)

2. Cells are seeded in 24-well plates at a density of 200,000 cells per well and incubated in 10% FBS-containing medium (1.0 mL) for 12 h.
3. The fluorescent dye-labeled L4/pLuci polyplexe is prepared at a DNA-dose of 20 μg/mL using the pLuci$^{Cy5}$ as described in Sect. 3.4. The ratio of pLuci$^{Cy5}$ in the total pLuci does is 5% (see Note 5).
4. The endocytosis inhibitor solutions of chlorpromazine (50 μM), filipin III (7.5 μM), wortmannin (5 μM) or cytochalasin D (5 μM) are pared in serum-free medium.
5. The cell medium in each well is replaced with fresh serum-free medium (1.0 mL) containing the endocytosis inhibitors of chlorpromazine (50 μM), filipin III (7.5 μM), wortmannin (5 μM) or cytochalasin D (5 μM), and incubated for 1 h. In parallel, the temperature effect of 4 °C is also performed. After replacement with fresh serum-free medium, the cell plate is placed in a 4 °C refrigerator and incubated for 1 h.
6. The L4/pLuci$^{Cy5}$ (50 μL, total pLuci equivalent 1 μg/mL in the medium) is added to each well and incubated for an additional 2 h.
7. The cells are washed three times with PBS, digested with 0.25% trypsin solution, rinsed with 1 mL 10% FBS-containing medium, and collected into a 5 mL polystyrene round bottom test tube.
8. The Cy5-positive cells are analyzed using` flow cytometry (BD FACS Calibur) (Fig. 10).

## 4 Notes

1. In the synthetic procedure, the temperature should not be higher than 50 °C to avoid the self-polymerization of the monomer.
2. With the acyl chains increasing, the polymers of L4, L5, and L6 are not easily precipitated in the ethyl ether. n-Hexane can be used.
3. Those polymers are easily hydrolyzed, so they must be kept at dry conditions and in a dark environment.
4. The prepared polyplexes should be used within 12 h to avoid the efficiency reduction of gene transfection.

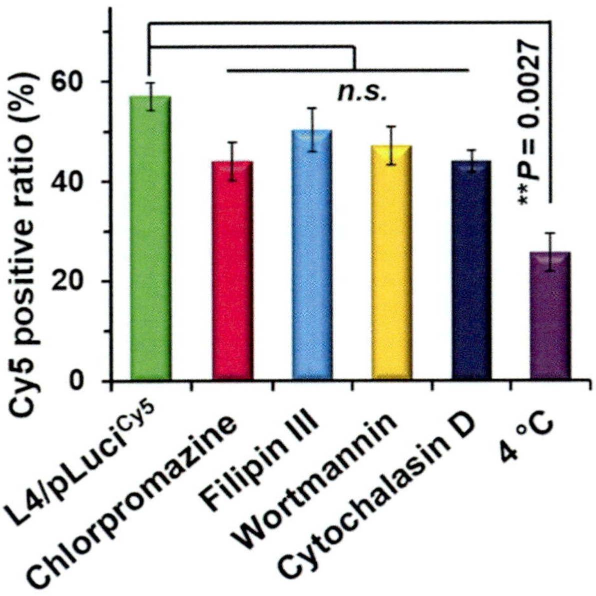


**Fig. 10** The effect of endocytosis inhibitors on cellular uptake of L4/pLuci$^{Cy5}$. Data are presented as mean ± SD of biological replicates, significances are determined by one-way ANOVA with Tukey's correction and 95% confidence intervals, *n.s.* means no significant difference, $^{**}$ $P < 0.01$

5. In the cellular uptake experiment, the ratio of pLuci$^{Cy5}$ in the total pLuci should not be more than 10%. The excessive amount of pLuci$^{Cy5}$ can result in false-positive results.

## 5 Conclusion

This protocol demonstrates the virus-mimicking vector capable of sticking onto the cell membrane and ejecting DNA into cytosol without entering the cells, bypassing endo-/lysosomal trapping-caused low transfection efficiency and avoiding the endocytosed carrier materials-caused adverse effects. The key to realizing this concept is an esterase-catalyzed charge-reversal polymer with proper acyl chains in N-[p-acyloxybenzyloxycarbonyl]ethyl-N-methyl ammonium of linear polyethyleneimine. The polymers with short acyl chains cannot make their polylexes stick on the cell membrane, while those with ultra-long acyl chains are insensitive to esterses and have slow charge-reversal rates once exposing to the cytosol, incapable of DNA-ejecting. The polymer with octanoyl chains, L4, has a balanced membrane-binding ability and esterase-triggered charge-reversal rate. So, once L4/DNA polyplexes contacts a cell, the pendant long octanoyl chains insert into the lipid-bilayer and tightly anchor the polyplexes onto the cytomembrane, exposing part of the polyplexes to abundant cytosolic esterases, which hydrolyze and turn the polymer neutral, liberalizing the DNA. The strong electrostatic repulsion among the anions squeezes the DNA into the cytosol.

## References

Bulcha JT, Wang Y, Ma H, Tai PW, Gao G (2021) Viral vector platforms within the gene therapy landscape. Signal Transduct Target Ther 6(1):1–24

Bus T, Traeger A, Schubert US (2018) The great escape: how cationic polyplexes overcome the endosomal barrier. J Mater Chem B 6(43):6904–6918

Chen H, Gu Z, An H, Chen C, Chen J, Cui R, Chen S, Chen W, Chen X, Chen X (2018) Precise nanomedicine for intelligent therapy of cancer. Sci China Chem 61(12):1503–1552

Chen Y, Aslanoglou S, Gervinskas G, Abdelmaksoud H, Voelcker NH, Elnathan R (2019) Cellular deformations induced by conical silicon nanowire arrays facilitate gene delivery. Small 15(47): 1904819

Curley CT, Mead BP, Negron K, Kim N, Garrison WJ, Miller GW, Kingsmore KM, Thim EA, Song J, Munson JM, Klibanov AL, Suk JS, Hanes J, Price RJ (2020) Augmentation of brain tumor interstitial flow via focused ultrasound promotes brain-penetrating nanoparticle dispersion and transfection. Sci Adv 6(18):eaay1344

Degors IMS, Wang C, Rehman ZU, Zuhorn IS (2019) Carriers break barriers in drug delivery: endocytosis and endosomal escape of gene delivery vectors. Acc Chem Res 52(7):1750–1760

Fang H, Chen J, Lin L, Liu F, Tian H, Chen X (2019) A strategy of killing three birds with one stone for cancer therapy through regulating the tumor microenvironment by H2O2-responsive gene delivery system. ACS Appl Bio Mater 11(51):47785–47797

Hardee CL, Arévalo-Soliz LM, Hornstein BD, Zechiedrich L (2017) Advances in nonviral DNA vectors for gene therapy. Genes 8(2):65

Li J, Yu X, Wang Y, Yuan Y, Xiao H, Cheng D, Shuai X (2014) A reduction and pH dual-sensitive polymeric vector for long-circulating and tumor-targeted siRNA delivery. Adv Mater 26(48): 8217–8224

Li Y, Zhang K, Liu P, Chen M, Zhong Y, Ye Q, Wei MQ, Zhao H, Tang Z (2019) Encapsulation of plasmid DNA by nanoscale metal-organic frameworks for efficient gene transportation and expression. Adv Mater 31(29):e1901570

Liu X, Xiang J, Zhu D, Jiang L, Zhou Z, Tang J, Liu X, Huang Y, Shen Y (2016) Fusogenic reactive oxygen species triggered charge-reversal vector for effective gene delivery. Adv Mater 28(9): 1743–1752

Liu J, Hu D, Zhou Q, Shen Y (2019) Design and challenge of cancer nanomedicine. Sci Sin Chim 49(9):1192–1202

Malik YS, Sheikh MA, Xing Z, Guo Z, Zhu X, Tian H, Chen X (2018) Polylysine-modified polyethylenimine polymer can generate genetically engineered mesenchymal stem cells for combinational suicidal gene therapy in glioblastoma. Acta Biomater 80:144–153

Mitchell MJ, Billingsley MM, Haley RM, Wechsler ME, Peppas NA, Langer R (2020) Engineering precision nanoparticles for drug delivery. Nat Rev Drug Discov 20:101–124

Molineux IJ, Panja D (2013) Popping the cork: mechanisms of phage genome ejection. Nat Rev Microbiol 11(3):194–204

Pollard H, Remy JS, Loussouarn G, Demolombe S, Behr JP, Escande D (1998) Polyethylenimine but not cationic lipids promotes transgene delivery to the nucleus in mammalian cells. J Biol Chem 273(13):7507–7511

Qiu N, Liu X, Zhong Y, Zhou Z, Piao Y, Miao L, Zhang Q, Tang J, Huang L, Shen Y (2016) Esterase-activated charge-reversal polymer for fibroblast-exempt cancer gene therapy. Adv Mater 28(48):10613–10622

Qiu C, Han H, Sun J, Zhang H, Wei W, Cui S, Chen X, Wang J, Zhang Q (2019) Regulating intracellular fate of siRNA by endoplasmic reticulum membrane-decorated hybrid nanoplexes. Nat Commun 10(1):2702

Qiu N, Wang G, Wang J, Zhou Q, Guo M, Wang Y, Hu X, Zhou H, Bai R, You M (2021) Tumor-associated macrophage and tumor-cell dually transfecting polyplexes for efficient interleukin-12 cancer gene therapy. Adv Mater 33(2):2006189

Shen Y, Xiang J, Shen Y (2020) A microfluidics-based stepwise assembly method for preparation of HA/PEI/DNA polyplexes. Acta Polym Sin 51(9):1029–1038

Sun W, Chen X, Xie C, Wang Y, Lin L, Zhu K, Shuai X (2018) Co-delivery of doxorubicin and anti-BCL-2 siRNA by pH-responsive polymeric vector to overcome drug resistance in in vitro and in vivo hepg2 hepatoma model. Biomacromolecules 19(6):2248–2256

Sun R, Qiu N, Shen Y (2019) Polymeric cancer nanomedicines: challenge and development. Acta Polym Sin 50(6):588–601

Tang X, Sheng Q, Xu C, Li M, Rao J, Wang X, Long Y, Tao Y, He X, Zhang Z, He Q (2021) pH/ATP cascade-responsive nano-courier with efficient tumor targeting and siRNA unloading for photothermal-immunotherapy. Nano Today 37:101083

Van Bruggen C, Hexum JK, Tan Z, Dalal RJ, Reineke TM (2019) Nonviral gene delivery with cationic Glycopolymers. Acc Chem Res 52(5):1347–1358

Vermeulen LM, Brans T, De Smedt SC, Remaut K, Braeckmans K (2018) Methodologies to investigate intracellular barriers for nucleic acid delivery in nonviral gene therapy. Nano Today 21:74–90

Wang H, Jiang Y, Peng H, Chen Y, Zhu P, Huang Y (2015) Recent progress in microRNA delivery for cancer therapy by nonviral synthetic vectors. Adv Drug Deliv Rev 81:142–160

Wang D, Tai PW, Gao G (2019) Adeno-associated virus vector as a platform for gene therapy delivery. Nat Rev Drug Discov 18(5):358–378

Wang D, Wang K, Cai Y (2020) An overview of development in gene therapeutics in China. Gene Ther 27(7):338–348

Wu M, Meng Q, Chen Y, Zhang L, Li M, Cai X, Li Y, Yu P, Zhang L, Shi J (2016) Large pore-sized hollow mesoporous organosilica for redox-responsive gene delivery and synergistic cancer chemotherapy. Adv Mater 28(10):1963–1969

Wu J, Chen J, Feng Y, Zhang S, Lin L, Guo Z, Sun P, Xu C, Tian H, Chen X (2020) An immune cocktail therapy to realize multiple boosting of the cancer-immunity cycle by combination of drug/gene delivery nanoparticles. Sci Adv 6(40):eabc7828

Yan H, Zhu D, Zhou Z, Liu X, Piao Y, Zhang Z, Liu X, Tang J, Shen Y (2018) Facile synthesis of semi-library of low charge density cationic polyesters from poly(alkylene maleate)s for efficient local gene delivery. Biomaterials 178:559–569

Zhou Z, Liu X, Zhu D, Wang Y, Zhang Z, Zhou X, Qiu N, Chen X, Shen Y (2017) Nonviral cancer gene therapy: delivery cascade and vector nanoproperty integration. Adv Drug Deliv Rev 115: 115–154

Zhou J, Shao Z, Liu J, Duan Q, Wang X, Li J, Yang H (2020) From endocytosis to nonendocytosis: the emerging era of gene delivery. ACS Appl Bio Mater 3(5):2686–2701

Zhu D, Yan H, Liu X, Xiang J, Zhou Z, Tang J, Liu X, Shen Y (2017) Intracellularly disintegratable polysulfoniums for efficient gene delivery. Adv Funct Mater 27(16):1606826

Zhuang X, Zhang H, Hu G (2019) Cancer and microenvironment plasticity: double-edged swords in metastasis. Trends Pharmacol Sci 40(6):419–429

# Rattle-Structured Rough Nanocapsules with In Situ-Formed Gold Nanorod Cores for Complementary Gene/Chemo/Photothermal Therapy

22

Kai Zhang, Nana Zhao, and Fu-jian Xu

## Contents



**Abstract**

The advent of nanotechnology has provided much promise and enormous breakthroughs for the design of versatile gene delivery systems with the high loading capacity and excellent biocompatibility. Tremendous observations suggest that the morphology of carriers influences their cellular uptake ability, and rough surface nanoparticles with higher cellular uptake efficiency compared with smooth surfaces. This protocol reports the design of a novel rattle-structured rough nanoplatform (Au@HSN-PGEA nanohybrids, AHPs) as drug/gene carriers, and evaluates its application in the gene/chemo/photothermal therapy of cancer. The AHPs are composed of gold nanorod cores and polycationic mesoporous silica shells with rough surface, endowing the high loading efficiency and NIR laser-responsive. Herein, the preparation procedure and characterization methods of AHPs are described in detail. Importantly, using sorafenib (SF) and

K. Zhang · N. Zhao (✉) · F.-j. Xu (✉)
Key Laboratory of Biomedical Materials of Natural Macromolecules, Beijing Laboratory of Biomedical Materials, Beijing University of Chemical Technology, Ministry of Education, Beijing, China

College of Materials Science and Engineering, Beijing University of Chemical Technology, Beijing, China
e-mail: zhaonn@mail.buct.edu.cn; xufj@mail.buct.edu.cn



H. Tian and X. Chen (eds.), *Gene Delivery*, Biomaterial Engineering,
https://doi.org/10.1007/978-981-16-5419-0_22

antioncogene p53 as model drugs, the drug/gene delivery effect of AHPs as carriers are systematically investigated and evaluated through fluorescence imaging and flow cytometry. Meanwhile, the gene transfection properties and photothermal effects of AHPs as well as the drug release behavior in response to NIR are also tested. Notably, the proposed versatile nanoplatform exhibits good photoacoustic capability for accurate tumor diagnosis. This work provides a facile strategy to design flexible platforms with high gene delivery performance and cellular internalization efficiency for complementary gene/chemo/photothermal therapy of cancers.

**Keywords**

Rough nanocapsule · Gene therapy · Gold nanorod · Drug · Complementary therapy

## 1 Overview

With the intensive study of the molecular mechanisms of various diseases and a comprehensive understanding of the complex interaction between nucleic acid and proteins, the repair of defective genes and the regulation of specific genes are considered as a new therapeutic strategy, which is called "gene therapy" (Song et al. 2004). Gene therapy is carried out by interfering with genes to controllably regulate the expression levels of specific proteins in cells (Ashrafizadeh et al. 2020). Compared with traditional therapeutic strategies for cancer therapy, including surgery, chemotherapy and radiotherapy, gene therapy exhibits unparalleled tumor-specific performance, which can achieve targeted therapy with the negligible damage to normal cells or organs (Mohammadinejad et al. 2020). To obtain highly efficient therapy of cancers, a safe and suitable gene vector is essential, which can protect nucleic acid from being degraded by nuclease during blood circulation, and achieve targeted delivery of genes to tumors. Consequently, off-target effects can be suppressed and the therapeutic efficiency of gene therapy can be significantly improved (Sung and Kim 2019).

As we all know, gene vectors are mainly divided into two types, viral vectors and non-viral vectors (Taghavi et al. 2016). Tremendous observations suggest that most of viral gene delivery systems hold high immunogenicity and possibility of recombinant oncogenes, which limits their applications in biomedical research (Kaygisiz and Synatschke 2020). Non-viral vectors have attracted much attention as alternative systems for gene delivery with numerous advantages, such as low host immunogenicity, high flexibility, and easy preparation (De Smedt et al. 2000). Notably, the emergence of nanotechnology provides great opportunities for the design and fabrication of novel and efficient non-viral gene delivery systems (Taghavi et al. 2020). To date, a variety of organic/inorganic nanoplatforms have been demonstrated to be promising gene carriers for efficient gene delivery and transfection (Zhao et al. 2019). These hybrid nanomaterials composed of cationic polymers and inorganic nanoparticles hold both high affinity of cationic polymers and the unique physicochemical properties of inorganic nanoparticles (Guo et al. 2019). Therefore, the development of novel and efficient multifunctional organic/inorganic hybrid nanomaterials as gene carriers opens up new avenues for cancer therapy and biomedical research.

Due to the favorable optical absorption in the near infrared (NIR) region, gold nanorods (Au NRs) are considered as attractive theranostic agents for accurate cancer diagnosis and efficient tumor treatment (Yang et al. 2015). Au NRs have been utilized as contrast agents of photoacoustic (PA) imaging for tumor visualization with high spatiotemporal resolution, and employed for photothermal therapy (PTT)-mediated cancer treatment (Zhao et al. 2016; Jung et al. 2016). Mesoporous silica nanoparticles exhibit good potential in gene delivery owing to their high specific surface area, controlled morphology, good biocompatibility and easy functionalization (Li et al. 2012). The integration of silica nanoparticles and Au NRs to construct a multifunctional nanoplatform for biomedical applications holds significant prospects. Especially, hetero-nanoparticles from hollow silica nanoparticles (HSNs) are beneficial for drug delivery since the hollow cavity can increase the loading capacity (Valtchev and Tosheva 2013). Meanwhile, the hollow cavity of HSNs can be used as chemical reactors to induce the production of Au NRs cores. Notably, the morphology of nanoplatform plays a critical role in the cellular uptake process and affects the intracellular delivery efficiency and clearance behavior (Kinnear et al. 2017). Compared with relatively smooth surface, the rough silica nanoparticles with spiky surfaces have been confirmed to possess a stronger plasmid DNA binding capacity and better transfection performance (Song et al. 2017). Therefore, the advantages of rough nanoparticles inspired us to propose more effective cancer treatment strategies by integrating multifunctional nanoplatforms and surface roughness. Herein, the protocol describes rattle-structured rough nanocapsules (Au@HSN-PGEA, AHPs) composed of *in-situ*-formed Au NR cores and polycationic mesoporous silica shells for PA imaging-guided complementary gene/chemo/photothermal therapy (Chen et al. 2018) (Fig. 1).

## 2 Protocol

### 2.1 Materials

#### 2.1.1 Synthesis of Rough Hollow Silica Nanoparticles (HSNs)

1. Resorcinol (Sigma-Aldrich Chemical Co., St Louis, MO)
2. Formaldehyde (Sigma-Aldrich Chemical Co., St Louis, MO)
3. Ethanol (Beijing Chemical Co., Beijing, China)
4. Ammonia (Beijing Chemical Co., Beijing, China)
5. Tetraethyl orthosilicate (TEOS) (Sigma-Aldrich Chemical Co., St Louis, USA)
6. Centrifuge (Eppendorf, Germany)

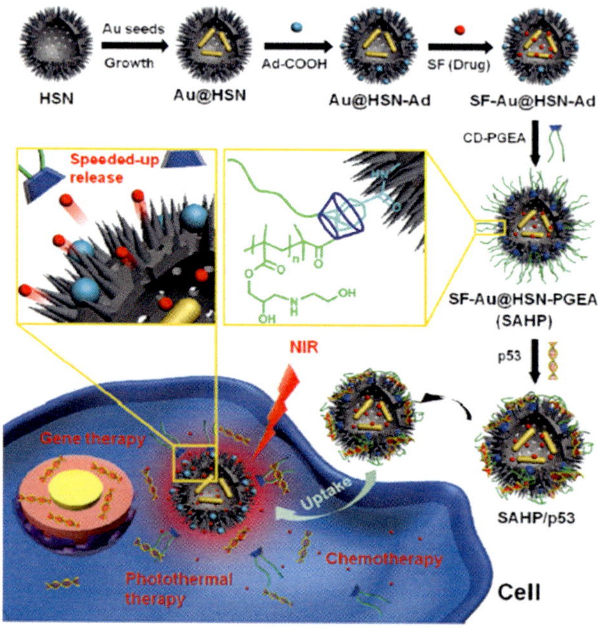


**Fig. 1** Schematic illustration of the preparation of SAHP and the resultant responsive drug/gene co-delivery process. (Adapted from reference Chen et al. (2018), with permission)

### 2.1.2 Synthesis of Rattle-Structured Rough Au@HSN

1. Cetyltrimethylammonium bromide (CTAB) (Sigma-Aldrich Chemical Co., St Louis, USA)
2. Chloroauric acid ($HAuCl_4$) (Sinopharm Group Co. Ltd., Beijing, China)
3. Sodium borohydride ($NaBH_4$) (Sigma-Aldrich Chemical Co., St Louis, MO)
4. Centrifuge (Eppendorf, Germany)
5. Ascorbic acid (AA) (Sinopharm Group Co. Ltd., Beijing, China)
6. Silver nitrate ($AgNO_3$) (Sigma-Aldrich Chemical Co., St Louis, MO)
7. Hydrochloric acid (Beijing Chemical Co., Beijing, China)

### 2.1.3 Synthesis of CD-PGEA

1. *β*-cyclodextrin (β-CD) (Sigma-Aldrich Chemical Co., St Louis, MO)
2. *N,N*-Dimethylformamide (DMF) (Beijing Chemical Co., Beijing, China)
3. 2-bromoisobutyryl bromide (BIBB) (Sigma-Aldrich Chemical Co., St Louis, MO)
4. Triethylamine (TEA) (Energy Chemical Co., Ltd., Shanghai, China)
5. Centrifuge (Eppendorf, Germany)
6. Ether
7. Dimethyl sulfoxide (DMSO) (Beijing Chemical Co., Beijing, China)
8. Glycidyl methacrylate (GMA) (Sigma-Aldrich Chemical Co., St Louis, MO)
9. *N,N,N′,N″,N″*-pentamethyldiethylenetriamine (PMDETA) (Sigma-Aldrich Chemical Co., St Louis, MO)
10. Copper (I) bromide (CuBr) (Sigma-Aldrich Chemical Co., St Louis, MO)

11. Methanol (Beijing Chemical Co., Beijing, China)
12. Ethanolamine (EA) (Sigma-Aldrich Chemical Co., St Louis, MO)
13. Freeze dryer application (Beijing Songyuan Huaxing official., China)

#### 2.1.4 Preparation of Rough Au@HSN-PGEA (AHPs)

1. Centrifuge (Eppendorf, Germany)
2. 3-aminopropyl triethoxysilane (APTES) (Energy Chemical Co., Ltd., Shanghai, China)
3. Triethylamine (TEA) (Energy Chemical Co., Ltd., Shanghai, China)
4. 1-ethyl-3-(3-dimethylaminopropyl) carbodiimide hydrochloride (EDAC) (Sigma-Aldrich Chemical Co., St Louis, MO)
5. N-hydroxysuccinimide (NHS) (Sigma-Aldrich Chemical Co., St Louis, MO)
6. Adamantanecarboxylic acid (Ad-COOH) (Energy Chemical Co., Ltd., Shanghai, China)
7. Dimethyl sulfoxide (DMSO) (Beijing Chemical Co., Beijing, China)
8. Freeze dryer application (Beijing Songyuan Huaxing official., China)

#### 2.1.5 BET Characterization of Material

1. $N_2$ gas stream

#### 2.1.6 Cytotoxicity Assay

1. HepG2 (American Type Culture Collection, Rockville, MD)
2. HEK293 (American Type Culture Collection, Rockville, MD)
3. Dulbecco's modification of Eagle's medium (DMEM)
4. Heat-inactivated fetal bovine serum (FBS)
5. Penicillin (Sigma-Aldrich Chemical Co., St. Louis, MO)
6. Streptomycin (Sigma-Aldrich Chemical Co., St. Louis, MO)
7. Phosphate buffered saline (PBS)
8. (4,5-Dimethylthiazol-2yl)-2,5-diphenyl tetrazolium bromide (MTT) (Sigma -Aldrich Chemical Co., St. Louis, MO)
9. Dimethyl sulfoxide (DMSO) (Beijing Chemical Co., Beijing, China)
10. 96-well microtiter plate (Nunc Co., Wiesbaden, Germany)
11. $CO_2$ incubator
12. Bio-Rad model 680 microplate reader

#### 2.1.7 In Vitro Gene Transfection Assay

1. Dulbecco's modification of Eagle's medium (DMEM)
2. Heat-inactivated fetal bovine serum (FBS)
3. Cell lysate (Promega C.o, Cergy Pontoise, France)
4. Phosphate buffered saline (PBS)
5. Commercial kit (Promega Co., Beijing, China)
6. HepG2 (American Type Culture Collection, Rockville, MD)
7. Plasmid pEGFP-N1 (BD Biosciences, San Jose, CA)
8. 24-well plates (Nunc Co, Wiesbaden, Germany)
9. Luminometer (Berthold Lumat LB 9507)

10. Leica DMIL fluorescence microscope
11. Flow cytometry (FCM) (Beckman Coulter, USA)

#### 2.1.8 Cellular Internalization

1. HepG2 (American Type Culture Collection, Rockville, MD)
2. Dulbecco's modification of Eagle's medium (DMEM)
3. YOYO-1
4. Culture medium
5. Phosphate buffered saline (PBS)
6. 4′6′- diamidino-2-phenylindole (DAPI)
7. 6-well plates (Nunc Co, Wiesbaden, Germany)
8. Flow cytometry (MoFlo XDP, Beckman, USA)
9. Leica DMI3000B fluorescence microscope

#### 2.1.9 SAHP/p53 Stability Characterization

1. p53
2. Laser particle size and potential analyzer (Malvern Instruments)

#### 2.1.10 Complementary Gene/Chemo/Photothermal Therapy In Vitro and In Vivo

1. 1.HepG2 (American Type Culture Collection, Rockville, MD)
2. BALB/c nude mice (6 weeks old, weight 15–18 g, Beijing Vital River Laboratory Animal Technology Co., Ltd., Beijing, China)
3. Phosphate buffered saline (PBS)
4. 96-well plates (Nunc Co., Wiesbaden, Germany)
5. 808 nm NIR laser

#### 2.1.11 Photoacoustic Imaging of AHPs *In Vitro* and *In Vivo*

1. AHP solutions
2. Prosthesis
3. BALB/c nude mice (6 weeks old, weight 15–18 g, Beijing Vital River Laboratory Animal Technology Co., Ltd., Beijing, China)
4. Isoflurane
5. Multispectral optoacoustic tomography imaging system (MSOT invision 256-TF, iThermedical, Germany)

#### 2.1.12 Photothermal Effect of AHP In Vitro and In Vivo

1. HepG2 (American Type Culture Collection, Rockville, MD)
2. Dulbecco's modification of Eagle's medium (DMEM)
3. Heat-inactivated fetal bovine serum (FBS)
4. Fluorescein diacetate (FDA) (Sigma-Aldrich Co., St Louis, MO)
5. Propidium iodide (PI) (Sigma-Aldrich Co., St Louis, MO)
6. Female BALB/c nude mice (6 weeks old, weight 15–18 g, Beijing Vital River Laboratory Animal Technology Co., Ltd., Beijing, China)
7. 96-well plates (Nunc Co, Wiesbaden, Germany)

8. NIR laser (Daheng New Epoch Technology Inc., Beijing, China)
9. AIR thermal camera (FLIR Systems Inc., Ohio, USA)
10. 24-well plates (Nunc Co, Wiesbaden, Germany)
11. Leica fluorescence microscope
12. Infrared camera

#### 2.1.13 Sorafenib Loading

1. 1.Sorafenib (SF) (AMQUAR Biological Technology Co., Ltd., Shanghai, China)
2. High-performance liquid chromatography (HPLC) system (Hitachi, Tokyo, Japan)
3. InertSustain C18 column (250 mm × 4.6 mm, 5-μm particle size, S/N 6GR98165)
4. Acetic acid
5. Acetonitrile

#### 2.1.14 NIR-Triggered Sorafenib Release

1. 808 nm NIR laser (Daheng Optoelectronics, China)
2. High-performance liquid chromatography (HPLC) system (Hitachi, Tokyo, Japan)
3. Dulbecco's modification of Eagle's medium (DMEM)
4. Heat-inactivated fetal bovine serum (FBS)

#### 2.1.15 Effects of NIR-Triggered Drug Release on HCC Cells

1. HepG2 (American Type Culture Collection, Rockville, MD)
2. (4,5-Dimethylthiazol-2yl)-2,5-diphenyl tetrazolium bromide (MTT) (Sigma-Aldrich Chemical Co., St. Louis, MO)
3. Propidium iodide (PI) (Sigma-Aldrich Co., St Louis, MO)
4. Fluorescence inverted microscope (Leica, Germany)
5. Fluorescein diacetate (FDA) (Sigma-Aldrich Co., St Louis, MO)

### 2.2 Methods

#### 2.2.1 Synthesis of Rough Hollow Silica Nanoparticles (HSNs)

1. Put formaldehyde (0.14 mL), resorcinol (0.1 g) and ammonia (3.36 mL) into a mixed solution of ethanol (70 mL) and water (9.64 mL), then stir the mixture at 27 °C for 6 h.
2. Add TEOS (0.5 mL) under the stirring and keep the procedure for 6 min.
3. Inject resorcinol (0.2 g) and formaldehyde (0.28 mL) to the mixture, and keep the stirring for a while. (**Note 1**)
4. Collect the product by centrifugation and dried.
5. Calcine in air at 550 °C for 2 h to obtain rough HSN.
6. View the morphology with transmission electron microscope (TEM) in Fig. 2 (**Note 2**).

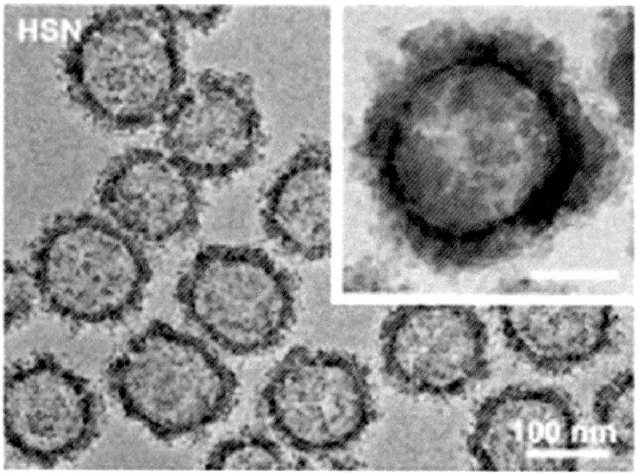


**Fig. 2** TEM images of HSNs and Au@HSN. Inset show the corresponding TEM images of higher magnification, scale bar: 50 nm. (Adapted from reference Chen et al. (2018), with permission)

Figure 2 shows that the particle size of the rough HSN is about 120–160 nm in diameter.

### 2.2.2 Synthesis of Rattle-Structured Rough Au@HSN

1. The HSN (30 mg) are ultrasonically dispersed in the aqueous solution containing CTAB (1.492 mL,0.1 mol/L).
2. Add $HAuCl_4$ (37.5 μL,0.01 mol/L) and $NaBH_4$ (90 μL,0.01 mol/L) into the HSN solution, and the mixture is stirred vigorously for 2 min.
3. Place the reaction mixture in a water bath at 27 °C for 2 h.
4. Centrifuge and purify product with aqueous solution containing CTAB (0.1 mol/L), and re-disperse the products in 750 μL of aqueous solution containing CTAB (0.1 mol/mL) as a seed solution.
5. Prepare the growth solution by adding the newly configured $AgNO_3$ (40 μL, 0.01 mol/L), $HAuCl_4$ (100 μL,0.01 mol/L), HCl (80 μL, 1 mol/L) and AA (64 μL,0.078 mol/L) into 2 mL of aqueous solution containing CTAB (0.2 mol/L)
6. Add 10 μL of seed solution to the growth solution, and place the mixture in a 27 °C water bath for 6 h.
7. The Au@HSN products obtained by centrifugation (**Note 3**).
8. View the morphology with transmission electron microscope (TEM) in Fig. 3 (**Note 2**).

Figure 3 shows the successful preparation of rattle-structured rough Au@HSN (comparable sizes of 130–170 nm) with uniform monodispersity. The encapsulated Au NR cores in the HSNs present 30 nm in length and ~10 nm in diameter.

### 2.2.3 Synthesis of CD-PGEA

1. Dissolve 2 g of β-CD in 10 mL of DMF, and then place the solution in an ice bath for 7 min with $N_2$ degassing.

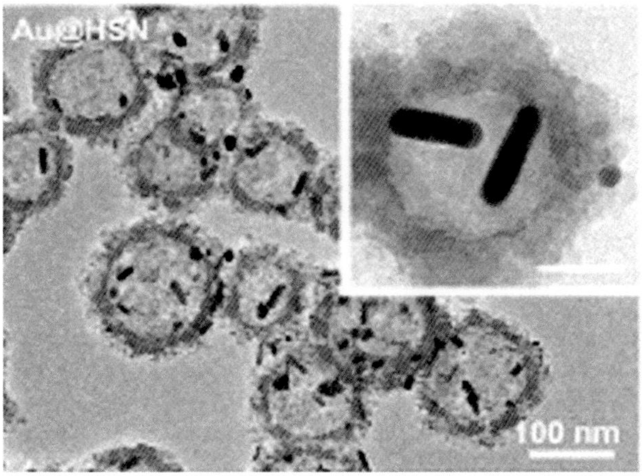


**Fig. 3** TEM images of Au@HSN. Inset show the corresponding TEM images of higher magnification, scale bar: 50 nm. (Adapted from reference Chen et al. (2018), with permission)

2. Put 4 mL of BIBB into 10 mL DMF and fully mix.
3. Dropwise add BIBB/DMF mixture into the above β-CD/DMF solution under $N_2$ conditions, and then add 2 mL of TEA to the mixed solution.
4. Place the mixed solution in an ice bath for 30 min, and then transfer to the room temperature for 24 h.
5. Centrifuge and obtain the supernatant, and then add ether to the supernatant to precipitate the product.
6. Dialyze and lyophilize the products to obtain CD-Br.
7. Dissolve CD-Br (0.2 g) in 2 mL of DMSO, and then add GMA (2.2 mL), PMDETA (116 μL) and CuBr (40.14 mg) in sequence to the CD-Br/DMSO solution and stir at 25 °C for 5 min.
8. Precipitate the product with methanol and obtain CD-PGMA through centrifugation and drying under vacuum.
9. Dissolve 0.1 g of CD-PGMA in 6 mL of DMSO and keep stirring for 30 min to form a homogeneous solution, and then add EA (4 mL) to the CD-PGMA solution (**Note 4**).
10. Stir the mixed solution at 50 °C for 12 h, and then dialyze by deionized water for 24 h.
11. The resultant CD-PGEA is collected by lyophilization.
12. Confirm the structure of the product with 1H NMR.

### 2.2.4 Synthesis of AHP

1. Disperse 10 mg of Au@HSN into 10 mL of ethanol/water solution (v/v = 9:1).
2. Add silane coupling agent (APTES) (300 μL) and triethylamine (500 μL) to the Au@HSN solution and maintain the reaction at room temperature overnight. Then the products are thoroughly washed with water and ethanol several times, and obtain the Au@HSN-$NH_2$.

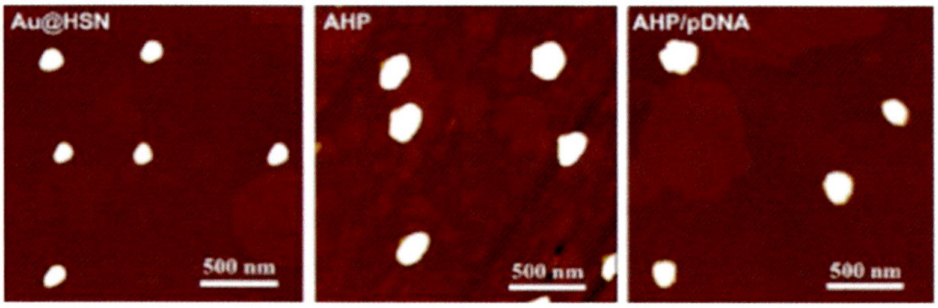


**Fig. 4** AFM images of Au@HSN, AHPs, and AHP/pDNA (N/P = 20). (Adapted from reference Chen et al. (2018), with permission)

3. Dissolve NHS (0.734 g), Ad-COOH (0.887 g), EDAC (1.427 g), and TEA (1.1 mL) into 6 mL of DMSO, and keep the incubation for 4 h at 37 °C.
4. Disperse 20 mg of Au@HSN-$NH_2$ into 4 mL of DMSO (4 mL), and add into the above solution, keeping the reaction for 48 h. Au@HSN-Ad is thoroughly washed by water (**Note 5**).
5. Add 0.5 mL of ethanol solution containing Au@HSN-Ad (1 mg/mL) into the CD-PGEA aqueous solution (5 mL,10 mg/mL), and shake at room temperature for 24 h.
6. Centrifuge to collect the precipitate, and obtain Au@HSN-PGEA (AHP) through freeze-drying.
7. View the morphology with atomic force microscopy imaging (AFM) in Fig. 4 (**Note 2**).

### 2.2.5 BET Characterization of Material

1. Weigh 50–100 mg of dried Au@HSN, Au@HSN-Ad, AHP, and SAHP (Sorafenib-loaded AHP), and degas at $10^{-3}$ Torr and 100 °C for 6 h.
2. $N_2$ absorption-desorption test is carried out accurately.
3. The surface area and pore diameter are calculated by the BET method, and the result are presented in Fig. 5.

Figure 5 shows the pore size distribution of Au@HSN (20 nm) and Au@HSN-Ad (16.2 nm). After modified by CD-PGEA and loaded with SF, the pore size distribution of AHP and SHAP decrease to 7.9 nm and 5.0 nm, respectively. These results suggest the successful preparation of AHP and SHAP.

### 2.2.6 Cytotoxicity Assay

1. Mix pristine AHP with different amounts and 0.33 μg of pDNA to obtain AHP/pDNA complexes with various N/P ratios.
2. Incubate HEK293 and HepG2 in DMEM cell medium containing 10% FBS, 100 units/mL penicillin, and 100 mg/mL streptomycin under 5% $CO_2$ atmosphere with 95% relative humidity at 37 °C.
3. Seed the cells in a 96-well microtiter plate at a density of $10^4$ cells per well and incubate in DMEM cell medium DMEM (100 μL) per well (**Note 6**).

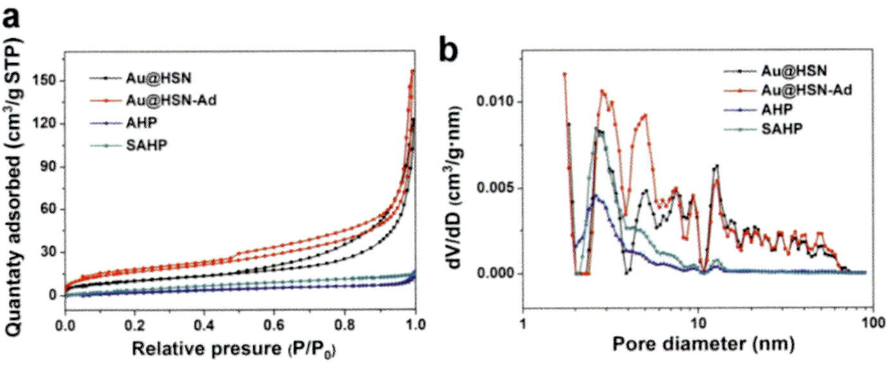


**Fig. 5** (**a**) Nitrogen sorption-desorption isotherms and (**b**) pore size distribution curves of Au@HSN-based nanoparticles. (Adapted from reference Chen et al. (2018), with permission)

4. Fresh medium containing AHP/pDNA complexes with different N/P ratios replace the culture media and further incubate for 24 h.
5. Add 10 μL of sterile-filtered MTT to each well for the incubation of 4 h.
6. add 100 μL of DMSO (**Note 7**).
7. Utilize Bio-Rad model 680 microplate reader to record the absorbance at 570 nm of each well. The results are presented in Fig. 6a.

Figure 6 shows that the AHP/pDNA complexes exhibit lower toxicity compared with branched PEI (25 kDa, "goldstandard" nonviral gene carriers) in both HEK293 and hepatoma HepG2 cell lines at various N/P ratios, indicating that the AHP can be used as a safe gene delivery.

### 2.2.7 In Vitro Gene Transfection Assay

1. Seed the cells into 24-well plates at a density of $5 \times 10^4$ cells per well, and incubate in DMEM medium (500 μL) for 24 h (**Note 8**).
2. Remove the culture medium and add 500 μL of fresh DMEM containing AHP/pDNA or sm-AHP (12.6–75.4 μg/mL), and incubate for another 4 h.
3. Transfer new fresh DMEM medium (500 μL, 10% FBS) to each well, and incubate for 20 h and transfect for 24 h.
4. Wash the cells with PBS twice, and add cell lysate (70 μL) to the cells.
5. Utilize luminometer and a commercial kit to quantify Luciferase gene expression.
6. The protein concentrations in the cells are analyzed by Bicinchoninic acid assay.
7. AHP mediated gene transfection is assessed as the above method.
8. The transfected cells are observed by Leica DMIL fluorescence microscope, and the percentage of EGFP-positive cells are determined by flow cytometry.

In Fig. 6b, the transfection efficiency of AHPs reaches to the maximum value at the N/P ratio of 20, which might be caused by the influences of pDNA condensation capability and cytotoxicity. Meanwhile, AHPs show a higher transfection efficiency than sm-AHP/pDNA, confirming the superiority of rough surface for gene transfection.

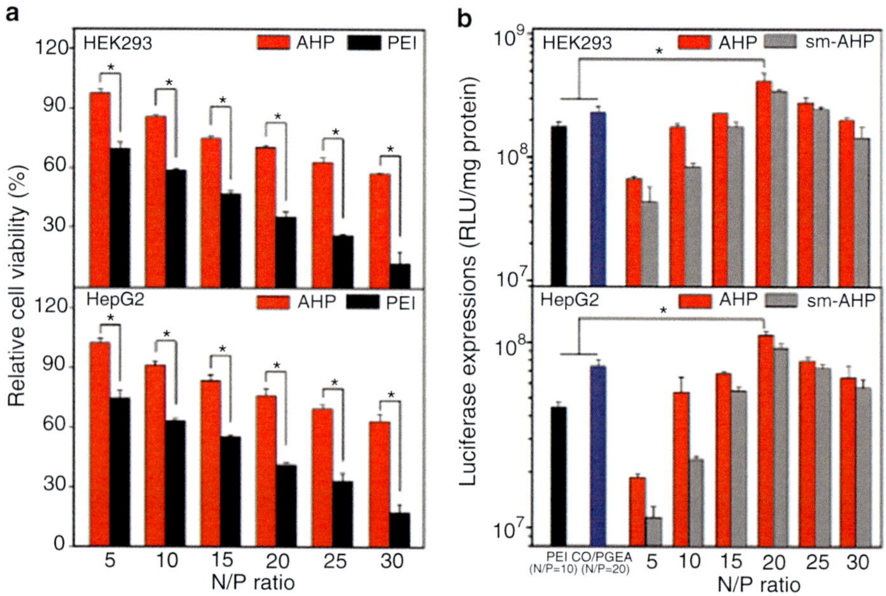


**Fig. 6** (**a**) MTT assay of HEK293 and HepG2 cell lines treated with AHP/pDNA and PEI/pDNA complexes at various N/P ratios. (**b**) Luciferase gene transfection assay of the AHP/pDNA and sm-AHP/pDNA complexes at different N/P ratios in comparison polyethylenimine (PEI) (25 kDa, at the optimal N/P ratio of 10) and CD-PGEA (at the optimal N/P ratio of 20) groups. (Adapted from reference Chen et al. (2018), with permission)

### 2.2.8 Cellular Internalization

1. Seed HepG2 cells in 6-well plates at a density of $8 \times 10^5$ cells per well in 3 mL of DMEM medium, and culture for 24 h.
2. Remove the DMEM medium, and add 3 mL of fresh DMEM medium (3 mL) with AHP (55.3 μg/mL) and smAHP (52.5 μg/mL) (optimal N/P = 20) to each plate for 4 h (pDNA (6 μg) is labeled by fluorescent dye YOYO-1).
3. Wash the cells three times by PBS, and collect the cells through trypsinize and centrifugation. Then re-disperse the cells in 1 mL of PBS. (**Note 9**)
4. Fluorescence intensities are evaluated by Flow cytometry. DAPI (200 μL, 0.15 mg/mL in PBS) stained cells for 10 min are imaged on a fluorescence microscope (Leica DMI3000B)
5. The green fluorescence signal from YOYO-1 labelled pDNA indicates the cellular uptake effect of the complex, and nuclei are marked as blue fluorescence by 4′,6-diamidino-2-phenylindole (DAPI). Figure 7 shows that the green fluorescence signals in AHP/pDNA complexes-treated HepG2 cells are much stronger than those in the sm-AHP/pDNA or CD-PGEA/pDNA complexes treated cells, indicating that AHP/pDNA exhibits an excellent cellular uptake capacity.

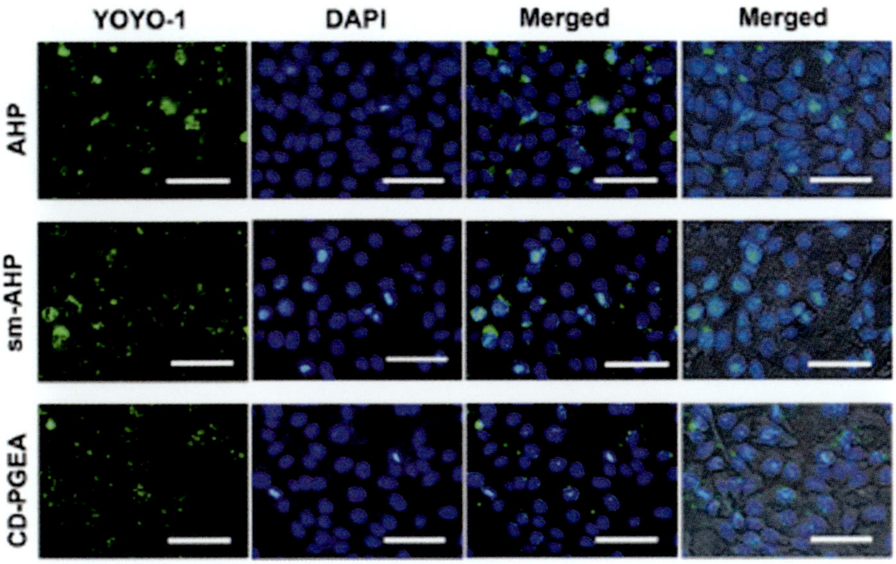


**Fig. 7** Fluorescent images of HepG2 cells treated with YOYO-labeled AHP/pDNA, sm-AHP/pDNA, and CD-PGEA/pDNA for 4 h. Scale bar: 50 (Adapted from reference Chen et al. (2018), with permission)

### 2.2.9 Photothermal Effect of AHP In Vitro and In Vivo

1. 808 nm NIR laser with a power density of 2 W/cm$^2$ are used as the light to irradiate the solutions (200 μL) in a 96-well plate for 5 min (Fig. 8b) (**Note 10**).
2. The temperature is recorded by AIR thermal camera at each time point.
3. Seed HepG2 in 24-well plates at a density of $5 \times 10^4$ cells per well, and incubate for 24 h with fresh DMEM (500 μL,10% FBS).
4. Transfer fresh medium containing AHP (500 μL, 33 μg/mL), and incubate for 4 h. Then, the cells are irradiated with 808 nm laser (2 W/cm$^2$) for 5 min.
5. Incubate the cells with FDA and PI in a dark room for 10 min. HepG2 cells without AHP under irradiation are regarded as control group. The fluorescent images are obtained from a Leica fluorescence microscope (Fig. 8c).
6. Graft HepG2 tumor pieces ($2 \times 2 \times 2$ mm$^3$ in size) into right hind leg of the nude mice by a trocar to construct the models for in vivo test. When the volumes of the tumors reach to 60–150 mm$^3$, the vivo experiments can start.
7. Intratumorally inject AHP solution (100 μL, 3.77 mg/mL). After 10 min, the tumors are treated with 808 nm NIR laser irradiation for 5 min, and an infrared camera are employed to monitor the whole-body infrared thermal images at different time points (Fig. 8d).

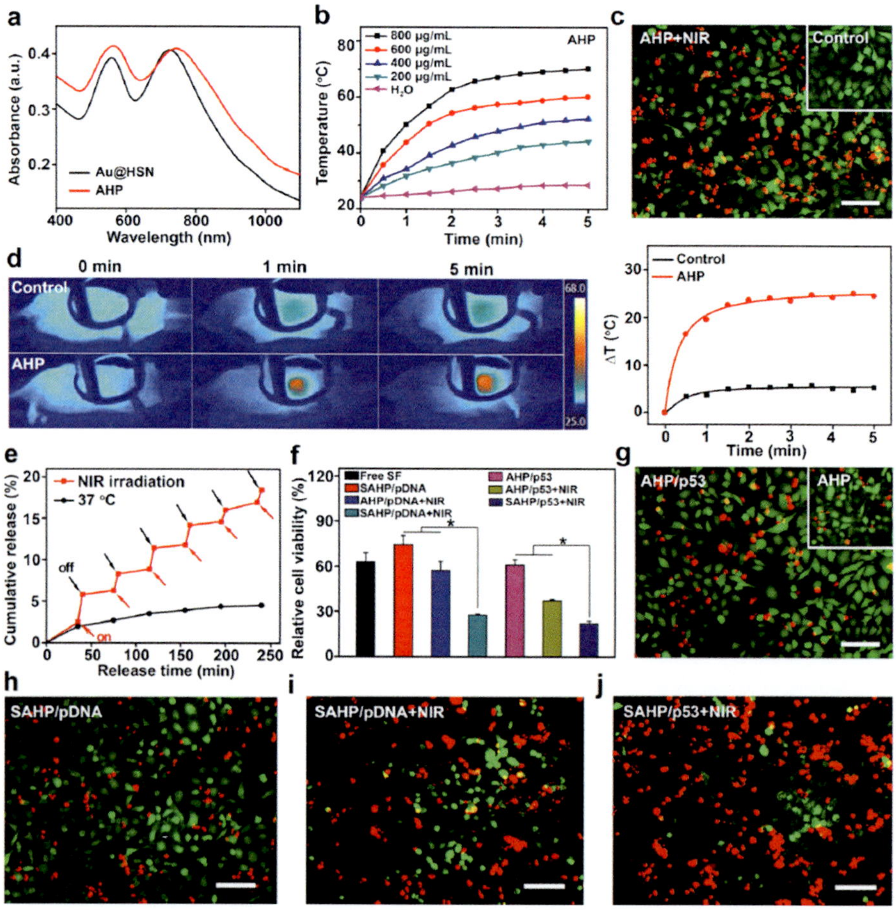


**Fig. 8** (**a**) UV-vis absorption spectra of Au@HSN and AHPs. (**b**) Temperature curves of AHP with different concentrations under a 808 nm laser irradiation (2 W/cm$^2$). (**c**) Fluorescent images of FDA-PI-stained HepG2 cells treated with AHPs or PBS after irradiation with an 808 nm laser. (**d**) Photothermal images and temperature plot of tumor-bearing mice with an injection of PBS and Au@HSN-PGEA after irradiation. (**e**) Cumulative release profile of SF from SAHPs with NIR irradiation at predetermined intervals. (**f**) MTT assay of HepG2 viabilities treated with free SF, SAHP/pDNA, AHP/pDNA+NIR, SAHP/pDNA+NIR, AHP/p53, AHP/ p53 + NIR, and SAHP/ p53 + NIR at the N/P ratio of 20. Corresponding fluorescent images of FDA-PI-stained HepG2 cells treated with AHP/ p53 (**g**), AHPs (inset in g), SAHP/pDNA (**h**), SAHP/pDNA+NIR (**i**), and SAHP/ p53 + NIR (**j**) at the N/P ratio of 20. Scale bar: 100 μm. (Adapted from reference Chen et al. (2018), with permission)

### 2.2.10 SF Loading

1. Disperse Au@HSN-Ad (10 mg) and SF (0.5 mL,10 mg/mL) in DMSO, and the mixture is continuously stirred at room temperature for 24 h.
2. The SF-loaded Au@HSN-Ad is collected by centrifugation, and thoroughly washed with DMSO and deionized water.

3. Dropwise add CD-PGEA aqueous solution (5 mL, 10 mg/mL) to 0.5 mL of ethanol containing SF-loaded Au@HSN-Ad, and the mixture is stirred at room temperature for 24 h to generate SF-loaded AHP (SAHP).
4. Utilize InertSustain C18 column for isocratic elution, and put in the mixture of methanol/acetonitrile/acetic acid (1%) (v/v/v = 38:35:27) to form the mobile phase.
5. Flow rate is chosen as 1.0 mL/min. Inject 100 μL of solution each time, and record the UV absorbance values at 254 nm.
6. Calculate drug loading and encapsulation efficiency according to the following equations: Loading content = (Weight of SF loaded in AHP)/(weight of SAHP). Entrapment efficiency = (Weight of SF loaded in AHP)/(Initial weight of SF).

### 2.2.11 NIR-Triggered SF Release

1. Disperse SAHP (100 μg/mL) in 1.5 mL DMEM containing 10% FBS, and place the mixture in a 37 °C water bath under stirring.
2. At fixed time intervals, remove the supernatant and analyze through HPLC (Compensate for an equal volume of DMEM solution).
3. Utilize 808 nm (2 W/cm$^2$) NIR laser to irradiate the solution for 5 min at regular intervals for determining the photothermal response to drug release.
4. Measure 750 μL of supernatant by HPLC, and compensate the residual mixture with 750 μL of DMEM containing 10% FBS.
5. After 35 min, collect 750 μL of supernatant and measure by HPLC again. The results are presented in Fig. 8e.

### 2.2.12 Effects of NIR-Triggered Drug Release on HCC Cells

1. Seed HepG2 into a 96-well plate at a density of $10^4$ cells per well in 100 μL of culture medium containing, and incubate for 24 h.
2. Replace the medium with 100 μL fresh DMEM medium, which contain free SF (0.02 μg), SAHP/pDNA (0.02 μg SF, 2.06 μg SAHP, 0.33 μg pDNA, N/P = 20) without NIR, AHP/pDNA (2.10 μg AHP, 0.33 μg pDNA, N/P = 20) with NIR and SAHP/pDNA (0.02 μg SF, 2.06 μg SAHP, 0.33 μg p53, N/P = 20) with NIR.
3. After incubation of 4 h, remove the medium. The cell viability is measured by MTT method after another 20 h of incubation.
4. The HepG2 cells are cultured for 4 h, and then received the 808 nm laser irradiation with an output power density of 2 W/cm$^2$ for 5 min.
5. Live/dead staining of HepG2 cells is performed by incubating with FDA and PI for 10 min in a dark room, and the fluorescence images are obtained using a Leica fluorescence microscope. The fluorescent images of the live/dead stained cells are presented in Fig. 8g, h, I, and j.

### 2.2.13 Evaluation of SAHP/p53 Stability

1. Mix SAHP and p53 with N/P of 20 to obtain SAHP/p53 complex.
2. Add SAHP/p53 complex into the medium containing 10% fetal bovine serum (FBS) to test the stability of SAHP/p53.
3. Test the particle size of the solution every 1 h within 6 h (Fig. 9).

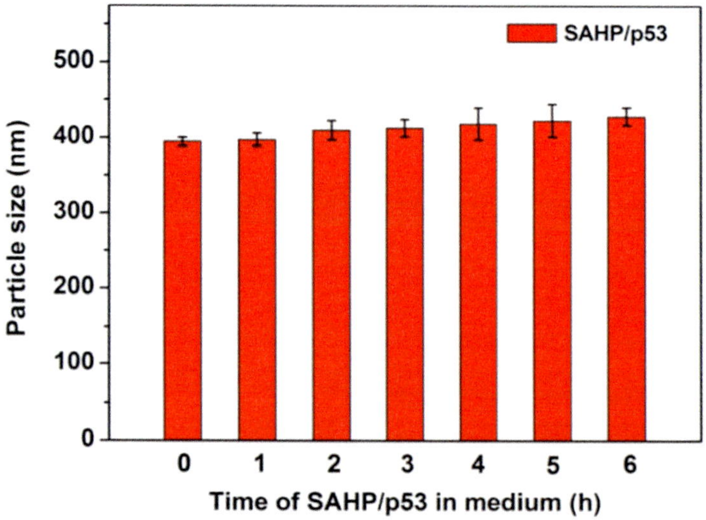


**Fig. 9** Particle sizes of SAHP/p53 complexes in medium with 10% fetal bovine serum (FBS) (mean ± SD, n = 3). (Adapted from reference Chen et al. (2018), with permission)

Figure 9 shows that the particle size of the SAHP/p53 complex remains constant in the FBS solution at an N/P ratio of 20 for 6 h, indicating the good stability of SAHP/p53

### 2.2.14 Complementary Gene/Chemo/Photothermal Therapy In Vitro and In Vivo

1. Seed HepG2 cells in 96-well plates at a density of $10^4$ cells per well in 100 μL of culture medium, and incubate for 24 h.
2. Add 100 μL of AHP/p53 complex (2.10 μg of AHP, 0.33 μg of p53, N/P = 20) into the wells and incubate for 4 h.
3. Remove medium, and add 100 μL of fresh culture medium for the incubation of 44 h. HepG2 cells with the co-incubation of pure p53 (0.33 μg) are regarded as the control group.
4. Incubate HepG2 cells with 100 μL of AHP/p53 (2.10 μg of AHP, 0.33 μg of p53, N/P = 20) and SAHP/p53 (0.02 μg of SF, 2.06 μg of SAHP, 0.33 μg of p53, N/P = 20) complexes for 4 h, respectively, to exploit the combined therapy effect of GT/PTT and gene/chemo/photothermal therapy in vitro,
5. Transfer the cells to fresh medium and receive the 808 nm NIR irradiation (2 W/$cm^2$, 5 min).
6. Divide the tumor bearing BALB/C nude mice into five groups at random with four mice in each group and receive different treatments, including (1) PBS (100 μL, control group, G1), (2) AHP + NIR (377 μg of AHP, G2), (3) AHP/p53 (377 μg of AHP, 15 μg of p53, N/P = 20, G3), (4) SAHP+NIR (370 μg of SAHP, G4), and (5) SAHP/p53 + NIR (370 μg of SAHP, 15 μg of p53, N/P = 20, G5).

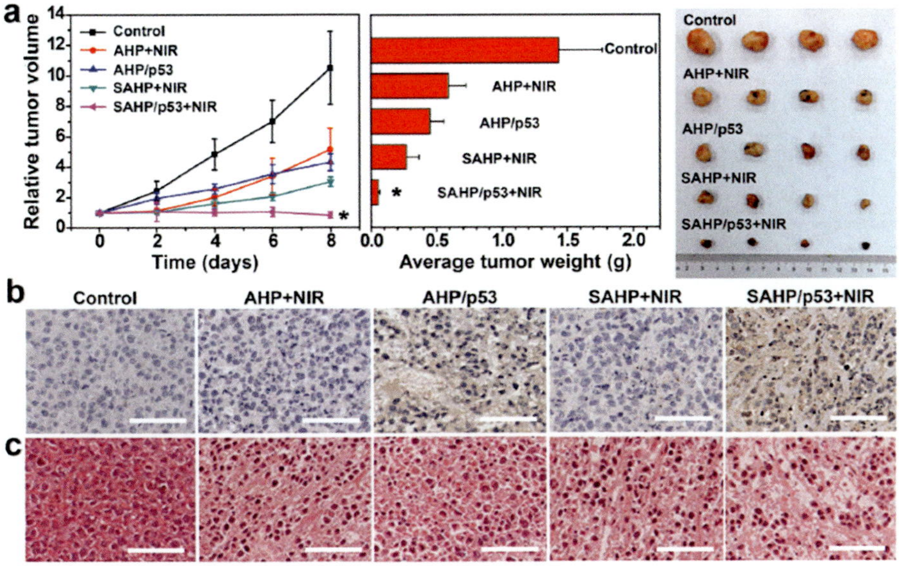


**Fig. 10** (**a**) Relative tumor volume, average tumor weights, and corresponding photographs of tumors after the mouse treatment with PBS, AHP + NIR, AHP/p53, SAHP+NIR, and SAHP/p53 + NIR, respectively. (**b**) P53 Immunohistochemical and (**c**) H&E-stained images of the tumors after different treatments. (Adapted from reference (Chen et al. (2018), with permission)

7. The mice are injected by nanomaterials four times for once every other day. After the first injection, the mice in G2, G4 and G5 groups are received 808 nm laser irradiation (2 W/cm$^2$, 5 min) only once.
8. Measure the sizes of tumors after treatment every 2 days.
9. After treatment, mice are euthanized, and the tumors are weighed, imaged, and dissected for H&E analysis and immunohistochemical analysis. The results are presented in Fig. 10.

Figure 10 shows that SAHP/p53 + NIR group received trimodal complementary therapy exhibit excellent tumor growth inhibition effect than the other groups. These results further validate the profound therapeutic efficacy of NIR-responsive complementary trimodal therapy.

### 2.2.15 PA Imaging of AHPs In Vitro and In Vivo

1. Put AHP solutions in prosthesis, and the PA images of the AHP are obtained through multispectral optoacoustic tomography imaging system.
2. Inject the AHP solutions into intratumor under isoflurane, and capture the PA images of the tumor-bearing mice before and 10 min after injection by multispectral optoacoustic tomography imaging system. The results are presented in Fig. 11b.

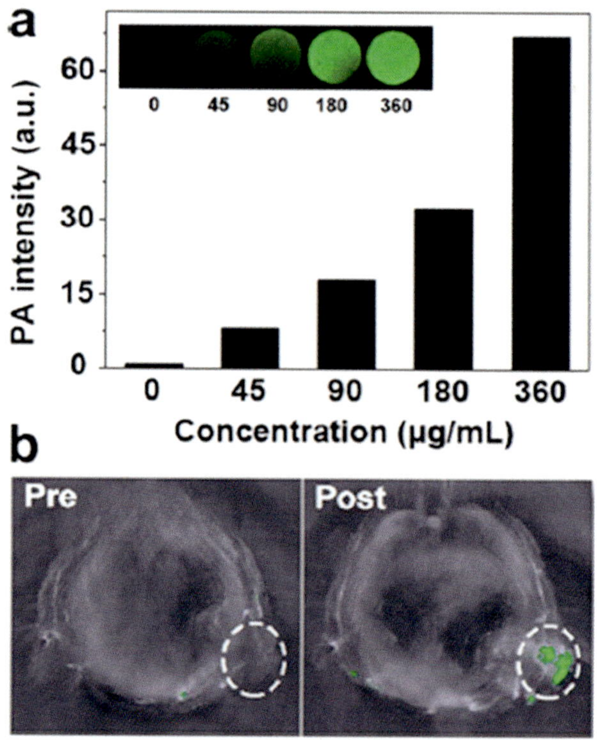


**Fig. 11** (**a**) PA images and the corresponding value of PA signal associated with different concentrations of AHP. (**b**) PA images of the tumor bearing mouse before and after injection of AHPs. (Adapted from reference Chen et al. (2018), with permission)

As shown in Fig. 11, the PA signal intensities of AHP gradually enhance with the increasing concentration of AHP. After injection of AHP for 10 min, a strong PA signal can be observed in the tumor tissue, indicating the significant accumulation of AHPs in the tumor tissues.

## 3 Discussion

There are common mistakes and necessary issues when following the above procedure. Some notes which can be used to solve possible problems have been provided as follows.

### 3.1 Note

1. Keep the continuous stirring for 18 h.
2. The nanoparticles are washed thoroughly and diluted enough before characterization using TEM and AFM.

3. The Au@HSN products are thoroughly and sequentially washed three times with aqueous solution containing CTAB (0.1 mol/L), water, and ethanol.
4. 4 mL of EA are dropwise added into the CD-PGMA solution.
5. The Au@HSN-$NH_2$ solution is dropwise added into the above solution, and keep the reaction for 48 h.
6. After incubation for 24 h, the cells can be used for the experiments.
7. MTT solution is completely removed, and then add 100 μL of DMSO.
8. The cells must be mixed well before seeded into the 24-well plates.
9. Cells solution must be gently agitated for a while, which can avoid to form the cell block.
10. The volumes of solution in the 96-well plate are consistent.

## 4 Conclusion

The protocol reports the design of a novel rattle-structured rough nanoplatform (Au@HSN-PGEA, AHPs) composed of *in-situ*-formed Au NR cores and polycationic mesoporous silica shells. Special morphology of AHPs endows the high loading efficiency and excellent transfection performance, realizing the efficient delivery of p53 gene and SF drug to the tumor location and elimination of solid tumors. Furthermore, the multifunctional nanoplatform exhibits good photoacoustic capability for accurate tumor diagnosis.

## References

Ashrafizadeh M, Fekri HS, Ahmadi Z, Farkhondeh T, Samarghandian S (2020) Therapeutic and biological activities of berberine: the involvement of Nrf2 signaling pathway. J Cell Biochem 121(2):1575–1585

Chen X, Zhang Q, Li J, Yang M, Zhao N, Xu F-J (2018) Rattle-structured rough nanocapsules with in-situ-formed gold nanorod cores for complementary gene/chemo/photothermal therapy. ACS Nano 12(6):5646–5656

De Smedt SC, Demeester J, Hennink WE (2000) Cationic polymer based gene delivery systems. Pharm Res 17(2):113–126

Guo K, Zhao X, Dai X, Zhao N, Xu F-J (2019) Organic/inorganic nanohybrids as multifunctional gene delivery systems. J Gene Med 21(5):e3084

Jung B-K, Lee YK, Hong J, Ghandehari H, Yun C-O (2016) Mild hyperthermia induced by gold nanorod-mediated plasmonic photothermal therapy enhances transduction and replication of oncolytic adenoviral gene delivery. ACS Nano 10(11):10533–10543

Kaygisiz K, Synatschke CV (2020) Materials promoting viral gene delivery. Biomater Sci 8(22): 6113–6156

Kinnear C, Moore TL, Rodriguez-Lorenzo L, Rothen-Rutishauser B, Petri-Fink A (2017) Form follows function: nanoparticle shape and its implications for nanomedicine. Chem Rev 117(17): 11476–11521

Li Z, Barnes JC, Bosoy A, Stoddart JF, Zink JI (2012) Mesoporous silica nanoparticles in biomedical applications. Chem Soc Rev 41(7):2590–2605

Mohammadinejad R, Dehshahri A, Sagar Madamsetty V, Zahmatkeshan M, Tavakol S, Makvandi P et al (2020) In vivo gene delivery mediated by non-viral vectors for cancer therapy. J Control Release 325:249–275

Song S, Goudy K, Campbell-Thompson M, Wasserfall C, Scott-Jorgensen M, Wang J et al (2004) Recombinant adeno-associated virus-mediated alpha-1 antitrypsin gene therapy prevents type I diabetes in NOD mice. Gene Ther 11(2):181–186

Song H, Yu M, Lu Y, Gu Z, Yang Y, Zhang M et al (2017) Plasmid DNA delivery: nanotopography matters. J Am Chem Soc 139(50):18247–18254

Sung YK, Kim SW (2019) Recent advances in the development of gene delivery systems. Biomater Res 23(1):8

Taghavi S, HashemNia A, Mosaffa F, Askarian S, Abnous K, Ramezani M (2016) Preparation and evaluation of polyethylenimine-functionalized carbon nanotubes tagged with 5TR1 aptamer for targeted delivery of Bcl-xL shRNA into breast cancer cells. Colloids Surf B Biointerfaces 140: 28–39

Taghavi S, Abnous K, Taghdisi SM, Ramezani M, Alibolandi M (2020) Hybrid carbon-based materials for gene delivery in cancer therapy. J Control Release 318:158–175

Valtchev V, Tosheva L (2013) Porous nanosized particles: preparation, properties, and applications. Chem Rev 113(8):6734–6760

Yang X, Yang M, Pang B, Vara M, Xia Y (2015) Gold nanomaterials at work in biomedicine. Chem Rev 115(19):10410–10488

Zhao N, Li J, Zhou Y, Hu Y, Wang R, Ji Z et al (2016) Hierarchical nanohybrids of gold nanorods and PGMA-based polycations for multifunctional theranostics. Adv Funct Mater 26(32):5848–5861

Zhao N, Yan L, Zhao X, Chen X, Li A, Zheng D et al (2019) Versatile types of organic/inorganic nanohybrids: from strategic design to biomedical applications. Chem Rev 119(3):1666–1762

# Preparation and Evaluation of Boronate-Linked Nanoassembly for Efficient Gene Delivery

# 23

Jing-Yi Zhu, Jun Feng, and Xian-Zheng Zhang

## Contents




J.-Y. Zhu · X.-Z. Zhang (✉)
Key Laboratory of Biomedical Polymers of Ministry of Education, Department of Chemistry, Wuhan University, Wuhan, P. R. China

Key Laboratory of Biomaterials of Guangdong Higher Education Institutes, Department of Biomedical Engineering, Jinan University, Guangzhou, P. R. China
e-mail: xz-zhang@whu.edu.cn

J. Feng (✉)
Key Laboratory of Biomedical Polymers of Ministry of Education, Department of Chemistry, Wuhan University, Wuhan, P. R. China
e-mail: fengjun@whu.edu.cn





H. Tian and X. Chen (eds.), *Gene Delivery*, Biomaterial Engineering,
https://doi.org/10.1007/978-981-16-5419-0_23

**Abstract**

Rapid transfection can not only maximize the bioavailability of vector-carried gene prior to exocytosis, but also well match chemotherapy for optimal combinational therapy in view of the rapid chemotherapeutic action. However, little attention has been paid to the "rapid" goal in vector-aided transfection process. This chapter describes a boronate-linked nanoassembly for the rapid transnuclear gene transport and efficient gene transfection in vitro and in vivo. The nanoassembly was constructed on the basis of the pH-reversible covalent boronic acid-diol coupling between 1,3-diol-rich oligoethylenimine (OEI-EHDO) and phenylboronic acid modified cholesterol (Chol-PBA). The obtained results demonstrate that the boronate-linked nanoassembly can lead to rapid and efficient nuclei-tropic delivery and transfection, which may largely rely on the lysosome-acidity induced assembly destruction followed by the easy liberation of gene payloads. Consequently, the nanoassembly-mediated transfection just at 8 h can afford the outcome comparable to that achieved at 48 h by the golden standard of PEI25K, and the transfection efficiency can remain at a high level during 48 h. In addition, the in vitro and in vivo results reveal the strong tolerance to the serum interference and the good biocompatibility of this hydroxyl-rich bio-decomposable nanoassembly.

**Keywords**

Bio-responsiveness · Boronate-linked nanoassembly · Lysosomal acidity · Rapid gene transfection · Transnuclear transport

# 1 Introduction

As well known, an elaborately designed gene delivery system is of great importance for the effective gene therapy. Numerous polycations have been exploited to condense therapeutic genes into the compact nanoparticles in order to protect genes from premature degradation and facilitate their passive accumulation in tumors through the enhanced permeability and retention (EPR) effects (Dhaliwal and Zheng 2019; Fang et al. 2020). Overall, the in vivo trials are highly restricted by several challenges, such as easy capture by negatively charged blood components (serum albumin, etc.) commonly followed by the clearance and embolism, premature release prior to cellular entry, insufficient gene release inside cells, and poor nuclear uptake of carried genes, although the in vitro outcome of gene transfection seems so attractive (Khandare et al. 2012; Mohammadinejad et al. 2020; Yin et al. 2014).

In order to achieve effective gene transfection inside target cells, stimuli-responsive gene delivery systems have been rapidly developed for temporal and/or spatial control over gene release during past decades (Shim and Kwon 2012; Wu et al. 2016). The controlled gene release can prevent DNA from premature release and enable desirable bioavailability of native DNA in the sites of interest (Zhang et al. 2020a; Zhu et al. 2017). These intelligent gene vectors can produce physico-chemical alternations in response to not only the internal signals associated with the transport mechanism and the pathological features but also the external stimulus commonly used for localized therapy (Ahmadi et al. 2020; Cai et al. 2020; Piotrowski-Daspit et al. 2020). In terms of tumor treatments, tumorous acidity is among the most investigated endogenous signals because the pH gradient from blood vessel to tumor tissues/organelles is closely related to the onset and progression of cancer disease (Boedtkjer and Pedersen 2020; Lo et al. 2020; Zhang et al. 2020b). Due to the "Warburg's effect," tumor environment is rich in lactic acid, giving rise to the acid tumor microenvironments (pH 6.5–7.2) (DeBerardinis and Chandel 2020; Heiden et al. 2009). Upon endocytosis of polycations, rapid endosomal acidification ($\sim$2–3 min) occurs due to the ATPase-mediated proton influx, resulting in a more acidic endo/lysosomal compartment (pH $\sim$ 4.5–6.0) (Forgac 2007).

Most of the studies show that more than 12 h is needed to enable the overwhelming distribution of the introduced genes in the cytoplasm (Li et al. 2015, 2020). It means that effective gene transfection may require more time because nuclear uptake of therapeutic genes is an essential prerequisite for the successful transcription and transfection. In principle, rapid gene transfection can maximize the gene bioavailability if the cellular efflux of DNA-entrapped complexes is considered (Deverman et al. 2018; Dobson 2006). Besides, rapid gene transfection is desired to well match the fast chemotherapy action when chemotherapy and gene therapy are combined for better therapy outcomes. Until now, however, very little attention has been paid to the "rapid" goal of gene therapy. We surmise if the carried genes are quickly liberated in target cells, the transfection may be accelerated. In our previous study,

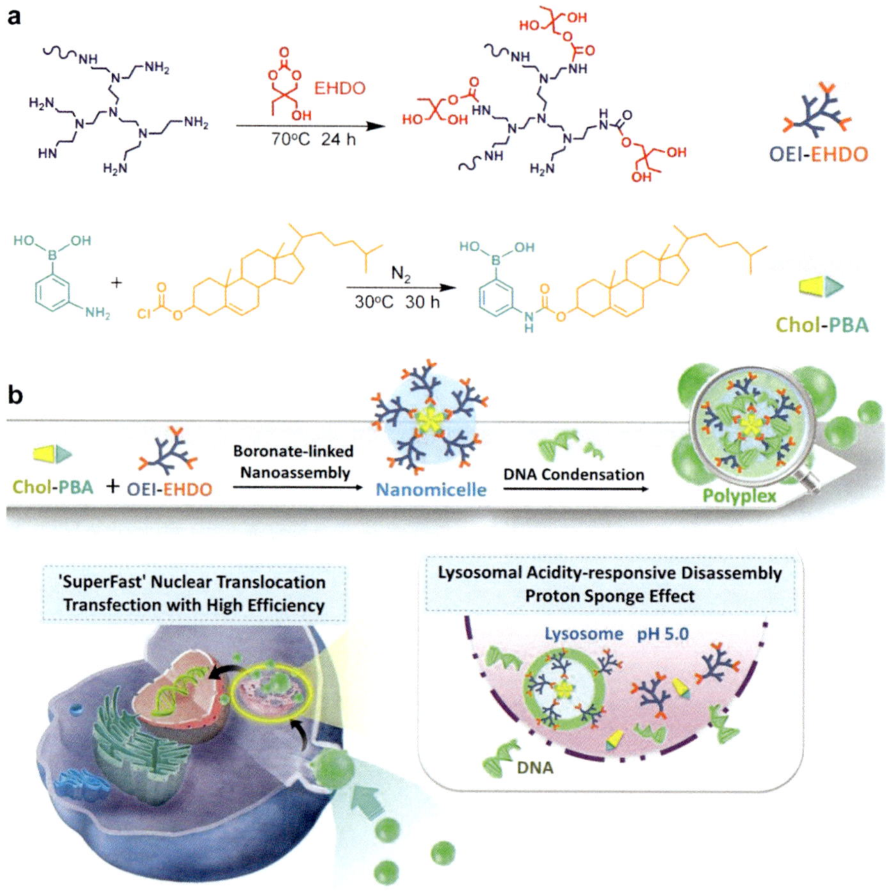


**Fig. 1** (**a**) Preparation and structures of OEI-EHDO and Chol-PBA. (**b**) Schematic diagram of OEI-EHDO/Chol-PBA nanoassembly mediated "Superfast" transnuclear gene translocation and efficient gene transfection depending on lysosomal-acidity-responsive disassembly. (Adapted from Zhu et al. (2016), with permission)

the self-assembled nanocarriers driven by pH-reversible covalent boronic acid/1,3-diol orthogonality can sensitively respond to endo/lysosomal acidity in favor of highly efficient accumulation of carried drugs in cell nuclei, leading to considerably enhanced pharmacological performance (Zhu et al. 2016).

Inspired by the encouraging findings, we intend to harness the boronic acid/1,3-diol orthogonality to establish an acid-responsive gene delivery system with the capability of rapid and efficient gene transfection, based on the spontaneous reaction between the phenylboronic acid conjugated cholesterol (Chol-PBA) and 1,3-diol enriched oligoethylenimine (OEI-EHDO) in aqueous conditions (Fig. 1) (Li et al. 2012; Zhu et al. 2015). The formation of boronate esters between the two resulted in the self-assembly into the amphiphilic micelles, thus giving the highly charged and acid-labile nanocarriers for the delivery of oppositely charged plasmid DNAs. The hydroxyl-rich surface on the obtained DNA/vector nanocomplexes benefited the serum-tolerant transfection due to the "hydroxylation effects," which we have previously proposed to effectively inhibit the nonspecific adsorption by blood components (Jia et al. 2014; Luo et al. 2011; Yang et al. 2014a, b). Cholesterol, an essential element existing in the membranes of eukaryotic cells and readily metabolized in the body, is used here as a good lipid anchor for improved cellular uptake (Kheirolomoom and Ferrara 2007). The boronate esters-linked micelles can remain stable at physiological pH conditions while being destructed in acid environments. The evaluations of "superfast"/efficient transnuclear gene transport and transfection are carried out in a series of cell lines and tumor-bearing BALB/c mice (Zhu et al. 2016).

## 2 Materials

### 2.1 Synthesis of EHDO-Modified Oligoethylenimine (OEI-EHDO)

1. Branched oligoethylenimine 1800 (OEI1800)
2. 5-ethyl-5-(hydroxymethyl)-1, 3-dioxan-2-oxo (EHDO)
3. Dimethyl sulfoxide (DMSO, analytical grade)
4. Diethyl ether (analytical grade)
5. Ethanol (analytical grade)
6. 25 mL and 250 mL round-bottom flask
7. Rotary vacuum evaporator
8. Bath-type sonicator
9. Circulating water multipurpose vacuum pump
10. Vacuum desiccator
11. Magnetic stirrer
12. Varian Unity 300 MHz spectrometer

### 2.2 Synthesis of Cholest-5-en-3-Ol(3b)-,(3-Boronophenyl) Carbamate (Chol-PBA)

1. 3-aminophenylboronic acid (PBA, 98%)
2. Cholesteryl chloroformate (Chol-Cl, 98%)
3. Distilled diethyl ether (analytical grade)
4. Nitrogen
5. N-methylimidazole
6. Deionized water
7. Sodium sulfate ($Na_2SO_4$)
8. Petroleum ether (analytical grade)
9. Ethyl acetate (analytical grade)

10. Acetonitrile (analytical grade)
11. Glass flask
12. Conical flask
13. Magnetic stirrer
14. Thin layer chromatography (TLC)
15. Silica gel chromatography
16. Rotary vacuum evaporator
17. Vacuum desiccator
18. Melting point apparatus
19. Varian Unity 100 MHz spectrometer
20. Shimadzu LC-6 AD liquid chromatograph equipped with an ultraviolet-visible detector (220 nm, Shimadzu SPD-20A) and GL Science Inertsil WR5-4173C18 (4.6 × 250 mm; 5 μm) column

### 2.3 Nanoassembly Preparation

1. EHDO-modified oligoethylenimine (OEI-EHDO)
2. Cholest-5-en-3-ol(3b)-,(3-boronophenyl)carbamate (Chol-PBA)
3. Tetrahydrofuran (THF) (analytical grade)
4. Deionized water
5. Filter funnel and paper
6. Glass flask
7. Magnetic stirrer
8. Rotary vacuum evaporator
9. Centrifuge
10. Lyophilizer

### 2.4 Determination of Grafting Degree

1. OEI-EHDO/Chol-PBA nanoparticles
2. Hydrochloric acid (HCl)
3. Chloroform (analytical grade)
4. 25 mL sample bottle
5. Separating funnel
6. Ultraviolet-visible (UV) spectrophotometer

### 2.5 Determination of Critical Micelle Concentration (CMC)

1. OEI-EHDO/Chol-PBA nanoparticles
2. Pyrene
3. Acetone (analytical grade)
4. Centrifuge tube

5. Drying oven
6. LS55 luminescence spectrometer (PerkinElmer) with a slit width of 5 nm

## 2.6 Visual Inspection on Nanoassembly in the Presence of Nile Red Dye

1. Nile Red dye
2. Tetrahydrofuran (THF)
3. EHDO-modified oligoethylenimine (OEI-EHDO)
4. Cholest-5-en-3-ol(3b)-,(3-boronophenyl)carbamate (Chol-PBA)
5. Cholesterol (Chol, 95%)
6. Magnetic stirrer
7. Camera

## 2.7 Variation of Nanoassembly at Different pHs

1. Nile Red dye
2. Tetrahydrofuran (THF)
3. OEI-EHDO/Chol-PBA nanoassembly
4. Hydrochloric acid (HCl)
5. Magnetic stirrer
6. Rotary vacuum evaporator
7. Filter funnel and paper
8. Camera

## 2.8 Preparation of Nanoassembly/DNA Complexes

1. pGL-3 plasmid
2. OEI-EHDO
3. OEI-EHDO/Chol-PBA nanoassembly
4. Phosphate-buffered saline (PBS) (137 mM NaCI, 2.7 mM KCl, 8 mM $Na_2HPO_4$, and 2 mM $KH_2PO_4$, pH 7.4)
5. Microcentrifuge tube

## 2.9 Agarose Gel Retardation Assay

1. Agarose
2. GelRed™
3. Tris-acetate (TAE) running buffer
4. Bromophenol blue
5. pGL-3 plasmid

6. Phosphate buffered saline (PBS) (137 mM NaCI, 2.7 mM KCl, 8 mM $Na_2HPO_4$, and 2 mM $KH_2PO_4$, pH 7.4)
7. Microcentrifuge tube
8. Vortex mixer
9. 37 °C incubator
10. Ultraviolet-visible lamp using a Vilber Lourmat imaging system (France)
11. Electrophoresis apparatus

## 2.10 Determination of Particle Size, Zeta Potential, and Morphology

1. pGL-3 plasmid
2. OEI-EHDO
3. OEI-EHDO/Chol-PBA nanoassembly
4. Deionized water
5. Phosphate-buffered saline (PBS) (137 mM NaCI, 2.7 mM KCl, 8 mM $Na_2HPO_4$, and 2 mM $KH_2PO_4$, pH 7.4)
6. Dynamic light scattering (DLS) analyzer (Malvern Nano Series Zen 3600 Zeta Sizer)
7. Transmission electron microscopy (JEOL JEM-100CXII instrument at an acceleration voltage of 80 KV)
8. Syringe and micropore filter (0.45 μm)
9. Copper grids coated with formvar films
10. 0.2% (w/v) phosphotungstic acid solution

## 2.11 Stability Study of Nanoassembly and its Complexes

1. pGL-3 plasmid
2. OEI-EHDO/Chol-PBA nanoassembly
3. Fetal bovine serum (FBS)
4. Syringe and micropore filter (0.45 μm)
5. Glucose
6. Bovine serum albumin (BSA)
7. Centrifuge
8. Ultraviolet-visible (UV) spectrophotometer
9. Shaker

## 2.12 Acid-Triggered Unpacking of Nanoassembly/DNA Complexes in the Presence of Heparin

1. Heparin
2. Ethylenediaminetetraacetic acid (EDTA) buffer

3. Phosphate-buffered saline (PBS) (137 mM NaCI, 2.7 mM KCl, 8 mM $Na_2HPO_4$, and 2 mM $KH_2PO_4$, pH 7.4)
4. Acetate buffer (0.2 M acetic acid, 0.2 M sodium acetate, pH 5.0)
5. Electrophoresis apparatus
6. Ultraviolet-visible lamp using a Vilber Lourmat imaging system

## 2.13 Cell Culture

1. African green monkey SV40-transformed kidney fibroblast cell line (COS7)
2. Mouse embryonic fibroblast cell line (3 T3)
3. Human liver hepatocellular carcinoma cell line (HepG2)
4. Human cervix carcinoma cells (HeLa)
5. Dulbecco's Modified Eagle's Medium (DMEM)
6. Trypsin EDTA
7. Penicillin
8. Streptomycin
9. Fetal bovine serum (FBS)
10. Cell culture flask (T-25, T-75)
11. $CO_2$ incubator
12. Vertical flow clean bench
13. Optical microscope

## 2.14 Amplification and Purification of Plasmid DNA

1. E. coli JM109
2. Terrific broth media (containing Beef extract and peptone)
3. EndoFree QiAfilterTM Plasmid Giga Kit (5)
4. Tris-EDTA (TE) buffer
5. Ultraviolet-visible (UV) spectrophotometer

## 2.15 In Vitro Gene Transfection

1. Human cervix carcinoma cells (HeLa)
2. Branched polyethyleneimine (Mw = 25 k) (PEI25K)
3. pGL-3 plasmid
4. 24-well culture plates
5. Dulbecco's Modified Eagle's Medium (DMEM)
6. Fetal bovine serum (FBS)
7. Phosphate-buffered saline (PBS) (137 mM NaCI, 2.7 mM KCl, 8 mM $Na_2HPO_4$, and 2 mM $KH_2PO_4$, pH 7.4)
8. Chemiluminometer (Lumat LB9507, EG&G Berthold, Germany)

9. BCA protein assay kit (Pierce)
10. Vortex mixer

## 2.16 Flow Cytometry

1. Human cervix carcinoma cells (HeLa)
2. 6-well culture plates
3. pGL-3 plasmid
4. Trypsin
5. Centrifuge tubes
6. Centrifuge
7. Flow cytometry (BD FACSAria™III, USA)

## 2.17 Confocal Laser Scanning Microscopy (CLSM)

1. Human cervix carcinoma cells (HeLa)
2. African green monkey SV40-transformed kidney fibroblast cell line (COS7)
3. Mouse embryonic fibroblast cell line (3 T3)
4. Human liver hepatocellular carcinoma cell line (HepG2)
5. pGL-3 plasmid
6. YOYO-1
7. Hoechst 33,342
8. Cholesterol (Chol, 95%)
9. Ethanol (analytical grade)
10. 35 mm confocal dishes
11. Dulbecco's Modified Eagle's Medium (DMEM)
12. Fetal bovine serum (FBS)
13. Confocal laser scanning microscope (Nikon C1-si TE2000, Japan)

## 2.18 $NH_4Cl$-Associated Interference of Endosomal Acidification Procession

1. Ammonium chloride ($NH_4Cl$)
2. Human cervix carcinoma cells (HeLa)
3. 24-well culture plates
4. 35 mm confocal dishes
5. YOYO-1
6. Hoechst 33,342
7. Phosphate-buffered saline (PBS) (137 mM NaCI, 2.7 mM KCl, 8 mM $Na_2HPO_4$, and 2 mM $KH_2PO_4$, pH 7.4)
8. Chemiluminometer (Lumat LB9507, EG&G Berthold, Germany)

9. BCA protein assay kit (Pierce)
10. Confocal laser scanning microscope (Nikon C1-si TE2000, Japan)

### 2.19 In Vitro Cytotoxicity Assays

1. Human cervix carcinoma cells (HeLa)
2. 96-well culture plates
3. 10% serum-containing DMEM
4. 3-(4, 5-dimethylthiazol-2-yl)-2, 5-diphenyltetrazolium bromide (MTT)
5. Microplate reader (BIO-RAD 550, USA)

### 2.20 In Vivo Animal Study

1. Female BALB/c mice (4–5 weeks old)
2. Hepatoma H22 cells
3. pGL-3 plasmid
4. pORF-LacZ plasmid
5. Ice-cold PBS
6. X-gal staining kit (InvivoGen, USA)
7. 3.7% formaldehyde
8. Paraffin
9. Light microscope coupled with a digital camera
10. IKA-Ultra-Turrax homogenizer
11. Promega cell lysis buffer
12. BCA protein assay kit (Pierce)

## 3 Methods

### 3.1 Preparation and Characterization of Boronate-Linked Nanoassembly

#### 3.1.1 Synthesis of EHDO-Modified Oligoethylenimine (OEI-EHDO)

1. Dissolve OEI1800 (0.27 g, 0.15 mM) and EHDO (0.09 g, 0.58 mM) in 5 mL of distilled dimethyl sulfoxide (DMSO) in a 25 mL round-bottom flask.
2. React at 70 °C for 24 h.
3. Pour the above reaction mixture into 150 mL of ether to isolate the insoluble crude product.
4. Dissolve the crude product in 5 mL of ethanol and precipitate in 150 mL of ether for three times.
5. Dry the product in vacuum.
6. Determine the substitution degree (DS: defined as the percentage of the reacted relative to the total amine amount within OEI1800) by comparing the areas of the

signal of the -$CH_3$ protons of EHDO (0.80 ppm) and that of the repeating units (-$CH_2CH_2NH$-) of OEI (2.49–2.61 ppm) in the $^1$H NMR spectrum.

### 3.1.2 Synthesis of Cholest-5-en-3-Ol (3b)-,(3-Boronophenyl) Carbamate (Chol-PBA)

1. Dissolve cholesterol chloroformate (1.8 g, 4.0 mM) and 3-aminophenylboronic acid (1.1 g, 8.0 mM) in 100 mL of dry distilled diethyl ether under the nitrogen protection at 30 °C.
2. Add N-methylimidazole (0.82 g, 10 mM) under stirring.
3. Monitor the reaction process by TLC.
4. Dilute the resulting cloudy solution with diethyl ether to 150 mL followed by washing with deionized water (4 × 50 mL) after 30 h reaction.
5. Dry the ether layer using $Na_2SO_4$.
6. Removed the solvent by rotary evaporation to give a white powder.
7. Purify the product using column chromatography (petroleum ether: ethyl acetate = 2:1).

### 3.1.3 Nanoassembly Preparation

1. Dissolve 15 mg of Chol-PBA in 80 μL of THF, and add to 20 mL of deionized water containing OEI-EHDO (3.0 mg/mL) under stirring for 24 h.
2. Remove the organic solvent by rotary evaporation.
3. Centrifuge and filter the above solution.
4. Lyophilize the obtained water solution to obtain the nanoassembly.

### 3.1.4 Determination of Grafting Degree

1. Define the grafting degree as the molar ratio of Chol-PBA to OEI-EHDO.
2. Dissolve 10 mg of nanoassembly in 10 mL of HCl solution (pH ~ 1.0) and stir over night.
3. Extract with 4 mL of chloroform.
4. Isolate the organic phase for UV-vis spectrum analysis.
5. Calculate the grating degree on the basis of the absorbance of Chol-PBA measured at 280 nm on the basis of the standard calibration curve experimentally obtained.

### 3.1.5 Determination of Critical Micelle Concentration (CMC)

1. Add 60 μL of pyrene solution in acetone ($1 \times 10^{-4}$ M in acetone) to 2 mL centrifuge tube and evaporate the acetone at 60 °C.
2. Add 1 mL of nanoassembly solution with a series of different concentrations to the above centrifuge tube containing the pyrene residue (All the sample solutions contain the equal and excessive pyrene at the same concentration of $6 \times 10^{-7}$ M).
3. Maintain the solutions at room temperature for 24 h to achieve the solubilization equilibrium of pyrene in the aqueous phase.
4. Record the excitation spectra at an emission wavelength of 393 nm on a LS55 luminescence spectrometer (PerkinElmer) with a slit width of 5 nm.

5. Set the intensity ratio ($I_{338}/I_{336}$) as a function against logarithm of polymer concentration.
6. Determine the critical micelle concentration (CMC) based on the intersection point at low concentration on the plot.

#### 3.1.6 Visual Inspection on Nanoassembly in the Presence of Nile Red Dye

1. Add 0.1 mL of THF solution containing the mixture of Nile Red (5 mM) and Chol-PBA (10 mM) dropwise into 3 mL of OEI-EHDO solution (3.0 mg/mL) under stirring for 24 h.
2. Perform the control experiment by using the mixture of PBA-free Chol and Nile Red instead.
3. Observe and photo the variation of the solution.

#### 3.1.7 Variation of Nanoassembly at Different pHs

1. Add 0.1 mL of Nile Red solution (2.0 mg/mL) in THF dropwise into 3 mL of the OEI-EHDO/Chol-PBA nanoassembly solution (~1.0 mg/mL) under stirring.
2. Rotary evaporate and filter the obtained solution.
3. Adjust the solution pH to 7.4 and 5.0, respectively.
4. Observe and photo the variation at different pH conditions at predefined time intervals (24 h, 48 h, 72 h, 96 h, 120 h) in Fig. 2.

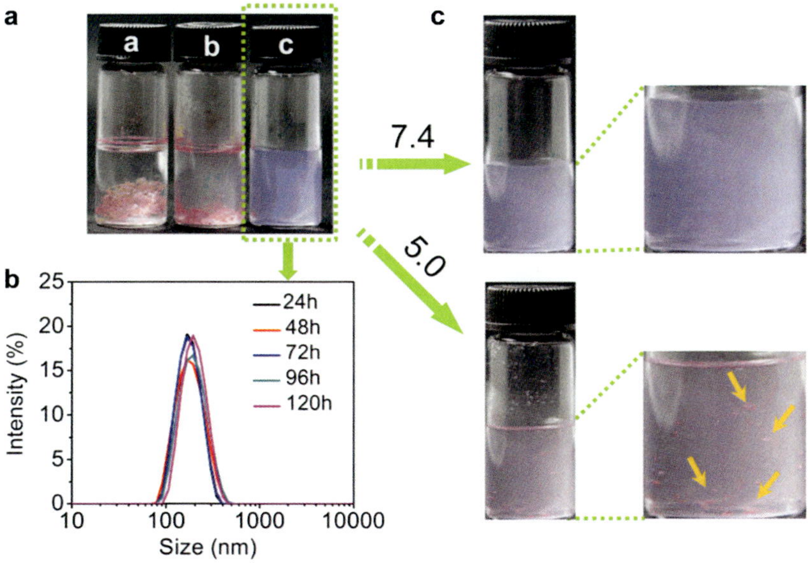


**Fig. 2** (**a**) Observation on the solutions of Nile Red-loaded OEI-EHDO/Chol (a), OEI/Chol-PBA (b), and OEI-EHDO/Chol-PBA nanoassembly (c) under identical conditions. Images were photoed after 24 h standing; (**b**) DLS profiles of OEI-EHDO/Chol-PBA solution in pH 7.4 buffer solution obtained at different time interval; (**c**) Observation on the solution of Nile Red-loaded OEI-EHDO/Chol-PBA nanoassembly at different pHs. (Adapted from Zhu et al. (2016), with permission)

### 3.1.8 Preparation of Nanoassembly/DNA Complexes

1. Prepare OEI-EHDO/Chol-PBA/pGL-3 complexes at different w/w ratios (weight ratio of polymer OEI-EHDO relative to pDNA) by adding appropriate volume polymer solution (in PBS buffer) to 1 μL of pGL-3 (100 ng/μL in water).
2. Prepare OEI-EHDO/pGL-3 complexes as described above.

### 3.1.9 Agarose Gel Retardation Assay

1. Dilute OEI-EHDO/pGL-3 and OEI-EHDO/Chol-PBA/pGL-3 complexes at different w/w ratios by PBS solution to the total volume of 8 mL.
2. Vortex for 30 s prior to incubation at 37 °C for 30 min.
3. Electrophorese on a 0.7% (W/V) agarose gel containing GelRedTM in Tris-acetate (TAE) running buffer at 80 V for 1 h.
4. Observe under an UV lamp using a Vilber Lourmat imaging system (France).

### 3.1.10 Particle Size and Zeta Potential Measurements

1. Prepare various DNA complexes with different w/w ratios.
2. Incubate at 37 °C for 30 min.
3. Dilute the complex by PBS to 1 mL prior to measurement.
4. Detect the particle size and zeta potential of various complexes.

### 3.1.11 Observation of the Morphology by TEM

1. Resuspend the OEI-EHDO/Chol-PBA nanoassembly in deionized water.
2. Filter through a micropore filter membrane (0.45 μm).
3. Use copper grids coated with formvar film to absorb the nanoparticles for 2 min in the nanoassembly suspension.
4. Take out copper grids and blot with filter paper.
5. Float these grids in 0.2% (w/v) phosphotungstic acid solution for 1 min, remove, blot with filter paper, and dry at room temperature.
6. Observe the specimens by TEM at 80 kV.

### 3.1.12 Stability Study

1. Detect the particle size and size distribution by DLS in 30% serum containing PBS or at a normal blood sugar concentration (~1.0 mg/mL) with 10% serum.
2. Add 1 mL of nanoassembly suspension (1.0 mg/mL) to 1 mL BSA solution (2.0 mg/mL).
3. Shake at 37 °C for 30 min, and centrifuge, collect the supernatant.
4. Determine the concentration of BSA in the supernatant from its characteristic UV absorbance (280 nm) using a calibration curve obtained from BSA solutions of known concentrations.
5. Calculate the protein adsorbed on the complexes with the following formula: $q = (C_0\text{-}C_1)V/m$, where $C_0$ and $C_1$ are the initial BSA concentration and the BSA concentration in the supernatant after adsorption experiments, respectively; V is the total volume of the solution (2 mL); and m is the weight of the polymer (1 mg) added into the solution

#### 3.1.13 Acid-Triggered Unpacking of Nanoassembly/DNA Complexes in the Presence of Heparin

1. Incubate the complexes (w/w ratio of 25) in 8 mL of pH 5.0 acetate buffer at 37 °C for 30 min.
2. Add appropriate volume heparin in EDTA buffer solution (4.0 mg/mL) to give heparin concentrations of 0, 0.2, 0.4, 0.6 mg/mL, respectively.
3. Incubate for another 1.5 h.
4. Add same amount of heparin to the complexes in pH 7.4 PBS buffer as control group.

### 3.2 Cell Culture

1. Passage HeLa, COS7, HepG2, and 3 T3 cells in the DMEM (10% fetal bovine serum, 10,000 U/mL penicillin-streptomycin).
2. Split the cells within 48 h after reaching full monolayer confluency in order to keep the cells in a healthy condition.

## 4 Maintain Cells at 37 °C in a Humidified Atmosphere Containing 5% $CO_2$

### 4.1 Amplification and Purification of Plasmid DNA

1. Amplify the pGL-3 plasmid in E. coli JM109 by acid-base titration at 37 °C overnight.
2. Purify the pGL-3 plasmid by an EndoFree QiAfilterTM Plasmid Giga Kit (5). 3. Dilute the purified plasmid with TE buffer solution and store at −20 °C.

## 5 Determine the Purity and Concentration of DNA by UV Absorbance at 260–280 Nm

### 5.1 In Vitro Gene Transfection

1. Seed HeLa Cells in 24-well plate at a density of $6 \times 10^4$ cells/well and incubate at 37 °C in the presence of 5% $CO_2$ for 24 h.
2. Prepare the complexes with w/w ratios ranging from 10 to 30.
3. Dilute the complexes solutions to 1 mL by DMEM containing 10% or 30% FBS.
4. Add the complexes to the cell wells and incubate for 4 h at 37 °C.
5. Wash the cells to remove the residual complexes and feed with fresh medium.
6. Measure the relative light units (RLU) by a chemiluminometer (Lumat LB9507, EG&G Berthold, Germany) at 44 h later.
7. Determine the total protein according to the BCA protein assay kit (Pierce). Luciferase activity was expressed as RLU/mg protein in Fig. 3.

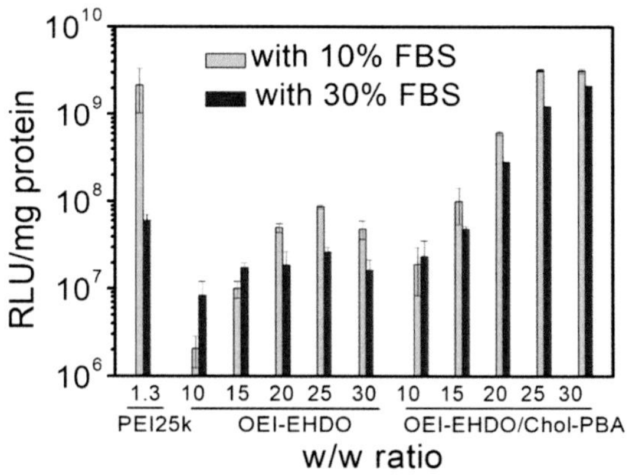


**Fig. 3** Transfection efficiency in HeLa cells mediated by nanoassembly/DNA complexes at various w/w ratios in the presence of 10% and 30% serum as compared with PEI25k and OEI-EHDO complexes. Data were shown as the mean ± S. D. (n = 3). (Adapted from Zhu et al. (2016), with permission)

## 5.2 Flow Cytometry

1. Seed HeLa cells in 6-well plate at a density of $6 \times 10^4$ cells/well and culture with 2 mL DMEM containing 10% FBS at 37 °C for 24 h.
2. Label pGL-3 plasmid with YOYO-1.
3. Prepare OEI-EHDO/pGL-3, OEI-EHDO/Chol-PBA/pGL-3, and PEI25K/pGL-3 complexes at the optimal w/w ratios of 20, 25, and 1.3, respectively, and then add to the plates after diluting the complexes to 2 mL with DMEM containing 10% or 30% FBS.
4. Remove the medium after 4 h incubation, and wash the cells three times with PBS.
5. Digest all the cells by trypsin and collect in centrifuge tubes upon centrifugation at 1000 rpm for 5 min.
6. Discard the supernatant and wash the bottom cells twice with PBS.
7. Filtrate the suspended cells and examine by flow cytometry (BD FACSAria™III, USA) in Fig. 4.
8. Calibrate the instrument with non-treated cells (negative control) to identify viable cells and determine the cells from a fluorescence scan performed with $1 \times 10^4$ cells using the FL1-H channel.

## 5.3 Confocal Laser Scanning Microscopy (CLSM)

1. Seed HeLa cells at a density of $2.5 \times 10^5$ cells per single dish and incubate at 37 °C for 24 h.
2. Label Plasmid pGL-3 with YOYO-1.

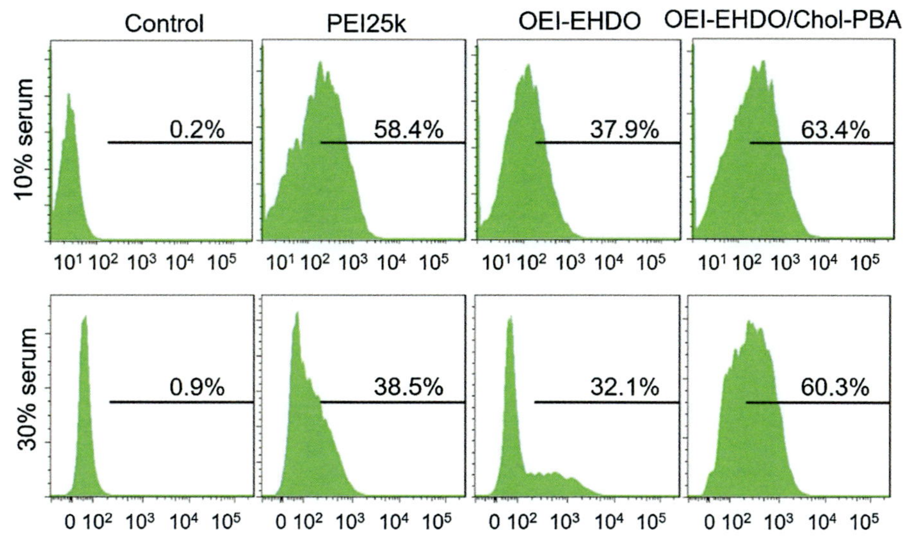


**Fig. 4** Flow cytometry profiles of three complexes prepared at their optimal transfection w/w ratios. (Adapted from Zhu et al. (2016), with permission)

3. Prepare various complexes at the optimal transfection w/w ratios, and co-incubate with cells for 8 h, and wash thrice with PBS.
4. Stain the cell nuclei by Hoechst 33342 for 10 min, and wash thrice with PBS.
5. Visualize the intracellular trafficking by a confocal laser scanning microscope (Nikon C1-si TE2000, Japan) and record by EZ-C1 software.
6. Add 25 μL of cholesterol solution in ethanol into the dish with the final cholesterol concentration of 4, 8, 16, 32 mg/μL, and add 25 μL of free ethanol for comparison.
7. Stand for 30 min, introduce OEI-EHDO/Chol-PBA/DNA complexes in DMEM containing 10% FBS for 4 h cell transfection. Use OEI-EHDO/DNA complexes as control group.
8. Photograph the cells by CLSM and record by EZ-C1 software.

### 5.4 $NH_4Cl$-Associated Interference of Endosomal Acidification Procession

1. Add OEI-EHDO/Chol-PBA/DNA complexes at various w/w ratios to the cell wells in the presence of $NH_4Cl$ (50 mM).
2. Transfect at 37 °C for 4 h, wash the cells, and replenish with fresh DMEM containing 10% FBS in the presence of $NH_4Cl$ (50 mM), and further incubate at 37 °C for 20 h.

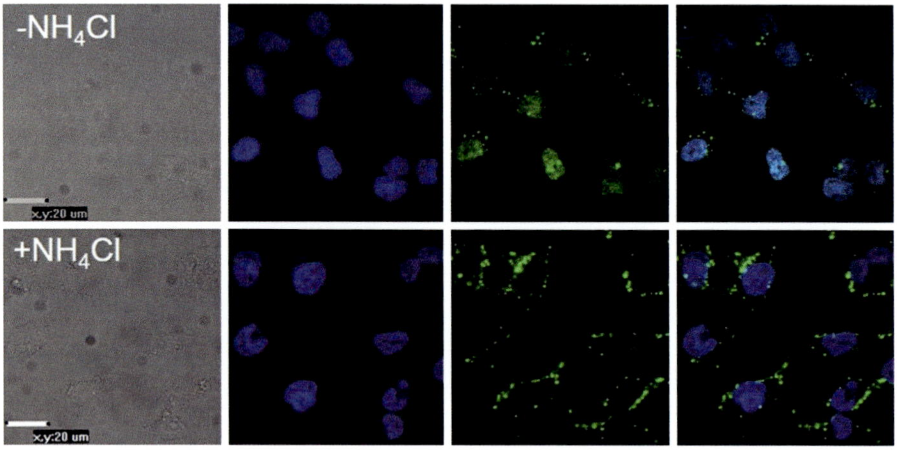


**Fig. 5** Confocal images of HeLa cells after co-incubation with OEIEHDO/Chol-PBA/pGL-3 complexes in the presence/absence of $NH_4Cl$ (50 mM). Plasmid pGL-3 was stained green by YOYO-1. Nuclei of cells were stained blue by Hoechst 33342. (Adapted from Zhu et al. (2016), with permission)

3. Perform the same treatment in the absence of $NH_4Cl$ as control group.
4. Dissolve OEI-EHDO/Chol-PBA/DNA complexes in DMEM containing 10% FBS, and add 1 mL of complexes solution into the single dish, and incubate at 37 °C for 8 h.
5. Wash cells several times with PBS, and stain cell nuclei with 1 mL of DMEM containing 10 μL Hoechst 33342 for 15 min, and wash the cells several times with PBS, and photograph the cells by CLSM, and record by EZ-C1 software in Fig. 5.

## 5.5 In Vitro Cytotoxicity Assays

1. Seed HeLa cells with a density of $6 \times 10^3$ cells/well in the 96-well plate and culture 24 h in 100 μL of DMEM containing 10% FBS.
2. Add the nanoassembly with various concentrations or complexes with various w/w ratios to each well, and culture at 37 °C for 4 h.
3. Replace the medium with 200 μL of fresh medium, and further culture the cells for 44 h.
4. Add 20 μL of MTT (5 mg/mL) solution to each well, and further culture for 4 h at 37 °C.
5. Remove the medium, and add 150 μL of DMSO, and measure the optical density (OD) at 570 nm with a microplate reader (BIO-RAD 550, USA).
6. Calculate the relative cell viability as follows: Relative cell viability (%) = $(OD570_{sample} - OD570_{background})/(OD570_{control} - OD570_{background}) \times$

100%, where $OD570_{sample}$ was obtained in the presence of nanoassembly, $OD570_{control}$ was obtained in the absence of nanoassembly, and $OD570_{background}$ was obtained in the absence of nanoassembly and cells.

### 5.6 In Vivo Animal Study

1. Purchase female BALB/c mice (4–5 weeks old) from the Wuhan University Center for Animal Experiment/A3-Lab.
2. Inject with hepatoma H22 cells.
3. Randomly divide the mice into five groups (six mice per group) when the tumors reach an approximate size of 100 $mm^3$.
4. Intratumorally inject with various samples (120 μL), including PBS buffer, naked DNA, OEI-EHDO/DNA complexes and OEI-EHDO/Chol-PBA/DNA complexes. The dosage of plasmid DNA (pORF-LacZ, pGL-3): 15 μg per mouse.
5. Two days later, sacrifice the mice by cervical vertebra-dislocation, and resect their tumors, wash them with ice-cold PBS.
6. Fix and stain the tumor tissues which injected pORF-LacZ formulations with X-gal staining kit (InvivoGen, USA) overnight.
7. Record photographically the stained tissues, and further fix them with 3.7% formaldehyde for 1 day.
8. Embed the samples into paraffin and cut into 5 μm thick sections, visualize under a light microscope coupled with a digital camera after H&E staining.
9. Homogenize the tumors injected with pGL-3 formulations using an IKA-Ultra-Turrax homogenizer in Promega cell lysis buffer.
10. Collect the supernatant via centrifugation (12,000 g/min) at 4 °C to quantify the luciferase activity and protein content in Fig. 6.
11. Express the transfection efficiency as RLU per mg protein.

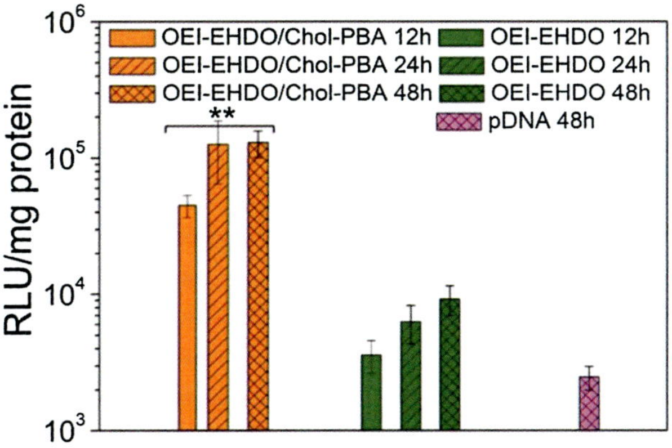


**Fig. 6** Luciferase expression in tumor after treatment with different complexes containing pGL-3 after the transfection at 12 h, 24 h, and 48 h (Adapted from Zhu et al. (2016), with permission). (** $p < 0.01$ as compared with the data of DNA)

## 5.7 Statistical Analysis

1. Present data as the mean ± standard deviation (SD).
2. Perform statistical analysis by Student's t test.
3. Consider a value of $p < 0.05$ to be statistically significant.

# 6 Notes

1. Boronic acid-diol orthogonality acts as a role of "joint" to spontaneously integrate hydrophilic cationic OEI-EHDO and hydrophobic Chol-PBA into one entity. The driving force relies on the unique feature of boronate bond that can readily form at neutral conditions without any catalysts.
2. The obtained OEI-EHDO should be sealed in dry place because it absorbs water easily.
3. Cholesterol chloroformate, 3-aminophenylboronic acid, N-methylimidazole, and diethyl ether should be strictly anhydrous.
4. During the nanoassembly preparation, THF solvent should be allowed to evaporate slowly under stirring.
5. To determine the grafting degree, the nanoassembly should be fully disintegrated in 10 mL of HCl (pH ~ 1.0) over night. The isolated Chol-PBA may be adhered to the bottle wall, which should be carefully extracted with chloroform three times.
6. Based on the hydrophilic and hydrophobic equilibrium, the molar ratio of OEI-EHDO/Chol-PBA in feed was set as 1:1 throughout the study.
7. The nanoassembly and their complexes solution should be passed through a 0.45 mm pore size filter (Shanghai Chemical Reagent Co.) prior to the measurement to avoid interference of the dust in the solution. To determine zeta potential, PBS buffer solution was replaced by deionized water.
8. The nanoassembly suspension should be fresh and diluted enough before characterization using DLS and TEM.
9. The cells must be mixed well when seeding into the wells. The cells are prone to settle down to the bottom of cell culture dish, and so the cells should be uniformly suspended prior to the seeding treatment.
10. Edge wells in plates should not be used in cell experiments in order to ensure the same growth rate with the cells in inner wells.
11. $NH_4Cl$ was well documented to effectively block the early-to-late endosomal acidification progression, and thus in the $NH_4Cl$-associated interference experiment, $NH_4Cl$ should be present in the whole process, including the cellular uptake and transfection process.
12. To stay in step with transfection experiment, the complexes should be added to co-incubate with cells for 4 h, and then the treated cells were exposed to the cytotoxicity assay.

13. Hepatoma H22 cells should be seeded on the basolateral compartment of the insert at a density of $1.0 \times 10^6$ cells per compartment. After about 5 days of incubation, the tumor model can be used for the following experiments.
14. Tumors injected with pORF-LacZ formulations should not be treated using iron-related equipment during X-gal staining process. This tumor staining experiment should be carried out at 37 °C overnight.
15. Tumor tissues injected with pGL-3 formulations should be homogenized with a homogenizer in Promega cell lysis buffer. The luciferase activity and protein content are measured according to the BCA protein assay kit.
16. The injection volume should be adjusted to 0.8 ml/100 g of mouse weight. The dosage of plasmid DNA (pORF-LacZ, pGL-3) was 15 μg per mouse.

## 7 Conclusion

This protocol presents a lysosome-targeting acidity-responsive nanoassembly on the basis of the spontaneous coupling between 1,3-diol-rich OEI-EHDO and phenylboronic acid modified Chol-PBA, aiming to achieve not only efficient but rapid transfection. The pH-reversible features of phenylboronate bond endow the nanoassembly with the rapid transnuclear entry of carried DNA. The in vitro and in vivo results demonstrate that the nanoassemblies can afford high transfection efficiency at as short as 8 h even comparable to that achieved at 48 h by the golden standard of PEI25K, and maintain the high transfection level during 48 h. The results manifest the high sensitivity to the lysosomal acidity, the strong tolerance to the serum interference, and good biocompatibility of this hydroxyl-rich bio-decomposable nanoassembly, suggesting its great potential as a rapid and efficient gene carrier for practical application.

## References


Ahmadi S, Rabiee N, Bagherzadeh M, Elmi F, Fatahi Y, Farjadian F, Baheiraei N, Nasseri B, Rabiee M, Dastjerd NT, Valibeik A, Karimi M, Hamblin MR (2020) Stimulus-responsive sequential release systems for drug and gene delivery. Nano Today 34:100914

Boedtkjer E, Pedersen SF (2020) The acidic tumor microenvironment as a driver of cancer. In M. T. Nelson & K. Walsh (Eds.). Annu Rev Physiol 82:103–126

Cai WQ, Luo TL, Mao LQ, Wang M (2020) Spatiotemporal delivery of crispr/cas9 genome editing machinery using stimuli-responsive vehicles. Angew Chem Int Ed 133(16):8679–8689

DeBerardinis RJ, Chandel NS (2020) We need to talk about the Warburg effect. Nat Metab 2(2): 127–129

Deverman BE, Ravina BM, Bankiewicz KS, Paul SM, Sah DWY (2018) Gene therapy for neurological disorders: Progress and prospects. Nat Rev Drug Discov 17(9):641–659

Dhaliwal A, Zheng G (2019) Improving accessibility of EPR-insensitive tumor phenotypes using EPR-adaptive strategies: designing a new perspective in nanomedicine delivery. Theranostics 9(26):8091–8108

Dobson J (2006) Gene therapy progress and prospects: magnetic nanoparticle-based gene delivery. Gene Ther 13(4):283–287

Fang J, Islam W, Maeda H (2020) Exploiting the dynamics of the EPR effect and strategies to improve the therapeutic effects of nanomedicines by using EPR effect enhancers. Adv Drug Deliv Rev 157:142–160

Forgac M (2007) Vacuolar ATPases: rotary proton pumps in physiology and pathophysiology. Nat Rev Mol Cell Biol 8(11):917–929

Heiden MGV, Cantley LC, Thompson CB (2009) Understanding the Warburg effect: the metabolic requirements of cell proliferation. Science 324(5930):1029–1033

Jia HZ, Zhu JY, Wang XL, Cheng H, Chen G, Zhao YF, Zeng X, Feng J, Zhang XZ, Zhuo RX (2014) A boronate-linked linear-hyperbranched polymeric nanovehicle for pH-dependent tumor-targeted drug delivery. Biomaterials 35(19):5240–5249

Khandare J, Calderon M, Dagia NM, Haag R (2012) Multifunctional dendritic polymers in nanomedicine: opportunities and challenges. Chem Soc Rev 41(7):2824–2848

Kheirolomoom A, Ferrara KW (2007) Cholesterol transport from liposomal delivery vehicles. Biomaterials 28(29):4311–4320

Li YP, Xiao WW, Xiao K, Berti L, Luo JT, Tseng HP, Fung G, Lam KS (2012) Well-defined, reversible boronate crosslinked nanocarriers for targeted drug delivery in response to acidic ph values and cis-diols. Angew Chem Int Ed 51(12):2864–2869

Li J, Zheng C, Cansiz S, Wu CC, Xu JH, Cui C, Liu Y, Hou WJ, Wang YY, Zhang LQ, Teng IT, Yang HH, Tan WH (2015) Self-assembly of DNA nanohydrogels with controllable size and stimuli-responsive property for targeted gene regulation therapy. J Am Chem Soc 137(4): 1412–1415

Li YW, Yue SZ, Cao JY, Zhu CZ, Wang YX, Hai X, Song WL, Bi S (2020) Ph-responsive DNA nanomicelles for chemo-gene synergetic therapy of anaplastic large cell lymphoma. Theranostics 10(18):8250–8263

Lo YL, Chang CH, Wang CS, Yang MH, Lin AMY, Hong CJ, Tseng WH (2020) Peg-coated nanoparticles detachable in acidic microenvironments for the tumor-directed delivery of chemo- and gene therapies for head and neck cancer. Theranostics 10(15):6695–6714

Luo XH, Huang FW, Qin SY, Wang HF, Feng J, Zhang XZ, Zhuo RX (2011) A strategy to improve serum-tolerant transfection activity of polycation vectors by surface hydroxylation. Biomaterials 32(36):9925–9939

Mohammadinejad R, Dehshahri A, Madamsetty VS, Zahmatkeshan M, Tavakol S, Makvandi P, Khorsandi D, Pardakhty A, Ashrafizadeh M, Afshar EG, Zarrabi A (2020) In vivo gene delivery mediated by non-viral vectors for cancer therapy. J Control Release 325:249–275

Piotrowski-Daspit AS, Kauffman AC, Bracaglia LG, Saltzman WM (2020) Polymeric vehicles for nucleic acid delivery. Adv Drug Deliv Rev 156:119–132

Shim MS, Kwon YJ (2012) Stimuli-responsive polymers and nanomaterials for gene delivery and imaging applications. Adv Drug Deliv Rev 64(11):1046–1058

Wu MY, Meng QS, Chen Y, Zhang LX, Li ML, Cai XJ, Li YP, Yu PC, Zhang LL, Shi JL (2016) Large pore-sized hollow mesoporous organosilica for redox-responsive gene delivery and synergistic cancer chemotherapy. Adv Mater 28(10):1963–1969

Yang B, Jia HZ, Wang XL, Chen S, Zhang XZ, Zhuo RX, Feng J (2014a) Self-assembled vehicle construction via boronic acid coupling and host-guest interaction for serum-tolerant DNA transport and pH-responsive drug delivery. Adv Healthc Mater 3(4):596–608

Yang B, Lv Y, Zhu JY, Han Y, Jia HZ, Chen WH, Feng J, Zhang XZ, Zhuo RX (2014b) A pH-responsive drug nanovehicle constructed by reversible attachment of cholesterol to pegylated poly(l-lysine) via catechol-boronic acid ester formation. Acta Biomater 10(8): 3686–3695

Yin H, Kanasty RL, Eltoukhy AA, Vegas AJ, Dorkin JR, Anderson DG (2014) Non-viral vectors for gene-based therapy. Nat Rev Genet 15(8):541–555

Zhang M, Guo XL, Wang MF, Liu KH (2020a) Tumor microenvironment-induced structure changing drug/gene delivery system for overcoming delivery -associated challenges. J Control Release 323:203–224

Zhang RJ, Liu RF, Liu C, Pan LN, Qi YT, Cheng J, Guo JW, Jia Y, Ding J, Zhang JX, Hu HY (2020b) A pH/ROS dual-responsive and targeting nanotherapy for vascular inflammatory diseases. Biomaterials 230:119605

Zhu JY, Lei Q, Yang B, Jia HZ, Qiu WX, Wang XL, Zeng X, Zhuo RX, Feng J, Zhang XZ (2015) Efficient nuclear drug translocation and improved drug efficacy mediated by acidity-responsive boronate-linked dextran/cholesterol nanoassembly. Biomaterials 52:281–290

Zhu JY, Zeng X, Qin SY, Wan SS, Jia HZ, Zhuo RX, Feng J, Zhang XZ (2016) Acidity-responsive gene delivery for "superfast" nuclear translocation and transfection with high efficiency. Biomaterials 83:79–92

Zhu JY, Wan SS, Zheng DW, Lei Q, Zhuo RX, Feng J, Zhang XZ (2017) Propelled transnuclear gene transport achieved through intracellularly redox-responsive and acidity-accelerative decomposition of supramolecular florescence-quenchable vectors. ACS Appl Mater Interfaces 9(1):255–265

# Preparation and Evaluation of Virus-Inspired Nanogenes for Host-Specific Transfection

# 24

Jing-Yi Zhu, Jun Feng, and Xian-Zheng Zhang

## Contents




J.-Y. Zhu · X.-Z. Zhang (✉)
Key Laboratory of Biomedical Polymers of Ministry of Education, Department of Chemistry, Wuhan University, Wuhan, P. R. China

Key Laboratory of Biomaterials of Guangdong Higher Education Institutes, Department of Biomedical Engineering, Jinan University, Guangzhou, P. R. China
e-mail: xz-zhang@whu.edu.cn

J. Feng (✉)
Key Laboratory of Biomedical Polymers of Ministry of Education, Department of Chemistry, Wuhan University, Wuhan, P. R. China
e-mail: fengjun@whu.edu.cn







H. Tian and X. Chen (eds.), *Gene Delivery*, Biomaterial Engineering,
https://doi.org/10.1007/978-981-16-5419-0_24

**Abstract**

Many viruses have a lipid envelope derived from the host cell membrane that contributes much to the host specificity and the cellular invasion. This chapter puts forward a virus-inspired technology that allows targeted genetic delivery free from man-made materials. Genetic therapeutics, metal ions, and biologically derived cell membranes are directly nanointegrated. Vulnerable genetic therapeutics contained in the formed "nanogene" can be well protected from unwanted attacks by blood components and enzymes. The surface envelope composed of cancer cell membrane fragments enables host-specific targeting of the nanogene at the source cancer cells and homologous tumors while effectively inhibiting recognition by macrophages. High-transfection efficiency highlights the potential of this technology for practical applications. Another attractive merit of this technology arises from the facile combination of special biofunction of metal ions with gene therapy. Typically, Gd(III)-involved nanogene generates a much higher *T*1 relaxation rate than the clinically used Gd-magnetic resonance imaging agent and exhibits the enhanced MRI contrast at tumors. This virus-inspired technology paves a new pathway for the disease-specific transport of genetic therapeutics and other biomacromolecules.

**Keywords**

Virus-mimetic biocarriage · Host-specific targeting · Cell membrane envelope · Gene transfection · MR imaging

## 1 Introduction

Great efforts have been made to advance the clinical translation of gene therapy by means of vector-aided delivery of genetic therapeutics, e.g., DNA and RNA (Degors et al. 2019; Guan and Rosenecker 2017; Wang et al. 2015). Viral vectors hold a leading position in the long history of gene therapy. However, clinical applications of viruses suffer seriously from mutagenesis, immunogenicity, the difficulty in large-scale manufacture, and the failure to load large genetic therapeutics (Challis et al. 2019; Thomas et al. 2003). Inorganic/organic man-made gene vectors have hence been extensively investigated to pursue nonviral candidates (He et al. 2019; Yang et al. 2015; Zhou et al. 2017). Nonviral gene delivery has made impressive progress in the past decade, and several products have come into market. However, translating the results from in vitro into preclinical therapies is hindered by the suboptimal performance of gene delivery vehicles in capturing, protecting, and delivering nucleic acid cargoes safely and efficaciously (Lostalé-Seijo and Montenegro 2018). Chemistry plays a key role in the development of innovative synthetic materials to overcome the challenges of producing next-generation gene delivery therapies and protocols. For example, Cheng et al. synthesized two different kinds of multifunctional peptide-conjugated AIE luminogens (AIEgens; AIE = aggregation-induced emission), $T_DNCP$ and $T_RNCP$, for real-time tracking and efficient and sequential targeted gene delivery into the nucleus (Cheng et al. 2019). Wang et al. designed a kind of heterogeneous membrane polymersomes with "boarding" and "debarkation" multi-functional gates via self-assembling from PEO-*b*-P(NIPAM-*stat*-CMA-*stat*-DEA) diblock copolymers for efficient gene delivery (Wang et al. 2018). However, complex chemistry, tedious process, difficult purification, and low yield have to be involved in the preparation of functional gene vectors (Zhu et al. 2017a). Moreover, man-made vectors always hardly meet the biofunctional requirement when applied in vivo. For example, clinical administration of nonviral gene vectors usually faces several prominent issues, including easy immune recognition, rapid clearance from the body, nonspecific uptake by tissues/cells, and high toxicity (Cheng et al. 2016b; Zhu et al. 2017b). In fact, the in vivo fate of almost all man-made vectors remains vague yet. All these concerns make it always ambiguous and questionable for the practical translation of nonviral gene therapy and prompt us to actively seek new strategies for the safe and effective gene therapy mediated by nonviral vectors.

As a kind of naturally present organism, viruses display a wide diversity of shapes, most of which have a diameter between 20 and 300 nm (Li and Samulski 2020; Thomas et al. 2003). Virus particles consist of nucleic acid surrounded with a protective coat of proteins. Of special note, quite a few of viruses, such as influenza virus, herpes virus, and HIV, have a lipid envelope derived from the host cell membrane that contributes much to the host specificity and the cellular invasion (Lorizate et al. 2013; Smith and Helenius 2004). The host-specific nature of certain cell membranes can find supporting evidences based on the recent work showing that the recombined cell membrane could endow nanoparticles with the improved biocompatibility, and more importantly, the natural targeting capability to the biologically related cells/tissues (Cheng et al. 2016b; Jiang et al. 2020; Sevencan et al. 2020; Zhu et al. 2016, 2017c, 2018, 2020). Inspired by the viral nanostructure with host-recognized lipid envelope, we hypothesize that by using biofunctional cell membrane, it might be accessible to achieve effective and disease-specific nonviral gene transfection without using any man-made materials. One challenge naturally emerges: How to integrate the genetic therapeutics with cell membrane because they are both negatively charged without the aid of artificial materials? Metal ions, which are vital in physiological activities of living organisms and also exist in some viruses, have found wide applications in therapy and diagnosis (Coughlin et al. 2014; Mjos and Orvig 2014; Thompson and Orvig 2003; Weekes and Orvig 2016). Metal ion-based nanoparticles or nanostructures are currently among the most fascinating nanomaterials. Interestingly, we note that multivalent metal ions, such as Zn(II), Ca(II), Mg(II), and Mn(II), have ever been employed to bridge DNA skeletons as the model for probing the mechanism of virus-DNA packaging and condensation in chromatin (Clever et al. 2007; Gao et al. 1993; Lim et al. 2015).

We herein report a virus-mimetic ternary nanoengineering built from genetic therapeutics, metal ions, and cell membrane in attempts to achieve host-specific gene therapy. Another advantage of this gene biocarriage strategy comes from a wide range of opportunities that gene therapy can be armed with the special functions of metal ions. Free metal ions possess high toxicity, which require the stable chelation using proper ligands (Sun et al. 2020). In principle, the complexation of metal ions in the nanoengineering would minimize the toxicity of metal irons.

In this protocol, we describe an example of theranostic "nanogene" by organically integrating Gd(III), DNA, and cracked cancer cell membrane (CCCM), as illustrated in Fig. 1. Gd(III) was used to shorten the distance among DNA skeletons via the electrostatic and coordinate interaction. Thereafter, Gd/DNA complexes were complexed with CCCMs to acquire the intact cell membrane envelope. Many kinds of cancer cells usually aggregate together beside the blood vessel endothelium, and the dispersed cancer cells intend to auto-aggregate into tumor spheroids, known as "homologous adhesion." Cancer cell membrane herein functions like the host-recognized lipid envelope of virus to drive the self-targeting of nanogenes to

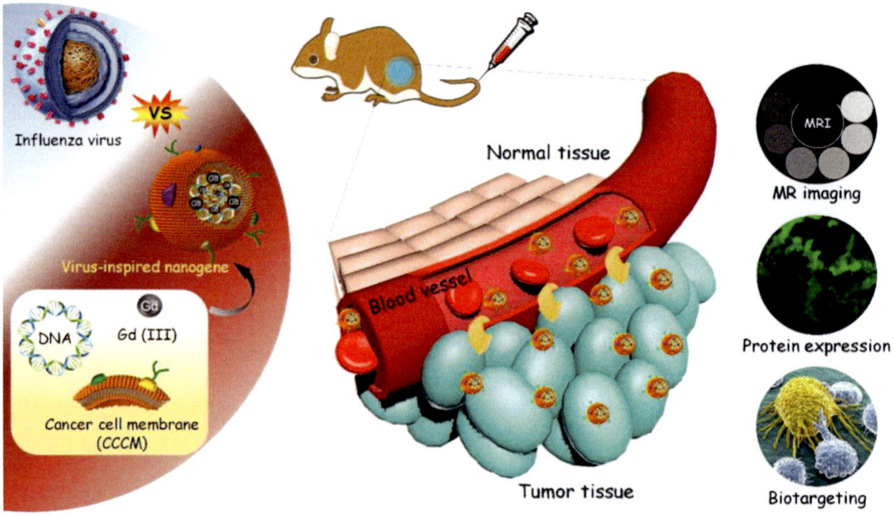


**Fig. 1** (**a**) Illustration of gene biocarriage concept by aid of cancer cell membrane and Gd(III) ion for host-specific transfection and enhanced magnetic resonance imaging (MRI). (Adapted from reference Zhu et al. (2018), with permission)

homologous tumors. It is expected that this engineering could provide improved biocompatibility, host-specific tumor targeting, and favorable transfection performance as well as bioaided MRI diagnosis. If established, this biocarriage technology may sharply pave a new avenue to advance the clinical translation of disease-specific genetic therapy, and also show promising applicability for other biomacromolecules, such as proteins and enzymes (Zhu et al. 2018).

# 2 Materials

## 2.1 Cell Culture and Amplification of Plasmid DNA

1. Human cervix carcinoma cell (HeLa)
2. African green monkey kidney cell (COS7)
3. Human squamous cell carcinoma (UM-SCC-7) cells
4. Mouse embryonic fibroblasts (3T3)
5. Raw 264.7 murine macrophages
6. Dulbecco's Modified Eagle's Medium (DMEM)
7. Fetal bovine serum (FBS)
8. Trypsin EDTA
9. Penicillin
10. Streptomycin
11. Cell culture flask (T-25, T-75)
12. $CO_2$ incubator
13. Vertical flow clean bench
14. Optical microscope
15. E. coli JM109
16. E. coli DH5α
17. Terrific broth media (containing beef extract and peptone)
18. EndoFree QiAfilter™ Plasmid Giga Kit (5) (QIAGEN, Germany)
19. Tris-EDTA (TE) buffer
20. Ultraviolet-visible (UV) spectrophotometer

## 2.2 Preparation of Cracked Cancer Cell Membrane (CCCM)

1. Cell culture dishes (10 cm in diameter)
2. Cell scraper
3. Centrifuge
4. Centrifuge tube
5. Phosphate-buffered saline (PBS) (137 mM NaCl, 2.7 mM KCl, 8 mM $Na_2HPO_4$, and 2 mM $KH_2PO_4$, pH 7.4)
6. Deionized water
7. Hypotonic lysing buffer
8. Phenylmethanesulfonyl fluoride (PMSF) (Beyotime Institute of Biotechnology)

9. High-speed refrigerated centrifuge
10. Ultralow temperature lab refrigerators (−80 °C)
11. Ultrapure water
12. Lyophilizer

## 2.3 Cancer Cell Membrane Protein Characterization

1. NuPAGE Novex 4–12% Bis-Tris minigel
2. Lithium dodecyl sulfate (LDS) loading buffer (Invitrogen)
3. 3-(N-morpholino) propane sulfonic acid (MOPS)
4. Sodium dodecyl sulfate (SDS)
5. MOPS-SDS running buffer (Invitrogen)
6. Coomassie blue (Invitrogen)

## 2.4 Agarose Gel Retardation Assay

1. Agarose
2. GelRed™
3. Tris-acetate (TAE) running buffer
4. Bromophenol blue
5. pGL-3 plasmid
6. Phosphate-buffered saline (PBS) (137 mM NaCI, 2.7 mM KCl, 8 mM $Na_2HPO_4$, and 2 mM $KH_2PO_4$, pH 7.4)
7. Microcentrifuge tube
8. Vortex mixer
9. 37 °C incubator
10. Ultraviolet-visible lamp using a Vilber Lourmat imaging system (France)
11. Electrophoresis apparatus

## 2.5 Optimization of Membrane Weight Ratio Within Gd/DNA@CCCM

1. Gadolinium ion ($Gd^{3+}$)
2. Plasmid DNA
3. Cracked cancer cell membrane (CCCM)
4. Centrifuge tube
5. Phosphate-buffered saline (PBS) (137 mM NaCI, 2.7 mM KCl, 8 mM $Na_2HPO_4$, and 2 mM $KH_2PO_4$, pH 7.4)
6. Microcentrifuge tube
7. Vortex mixer

## 2.6 Preparation of CCCM-Coated Gd/DNA (Gd/DNA@CCCM)

1. Gd/DNA complexes (w/w: 10)
2. HeLa CCCM
3. Deionized water
4. Phosphate-buffered saline (PBS) (137 mM NaCI, 2.7 mM KCl, 8 mM $Na_2HPO_4$, and 2 mM $KH_2PO_4$, pH 7.4)
5. Dynamic light scattering (DLS) analyzer (Malvern Nano Series Zen 3600 Zeta Sizer)
6. Syringe and micropore filter
7. Water-phase filters (2.0 μm, 0.8 μm, and 0.45 μm)

## 2.7 Transmission Electron Microscopy (TEM) Observation

1. Gd/DNA@CCCM suspension
2. Transmission electron microscopy (JEOL JEM-100CXII instrument at an acceleration voltage of 80 KV)
3. Copper grids coated with formvar films
4. 0.2% (w/v) phosphotungstic acid solution

## 2.8 Protein Adsorption Assay

1. pGL-3 plasmid
2. Gd/DNA@CCCM complexes solution (1.0 mg/mL)
3. Bovine serum albumin (BSA)
4. Centrifuge
5. Ultraviolet-visible (UV) spectrophotometer
6. Shaker

## 2.9 Stability of Gd/DNA@CCCM in the Presence of Heparin and/or DNase

1. pGL-3 plasmid
2. Gd/DNA@CCCM complexes
3. Gd/DNA complexes
4. Phosphate-buffered saline (PBS) (137 mM NaCI, 2.7 mM KCl, 8 mM $Na_2HPO_4$, and 2 mM $KH_2PO_4$, pH 7.4)
5. Ethylenediaminetetraacetic acid (EDTA) buffer
6. Heparin
7. DNase

8. Microcentrifuge tube
9. Vortex mixer
10. Electrophoresis apparatus

## 2.10 Stability of Gd/DNA@CCCM under 10% Serum Conditions

1. pGL-3 plasmid
2. Gd/DNA@CCCM complexes
3. Gd/DNA complexes
4. Fetal bovine serum (FBS)
5. Phosphate-buffered saline (PBS) (137 mM NaCI, 2.7 mM KCl, 8 mM $Na_2HPO_4$, and 2 mM $KH_2PO_4$, pH 7.4)
6. Dynamic light scattering (DLS) analyzer (Malvern Nano Series Zen 3600 Zeta Sizer)
7. Syringe and micropore filter (0.45 μm).

## 2.11 *In Vitro* Targeting Recognition Toward Homotypic Cancer Cells

1. Human cervix carcinoma cell (HeLa)
2. African green monkey kidney cell (COS7)
3. Human squamous cell carcinoma (UM-SCC-7) cells
4. Mouse embryonic fibroblasts (3T3)
5. pGL-3 plasmid
6. Gd/DNA@CCCM complexes
7. Gd/DNA complexes
8. YOYO-1
9. Hoechst 33,342
10. 35 mm confocal dishes
11. Dulbecco's Modified Eagle's Medium (DMEM)
12. Fetal bovine serum (FBS)
13. Confocal laser scanning microscope (Nikon C1-si TE2000, Japan)
14. 6-well culture plates
15. Trypsin
16. Centrifuge tubes
17. Centrifuge
18. Flow cytometry (BD FACSAria™III, USA)

## 2.12 *In Vitro* Macrophage Uptake Study

1. Raw 264.7 macrophage cells
2. pGL-3 plasmid
3. Gd/DNA@HeLa CCCM complexes

4. Gd/DNA complexes
5. YOYO-1
6. Hoechst 33,342
7. Trypsin
8. Phosphate-buffered saline (PBS) (137 mM NaCI, 2.7 mM KCl, 8 mM $Na_2HPO_4$, and 2 mM $KH_2PO_4$, pH 7.4)
9. 35 mm confocal dishes
10. 6-well culture plates
11. Confocal laser-scanning microscope (Nikon C1-si TE2000, Japan)
12. Flow cytometry (BD FACSAria™III, USA)

## 2.13 Luciferase Assay

1. HeLa cells
2. COS7 cells
3. UM-SCC-7 cells
4. Branched polyethyleneimine (Mw = 25 k) (PEI25K)
5. pGL-3 plasmid
6. Gd/DNA complexes
7. Gd/DNA@HeLa CCCM complexes
8. Gd/DNA@UM-SCC-7 CCCM complexes
9. 24-well culture plates
10. Dulbecco's Modified Eagle's Medium (DMEM)
11. Fetal bovine serum (FBS)
12. Phosphate-buffered saline (PBS) (137 mM NaCI, 2.7 mM KCl, 8 mM $Na_2HPO_4$, and 2 mM $KH_2PO_4$, pH 7.4)
13. Lysis buffer (Pierce)
14. Chemiluminometer (Lumat LB9507, EG&G Berthold, Germany)
15. BCA protein assay kit (Pierce)
16. Vortex mixer

## 2.14 Green Fluorescent Protein Assay

1. pGL-3 plasmid
2. Gd/DNA complexes
3. Gd/DNA@HeLa CCCM complexes
4. 24-well culture plates
5. Inverted microscope (IX 70, Olympus, Japan)

## 2.15 Cytotoxicity Assay

1. Human cervix carcinoma cells (HeLa)
2. 96-well culture plates

3. 10% serum-containing DMEM
4. 3-(4, 5-dimethylthiazol-2-yl)-2, 5-diphenyltetrazolium bromide (MTT)
5. Microplate reader (BIO-RAD 550, USA)

### 2.16 *In Vivo* Gene Transfection Study

1. Female BALB/c mice (4–5 weeks old)
2. HeLa cells
3. pGL-3 plasmid
4. pEGFP-C1 plasmid
5. pORF-LacZ plasmid
6. Ice-cold PBS
7. X-gal staining kit (InvivoGen, USA)
8. 4% formaldehyde
9. Paraffin
10. Hematoxylin
11. Eosin
12. Light microscope coupled with a digital camera
13. IKA-Ultra-Turrax homogenizer
14. Promega cell lysis buffer
15. BCA protein assay kit (Pierce)
16. Microscope (BX60, Olympus, Japan)

### 2.17 *In Vitro* and *In Vivo* MR Imaging

1. Gd/DNA complexes
2. Gd/DNA@HeLa CCCM complexes
3. Deionized water
4. Phosphate-buffered saline (PBS) (137 mM NaCI, 2.7 mM KCl, 8 mM $Na_2HPO_4$, and 2 mM $KH_2PO_4$, pH 7.4)
5. Female BALB/c nude mice
6. NMR tubes
7. 7 T Magnetic Resonance Imaging (BioSpec 4.7/30)

## 3 Methods

### 3.1 Preparation and Characterization of Virus-Inspired Nanogenes

#### 3.1.1 Cell Culture

1. Incubate HeLa, COS7, UM-SCC-7, Raw 264.7 murine macrophages, and 3 T3 cells in the DMEM (10% fetal bovine serum, 10,000 U/mL penicillin-streptomycin).

2. Split the cells within 48 h after reaching full monolayer confluency in order to keep the cells in a healthy condition.
3. Maintain cells at 37 °C in a humidified atmosphere containing 5% $CO_2$.

### 3.1.2 Amplification of Plasmid DNA

1. Transform the pGL-3 plasmid in E. coli JM109.
2. Transform the pEGFP-C1 and pORF-LacZ plasmids in E. coli DH5α.
3. Amplify three plasmids in terrific broth media at 37 °C overnight.
4. Purify three plasmids by an EndoFree QiAfilter™ Plasmid Giga Kit (5).
5. Dilute the purified plasmid with TE buffer solution, and store at −20 °C.
6. Determine the purity and concentration of DNA by UV absorbance at 260–280 nm.

### 3.1.3 Preparation of Cracked Cancer Cell Membrane (CCCM)

1. Culture cells in cell culture dishes, and detach cells with a cell scraper.
2. Isolate and collect cells through centrifugation treatment.
3. Resuspend the collected cell pellets in cooled PBS (pH = 7.4), and centrifugate at 700 g for 5 min.
4. Resuspend the obtained cell pellets in a hypotonic lysing buffer containing membrane protein extraction reagent and phenylmethanesulfonyl fluoride (PMSF), and incubate in ice-bath for 10–15 min.
5. Break the cells in the above solution using a freeze-thaw method, and centrifuge at 700 g for 10 min at 4 °C.
6. Centrifuge the above supernatant at 14,000 g for 30 min to collect the cracked cell membrane.
7. Lyophilize the products of cell membrane, and store at −80 °C.
8. Rehydrate the lyophilized membrane materials in PBS (pH = 7.4) or ultrapure water prior to use.

### 3.1.4 Cancer Cell Membrane Protein Characterization

1. Heat the samples of cracked cancer cell membrane (CCCM) in lithium dodecyl sulfate (LDS) loading buffer to 90 °C for 10 min.
2. Add 20 μL of sample into each well of a NuPAGE Novex 4–12% Bis-Tris minigel.
3. Use 3-(N-morpholino) propane sulfonic acid (MOPS) sodium dodecyl sulfate (SDS) as running buffer.
4. Stain proteins using Coomassie Blue (Invitrogen).
5. Destain in water overnight prior to imaging.

### 3.1.5 Agarose Gel Retardation Assay

1. Prepare the Gd/DNA complexes at various w/w ratio of 5, 10, 20, 30, 40, 50, and 60 by adding a different volume of Gd solution (1.0 mg/mL) into the solution containing 1.0 μg of DNA.
2. Dilute the mixture with PBS solution to 8 μL and vortexed for 30 s followed by 30 min incubation at 37 °C.

3. Perform electrophoresis on a 0.7% (W/V) agarose gel-containing GelRed™ in Tris-acetate (TAE) running buffer at 80 V for 1 h.
4. Photo the gel under a UV lamp using a Vilber Lourmat imaging system.

### 3.1.6 Preparation of CCCM-Coated Gd/DNA (Gd/DNA@CCCM)

1. Prepare the Gd/DNA complexes at w/w ratio of 10.
2. Add the complex solution dropwise into 1.0 mL of the dilute dispersion of HeLa CCCM (10 μg/mL) under vortexing.
3. Extrude the mixture through 2.0 μm, 0.8 μm, and 0.45 μm water-phase filters, respectively.
4. Determine the particle size and zeta potential of Gd/DNA@CCCM.

### 3.1.7 Transmission Electron Microscopy (TEM) Observation

1. Resuspend the Gd/DNA@CCCM in deionized water.
2. Filter through a micropore filter membrane (0.45 μm).
3. Use copper grids coated with formvar film to absorb the suspension for 2 min.
4. Take out copper grids, and blot with filter paper.
5. Float these grids in 1% uranium acetate solution for 1 min, remove, blot with filter paper, and dry at room temperature.
6. Observe the specimens by TEM at 80 kV. 1% uranium acetate.

### 3.1.8 Protein Adsorption Assay

1. Add 1 mL of Gd/DNA@CCCM solution (1.0 mg/mL) into 1 mL BSA solution (2.0 mg/mL).
2. Shake at 37 °C for 30 min, expose the mixture to centrifugation treatment, and collect the supernatant.
3. Determine the content of BSA in the supernatant by UV absorbance (280 nm) using a calibration curve for BSA solutions.
4. Calculate the protein adsorbed on the complexes as follows:
5. $Q = (C_0 - C_1)\ V/m$, where $C_0$ and $C_1$ are the initial BSA concentration and the BSA concentration in the supernatant after adsorption tests, respectively; V is the total volume of the solution (2 mL); and m is the weight of the vector (1 mg) added into the solution.

### 3.1.9 Stability Study

1. Prepare Gd/DNA@CCCM with the optimal w/w ratio (CCCM/Gd/DNA = 1: 1:0.1, DNA: 0.1 μg) in 8 μL of PBS (pH = 7.4).
2. Treat the above solution with 1 μL of EDTA buffer solution (0.5 M) containing 2.0 mg/mL heparin for 2 h.
3. Expose to agarose gel electrophoreses.
4. Incubate the Gd/DNA@CCCM complexes at 37 °C for 30 min, and dilute with PBS buffer containing 10% serum to 1.0 mL.
5. Monitor the particle size on a Nano-ZSZEN3600 (Malvern Instruments).

## 3.2 *In Vitro* Homotypic Targeting Study

1. Seed HeLa and UM-SCC-7 cells at a density of $2.5 \times 10^5$ cells per single dish and incubate at 37 °C for 24 h.
2. Replace the medium with fresh medium containing Gd/DNA@CCCM (CCCM/Gd/DNA = 1:1:0.1, DNA: 1.0 μg) or Gd/DNA (Gd/DNA = 1:0.1, DNA: 1.0 μg).
3. Incubate for 4 h, discard the medium, and wash the cells thrice with PBS.
4. Further incubate in 1 mL of DMEM containing 10 μL Hoechst 33342 for 15 min, photograph the cells by CLSM, and record by EZ-C1 software in Fig. 2.
5. Seed HeLa cells in 6-well plates at a density of $6 \times 10^4$ cells per well, and incubate for 24 h in 2 mL of DMEM containing 10% FBS at 37 °C.
6. Incubation cells with Gd/DNA@CCCM (CCCM/Gd/DNA = 1:1:0.1, DNA: 1.0 μg) or Gd/DNA (Gd/DNA = 1:0.1, DNA: 1.0 μg) for 4 h, wash the cells thrice with PBS, and digest by trypsin.
7. Collect the cell pellets by centrifugation treatment (1000 rpm, 5 min), and wash twice with PBS.
8. Filtrate the cell suspensions, and examine the cells by flow cytometry (BD FACSAria™ III, USA).
9. Perform the identical treatment in COS7, UM-SCC-7, and 3 T3 cells.

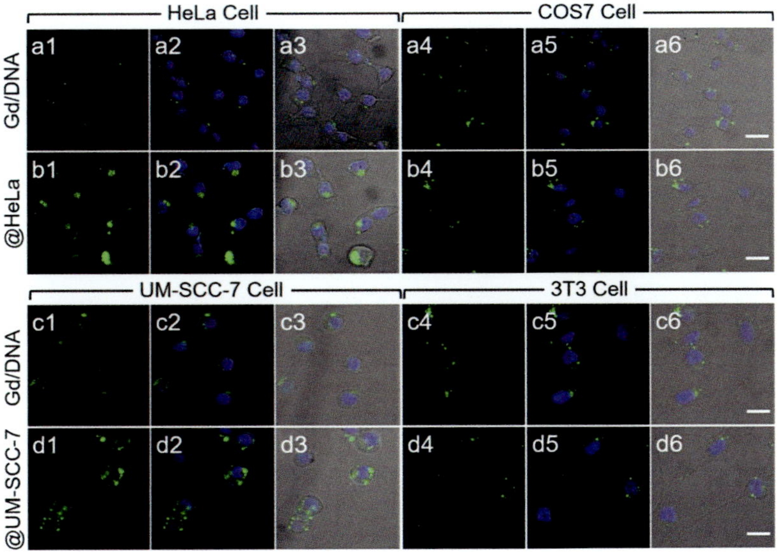


**Fig. 2** CLSM images of four cell lines including HeLa, COS7, UM-SCC-7, and 3 T3 cells upon 4-h coincubation with Gd/DNA@HeLa and Gd/DNA@UM-SCC-7, respectively. Cells treated with Gd/DNA were served as controls (a1-a3, a4-a6, c1-c3, and c4-c6). Nuclei were stained blue with Hoechst 33342. DNA was stained green with YOYO-1. Scale bars: 20 μm. (Adapted from reference Zhu et al. (2018), with permission)

## 3.3 *In Vitro* Macrophage Uptake Study

1. Seed Raw 264.7 macrophage cells at a density of $2.5 \times 10^5$ cells per single dish in 1 mL of DMEM supplemented with 10% FBS, and incubate at 37 °C for 24 h.
2. Replace the medium with the fresh medium containing Gd/DNA@HeLa (HeLa CCCM/Gd/DNA = 1:1:0.1, DNA: 1.0 μg) or Gd/DNA (Gd/DNA = 1:0.1, DNA: 1.0 μg).
3. Incubate for 4 h, rinse the cells thrice with PBS, and then stain with 1 mL of DMEM containing 10 μL Hoechst 33342 at 37 °C for 15 min.
4. Photograph the cells by CLSM.
5. Seed Raw 264.7 macrophage cells in 6-well plates with a density of $6 \times 10^4$ cells/well, and culture in 2 mL of DMEM containing 10% FBS for 24 h.
6. Incubate the cells with Gd/DNA@HeLa (HeLa CCCM/Gd/DNA = 1:1:0.1, DNA: 1.0 μg) or Gd/DNA (Gd/DNA = 1:0.1, DNA: 1.0 μg) for 4 h.
7. Wash the cells with PBS, digest using trypsin, and collect by centrifugation treatment (1000 rpm, 5 min).
8. Wash the cell pellets twice with PBS, resuspend in PBS, and filtrate prior to examination by flow cytometry (BD FACSAria™ III, USA).

## 3.4 Luciferase Assay

1. Seed the cells in 24-well plates ($6 \times 10^4$ cells/well) and incubated in DMEM containing 10% FBS for 24 h at 37 °C.
2. Decant the medium, and add the fresh medium containing Gd/DNA@HeLa (HeLa CCCM/Gd/DNA = 1:1:0.1, DNA: 1.0 μg) into the cell wells. Use Gd/DNA (Gd/DNA = 1:0.1, DNA: 1.0 μg), Gd/DNA@UM-SCC-7 (UM-SCC-7 CCCM/Gd/DNA = 1:1:0.1, DNA: 1.0 μg), and naked DNA (1.0 μg) as control groups. Use PEI25K (PEI25K/DNA = 1.3:1, DNA: 1.0 μg) as positive control.
3. 4 h later, replace the media with fresh DMEM containing 10% FBS, and further culture the cells for 48 h.
4. Decant the medium, wash the cells thrice with PBS, and then lyse by adding 200 μL of reporter lysis buffer.
5. Expose the above cells to the repeated freeze-thaw treatment.
6. Measure the relative light units (RLUs) by chemiluminometer (Lumat LB9507, EG&G Berthold, Germany).
7. Measure the cellular protein using the BCA protein assay kit (Pierce), and express the luciferase activity as RLU/mg Protein in Fig. 3.

## 3.5 Green Fluorescent Protein Assay

1. Prepare Gd/DNA@HeLa and Gd/DNA same as that for the luciferase assay.
2. Observe the cells expressing GFPs by an inverted microscope (IX 70, Olympus, Japan).

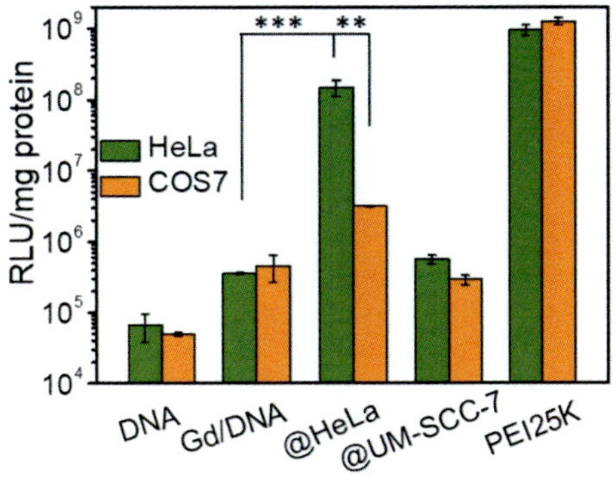


**Fig. 3** *In vitro* serum-free transfection in HeLa and COS7 cells mediated by naked DNA, Gd/DNA, Gd/DNA@HeLa, Gd/DNA@UM-SCC-7, and PEI25K. $^{**}p < 0.01$, $^{***}p < 0.001$. (Adapted from reference Zhu et al. (2018), with permission)

3. Obtain the images at a magnification of 100×, and record with CoolSNAP-Pro (4.5.1.1) version software.

## 3.6 Cytotoxicity Assay

1. Seed HeLa cells in 96-well plates at a density of $5 \times 10^3$ cells per well and incubate for 24 h.
2. Replace the medium with fresh medium containing different samples including Gd/DNA@HeLa, Gd/DNA, and free Gd ions, and continue to incubate for 4 h.
3. Decant the medium, and replace with fresh medium for further 48 h incubation.
4. Add MTT (5 mg/mL) into each well (20 μL per well), and incubate for another 4 h.
5. Decant the supernatant, and add dimethyl sulfoxide (DMSO, 150 μL per well) into each well to dissolve the formazan of MTT.
6. Measure the absorption at 570 nm using an ELISA plate reader (Bio-Rad, Microplate Reader 550), and calculate cell viability.

## 3.7 *In Vivo* Gene Transfection Study

1. Purchase 4–5-weeks-old female BALB/c mice from the Wuhan University Center for Animal Experiment/A3-Lab.
2. Subcutaneously inject with 100 μL of HeLa cells ($1 \times 10^6$) in the lateral of the right hind limb.
3. Randomly divide the mice into four groups (6 mice per group) when the tumors reach about 100 $mm^3$.
4. Intravenously inject with various formulations (100 μL) including Gd/DNA, Gd/DNA@HeLa, Gd/DNA@HepG2, and Gd/DNA@UM-SCC-7. The dosage of plasmid DNA (pORF-LacZ, pGL-3): 15 μg per mouse.
5. 48 h postinjection, sacrifice the mice, and exfoliate each tumor.

6. Wash the tumor tissues of mice that were injected pORF-LacZ formulations with ice-cold PBS buffer, fix, and stain with X-gal staining kit (InvivoGen, USA) for 12 h.
7. Record the stained tissues photographically.
8. Fix with 4% formaldehyde for 24 h, and then embed in paraffin, and section.
9. Fix sections with 5 μm thickness on glass slides, and finally stain with eosin, and examine by light microscopy for observing the pORF-LacZ expression.
10. Freeze the tumors injected with pEGFP-C1 formulations, and cut into 5 μm-thick cryosections.
11. Observe the in vivo EGFP expression by CLSM.
12. Homogenize tumors injected with pGL-3 formulations using an IKA-Ultra-Turrax homogenizer in Promega cell lysis buffer.
13. Collect the supernatant by centrifugation treatment (12,000 g/min) at 4 °C. 13. Express the transfection efficiency as RLU per mg protein.
14. Sacrifice the mice, collect the organs of heart, liver, spleen, lung, kidney, and tumor tissues, fix them in 4% formalin, embed in paraffin, and then section. 15. Place the sections with 5 μm thickness on polylysine-coated slides, and finally stain with hematoxylin and eosin.
15. Picture the stained slides under a microscope (BX60, Olympus, Japan) at 200× magnifications.
16. Upon deparaffinization and rehydration treatment, incubate the tumor sections with 20 μg/ml proteinase-K solution for 10 min at 37 °C, followed by 3% $H_2O_2$ in methanol for 10 min at 25 °C to block endogenous peroxidase activity.
17. Incubate with terminal deoxynucleotidyl transferase (TdT)/biotinylated dNTP and peroxidase-conjugate streptavidin for 60 and 30 min at 37 °C, respectively.
18. Wash the slides with PBS, incubate in 0.1% DAB solution, and counterstain with hematoxylin.
19. Replace the TdT solution with distilled water as negative control.
20. Observe the slides, and score with a bright-field Zeiss Axioscop Plus microscope at 200× magnifications.

## 3.8 *In Vitro* and *In Vivo* MR Imaging

1. Disperse Gd/DNA@HeLa and Gd/DNA in deionized water under ultrasonic vibration to provide a series of solutions with Gd ion concentration ranging from 0.005 to 0.25 mM.
2. Transfer the sample solutions into NMR tubes, and place in a 7 T Magnetic Resonance Imaging (BioSpec 4.7/30).
3. Compute the T1 relaxation time of the samples using Paravision 5.0.
4. Plot the T1 relaxation rates (1/T1) versus Gd concentration, and determine the T1 relaxivity on the basis of a linear fit in Fig. 4a.
5. Conduct the in vivo MR-imaging experiment on Female BALB/c mice bearing a HeLa xenograft tumor on right hind limb.
6. Anesthetize the mice with isoflurane prior to Gd/DNA@HeLa injection via tail vein.

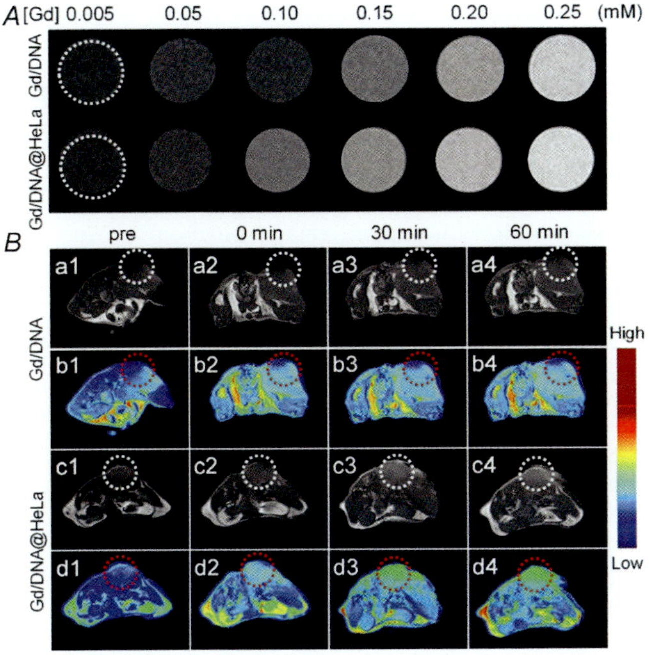


**Fig. 4** (**a**) T1-MR images of Gd/DNA and Gd/DNA@HeLa in DI water at different Gd concentrations; (**b**) representative 2D axial T1-weighted spin-echo MR images and representative color-coded maps of MR images before injection (pre), and at 0, 30, and 60 min postinjection. The circles point to the tumors. (Adapted from reference Zhu et al. (2018), with permission)

7. Scan the mice before and after administration with 200 μL of Gd/DNA@HeLa in PBS at a [Gd] dose of 15.5 mg/kg mouse.
8. Record the T1-weighted MR image of the tumor on the 7 T Magnetic Resonance Imaging (BioSpec 4.7/30) in Fig. 4b.

### 3.9 Statistical Analysis

1. Present data as the mean ± standard deviation (SD).
2. Perform statistical analysis by Student's t test.
3. Consider a value of $p < 0.05$ to be statistically significant.

## 4 Notes

1. In principle, multivalent ion (e. g., Gd(III)) is able to shorten the distance among DNA skeletons and condense DNA via the electrostatic/coordinate interaction and the surface charge shielding of DNA molecules (Gao et al. 1993).

2. The cells should be healthy before large scale proliferation for cell membrane extraction. The whole process of cell membrane collection should be carried out on the ice to retain the activity of membrane proteins.
3. After further breaking by freeze-thaw method, the cells should be exposed to microscopical observation, and if a shiny ring around the nuclei or intact cell morphology is observed, the freeze-thaw treatment should be repeated until more than 70% of the cells are disrupted.
4. The solution of Gd/DNA mixture should be dropwise introduced into the CCCM dispersion under mild stirring for homogeneous mixing, and then the mixture solution is subjected to the treatment with consecutive extrusion through a series of water-phase filters with the reducing pore size (2.0 μm, 800.0, and 450.0 nm).
5. Though Gd/DNA with the w/w ratio of 10 could not effectively retard the migration of DNA, this ratio is still utilized for the following experiments due to the concern of Gd-induced toxicity, and further coating with cell membrane is able to completely retard the migration of DNA.
6. The Gd/DNA@CCCM complexes solution should be passed through a 0.45 mm pore size filter (Shanghai Chemical Reagent Co.) prior to the DLS measurement to avoid interference of the dust in the solution. To determine zeta potential, PBS buffer solution was replaced by deionized water.
7. The Gd/DNA@CCCM complexes solution should be fresh before characterization using TEM. Gd/DNA@CCCM complexes are first negatively stained with 1% uranium acetate prior to observation under transmission microscope.
8. The cells must be mixed well when seeding into the wells. The cells are prone to settle down to the bottom of cell culture dish, and thus the cells should be uniformly suspended prior to the seeding treatment.
9. For cytotoxicity assay, edge wells in plates should not be used in cell experiments in order to ensure the same growth rate with the cells in inner wells.
10. HeLa cells should be seeded on the basolateral compartment of the insert at a density of $1.0 \times 10^6$ cells per compartment. After about 5 days of incubation, the tumor model can be used for the following experiments.
11. Tumors injected with pORF-LacZ formulations should not be treated using iron-related equipment during X-gal staining process. This tumor-staining experiment should be carried out at 37 °C overnight.
12. The injection volume should be adjusted to 0.8 ml/100 g of mouse weight. The dosage of plasmid DNA (pORF-LacZ, pGL-3) was 15 μg per mouse.

## 5 Conclusion

This protocol describes a virus-mimetic nanoengineering based on DNA, Gd(III) ions, and biologically derived CCCM for the host-specific genetic therapy. This nanogene has demonstrated the strong ability to protect DNA payload from the unwanted biological threats (phagocytosis, protein adsorption, competitive extraction by blood components, enzymatic digestion, etc.), the host-specific biotargeting to the source cancer cells and the homologous tumors, as well as the high serum-tolerant transfection efficiency. In addition, this Gd(III)-based nanogene exhibited much higher $T_1$ relaxation rate than the clinically used MRI agents and eventually generated the enhanced MRI contrast at tumor sites. This study paves a sharply new and feasible pathway for the practical translation of gene therapy while overcoming the common problems associated with nonviral gene vectors. Noticeably, this innovative technology offers unique chances to combine genetic therapy together with the special functions arising from metal ions, not limited to Gd(III) ion as discussed in this chapter. Theoretically speaking, this strategy could expand to the transport of other biomacromolecules, such as proteins and enzymes. Further studies to identify the mechanism for the host-specific recognition of cell membranes open up a wide range of opportunities for the applications of disease-specific therapy and diagnosis.

## References

Challis RC, Kumar SR, Chan KY, Challis C, Beadle K, Jang MJ, Kim HM, Rajendran PS, Tompkins JD, Shivkumar K, Deverman BE, Gradinaru V (2019) Systemic AAV vectors for widespread and targeted gene delivery in rodents. Nat Protoc 14(2):379–414

Cheng YL, Yumul RC, Pun SH (2016a) Virus-inspired polymer for efficient in vitro and in vivo gene delivery. Angew Chem Int Ed Engl 55(39):12013–12017

Cheng H, Zhu JY, Li SY, Zeng JY, Lei Q, Chen KW, Zhang C, Zhang XZ (2016b) An $O_2$ self-sufficient biomimetic nanoplatform for highly specific and efficient photodynamic therapy. Adv Funct Mater 26(43):7847–7860

Cheng Y, Sun C, Liu R, Yang JL, Dai J, Zhai TY, Lou XD, Xia F (2019) A multifunctional peptide-conjugated AIEgen for efficient and sequential targeted gene delivery into the nucleus. Angew Chem Int Ed Engl 58(15):5049–5053

Clever GH, Kaul C, Carell T (2007) DNA – metal base pairs. Angew Chem Int Ed Engl 46(33): 6226–6236

Coughlin AJ, Ananta JS, Deng NF, Larina IV, Decuzzi P, West JL (2014) Gadolinium-conjugated gold nanoshells for multimodal diagnostic imaging and photothermal cancer therapy. Small 10(3):556–565

Degors IMS, Wang CF, Rehman ZU, Zuhorn IS (2019) Carriers break barriers in drug delivery: endocytosis and endosomal escape of gene delivery vectors. Acc Chem Res 52(7):1750–1760

Gao YG, Sriram M, Wang AHJ (1993) Crystallographic studies of metal ion-DNA interactions: different binding modes of cobalt(II), copper(II) and barium(II) to N7 of guanines in Z-DNA and a drug-DNA complex. Nucleic Acids Res 21(17):4093–4101

Guan S, Rosenecker J (2017) Nanotechnologies in delivery of mRNA therapeutics using nonviral vector-based delivery systems. Gene Ther 24(3):133–143

He XW, Yin F, Wang DY, Xiong LH, Kwok RTK, Gao PF, Zhao Z, Lam JWY, Yong KT, Li ZG, Tang BZ (2019) AIE featured inorganic-organic core@shell nanoparticles for high-efficiency siRNA delivery and real-time monitoring. Nano Lett 19(4):2272–2279

Jiang Y, Krishnan N, Zhou JR, Chekuri S, Wei XL, Kroll AV, Yu CL, Duan YO, Gao WW, Fang RH, Zhang LF (2020) Engineered cell-membrane-coated nanoparticles directly present tumor antigens to promote anticancer immunity. Adv Mater 32(30):2001808

Li CW, Samulski RJ (2020) Engineering adeno-associated virus vectors for gene therapy. Nat Rev Genet 21(4):255–272

Lim KS, Lee DY, Valencia GM, Won YW, Bull DA (2015) Nano-self-assembly of nucleic acids capable of transfection without a gene carrier. Adv Funct Mater 25(34):5445–5451

Lorizate M, Sachsenheimer T, Glass B, Habermann A, Gerl MJ, Krausslich HG, Brugger B (2013) Comparative lipidomics analysis of HIV-1 particles and their producer cell membrane in different cell lines. Cell Microbiol 15(2):292–304

Lostalé-Seijo I, Montenegro J (2018) Synthetic materials at the forefront of gene delivery. Nat Rev Chem 2(10):258–277

Mjos KD, Orvig C (2014) Metallodrugs in medicinal inorganic chemistry. Chem Rev 114(8): 4540–4563

Sevencan C, McCoy RSA, Ravisankar P, Liu M, Govindarajan S, Zhu JY, Bay BH, Leong DT (2020) Cell membrane nanotherapeutics: from synthesis to applications emerging tools for personalized cancer therapy. Adv Ther 3(3):1900201

Smith AE, Helenius A (2004) How viruses enter animal cells. Science 304(5668):237–242

Sun C, Lin HY, Gong XQ, Yang ZX, Mo Y, Chen XY, Gao JH (2020) DOTA-branched organic frameworks as giant and potent metal chelators. J Am Chem Soc 142(1):198–206

Thomas CE, Ehrhardt AE, Kay MA (2003) Progress and problems with the use of viral vectors for gene therapy. Nat Rev Genet 4(5):346–358

Thompson KH, Orvig C (2003) Boon and bane of metal ions in medicine. Science 300(5621): 936–939

Wang HY, Jiang YF, Peng HG, Chen YZ, Zhu PZ, Huang YZ (2015) Recent progress in microRNA delivery for cancer therapy by non-viral synthetic vectors. Adv Drug Deliv Rev 81:142–160

Wang FYK, Gao JY, Xiao JG, Du JZ (2018) Dually gated polymersomes for gene delivery. Nano Lett 18(9):5562–5568

Weekes DM, Orvig C (2016) Harnessing the bone-seeking ability of Ca(II)-like metal ions in the treatment of metastatic cancer and resorption disorders. Chem Soc Rev 45(8):2024–2031

Yang JP, Zhang Q, Chang H, Cheng YY (2015) Surface-engineered dendrimers in gene delivery. Chem Rev 115(11):5274–5300

Zhou ZX, Liu XR, Zhu DC, Wang Y, Zhang Z, Zhou XF, Qiu N, Chen XS, Shen YQ (2017) Nonviral cancer gene therapy: delivery cascade and vector nanoproperty integration. Adv Drug Deliv Rev 115:115–154

Zhu JY, Zheng DW, Zhang MK, Yu WY, Qiu WX, Hu JJ, Feng J, Zhang XZ (2016) Preferential cancer cell self-recognition and tumor self-targeting by coating nanoparticles with homotypic cancer cell membranes. Nano Lett 16(9):5895–5901

Zhu JY, Wan SS, Zheng DW, Lei Q, Zhuo RX, Feng J, Zhang XZ (2017a) Propelled transnuclear gene transport achieved through intracellularly redox-responsive and acidity-accelerative decomposition of supramolecular florescence-quenchable vectors. ACS Appl Mater Interfaces 9(1):255–265

Zhu DC, Yan HJ, Liu X, Xiang JJ, Zhou ZX, Tang JB, Liu XR, Shen YQ (2017b) Intracellularly disintegratable polysulfoniums for efficient gene delivery. Adv Funct Mater 27(16):1606826

Zhu JY, Zhang MK, Zheng DW, Yang B, Ma N, Li RQ, Feng J, Zhang XZ (2017c) A biohybrid lurker-to-attacker strategy to solve inherent dilemma of positively charged delivery nanoparticles. Chem Mater 29(5):2227–2231

Zhu JY, Zhang MK, Ding XG, Qiu WX, Yu WY, Feng J, Zhang XZ (2018) Virus-inspired nanogenes free from man-made materials for host-specific transfection and bio-aided MR imaging. Adv Mater 30(22):1707459

Zhu JY, Sevencan C, Zhang MK, McCoy RSA, Ding XG, Ye JJ, Xie JP, Ariga K, Feng J, Bay BH, Leong DT (2020) Increasing the potential interacting area of nanomedicine enhances its homotypic cancer targeting efficacy. ACS Nano 14(3):3259–3271

# Calcium Carbonate-Based Nanoparticles for Gene Delivery

# 25

Asim Mushtaq, M. Zubair Iqbal, and Xiangdong Kong

## Contents




**Abstract**

Gene therapy is an advanced treatment to cure many complex diseases and attained significant interest to stop the defective mutations at gene level. However, delivering the considerable concentration of right molecule to the desired cells or tissues and overcome multidrug resistance (MDR) are challenging tasks in gene therapy. To date, several viral and nonviral vectors for gene delivery systems have been developed and possess some serious unresolved concerns. Inorganic nanoparticles (NPs) have been used as potential alternative nonviral carriers for gene delivery systems with improved transfection efficiency. Among nonviral carriers, calcium ($Ca^{2+}$) incorporated with inorganic anions ($CO_3^{2-}$ and $PO_4^{3-}$) has promising advantages in terms of gene loading and biocompatibility. Particularly, $CaCO_3$ is a natural mineral which is widely available in hard tissues and by varying the ratio of $Ca/CO_3^{2-}$, DNA and drugs could be loaded with high encapsulation efficiency. Therefore, this chapter will discuss the synthesis of $CaCO_3$-based nanocomposites with respect to gene delivery applications. This



A. Mushtaq · M. Z. Iqbal · X. Kong (✉)
Institute of Smart Biomedical Materials, School of Materials Science and Engineering, Zhejiang Sci-Tech University, Hangzhou, China

Zhejiang-Mauritius Joint Research Center for Biomaterials and Tissue Engineering, Hangzhou, China
e-mail: kongxd@zstu.edu.cn







H. Tian and X. Chen (eds.), *Gene Delivery*, Biomaterial Engineering,
https://doi.org/10.1007/978-981-16-5419-0_26

chapter beautifully elaborates the wide range of primary materials for the fabrication of $CaCO_3$, coating substance for the functionalization, and various gene loading/unloading mechanisms under various factors for gene delivery with impactful discussion.

**Keywords**

Calcium carbonate · Gene delivery · Composites · DNA · siRNA · Nanoparticles

## 1 Overview

Gene therapy has gained prominent position in the field of molecular genetics during last decades (Mintzer and Simanek 2009). It is focused on transferring of therapeutic gene to the target cell with a carrier (Moss 2014). Gene therapy has become more prevalent due to accomplishment in the treatment of choroideremia (Fischer et al. 2020), blood diseases (Kohn 2019) like hemophilia (Sharma et al. 2020), chronic (Wierda et al. 2010) and acute leukemia (Chapuis et al. 2019), Parkinson's disease (Axelsen and Woldbye 2018), multiple myeloma (Dupéré-Richer and Licht 2018), X-linked severe combined immunodeficiency (Pai and Thrasher 2020), adrenoleukodystrophy (Mallack et al. 2019), and cancer (Yahya and Alqadhi 2021). There are two categories of gene therapy, one is somatic cell gene therapy (SCGT) and other is through germline gene therapy (GGT) (Wirth et al. 2013). Furthermore, the insertion of imported genome to the target cell is carried out by viral as well as nonviral delivery systems (Nayerossadat et al. 2012). Nonviral mode of gene therapy is advantageous over viral gene therapy because of its less pathogenicity, cost effective, easy production, and especially the biosafety (Ramamoorth and Narvekar 2015). The development of nanotechnology has supported the nonviral gene delivery (Labhasetwar 2005). Researchers are utilizing the polymer-based nanomaterials, inorganic and organic nanoparticles, magnetic nanoparticles, nanocomposites, and quantum dots for efficient and targeted gene delivery (Anis 2019). Calcium and calcium-based materials play an important role in human health. These are essential for teeth and bones, rhythmic heart beat and muscle contraction, fluid stability of cell, coagulation of blood, oocyte stimulation, neural impulses and transmission, growth and development (Pravina et al. 2013). Nowadays, calcium-based compounds (calcium oxides, calcium phosphates, calcium oxides) are gaining the attention of researchers in the treatment of human diseases and disorders via drug and gene delivery owing to their high biocompatibility, low cytotoxicity, and excellent drug and gene loading capacity. Generally, $CaCO_3$-based compounds are found to be very efficient for advanced biomedical applications, including combined photothermal therapy, targeted delivery agent for therapeutics, drugs, genes, antibodies, and various kinds of enzymes, due to their easy manufacturing, cost effectiveness, biodegradability, and biocompatibility (Kong et al. 2016). Among these categories, $CaCO_3$ is reported as a promising material for efficient gene delivery (Kong et al. 2012).

This chapter describes about synthetic routes of $CaCO_3$-based nanomaterials with a variety of modifications for efficient gene delivery.

# 2 Protocol

## 2.1 Materials

### 2.1.1 $CaCO_3$ NPs: Vascular Endothelial Growth Factor-C siRNA (He et al. 2008)

1. Calcium chloride ($CaCl_2$).
2. Sodium dodecyl sulfate (SDS) (99% pure).
3. Pluronic® F-68.
4. Sodium carbonate ($Na_2CO_3$).
5. Sodium citrate.
6. Ethanol (75%).
7. Uranyl acetate solution (0.04% in methanol).
8. Plasmid DNA (pEGFP-N1 DNA).
9. Dulbecco's modified Eagle medium (DMEM).

### 2.1.2 Coprecipitation for the Synthesis of $CaCO_3$-Plasmid DNA (Chen et al. 2011)

1. Calcium chloride ($CaCl_2$).
2. Sodium carbonate ($Na_2CO_3$).
3. Plasmid DNA for luciferase (pGL3-Luc).
4. QIAfilter Plasmid Mega Kit (QIAGEN).
5. Dulbecco's modified Eagle medium (DMEM).
6. Fetal bovine serum (FBS).

### 2.1.3 KALA-Modified $CaCO_3$-DNA (Zhao et al. 2012)

1. KALA peptide (WEAKLAKALAKALAKHLAKALAKALKACEA) ($M_w$ = 3131gmol$^{-1}$).
2. Plasmid luciferase (pGL3-Luc).
3. Plasmid (p53).
4. Calcium chloride ($CaCl_2$).
5. Sodium carbonate ($Na_2CO_3$).
6. Dulbecco's modified Eagle medium (DMEM).
7. Fetal bovine serum (FBS).

### 2.1.4 Alginate-$CaCO_3$ Hybrid (Zhao et al. 2012)

1. Calcium chloride ($CaCl_2$).
2. Sodium carbonate ($Na_2CO_3$).
3. Sodium alginate (viscosity = Pa.s, 1% solution$_{(aq)}$).
4. cDNA (p53),
5. Dulbecco's modified Eagle medium (DMEM).

6. Fetal bovine serum (FBS).
7. QIAfilter Plasmid Mega Kit (QIAGEN).

#### 2.1.5 Nanostructured $CaCO_3$-DNA (Chen et al. 2012)

1. Calcium chloride ($CaCl_2$).
2. Sodium carbonate ($Na_2CO_3$).
3. cDNA (pDsRed2-N1-p53),
4. Dulbecco's modified Eagle medium (DMEM).
5. Fetal bovine serum (FBS).
6. QIAfilter Plasmid Mega Kit (QIAGEN).

#### 2.1.6 $CaCO_3$ Particles: Plasmid pEGFP-C1-p53 (Kong et al. 2012)

1. Sodium polyacrylate (PAAS).
2. Calcium carbonate di-hydrate ($CaCl_2.2H_2O$).
3. Sodium dodecyl sulfate (SDS).
4. Plasmid (pEGFP-C1-p53).
5. Dulbecco's modified Eagle medium (DMEM).
6. Fetal bovine serum (FBS).

#### 2.1.7 Protamine Sulfate $CaCO_3$-DNA Nanoparticles (Wang et al. 2014)

1. Protamine sulfate.
2. Calcium chloride ($CaCl_2$).
3. Sodium carbonate ($Na_2CO_3$).
4. Plasmids (pGL3-Luc, pEGFP-C1).
5. Sodium hydrogen carbonate ($NaHCO_3$).
6. Dimethyl sulfoxide (DMSO).
7. Dulbecco's modified Eagle medium (DMEM).
8. Fetal bovine serum (FBS).
9. QIAfilter Plasmid Mega Kit (QIAGEN).

#### 2.1.8 KALA-Protamine Sulfate-$CaCO_3$-DNA Nanoparticles (Wang et al. 2014)

1. Calcium chloride ($CaCl_2$).
2. Sodium carbonate ($Na_2CO_3$).
3. KALA (WEAKLAKALAKALAKHLAKALAKALKACEA).
4. Molecular probes (Hoechst 33258 and YOYO-1 iodide, Lipofectamine 2000).
5. Plasmid (pGL3-Luc).
6. Dulbecco's modified Eagle medium (DMEM).
7. Fetal bovine serum (FBS).
8. QIAfilter Plasmid Mega Kit (QIAGEN).

#### 2.1.9 Calcium Carbonate-Calcium Phosphate-DNA NPs (Zhao et al. 2014)

1. Calcium chloride ($CaCl_2$).
2. Sodium carbonate ($Na_2CO_3$).
3. Sodium phosphate tribasic dodecahydrate.

4. 3-(4,5-Dimethylthiazol-2-yl)-2,5-diphenyltetrazolium bromide (MTT)
5. Dimethyl sulfoxide (DMSO).
6. Plasmid luciferase (pGL3-Luc).
7. Dulbecco's modified Eagle medium (DMEM).
8. Fetal bovine serum (FBS).
9. QIAfilter Plasmid Mega Kit (QIAGEN).

#### 2.1.10 Polyethyleneimine-$CaCO_3$-DNA Nanoparticles (Chen et al. 2016)

1. Calcium chloride ($CaCl_2$).
2. Sodium carbonate ($Na_2CO_3$).
3. Polyethyleneimine.
4. Arginine.
5. p53 antibody,
6. Dulbecco's modified Eagle medium (DMEM).
7. Fetal bovine serum (FBS).

#### 2.1.11 Lipid-Coated Calcium Carbonate/Phosphate Hybrid (LCC) NPs (Wu et al. 2017)

1. Calcium chloride ($CaCl_2$).
2. Sodium hydrogen carbonate ($NaHCO_3$).
3. Cyclohexane.
4. Igepal-CO520.
5. Trichloromethane ($CHCl_3$).
6. Ethanol.
7. Phospholipids (DOPA, DOPC/Cholesterol).
8. dsDNA,
9. Cyanine 5 (cy5).

#### 2.1.12 $MnO_2$-$CaCO_3$-ICG/siRNA Nanoplatform (Liu et al. 2019)

1. Manganese dioxide ($MnO_2$).
2. Calcium chloride ($CaCl_2$).
3. Indocyanine green (ICG).
4. Sodium carbonate ($Na_2CO_3$).
5. Polycyclic aromatic hydrocarbons (PAH).
6. PD-L1 siRNA (5'-GGC GUU UAC UGC UGC AUA ATT-3′).
7. Polyacrylamide gel.

## 2.2 Methods

### 2.2.1 $CaCO_3$ NPs: Vascular Endothelial Growth Factor-C siRNA

#### Preparation of $CaCO_3$ NPs

1. Blend 50 ml $CaCl_2$, 10 ml SDS (1%), and 10 ml PF-68 (1%) with constant stirring at 300 rpm for 24 h to get a microemulsion A.

2. Similarly, blend 50 ml $Na_2CO_3$ (0.025 M), 50 ml sodium citrate (0.025 M), 10 ml PF-68 (1%), and 10 ml SDS (1%) with constant stirring at 300 rpm for 24 h to make a microemulsion B.
3. After this, mix the emulsion B with emulsion A, with the speed of 10 ml $h^{-1}$ and stir continuously (350 rpm) at 35 °C follow by the stirring for 72 h.
4. Centrifuge the nanoparticles with the speed of 15,000 rpm for 15 min.
5. Wash the nanoparticles three times with ethanol (75%) and disperse in 15 ml double distilled water.
6. Do the freeze-drying and save the $CaCO_3$ nanoparticles for further use.

#### Preparation of $CaCO_3$-DNA Complex

1. Mix the suspension of $CaCO_3$ with plasmid DNA at various ratios (5,1, 10:1, 15:1).
2. Keep the mixture in suspension for 30 min at 25 °C.
3. Centrifuge the mixture for 10 min at 10000 rpm.
4. Identify the unbound DNA from supernatant by gel electrophoresis.

#### $CaCO_3$-DNA Protection Analysis

1. Mix 4 μg pEGFP-N1 DNA with RPMI 1640 complete media having FBS (10% w/v) and incubate for 12 h at 37 °C.
2. Similarly, incubate $CaCO_3$-DNA complex (4 μg DNA and 60 μg $CaCO_3$) with FBS, for 12 h at 37 °C follow by centrifugation for 10 min at 10000 rpm.
3. Discard the supernatant and resuspend the particles with TE (pH 10).
4. Detect $CaCO_3$ nanoparticles by gel electrophoresis (agarose gel).

#### In Vitro Transfection

1. Take the $CaCO_3$-DNA complex (2 μg pEGFP-N1 DNA and 30 μg $CaCO_3$).
2. SGC-7901 cells seeding is carried out in 12-well plate with $2 \times 10^5$ cell density per well.
3. Keep the cells overnight to attain 70–80% convergence.
4. Transfect the cells by adding $CaCO_3$-DNA complex in each well having bovine serum (10% w/v) and keep for 24 h.
5. Use liposomes facilitated pEGFP-N1 DNA (10:2 μg) and apply on separate cells (SGC-7901) to get a positive control.
6. Green fluorescent protein (GFP) expression is examined by using confocal laser scanning microscopy after 24 h incubation.

#### $CaCO_3$-siRNA Transfection for Gastric Cell Line SGC-7901

1. Culture the SGC-7901 cells in 160 mm dish having RPMI 1640 and FBS (10%), $CO_2$ (5%) at 37 °C.
2. After 70% growth of cells, add $CaCO_3$-siRNA complex (75:5 μg).
3. Analyze the transfection efficiency after 48 h incubation.

### 2.2.2 Coprecipitation for the Preparation of $CaCO_3$-Plasmid DNA

#### Formulation of $CaCO_3$-DNA Complex

1. Take 10 μg of plasmid DNA and dilute to 125 μl with water (deionized).
2. Add 120 μl of $CaCl_2$ (0.5 M) with gentle stirring at room temperature.
3. Do the dropwise addition of mixture to the 255 μl solution of $Na_2CO_3$ (variable concentrations from 0.1 μmol to 80 μmol).
4. The solution of $CaCO_3$-DNA coprecipitates will be obtained at 25 °C.
5. Incubate the solution for 5 min before transfection.

#### In Vitro Transfection

1. Seed the cells in 24-well plate ($5 \times 10^4$ cells/well) having 1 ml DMEM medium and FBS (10%) and incubate for 24 h at 37 °C.
2. Add 100 μl of solution of $CaCO_3$-DNA coprecipitates in each well and incubate for 48 h.
3. For luciferase gene expression analysis, eliminate the medium gently by rinsing the cells with PBS (0.1 M, 7.4 pH).
4. Incubate 20 μl cell lysate with 100 μl luciferin (Promega) and determine the luciferase action by luminometer.
5. Measure the cell lysate protein content by BCA protein kit.

### 2.2.3 KALA-Modified $CaCO_3$-DNA

#### Preparation of $CaCO_3$-KALA-DNA

1. Make a mixture of 16 μl $CaCl_2$ (0.5 M), 1 μg $\mu l^{-1}$ KALA (different amount, 1, 2, 5, and 10 μg), and 1 μl DNA solution (having 1 μg pGL3-Luc), and dilute the mixture with deionized water to get 50 μl volume of mixture.
2. Dilute 16 μl solution of $Na_2CO_3$ (0.01 M) with deionized water up to 50 μl volume.
3. Mix these two solutions quickly with continuous stirring to get $CaCO_3$-KALA-DNA NPs.
4. Use this solution immediately for gene transfection.

#### In Vitro Transfection

1. Do the cells seeding in 24-well plate ($5 \times 10^4$ cells per well) having 1 ml DMEM and FBS (10%) followed by the incubation for 24 h.
2. Add freshly prepared $CaCO_3$-KALA-DNA solution (100 μl having 1 μg pGL3-Luc) to each well and incubate at 37 °C.
3. Observe the gene expression after 48 h.
4. To analyze luciferase gene expression, remove the medium gently by rinsing the cells with PBS (0.1 M, 7.4 pH).
5. Incubate 20 μl cell lysate with 100 μl luciferin (Promega) and determine the luciferase action by luminometer.
6. Determine the cell lysate protein part by BCA protein analysis kit.

7. After the treatment with NPs, stain the HeLa cells with FITC and PI and incubate for 48 h to take confocal images.

### 2.2.4 Alginate-$CaCO_3$ Hybrid

**Preparation of Aginate-$CaCO_3$-DNA/DOX**

1. Use deionized water for the preparation of solutions of $CaCl_2$, $Na_2CO_3$, sodium alginate, DNA, and DOX separately.
2. Mix 1 μg/μl solution of DNA, 16 μl solution of $CaCl_2$ (0.5 M), DOX solution with different concentration of DOX (0.1–0.4 μg), and dilute the mixture with deionized water to get 20 μl volume.
3. Besides this, mix 1 μg sodium alginate with 16 μl solution of $Na_2CO_3$ (0.01 M) and dilute up to 20 μl with deionized water.
4. Blend these two mixtures quickly with continuous stirring to form Aginate-$CaCO_3$-DNA/DOX NPs.
5. Dilute the NPs solution with deionized water up to 100 μl.
6. Immediately use this solution for drug and gene delivery. A schematic illustration is presented in Fig. 1.

**Evaluation of Encapsulation Efficiency and Amount Loaded of DOX and DNA**

1. Take 500 μl of NPs solution having 1 μg DOX and 10 μg DNA.
2. Centrifuge the solution at 4 °C with the speed of 18,000 rpm for 1 h.
3. Separate the supernatant to check the amount of free DNA by Quant-iT dsDNA analysis kit using spectrofluorophotometer.
4. Similarly, the amount of free DOX is calculated from supernatant by using UV/vis spectrophotometer at 485 nm.
5. Following formulas are used to calculate the loading amount and encapsulation efficiency of DNA or DOX.

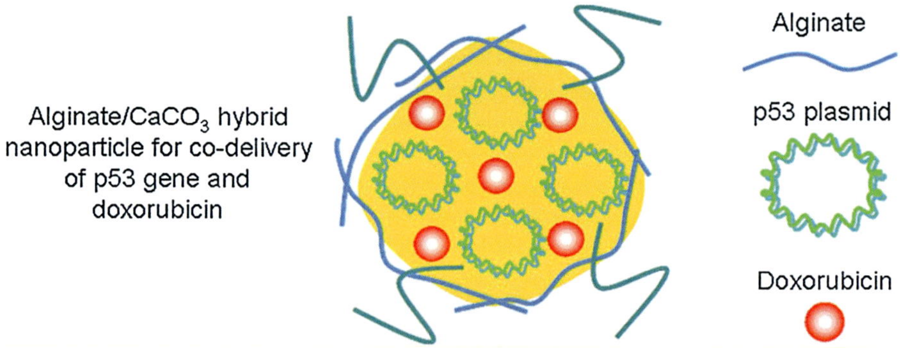


**Fig. 1** Schematic diagram of alginate-$CaCO_3$-DNA/DOX NPs for co-delivery of gene (p53) and DOX. (Reprinted with the permission of Zhao et al. (2012))

$$\text{Loading amount\%} = (W_T - W_F)/W_{NPs} \times 100$$
$$\text{Encapsulation efficiency\%} = (W_T - W_F)/W_T \times 100$$

In these equations, $W_F$ is weight of free DOX or DNA, $W_T$ is total weight of DOX or DNA, and $W_{NPs}$ is weight of NPs.

#### In Vitro Release of Drug

1. Take 4 ml of NPs solution (having 8 μg of DOX and 80 μg of DNA) and shake it in water bath at 37 °C.
2. After specific periods, centrifuge the sample at 4 °C with speed of 18,000 rpm for 1 h.
3. Determine the amount of free DOX from supernatant at 485 nm absorbance by using UV/vis spectrophotometer.
4. Repeat three times and measure the mean standard deviation.

#### In Vitro Cell Inhibition Analysis

1. Seed the HeLa cells in 24-well plate ($5 \times 10^4$ cells per well) contains DMEM and FBS (10%) and incubate it for 24 h at 37 °C.
2. Then add freshly prepared solution of NPs in each cell and incubate it for 48 h at 37 °C.
3. Eliminate the medium having particular agent and add 1 ml of medium and MTT (60 μl, 5 mg/ml) and incubate for 4 h at 37 °C.
4. Separate the supernatant carefully and dissolve formazan crystals by adding 850 μl DMSO in each well.
5. Measure the absorbance at 570 nm by using microplate reader and get the OD value. Furthermore, calculate cell inhibition by using following formula.

$$\text{Cell inhibition rate\%} = (1 - OD_{treated}/OD_{control}) \times 100$$

Here $OD_{treated}$ is calculated after the therapy of cells with a specific agent, and $OD_{control}$ is calculated from the cells with no therapy.

### 2.2.5 Nanostructured $CaCO_3$-DNA

#### Preparation of $CaCO_3$-DNA NPs

1. Make the solution of plasmid DNA with deionized water (10 μg in 125 μl).
2. Prepare $CaCl_2$ solution by dissolving 60 μmol of $CaCl_2$ in deionized water to get the volume of 120 μl.
3. Mix these solutions gently at room temperature.
4. After that, add the blend dropwise to the $Na_2CO_3$ aqueous solution (255 μl) having 1.6 μmol sodium carbonate. This will give the $CaCO_3$-DNA NPs solution.

5. To make the $CaCO_3$-DNA-DOX NPs solution, add 1 μg DOX while making $CaCl_2$ solution as discussed in step 2. Remaining process will be same as described above.

**Calculation of Encapsulation Efficiency and Loading Content**

1. Centrifuge the 500 μl solution of NPs for 1 h at 4 °C with 18,000 rpm speed.
2. Calculate the amount of free DNA in supernatant by using Quant-iT dsDNA kit.
3. Furthermore, determine the value of free DOX by taking the absorbance at 485 nm using UV/vis spectrophotometer.

**Calculation of in Vitro Drug Release**

1. Take 4 ml of NPs solution in dialysis bag (having 8 μg DOX and 80 μg DNA) and immersed in PBS (30 ml) at pH 7.4 and continue to shake by using water bath at 37 °C.
2. After specific intervals, take out 4 ml of solution from dialysis bag and replace by 4 ml PBS.
3. Use UV/vis spectrophotometer for the determination of drug concentration by taking absorbance at 485 nm.

**In Vitro Cell Inhibition Evaluation**

1. Seed the HeLa cells in 24-well plate ($5 \times 10^4$ cells per well) having 1 ml DMEM medium and 10% FBS. Then incubation of the culture for 24 h at 37 °C.
2. Add 100 μl of NPs solution (containing 0.2 μg DOX and 2 μg DNA) to each well and incubate at 37 °C.
3. Follow the MTT assay for the calculation of cell inhibition rate.

**Cell Apoptosis Study**

1. Analyze the cell apoptosis with FITC Annexin V.
2. Wash the HeLa cells (coprecipitated with NPs solution) with PBS (cold) and 1 × annexin binding buffer.
3. Add 1 × annexin binding buffer (100 μl), annexin V (5 μl), and PI (Invitrogen) (1 μl) to the cells.
4. After 15 min incubation, wash the cells with 1 × annexin binding buffer and observe under confocal laser scanning microscope at magnification of 400 and excitation at 488 nm.

### 2.2.6 $CaCO_3$ Particles: Plasmid pEGFP-C1-p53

**Preparation of $CaCO_3$ Particles**

1. Prepare 0.1 M solutions of $CaCl_2$ and $Na_2CO_3$.
2. Make mixture A by adding PAAS solution (1.0 g/L) into $CaCl_2$ solution.
3. Similarly, make mixture B with the addition of PAAS (1.0 g/L) and SDS solution (10 mM) to $Na_2CO_3$ solution.
4. Blend these two mixtures (A and B) for 1 h with stirring (200 rpm) at 80 °C.

5. Separate the powder of $CaCO_3$ by filtration and do the drying in vacuum desiccator for 24 h at 80 °C.

**Plasmid pEGFP-C1-p53 Construction**

1. The isolation of p53 gene is brought out with reverse transcriptase polymerase chain reaction (RT-PCR).
2. For RNA extraction, use human hepatocyte cell line (QSG7701) with Trizol reagent and use Rever Tra Ace® qPCR RT kit for synthesis of cDNA.
3. Use dipetalogastin cDNA as a template for PCR.
4. Perform PCR for 30 cycles possessing denaturation 50 s at 98 °C followed by annealing 50 s at 58 °C and extend for 1 min 30s at 68 °C.
5. Purify the PCR outcomes by 1.0% agarose gel electrophoresis with digestion by BamH I and XhoI I, sub-cloning is carried out in the vector pEGF-C1 with the help of DNA ligase and transmuted in *E. coli* DH 5α.
6. Verify pEGFP-C1-p53 recombinant plasmid by double enzyme cleavage and PCR. BigDye chemistry is utilized for the confirmation of DNA sequencing with ABI 3730.

**Preparation of Plasmid-Loaded $CaCO_3$**

1. Take 10 mg of $CaCO_3$ powder and suspend in DMEM by utilizing microtip probe sonicator on ice bath with 90 W output energy for 5 min.
2. Add various quantity of pEGFP-C1-p53 (1.0 μg to 10.0 μg) in the suspension and incubate for 15 min to 60 min at 25 °C.
3. Perform gel electrophoresis after the dispersion of gene-loaded particles in water. Also use 15 K Trance DNA marker ethidium bromide stain for visualization.

**In Vitro Transfection**

1. The seeding of HeLa cells is carried out in 6-well plate ($1 \times 10^5$ cells per well) comprising of DMEM medium along with incubation at 37 °C under 5% $CO_2$ humidified environment.
2. Add 50 μl solution of pEGFP-C1-$CaCO_3$ and incubate for 48 h.
3. Similarly, pEGFP-C1-effectene and pEGFP-C1 are used as reference.
4. Fluorescence microscope and flow cytometry are used for the cell examination.

**Cell Viability, Cytotoxicity, and Apoptosis Assay**

1. Treat the cells cultured in 96-well plate through pEGFP-C1-$CaCO_3$ for cell viability test.
2. Utilize pEGFP-C1-effectene and pEGFP-C1 as references.
3. Investigate cell viability by MTT test.
4. To measure the cytotoxicity, cells are cultivated in 24-well plate along with the treatment by various samples (pEGFP-C1-$CaCO_3$, pEGFP-C1-effectene, pEGFP-C1, pEGFP-C1-p53-$CaCO_3$, pEGFP-C1-p53-effectene, and pEGFP-C1-p53) and incubate for 72 h.
5. Take off the medium from culture and rinse the adherent cells by means of PBS (4%) at 25 °C for a period of 10 min.

6. As fixation is completed, wash the cells and add 1% crystal violet stain (solution in 70% ethanol). Incubate it for 15 min.
7. Final washing is carried out by water and air-dried, and then perform the scanning.
8. The apoptosis assay is carried out by the cells seeded in 6-well plate with the treatment of various samples as discussed in point 4, and cells are stained by molecular probe Hoechst 33342 (1 μg/ml for 10 min) after 29 h.
9. Wash up the cells with PBS and take the observations by fluorescence microscope.

#### Identification of p53 Gene Expression

1. Separate the proteins on polyacrylamide gel and transfer to the nitrocellulose with a buffer system of methanol (20%), 192 m*M* glycine, and 25 m*M* Tris-HCl (8.3 pH).
2. Add blocking buffer for minimum 45 min and incubate protein p53 with antibodies.
3. Detection is carried out by adding anti-rabbit IR dye 700 with dilution (1:1000), and observations are taken by IR imaging system (LI-COR, Odyssey).

### 2.2.7 Protamine Sulfate $CaCO_3$-DNA Nanoparticles

#### Preparation of PS-$CaCO_3$-DNA NPs

1. Dilute 1 μg plasmid DNA solution to 10 μl.
2. Pour 16 μl solution of $CaCl_2$ (0.5 M) dropwise and dilute the mixture with deionized water to get 60 μl volume.
3. Next, make the mixture of 16 μl solution of $Na_2CO_3$ (0.01 M) and solution of protamine sulfate (PS) with specific amount (0.05, 0.1, 0.15,0.2, 0.5, and 1 μg) and dilute the mixture to make 40 μl volume.
4. Gently blend these two mixtures to get 100 ul solution of PS-$CaCO_3$-DNA NPs and use freshly prepared NPs for transfection.

#### Encapsulation Efficiency of DNA

1. For the DNA encapsulation efficiency, centrifuge the NPs solution for 1 h at 4 °C with speed of 18,000 rpm.
2. Calculate the value of free DNA from supernatant by Quant-iT Pico Green® dsDNA analysis kit and spectrofluorophotometer.

#### In Vitro Luciferase Plasmid Transfection

1. Culture the cells in 24-well plate ($5 \times 10^4$ cells in each well) containing the 1 ml DMEM medium and FBS (10%).
2. Incubate the cells for 24 h with addition of 2 mg $ml^{-1}$ $NaHCO_3$ and 100 U $ml^{-1}$ of penicillin or streptomycin.
3. Then add 100 μl of NPs solution (containing 1 μg pGL3-Luc) in each well and incubate for 48 h at 37 °C.

4. Investigate the gene expression by eradicating the medium gently and rinsing the cells with PBS (0.1 M, 7.4 pH).
5. Incubate 20 μl cell lysate with 100 μl luciferin (Promega) and determine the luciferase action by luminometer.
6. BCA protein analysis kit is utilized to determine the cell lysate protein part.
7. Furthermore, carry out the flow cytometry analysis of 293 T cells after treatment.

#### Cell Viability Assay

1. Take co-incubated 293 T cells and NPs after 48 h and remove the medium.
2. Pour 1 ml fresh medium and MTT (60 ul, 5 mg $ml^{-1}$) in each well and develop for 4 h at 37 °C.
3. Take off the supernatant and add 850 μl DMSO to vanish formazan crystals.
4. Compute the absorbance at 570 nm by microplate reader to get OD value.

### 2.2.8 KALA-Protamine Sulfate-$CaCO_3$-DNA Nanoparticles

#### Synthesis of KALA-PS-$CaCO_3$-DNA NPs

1. Dilute 1 ug plasmid DNA solution to 10 μl and mix it with 16 μl solution of $CaCl_2$ (0.5 M) dropwise and make the volume of mixture to 60 μl with deionized water.
2. Take 0.15 μg PS, KALA (0.1, 0.2, 0.5, 1, 2, and 5 μg), and 16 μl $Na_2CO_3$ solution (0.01 M). Mix all the materials and dilute to 40 μl by deionized water.
3. Blend these two mixtures gently to get 100 μl solution of KALA-PS-$CaCO_3$-DNA NPs.
4. Determine the encapsulation efficiency by the protocol of Quant-iT Pico Green® dsDNA Assay Kit.

#### In Vitro Transfection and Cell Viability

1. Seed the cells in 24-well plate ($5 \times 10^4$ cells per plate) containing 1 ml DMEM medium and 10% FBS. Then incubate it for 24 h.
2. Add specific amount of KALA-PS-$CaCO_3$-DNA NPs, as 20 μl (having 0.2 μg DNA), 50 μl (having 0.5 μg DNA), and 100 μl (having 1 μg DNA), in each well and incubate for 48 h at 37 °C.
3. Eliminate the medium and rinse the cells with the solution of PBS (0.1 M, 7.4 pH).
4. Determine the luciferase activity after the lysis of cells through lysis buffer (200 μl each well). Luciferase activity is detected by co-incubated cell lysate (20 μl) and luciferin substrate (100 μl) in luminometer.
5. Utilize BCA protein analysis kit for the identification of protein content in cell lysate, and optical density (OD) is calculated by microplate reader at 570 nm.
6. Take three independent measurements for the calculation of standard deviation (SD).
7. Cell viability assay is carried out by taking the incubated sample with HeLa cells after 48 h and remove the medium to replace it with 1 ml MTT (60 μl, 5 mg $ml^{-1}$) comply with 4 h incubation at 37 °C.

8. Remove supernatant and add 850 μl DMSO to dissolve formazan crystals and take the absorbance at 570 nm with microplate reader.

### 2.2.9 Calcium Carbonate-Calcium Phosphate-DNA NPs

**Synthesis of $CaCO_3$-CaP-DNA NPs**

1. Take 1 ug pGL3-Luc (1 μg/μL) and add to 16 μl solution of $CaCl_2$ (0.5 M) and dilute it by deionized water to attain the volume 50 μl.
2. Prepare mixture of $Na_2CO_3$ (0.01 M) and $Na_3PO_4$ (0.01 M) (specific volume proportion 31, 15, 10, 7, 3, and 1, correspondingly) to get 16 μl solution and dilute to obtain 50 μl volume.
3. Blend these two mixtures rapidly under consistent stirring to get $CaCO_3$-CaP-DNA NPs.

**DNA Encapsulation Efficiency**

1. Take 500 μl $CaCO_3$-CaP-DNA NPs solution (having 5 μg pGL3-Luc) and centrifuge it with the speed of 18,000 rpm for 1 h at 4 °C.
2. Follow the protocol of Quant-iT Pico Green® dsDNA Assay Kit and spectrofluorometer to calculate quantity of available DNA in supernatant and encapsulation efficiency.

**In Vitro Transfection and Gene Expression**

1. Apply 24-well plate for cell culturing ($5 \times 10^4$ cells per well) with 1 ml DMEM medium and FBS (10%) followed by the incubation for 24 h.
2. Pour 100 μl NPs solution (with 1 μg pGL3-Luc) in each well and incubate for 48 h at 37 °C and use it for gene expression.
3. Apply cell lysate protocol for determination of gene expression, BCA protein analysis kit for protein content and microplate reader to observe optical density (OD) at 570 nm and cytotoxicity under MTT assay protocol.
4. To examine the influence of NPs on the cell growth after transfection for 48 h, take images by inverted microscope as shown in Fig. 2.

**Cellular Uptake Assay**

1. Mix 1 μg pGL3-Luc and 2.5 μl YOYO-1 solution (10 μM) and incubate at 37 °C for 15 min.
2. Use YOYO-1 labeled pGL3-Luc for the synthesis of NPs and follow the standard cell seeding protocol.
3. After successful removal of the medium and washing with PBS, stain the cell nuclei with solution of Hoechst 33258 for 20 min at 37 °C.
4. Wash the cells with PBS and incubate with 200 μl PBS.
5. Envisage the cells via confocal laser scanning microscope with 1000 magnification.

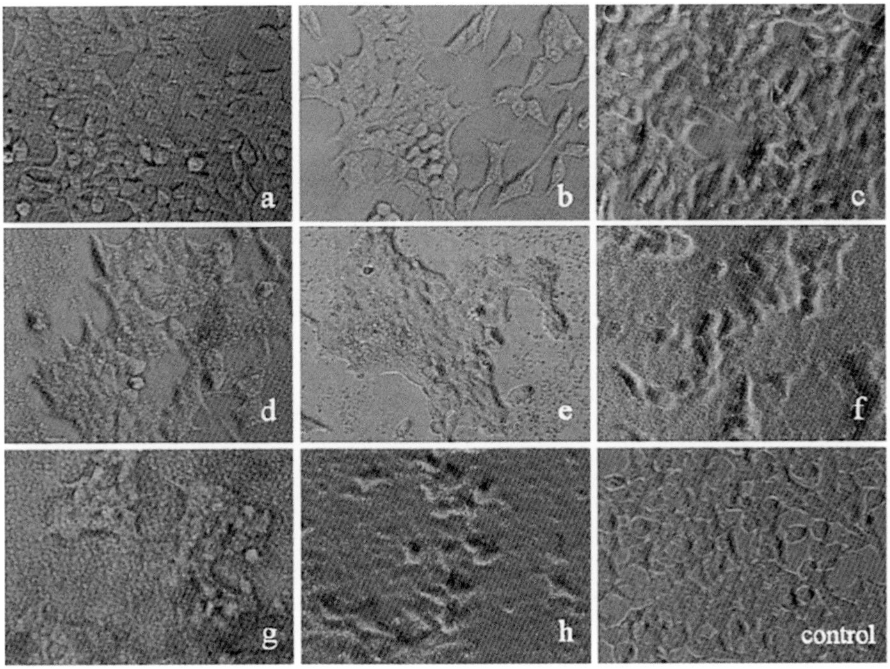


**Fig. 2** 293 T cells images after 48 h transfection facilitated by various transfer approaches: (**a**) $CaCO_3$/DNA NPs, (**b–g**) $CaCO_3$/CaP/DNA NPs having $CO_3^{2-}/PO_4^{3-}$ molar proportions of 31, 15, 10, 7, 3, and 1, correspondingly, and (**h**) CaP/DNA coprecipitates. Control are the cells with no treatment. (Reprinted with the permission of Zhao et al. (2014))

### 2.2.10 Polyethyleneimine-$CaCO_3$-DNA Nanoparticles

#### Preparation of $CaCO_3$ NPs

1. Mix $Na_2CO_3$ solution (60 mM) and arginine solution (2%) with 1:1 ratio.
2. Add the mixture dropwise to $CaCl_2$ solution (60 mM) with strong stirring about 15 min.
3. Separate the precipitates of arginine-$CaCO_3$ (ACa) NPs by centrifugation and wash with $C_2H_5OH$ and water (deionized) and dry at 60 °C.

#### Preparation of PEI-ACa-DNA NPs

1. Mix ACa with polyethyleneimine (PEI) mixture and develop for 40 min at 37 °C.
2. Add a decided amount of plasmid DNA to the PEI-ACa solution and incubate for 15–30 min for the preparation of PEI-ACa-pEGFP-C1-p53 and PEI-ACa-pEGFP-C1.
3. Use freshly prepared particles for further study.

#### In Vitro Transfection of NPs

1. Cultivate the cells in DMEM medium (1 ml) and FBS (10%) on 24-well plate ($5 \times 10^4$ cells each well) and incubate for 24 h.
2. Add 50 μl PEI-ACa-DNA NPs solution (having 2.5 μg of pEGFP-C1) and incubate at 37 °C.
3. Determine the gene expression after 24 h, 48 h, and 72 h with the help of fluorescence microscope.

#### p53 Gene Expression and Cell Growth Inhibition

1. Culture H1299 cells on 96-well plate ($5 \times 10^4$ cells each well) with 100 μl DMEM and 10% FBS and raise for 24 h at 37 °C. Also seed the cells on polystyrene plate to use as a control.
2. Apply solution of NPs with specific agent and incubate for 24 h, 48 h, and 72 h at 37 °C.
3. After decided time, apply cells extract to SDS-PAGE and electroblot to nitrocellulose membrane with the buffer system (Tris HCl (25 mM) 8.3 pH, glycine (192 mM), and methanol (20%)).
4. Block the membrane with blocking buffer and develop overnight with antibody at 4 °C.
5. Wash the membrane and again develop for 1 h at 25 °C with IR Dye 700 anti-rabbit IgG (Lincoln, NA).
6. Wash the membrane and do the analysis under Odyssey IR imaging system.
7. Follow the MTT assay protocol for the evaluation of cell inhibition. Furthermore, Hoechst 33342 staining procedure is used for cell apoptosis study and observations are recorded by fluorescence microscope.
8. Observe the protein expression by Western blotting protocol as presented in Fig. 3.

### 2.2.11 Lipid-Coated Calcium Carbonate/Phosphate Hybrid (LCC) NPs

#### Preparation of LCC NPs with Various Ratios of C/P

1. Take 150 μl solution of $CaCl_2$ (2.5 M) 7.0 pH and pour into 5 ml solution of igepal-CO520/cyclohexane (3:7; v/v) with constant stirring to make an emulsion (water-in-oil).
2. Similarly, take 150 μl solution of $NaHCO_3/Na_2HPO_4$ (25 mM) 9.0 pH and pour into 5 ml solution of igepal-CO520/cyclohexane (3:7; v/v) in addition to 50 μl DOPA (20 mM) in trichloromethane.
3. Fix the $NaHCO_3/Na_2HPO_4$ (C/P) molar ratio according to 0/4, 1/3, 2/2, and 3/1, respectively.
4. Then blend second emulsion with first emulsion dropwise assisted by constant stirring for 20 min.
5. Add equal volume of ethanol to the mixture and stir for 5 min.
6. Separate the hybrid NPs by 20 min centrifugation of mixture with the speed of 12,500 rpm and wash the particles three times with absolute ethanol.

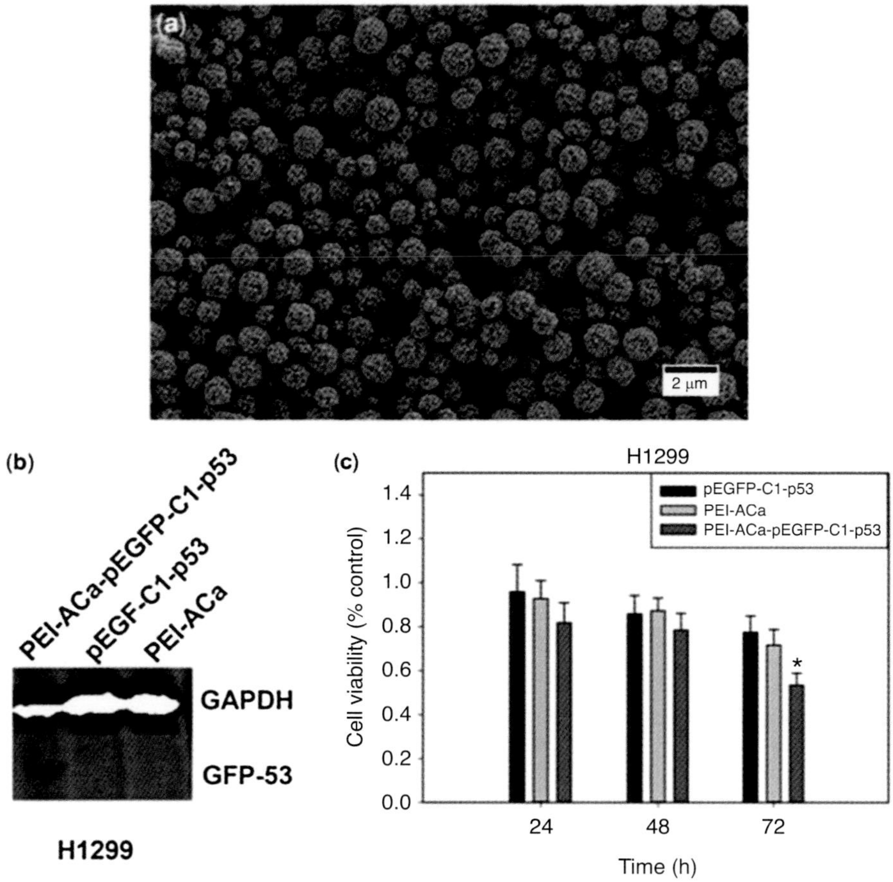


**Fig. 3** (**a**) SEM image of $CaCO_3$ particles, (**b**) protein expression (GFP-p53) determined by Western blot, and (**c**) H1299 cells growth inhibition and percentage cell viability. (Reprinted with the permission of Chen et al. 2016))

7. Disperse hybrid NPs in 1 ml trichloromethane ($CHCl_3$) and blend with 70 μl cholesterol/DOPC (20 mM).
8. Evaporate the solvent with low pressure and hydrate the lipid film with water or PBS to generate LCC NPs.

### Encapsulation of siRNA

1. Use same procedure for the encapsulation of dsDNA/siRNA, as mix the half quantity of dsDNA/siRNA together with aqueous solutions prior to emulsification.
2. Change the concentration of dsDNA from 1 to 4 nmol to estimate the payload by performing batch experiments. On the other hand, fix C/P payload to 1/3.

3. Utilize fluorescent plate read to calculate cy5-labelled dsDNA payload.
4. Treat LCC NPs with lysis buffer for 10 min at 65 °C before measurement.

**Colloidal Stability Assay**

1. Take 50 μl of LCC NPs suspension and dilute by DMEM having FBS (10%) and incubate it for 4 h.
2. Rinse the cells three intervals via PBS and stain for 30 min with 2 μM lysosensor-DND 189 for the visual representation of endosomes and lysosomes in cytoplasm.
3. Do the fixing for 20 min with PFA (4%) after washing the cells carefully with PBS.
4. Use 4′6-diamidino-2-phenylindole mounting medium fluo-sheild to mount cover slips on cell slides and take the observations under confocal laser scanning microscope with 40× lens and zoom at 2.0×.

**PD-L1 Expression**

1. PD-L1 protein expression is quantified by cultivation of FACS, B16F10 cells in 12-well plate ($5 \times 10^4$ cells in each well) and incubate overnight.
2. Replace the medium by 500 μl DMEM having LCC-PD-L1 siRNA (40 nM siRNA) and transfect for 4 h.
3. Remove the medium and add fresh DMEM medium with FBS (10%) and continue to seed for 48 h.
4. Stain the PD-L1 expression by PD-L1 anti-mouse antibodies.
5. Use the untreated cells having no antibody as a positive cells gate and the untouched cells with PD-L1 antibody stain as a positive control.
6. Similarly, pursue MTT analysis protocol for the measurement of cell viability and check absorbance at 490 nm with the help of microplate reader.

### 2.2.12 $MnO_2$-$CaCO_3$-ICG/siRNA Nanoplatform

**Synthesis of $MnO_2$ NPs**

1. Take 20 μl potassium permanganate ($KMnO_4$) solution (23.6 mg $ml^{-1}$) and mix with 12 ml PAH aqueous solution (8.43 μg $ml^{-1}$) and subjected to ultrasound for 30 s.
2. Keep the mixture at 25 °C without disturbance and after 5 min, light purple color will change to yellowish brown color suggesting the creation of $MnO_2$ NPs.
3. Store the $MnO_2$ NPs at 4 °C for further use.

**Preparation of $MnO_2$-$CaCO_3$-ICG/siRNA Nanoplatform**

1. Take 50 ml of $MnO_2$ NPs and ultracentrifuge for 30 min with 13,000 rpm speed and wash twice with deionized water.
2. Re-disperse the NPs in 10 ml deionized water in addition to 2 mg $CaCl_2$ and 100 μg ICG and keep under mild stirring overnight.

3. Remove the extra chemicals by centrifugation.
4. Disperse the precipitates in 20 ml deionized water possessing ICG (5 μg $ml^{-1}$) and $Na_2CO_3$ (50 μg $ml^{-1}$) and leave in dark for 24 h with mild stirring.
5. Finally, wash carefully with deionized water followed by centrifugation to get Mn@$CaCO_3$-ICG.
6. Next, take 20 ml of Mn@$CaCO_3$-ICG solution and add 20 ul PAH (23.6 mg $ml^{-1}$) with slow stirring for 6 h, after this, wash carefully with deionized water and centrifuge.
7. Disperse these precipitates in 20 ml aqueous solution of siRNA (50 nmol) with constant shaking for 3 h to obtain Mn@$CaCO_3$-ICG@siRNA.
8. Lastly, observe siRNA binding ratio with polyacrylamide gel electrophoresis.

**Biocompatibility and Cellular Uptake**

1. Culture Lewis lung tumor cell in 96-well plate and treat with nanoplatform according to the standard cell culturing protocol and evaluate by CCK8 assay.
2. Use real-time cell analyzer to observe the effect of nanoprobe on viability as well as cell proliferation.
3. Similarly, after culturing of cells and treatment with nanoprobes, stain the cells with Hoechst 33342 and get the confocal fluorescence images.
4. Furthermore, follow the Western blot assay after 48 h incubation of Mn@$CaCO_3$-ICG@siRNA to observe PD-L1 knock over.
5. Finally, in vivo fluorescence, MR, as well as CT imaging will help to study the efficiency of nanoplatform. As ICG excite by 710 nm to give NIR fluorescence imaging and presence of Mn in nanoplatform will support the MR imaging. Moreover, Mn@$CaCO_3$-ICG@siRNA nanoplatform is also feasible for PDT and PTT.
6. A complete schematic illustration is shown in Fig. 4.

## 3 Discussion

There are a few common shortcomings that can be improved as discussed in following notes.

1. Shape, size, and homogeneity of the particles is very important for effective gene delivery. This can be solved by constant check and balance of synthesis conditions, procedures, and grading system by careful handling.
2. Use of biocompatible polymers as a coating material on NPs can enhance the gene loading and unloading efficiency.
3. Light-sensitive substrates should be treated without light and especially time must be controlled strictly according to the protocol.
4. While culturing the cells and changing the medium, extra care is required, because minor mistakes can lead to false results.
5. Must choose proper stain according to the requirement of material.

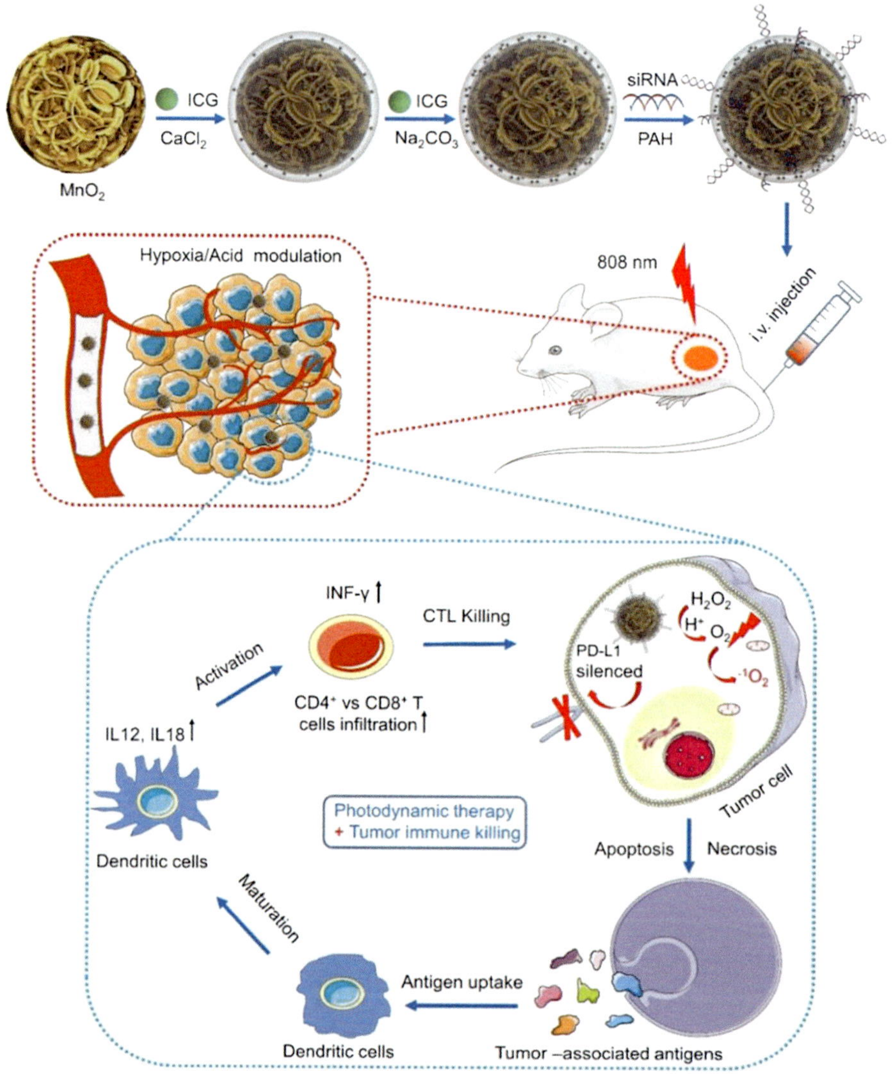


**Fig. 4** Schematic diagram presenting the route of synthesis to in vivo nanoprobe-mediated photodynamic immunotherapy of tumor. (Reprinted with the permission of Liu et al. (2019))

6. MTT assay is not valid for all kind of materials (especially for some plant extracts), so other tests can also be used to check cell viability.
7. Handling of ICG requires extra care, because it is a light- and heat-sensitive material.
8. RNA interference is sequence specific and gene silencing (post-transcription). Gene silencing is prompted by RNA (double stranded) and it helps in degradation of target mRNA (Mandriota et al. 2001).

9. Transfect pGenesil-1 siRNA VEGF-C expression plasmid into SGC-7901 cells with $CaCO_3$ NPs method to estimate efficiency of VEGF-C siRNA.
10. Gene expression is seriously affected by ratio of $Ca^{2+}$ and $CO_3^{2-}$ because the size of composite of $CaCO_3$-DNA depends upon $Ca^{2+}$ and $CO_3^{2-}$ ratio. So, there should be careful handling and calculated ratio of ions.
11. Suitable modifications (like KALA, ICG, inorganic and organic NPs) with $CaCO_3$ NPs help to enhance the efficiency of gene delivery.

## 4 Conclusion

$CaCO_3$ is found to be the attractive candidate for the gene and drug delivery applications due to its high biocompatibility, easy degradation, high loading capacity, and accessibility to modify with suitable reagents. The study outcomes highlighted the efficiency of $CaCO_3$ NPs as well as the $CaCO_3$ nanocomposites in gene delivery applications. This chapter summarizes the synthetic routes for the manufacturing of $CaCO_3$ NPs, $CaCO_3$-siRNA, $CaCO_3$-DNA, $CaCO_3$-p53, KALA-modified $CaCO_3$, alginate-modified $CaCO_3$/plasmid DNA, $CaCO_3$ particles – plasmid pEGFP-C1-p53, protamine sulfate $CaCO_3$-DNA, lipid-coated calcium carbonate/phosphate hybrid (LCC) NPs, $MnO_2$-$CaCO_3$-ICG/siRNA nanoplatform, polyethyleneimine-$CaCO_3$-DNA nanoparticles, and KALA-protamine sulfate-$CaCO_3$-DNA nanoparticles. Furthermore, there is the discussion about the efficiency, fundamental tests, and reliability of these nanoplatforms in gene delivery.

## References

Anis HA (2019) Gene therapy in the era of nanotechnology/a review of current data. J Cancer Prev Curr Res 10:1–2. https://doi.org/10.15406/jcpcr.2019.10.00380

Axelsen TM, Woldbye DPD (2018) Gene therapy for Parkinson's disease, an update. J Parkinsons Dis 8:195–215. https://doi.org/10.3233/JPD-181331

Chapuis AG, Egan DN, Bar M et al (2019) T cell receptor gene therapy targeting WT1 prevents acute myeloid leukemia relapse post-transplant. Nat Med 25:1064–1072. https://doi.org/10.1038/s41591-019-0472-9

Chen C, Han H, Yang W et al (2016) Polyethyleneimine-modified calcium carbonate nanoparticles for P 53 gene delivery. Regen Biomater 3:57–63. https://doi.org/10.1093/RB/RBV029

Chen S, Li F, Zhuo RX, Cheng SX (2011) Efficient non-viral gene delivery mediated by nanostructured calcium carbonate in solution-based transfection and solid-phase transfection. Mol BioSyst 7:2841–2847. https://doi.org/10.1039/c1mb05147d

Chen S, Zhao D, Li F et al (2012) Co-delivery of genes and drugs with nanostructured calcium carbonate for cancer therapy. RSC Adv 2:1820–1826. https://doi.org/10.1039/c1ra00527h

Dupéré-Richer D, Licht JD (2018) Epigenetic regulatory mutations and epigenetic therapy for multiple myeloma. Curr Opin Hematol 24:336–344. https://doi.org/10.1097/MOH.0000000000000358

Fischer MD, Ochakovski GA, Beier B et al (2020) Changes in retinal sensitivity after gene therapy in choroideremia. Retina 40:160–168. https://doi.org/10.1097/IAE.0000000000002360

He XW, Liu T, Chen YX et al (2008) Calcium carbonate nanoparticle delivering vascular endothelial growth factor-C siRNA effectively inhibits lymphangiogenesis and growth of gastric cancer in vivo. Cancer Gene Ther 15:193–202. https://doi.org/10.1038/sj.cgt.7701122

Kohn DB (2019) Gene therapy for blood diseases. Curr Opin Biotechnol 60:39–45. https://doi.org/10.1016/j.copbio.2018.11.016

Kong X, Xu S, Wang X et al (2012) Calcium carbonate microparticles used as a gene vector for delivering p53 gene into cancer cells. J Biomed Mater Res – Part A 100(A):2312–2318. https://doi.org/10.1002/jbm.a.34155

Kong F, Zhang H, Zhang X et al (2016) Biodegradable photothermal and pH responsive calcium carbonate@phospholipid@acetalated dextran hybrid platform for advancing biomedical applications. Adv Funct Mater 26:6158–6169. https://doi.org/10.1002/adfm.201602715

Labhasetwar V (2005) Nanotechnology for drug and gene therapy: the importance of understanding molecular mechanisms of delivery. Curr Opin Biotechnol 16:674–680. https://doi.org/10.1016/j.copbio.2005.10.009

Liu Y, Pan Y, Cao W et al (2019) A tumor microenvironment responsive biodegradable $CaCO_3$/$MnO_2$-based nanoplatform for the enhanced photodynamic therapy and improved PD-L1 immunotherapy. Theranostics 9:6867–6884. https://doi.org/10.7150/thno.37586

Mallack EJ, Turk B, Yan H, Eichler FS (2019) The landscape of hematopoietic stem cell transplant and gene therapy for x-linked adrenoleukodystrophy. Curr Treat Options Neurol 21:61. https://doi.org/10.1007/s11940-019-0605-y

Mandriota SJ, Jussila L, Jeltsch M et al (2001) Vascular endothelial growth factor-C-mediated lymphangiogenesis promotes tumour metastasis. EMBO J 20:672–682. https://doi.org/10.1093/emboj/20.4.672

Mintzer MA, Simanek EE (2009) Nonviral vectors for gene delivery. Chem Rev 109:259–302. https://doi.org/10.1021/cr800409e

Moss JA (2014) Gene therapy review. Radiol Technol 86:154–155

Nayerossadat N, Ali P, Maedeh T (2012) Viral and nonviral delivery systems for gene delivery. Adv Biomed Res 1:27. https://doi.org/10.4103/2277-9175.98152

Pai SY, Thrasher AJ (2020) Gene therapy for X-linked severe combined immunodeficiency: historical outcomes and current status. J Allergy Clin Immunol 146:258–261. https://doi.org/10.1016/j.jaci.2020.05.055

Pravina P, Sayaji D, Avinash M (2013) Calcium and its role in human body. Int J Res Pharmaceut Biomed Sci 4:659–668

Ramamoorth M, Narvekar A (2015) Non viral vectors in gene therapy – an overview. J Clin Diagn Res 9:1–6. https://doi.org/10.7860/JCDR/2015/10443.5394

Sharma A, Easow Mathew M, Sriganesh V, Reiss UM (2020) Gene therapy for haemophilia. Cochrane Database Syst Rev 2020:CD010822. https://doi.org/10.1002/14651858.CD010822.pub4

Wang CQ, Gong MQ, Wu JL et al (2014) Dual-functionalized calcium carbonate based gene delivery system for efficient gene delivery. RSC Adv 4:38623–38629. https://doi.org/10.1039/c4ra05468g

Wang CQ, Wu JL, Zhuo RX, Cheng SX (2014) Protamine sulfate-calcium carbonate-plasmid DNA ternary nanoparticles for efficient gene delivery. Mol BioSyst 10:672–678. https://doi.org/10.1039/c3mb70502a

Wierda WG, Castro JE, Aguillon R et al (2010) A phase i study of immune gene therapy for patients with CLL using a membrane-stable, humanized CD154. Leukemia 24:1893–1900. https://doi.org/10.1038/leu.2010.191

Wirth T, Parker N, Ylä-Herttuala S (2013) History of gene therapy. Gene 525:162–169. https://doi.org/10.1016/j.gene.2013.03.137

Wu Y, Gu W, Tang J, Xu ZP (2017) Devising new lipid-coated calcium phosphate/carbonate hybrid nanoparticles for controlled release in endosomes for efficient gene delivery. J Mater Chem B 5:7194–7203. https://doi.org/10.1039/c7tb01635b

Yahya EB, Alqadhi AM (2021) Recent trends in cancer therapy: a review on the current state of gene delivery. Life Sci 269:119087. https://doi.org/10.1016/j.lfs.2021.119087

Zhao D, Liu CJ, Zhuo RX, Cheng SX (2012) Alginate/$CaCO_3$ hybrid nanoparticles for efficient codelivery of antitumor gene and drug. Mol Pharm 9:2887–2893. https://doi.org/10.1021/mp3002123

Zhao D, Wang CQ, Zhuo RX, Cheng SX (2014) Modification of nanostructured calcium carbonate for efficient gene delivery. Colloids Surf B Biointerfaces 118:111–116. https://doi.org/10.1016/j.colsurfb.2014.03.007

Zhao D, Zhuo RX, Cheng SX (2012) Modification of calcium carbonate based gene and drug delivery systems by a cell-penetrating peptide. Mol BioSyst 8:3288–3294. https://doi.org/10.1039/c2mb25233c

# A Codelivery System of Anticancer Drug Doxorubicin and Tumor-Suppressor Gene p53 Based on Polyphosphoester for Lung Cancer Therapy

26

Peihong Ni, Jie Liu, Jinlin He, and Mingzu Zhang

## Contents




**Abstract**

In order to obtain nanoparticles loaded with both the anticancer drug doxorubicin (DOX) and p53 gene, a pH-responsive doxorubicin prodrug and polycationic carrier can be respectively prepared through a combination of ring-opening



P. Ni (✉) · J. Liu · J. He · M. Zhang
College of Chemistry, Chemical Engineering and Materials Science, State and Local Joint Engineering Laboratory for Novel Functional Polymeric Materials, Jiangsu Key Laboratory of Advanced Functional Polymer Design and Application, Suzhou Key Laboratory of Macromolecular Design and Precision Synthesis, Soochow University, Suzhou, P. R. China
e-mail: phni@suda.edu.cn






H. Tian and X. Chen (eds.), *Gene Delivery*, Biomaterial Engineering,
https://doi.org/10.1007/978-981-16-5419-0_27

polymerization (ROP) and "click" reaction. First, poly(ethylene glycol)monomethyl ether (mPEG) is used to initiate the ring-opening polymerization of a cyclic phosphoester monomer, 2-(but-3-yn-1-yloxy)-2-oxo-1,3,2-dioxaphospholane (abbreviated as BYP), resulting in a block copolymer precursor (mPEG-*b*-PBYP) containing alkynyl groups in the side chain. In another reaction, a pH-responsive doxorubicin derivative (DOX-*hyd*-$N_3$) containing an azide group and an acid-sensitive hydrazone bond (-*hyd*-) is synthesized. Subsequently, the polymeric prodrug mPEG-*b*-PBYP-*hyd*-DOX is prepared by Cu(I)-catalyzed alkyne-azide cycloaddition (CuAAC) "click" reaction between the alkynyl group of mPEG-*b*-PBYP and the azide group of DOX-*hyd*-$N_3$. And the polycationic carrier (abbreviated as mPEG-*b*-PBYP-*g*-DAE) is obtained *via* the thiol-yne "click" reaction between mPEG-*b*-PBYP and 2-dimethylaminoethanethiol hydrochloride (DAE). The structures of mPEG-*b*-PBYP-*hyd*-DOX and mPEG-*b*-PBYP-*g*-DAE are characterized by magnetic resonance spectroscopy (NMR), gel permeation chromatography (GPC), ultraviolet-visible spectrophotometer (UV-vis), Fourier transform infrared spectroscopy (FT-IR), and high-performance liquid chromatography (HPLC) analyses. The two kinds of polymers can self-assemble into mixed micelles in aqueous solution, which are then combined with p53 gene by electrostatic interaction to form nanoparticles coencapsulated with the DOX and p53 gene. The size and morphology of the mixed micelles are characterized by dynamic light scattering (DLS) and transmission electron microscopy (TEM). And the release of DOX from the nanoparticles is studied by fluorescence spectrophotometer. The gene condensation ability of the mixed micelles is tested by zeta potential and gel retardation assay. Furthermore, *in vitro* cell experiments have proved the biocompatibility of the polymer precursor, the effect of nanoparticles on cancer cell inhibition, and the process of effective release of DOX and p53 gene after the nanoparticle enters the A549 cells by endocytosis. Meanwhile, the gene transfection effect of nanoparticles at different N/P ratios can be observed by confocal laser-scanning microscope. These results demonstrate that the DOX/p53 gene-coloaded nanoparticles have broad application prospects in the treatment of lung cancer.

**Keywords**

Drug/p53 gene codelivery · Polyphosphoester · Polymeric prodrug · Self-assembly

## 1 Introduction

Lung cancer is a major threat to human health, and its mortality rates have been at the forefront of cancer mortality rates over the past few years (Torre et al. 2015; Jemal et al. 2011). Chemotherapy is one of the most common treatments for lung cancer. However, due to the complexity of cancer pathology and the rapid metastasis of lung cancer, it is difficult to develop a treatment with a single therapeutic element that produces the desired results (Yang et al. 2015; Zhang et al. 2016). In recent years, a combination therapy of anticancer drugs and the p53 gene has become a newly developed approach for lung cancer treatment. The p53 gene is one of the most important tumor suppressor genes and is widely used in cancer therapy (Tseng et al. 2015; Zeng et al. 2010). Mutations or deletions of p53 could result in genetic instability and insensitivity to chemotherapy and the radiation therapy of cancer cells (Wang et al. 2014; Szymañska and Hainaut 2003; Lane et al. 2010). Preclinical and clinical studies have shown that the introduction of a wild-type p53 gene could inhibit tumor growth, promote apoptosis, and increase tumor chemosensitivity (Tseng et al. 2015; Fisher et al. 2001; Li et al. 2015a; Kim et al. 2014; Chenau et al. 2009). Based on these factors, researchers have proposed that the introduction of an exogenous p53 gene can increase the sensitivity of lung cancer cells to chemotherapeutic drugs (e.g., doxorubicin, camptothecin , and paclitaxel) and improve the bioavailability of drugs (Li et al. 2015b; Xu et al. 2013). Therefore, the combination therapy of p53 gene and doxorubicin (DOX) can be used as a new treatment for lung cancer (Zhao et al. 2012).

In order to improve the stability of hydrophobic drugs, prolong the cycle time of drugs *in vivo,* and reduce the toxic side effects of small-molecule drugs, a variety of strategies for the attachment of anticancer drugs to water-soluble polymers have been proposed to form polymeric prodrugs (Delplace et al. 2014). At the same time, a series of sensitive linking groups can be used to covalently link drugs and polymers to release an active drug quickly (Bildstein et al. 2011), for example, acidic-cleavable groups (Pang et al. 2016) (such as acetals (Huang et al. 2015), hydrazones (Ding et al. 2014; Zan et al. 2014), and oximes (Jin et al. 2011)) and redox-sensitive groups (such as disulfides) (Zhang et al. 2015).

The properties of polymeric carriers play a key role in the simultaneous delivery of drugs and the p53 gene. Polyphosphoesters have side chains to be easily modified, and their degradation products are similar to teichoic acid and nucleic acid (Steinbach and Wurm 2015). PPEs have separately been used as drug or gene carriers (Cao et al. 2016; Chan et al. 2016; Zhang et al. 2012a; Lim et al. 2015). Herein, we present a synergistic release system that can be obtained by integrating the tumor-sensitive groups with a biodegradable polyphosphoester and antineoplastic agents. We synthesized an amphiphilic block copolymer precursor mPEG-*b*-PBYP using poly(ethylene glycol)monomethyl ether (mPEG) as the initiator and a cyclic phosphoester compound (BYP) containing alkynyl group as the monomer. A pH-sensitive doxorubicin prodrug, mPEG-*b*-PBYP-*hyd*-DOX, was prepared by the CuAAC "click" reaction between mPEG-*b*-PBYP and a hydrazine-containing doxorubicin derivative (DOX-*hyd*-$N_3$). In another reaction, the precursor was used to prepare a polycationic carrier, mPEG-*b*-PBYP-*g*-DAE, *via* a thiol-yne "click" reaction. The resulting prodrug and polycationic carriers self-assembled into hybrid micelles, which were expected to achieve triggered release in a tumor cell microenvironment. Because of the acidic environment and the higher level of phosphodiesterase I (PDE I) in tumor cells in comparison to normal tissues, the hydrazone bond of the prodrug and polyphosphoester linkage in the precursor polymer chain could be degraded rapidly and release doxorubicin and p53 gene, which inhibit the growth of tumor cells. The nanoparticles have significant advantages as follows: (1) desired combination therapy effect of drug and gene; (2) simple preparation and purification process; and (3) responsive to stimulation, so as to achieve quick release in the tumor tissue and inhibit the growth of the tumor cell effectively (Liu et al. 2018).

## 2 Materials

2-(But-3-yn-1-yloxy)-2-oxo-1,3,2-dioxaphospholane (BYP) was prepared and purified according to the literature. The DOX derivative DOX-*hyd*-$N_3$ was prepared according to a previously reported method. All other chemicals were purchased and used as received without further purification as follows: poly(ethylene glycol)monomethyl ether (mPEG$_{113}$-OH, $M_n \approx 5000$ g mol$^{-1}$, $Đ = 1.06$, Sigma-Aldrich), doxorubicin hydrochloride (DOX·HCl, 99%, Beijing Zhongshuo Pharmaceutical Technology Development), 6-bromohexanoic acid (98%), *N,N,N′,N″,N″*-pentamethyl diethylenetriamine (PMDETA, 98%, Sigma-Aldrich), 1,8-diazabicyclo-[5,4,0]-ene (DBU, 98%, TCI), 2,2-dimethoxy-2-phenylacetophenone (DMPA, 99%, Shanghai Yuanye Bio Technology), 2-dimethylaminoethanethiol hydrochloride (DAE, 95%, Energy Chemical), 6× DNA loading buffer (Shanghai Yuanye Bio Technology), 3-(4,5-dimethylthiazol-2-yl)-2,5-diphenyl tetrazolium bromide (MTT, 98%, Sigma-Aldrich), and bisbenzimide Hoechst 33342 trihydrochloride (H 33342, 98%, Sigma-Aldrich). Hydrazone hydrate 85% (A.R.), glacial acetic acid (AcOH, A.R.), sodium azide ($NaN_3$, 98%), acetonitrile (HPLC grade), and agarose (BR) were purchased from Sinopharm Chemical Reagent and were used as received. Cuprous bromide (CuBr, 95%, Sinopharm Chemical Reagent) was purified by washing sequentially with acetone, glacial acetic acid, and ethanol three times, followed by drying under vacuum at room temperature for 24 h. Dichloromethane ($CH_2Cl_2$) and *N,N*-dimethylformamide (DMF) were refluxed with $CaH_2$ and distilled before use. Milli-Q water (18.2 MΩ cm) was generated using a water purification system (Simplicity UV, Millipore). All other chemicals were of analytical reagent grade and were used as received, unless otherwise mentioned.

## 3 Methods

### 3.1 Preparation of pH-Responsive Doxorubicin Derivative DOX-*hyd*-$N_3$

Azide-modified DOX (DOX-*hyd*-$N_3$) was prepared and purified according to the previously reported methods (Chen et al. 2012; Li et al. 2015c), and the synthetic routes are shown in Scheme 1. In a 50 mL dry round-bottomed flask, 6-bromohexanoic acid (2.35 g, 11.24 mmol) and sodium azide ($NaN_3$, 1.83 g, 28.15 mmol) were added in 15 mL DMF, and the reaction was carried out for 12 h at 60 °C. The mixture was filtered with a short column of neutral aluminum oxide to remove the salt, and DMF was then removed under reduced pressure. Subsequently, the crude product was dissolved in 20 mL $CH_2Cl_2$ and washed three times with

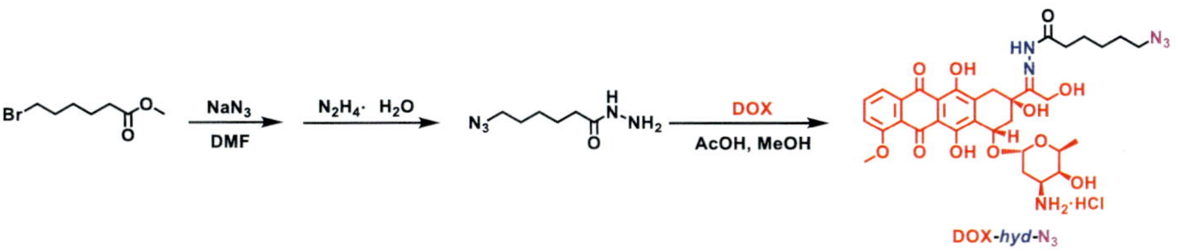


**Scheme 1** Synthetic route of hydrazine-containing and azide-modified DOX (DOX-*hyd*-$N_3$)

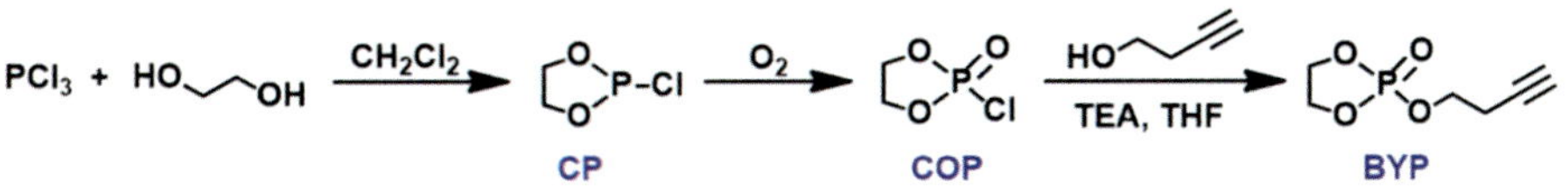


**Scheme 2** Synthetic route of 2-(but-3-yn-1-yloxy)-2-oxo-1,3,2-dioxaphospholane (BYP)

40 mL Milli-Q water. The organic layer was collected, dried over anhydrous $Na_2SO_4$ for 2 h, and evaporated to give a product. After drying under vacuum at 25 °C for 24 h, 6-azidohexanoic acid methyl ester was obtained (1.14 g, yield: 66.8%).

6-Azidohexanoic acid methyl ester (0.54 g, 3.17 mmol), hydrazine hydrate 85% (4.70 g, 79.4 mmol), and 20 mL THF were added into a round-bottomed flask, stirred evenly, and refluxed for 12 h at 80 °C. After removing the solvent by rotary evaporation, the crude product was dissolved in $CH_2Cl_2$ and washed with NaCl aqueous solution twice. The organic phase was dried over anhydrous $Na_2SO_4$. The filtrate was concentrated and dried under vacuum at 25 °C for 24 h to get the 6-azidehexanohydrazine (0.29 g, yield: 53.5%).

Finally, 6-azidehexanohydrazine (102 mg, 0.60 mmol), DOX·HCl (115.9 mg, 0.20 mmol), anhydrous $Na_2SO_4$ (103 mg, 0.73 mmol), and 30 mL anhydrous methanol ($CH_3OH$) were added into a round-bottom flask with condensation reflux device. Two or three drops of glacial acetic acid were then added, fully stirred evenly, and reacted at 60 °C for 24 h in the dark. At the end of the reaction, the product was precipitated three times with diethyl ether, and the precipitate was obtained by centrifugation. After 24 h of vacuum drying, the red powder product was obtained (DOX-*hyd*-$N_3$, 93.5 mg, yield: 62.4%).

## 3.2 Preparation of Alkynyl-Containing Block Copolymer Precursor mPEG-*b*-PBYP

### 3.2.1 Preparation of Cyclic Phosphoester Monomer BYP

2-(But-3-yn-1-yloxy)-2-oxo-1,3,2-dioxaphospholane (BYP) was prepared and purified by a modified literature protocol (Libiszowski et al. 1978; Steinbach et al. 2013; Zhang et al. 2012b) (Scheme 2).

#### Preparation of 2-Chloro-1,3,2-Dioxaphospholane (CP)

First, a 500 mL three-necked flask equipped with a stir bar, a serpentine condenser, an elbow, and a constant pressure-dropping funnel was put into a 120 °C oven to dry for more than 12 h. Before use, take out the above glass instruments and place them in a desiccator to cool to room temperature. 150 mL of anhydrous $CH_2Cl_2$ was added to the dry three-necked flask, followed by phosphorus trichloride (221.5 g, 1.60 mol) that was obtained from new distillation. Ethylene glycol (102.9 g, 1.66 mol) was added into the constant-pressure-dropping funnel, and then the gas-receiving device was introduced on the condenser into the configured alkali solution. Turn on the knob of the constant-pressure-dropping funnel while stirring, and slowly drip into the ethylene glycol. After the solution was dripped completely, the reaction was continued at room temperature for 1 h. After the completion of the reaction, most of $CH_2Cl_2$ was first removed under reduced pressure with a water pump, and then vacuum distilled using an oil pump to obtain a colorless liquid CP.

#### Preparation of 2-Chloro-2-Oxo-1,3,2-Dioxaphospholane (COP)

A 250 mL three-necked flask equipped with a stir bar was put into an oven at 120 °C to dry for more than 12 h. Before use, take out the device and place it in a desiccator to cool to room temperature. The CP distilled in the previous step was added to the dry three-necked flask, and then 100 mL of freshly distilled benzene was added as a solvent. Dry oxygen was slowly introduced while stirring at room temperature for 72 h. After the completion of the reaction, most of benzene was first removed under reduced pressure with a water pump, and then vacuum distilled using an oil pump to obtain a colorless liquid COP. Since COP can easily react with water in the air, it is necessary to fill a storage bottle with nitrogen and store it at −20 °C. In some countries, COP is also commercially available.

#### Preparation of 2-(but-3-yn-1-yloxy)-2-Oxo-1,3,2-Dioxaphospholane (BYP)

The monomer BYP with high yield and purity was obtained through a one-step esterification reaction between two commercially available compounds, 3-butyn-1-ol and COP, followed by simple filtration and vacuum distillation. The specific operation is as follows.

A 250 mL three-necked flask equipped with a stir bar, a serpentine condenser, an elbow, and a constant-pressure-dropping funnel was put into an oven at 120 °C to dry for more than 12 h. Before use, take out the above glass instruments and place them in a desiccator to cool to room temperature. Under the protection of a nitrogen atmosphere, 100 mL of dry THF was added to the three-necked flask, and another 20 mL of dry THF was added to the constant-pressure-dropping funnel. COP (19.26 g, 0.14 mmol) was then transferred to the constant-pressure-dropping funnel using a dry syringe. 3-butyn-1-ol (9.50 g, 0.14 mmol) and triethylamine (15.04 g, 0.15 mmol) were weighed and added into the three-necked flask, and the solution was stirred well, filled with nitrogen three times, and transferred to a −10 °C bath. After the solution became cool, COP was slowly dripped from the funnel into the reaction flask. After the addition is complete, the reaction was continued for 12 h. The triethylamine hydrochloride formed from the reaction was filtered off with a sand core funnel, and the filtrate was concentrated by rotary evaporation to obtain a crude product. Finally, the crude product was distilled under vacuum to obtain a colorless liquid BYP. Due to the high activity of BYP, it is necessary to fill the storage bottle with nitrogen and store it at −20 °C.

### 3.2.2 Preparation of Diblock Copolymer Precursor mPEG-*b*-PBYP

mPEG-*b*-PBYP was synthesized by the ROP reaction according to previous publications (Chen et al. 2012; Lim et al. 2013). mPEG (0.82 g, 0.16 mmol) was added to a 50 mL dry flask and azeotropic distilled with anhydrous toluene two times, and 7 mL of anhydrous $CH_2Cl_2$ was added to dissolve mPEG. BYP (2.12 g, 11.9 mmol) and DBU (0.049 g, 0.32 mmol) were then added to the flask, followed by three exhausting-refilling nitrogen cycles; the reaction was conducted at 25 °C for 30 min. The solvent was concentrated and precipitated with 100 mL of cold diethyl ether/methanol (10/1, v/v) twice. The white sticky solid was collected and dried under vacuum at 25 °C to a constant weight (mPEG-*b*-PBYP, 2.64 g, yield: 89.8%).

## 3.3 Preparation of pH-Responsive Doxorubicin Prodrug mPEG-*b*-PBYP-*hyd*-DOX

The acid-cleavable prodrug mPEG-*b*-PBYP-*hyd*-DOX was prepared via CuAAC "click" reaction between the diblock copolymer precursor mPEG-*b*-PBYP and DOX-*hyd*-$N_3$, as shown in Scheme 3. A 50 mL dry flask was charged with mPEG-*b*-PBYP (387.7 mg, 0.02 mmol), DOX-*hyd*-$N_3$ (293.3 mg, 0.4 mmol), and 10 mL anhydrous DMF, and stirred evenly. Subsequently, CuBr (64.3 mg, 0.45 mmol) and *N*,*N*,*N′*,*N″*,*N″*-pentamethyl diethylenetriamine (PMDETA) (155.3 mg, 0.90 mmol) were added under a nitrogen atmosphere, followed by three exhausting-refilling nitrogen cycles. The reaction mixture was then stirred at 45 °C for 48 h. The crude products were further dialyzed (MWCO 7000) against Milli-Q water for 24 h. The purple floc was obtained after lyophilization (mPEG-*b*-PBYP-*hyd*-DOX, 489.6 mg, yield: 68.4%).

## 3.4 Preparation of Polycationic Carrier mPEG-*b*-PBYP-*g*-DAE

The polycationic gene vector mPEG-*b*-PBYP-g-DAE was prepared *via* the thiol-yne "click" reaction between mPEG-*b*-PBYP and 2-dimethylaminoethanethiol hydrochloride (DAE), as shown in Scheme 4. mPEG-*b*-PBYP (396.3 mg, 0.02 mmol) and DAE (907.0 mg, 6.40 mmol) were added to a quartz glass flask and dissolved in 15 mL of anhydrous methyl alcohol, followed by the addition of photoinitiator, 2,2-dimethoxy-2-phenylacetophenone (DMPA) (107.7 mg, 0.48 mmol). The reaction was stirred under

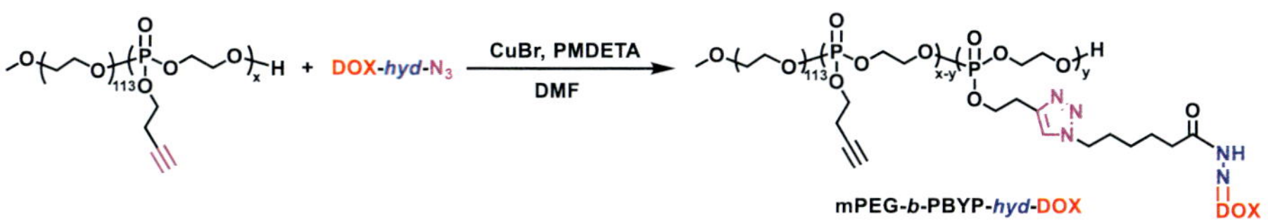


**Scheme 3** Synthetic route of mPEG-*b*-PBYP-*hyd*-DOX

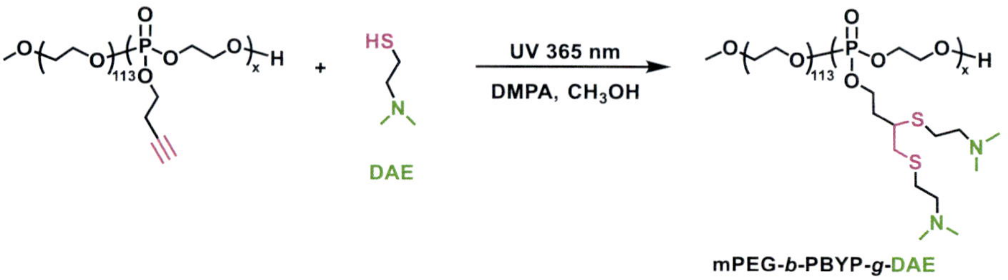


**Scheme 4** Synthetic route of mPEG-*b*-PBYP-*hyd*-DAE

365 nm UV irradiation for 1 h. The crude products were further dialyzed (MWCO 7000) against Milli-Q water for 24 h. The white sticky solid was obtained after lyophilization (mPEG-*b*-PBYP-*g*-DAE, 562.3 mg, yield: 66.2%).

## 3.5 Characterization of Chemical Structure and Molecular Weights

1. The polymer structures were characterized by nuclear magnetic resonance spectroscopy ($^1$H NMR, $^{13}$C NMR) using a 400 MHz/600 MHz NMR instrument (INOVA-400/INOVA-600, Varian) with $CDCl_3$ as the solvent and tetramethylsilane (TMS) as the internal reference.
2. Fourier transform infrared (FT-IR) spectra were recorded on a Bruker TENSOR-27 FT-IR spectrometer using the KBr disk method.
3. Gel permeation chromatography (GPC) analysis was conducted on a HLC-8320 (Tosoh) equipped with a refractive-index detector (TOSOH), using a TSKgel guard column SuperMP-N column (4.6 × 20 mm) and two TSKgel SuperMultiporeHZ-N columns (4.6 × 150 mm) with measurable molecular weights ranging from $5.0 \times 10^2$ to $1.9 \times 10^5$ g mol$^{-1}$. The tests were performed at 40 °C using polystyrene as the standard and DMF including 0.1 wt% LiBr as the eluent with a flow rate of 0.6 mL min$^{-1}$.
4. The DOX derivative and polymeric prodrugs were analyzed by high performance liquid chromatography (HPLC) (UltiMate 3000, Thermo Fisher Scientific) at 30 °C with acetonitrile/Milli-Q water (50/50, v/v) as the mobile phase at a flow rate of 1.0 mL min$^{-1}$ at 488 nm.
5. The ultraviolet-visible (UV-vis) absorption spectra are recorded on a UV-vis spectrophotometer (Cary 60 UV-vis, Agilent Technologies), and the fluorescence spectra were recorded on a fluorescence spectrophotometer (Cary Eclipse, Agilent Technologies).

## 3.6 Measurement of Critical Aggregation Concentration (CAC) of Copolymers

The critical aggregation concentration (CAC) was measured by a fluorescence probe method on a fluorescence spectrophotometer, and pyrene was used as the probe.

Typically, a predetermined pyrene solution in acetone was added into a series of ampoule bottles, and then acetone was removed under reduced pressure. The bottles were separately added with 5 mL of the copolymer solution with different concentrations. Then the mixture was sonicated for 20 min and stirred for 48 h at room temperature before measurement. The solutions were analyzed on a fluorescence spectrophotometer. The excitation wavelength was 335 nm, and the emission spectra were recorded ranging from 350 nm to 500 nm with a 2.5 nm slit width at medium voltage. From the emission spectra, the intensity ratio ($I_3/I_1$) of the third bond (383 nm, $I_3$) to the first bond (372 nm, $I_1$) was analyzed as the function of the logarithm concentration of the copolymer solution. The CAC value was determined by the intersection of the two lines in the plot of intensity ratio ($I_3/I_1$) versus the copolymer concentration.

## 3.7 Preparation and Characterization of Hybrid Micelles

A modified dialysis method was used for the self-assembly of the polymeric prodrug and polycationic vector. The polymers mPEG-*b*-PBYP-*hyd*-DOX (12.5 mg) and mPEG-*b*-PBYP-*g*-DAE (12.5 mg) were codissolved in 2.0 mL of DMSO and stirred for 4 h at room temperature. Milli-Q water (18 mL) was then added dropwise at a rate of 2 mL $h^{-1}$ with moderate stirring. After the dropwise addition, the mixture was dialyzed (MWCO 7000) against Milli-Q water for 24 h to remove DMSO. Finally, the hybrid micelle solution was diluted to 25 mL with Milli-Q water to a concentration of 1 mg $mL^{-1}$. Scheme 5 shows the preparation process and structure diagrams of the mixed micelles and the p53 gene complex.

The hybrid micelles/p53 gene complex at various weight ratios were formed by adding the same amount of the p53 gene into the hybrid micelle solutions of different concentrations and vortexing for 10 s. The solutions were then allowed to stand at room temperature for 30 minutes to form the nanoparticles containing DOX and the p53 gene. The N/P ratio refers to the weight ratio of all the copolymers to p53 gene in this study, and the calculations were performed based on Eq. (1)

$$\text{N/P ratio} = \frac{m_{(\text{mPEG-}b\text{-PBYP-}hyd\text{-DOX})} + m_{(\text{mPEG-}b\text{-PBYP-}g\text{-DAE})}}{m_{\text{p53 gene}}} \quad (1)$$

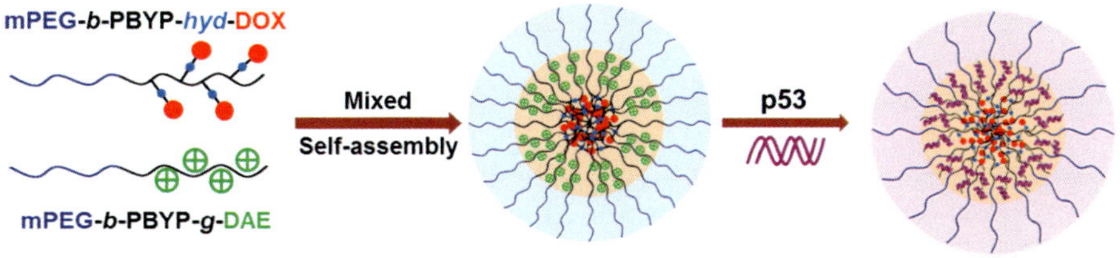


**Scheme 5** Preparation of hybrid micelles and hybrid micelles/p53 gene complex

where $m_{(\text{mPEG-}b\text{-PBYP-}hyd\text{-DOX})}$ and $m_{(\text{mPEG-}b\text{-PBYP-}g\text{-DAE})}$ represent the weights of the prodrug and the polycation carrier, respectively, while $m_{\text{p53gene}}$ represents the weight of p53 gene.

The average diameter, particle size distribution (size PDI), and zeta potential of the hybrid micelles and hybrid micelles/p53 gene nanoparticles at different N/P ratios were characterized by a dynamic light-scattering instrument (Zetasizer Nano ZS, Malvern, 90° collecting optics) at 25 °C. The morphologies of the nanoparticles self-assembled from the hybrid micelles were observed using a transmission electron microscope (TEM) instrument (HT7700, Hitachi) operated at 120 kV.

## 3.8 *In Vitro* Drug Release

The release of the DOX from the hybrid micelles containing the mPEG-*b*-PBYP-*hyd*-DOX prodrug was investigated in phosphate buffer solution under different conditions: pH 7.4, pH 6.0, pH 5.0, and pH 7.4 with PDE I (0.25 mg $mL^{-1}$), respectively. The prepared hybrid micelles (5 mL) were transferred into a dialysis bag (MWCO 12,000–14,000) and were soaked in 30 mL of phosphate buffer solution. Then, the solutions were placed into a constant temperature oscillation device at 37.5 °C. At set intervals, 5 mL of the solution was taken out and placed into a tube and stored in the dark, and then an equal volume of fresh buffer solution was added. The concentration of the released DOX was measured using a fluorescence spectrophotometer at an excitation wavelength of 480 nm and an emission wavelength of 520 nm to 620 nm, with the slit width set to 10 nm.

## 3.9 Gel Retardation Assay

The binding ability of the p53 gene and hybrid micelles was characterized by gel retardation assay. Hybrid micelle/p53 gene complexes of different N/P ratios were prepared as described above. A solution containing 10 μL of complex and 2 μL of 6× loading buffer was added into each well on a 1% agarose gel containing gel red (0.1 μL $mL^{-1}$) and ran in 0.5× Tris-boric acid-EDTA (TBE) running buffer at 90 V for 40 min. The results were visualized under UV (365 nm) light.

## 3.10 Cell Culture and Gene Supplier

L929 cells (mouse fibroblasts cells), A549 cells (human lung cancer cells), and H1299 cells (human lung cancer cells, derived from a metastatic state, in the absence of the p53 gene) were cultured in Roswell Park Memorial Institute (RPMI) 1640 medium with 10% fetal bovine serum (FBS) and 1% penicillin-streptomycin solution in a humidified atmosphere of 37 °C and 5% $CO_2$. The p53, GFP, and p53-GFP genes were obtained from Dr. Guanghui Wang at the College of Pharmaceutical Science at Soochow University.

## 3.11 *In Vitro* Cytotoxicity Assay

The cell toxicity of the hybrid micelles was characterized by MTT assay, using free DOX and free p53 genes as the controls, respectively. A549 cells and H1299 cells were seeded into 96-well plates at a density of $6 \times 10^3$ cells per well in 100 μL of RPMI 1640 medium containing 10% serum and 1% penicillin-streptomycin solution and incubated under a humidified atmosphere of 37 °C and 5% $CO_2$ for 12 h. Then, the nanoparticles at different concentrations were added into the treated wells. At the same time, the same volume of pure medium was added to the control wells and then incubated for another 48 h. Then, 25 μL of MTT solution (5 mg $mL^{-1}$ in PBS) prepared in advance was added into each well. After incubation for 4 h, the RPMI 1640 medium was removed and 150 μL DMSO was added into each well to dissolve the produced purple formazan. Finally, the optical density (OD) value at 570 nm of each well was measured using a microplate reader (Bio-Rad 680, USA). The cell viability was calculated using the formula: cell viability (%) = $(OD_{treated}/OD_{control}) \times 100$, where $OD_{treated}$ and $OD_{control}$ represent the OD values of the treated wells in the presence of samples and the control wells in the absence of samples, respectively. Data were presented as the average values with standard deviations.

## 3.12 *In Vitro* Transfection

*In vitro* transfection was performed in A549 cells. Cells ($15 \times 10^4$ cells) were seeded in Φ 35 mm glass bottom cell culture dishes and incubated for 12 h in 1 mL of RPMI 1640 medium at 37 °C under a 5% $CO_2$ atmosphere. The hybrid micelles were blended with the DNA of a green fluorescence protein (GFPDNA, 3 μg $mL^{-1}$ in PBS) at various N/P ratios for 30 min at 25 °C to form nanoparticles containing DOX and GFP-DNA. Subsequently, the samples were added to each well, gently mixed, and incubated for 6 h. After that, the RPMI 1640 medium containing the samples was removed and 1 mL of fresh medium was added. Then, the cells were incubated for 48 h at 37 °C under a 5% $CO_2$ atmosphere. Finally, the results of the transfection were captured by a live cell imaging system (CELL'R, Olympus).

## 3.13 Measurement of Cellular Uptake

The cell endocytosis and intracellular release behaviors of the nanoparticles against A549 cells were visualized with a live cell imaging system. First, A549 cells ($15 \times 10^4$ cells) were seeded in a Φ 35 mm glass bottom cell culture dish for 12 h. Then, the medium was removed, and the cells were washed three times with PBS and stained with H 33342 (10 mg $L^{-1}$) for 30 min and were then washed three times with PBS. Subsequently, the medium was replaced by fresh RPMI 1640 medium containing the hybrid micelle/p53-GFP gene complex (13.5 mg $L^{-1}$ of DOX, 3 mg $L^{-1}$ of p53-GFP genes). The culture dish was mounted into the incubation system of the live cell imaging system at 37 °C under 5% $CO_2$ atmosphere for 6 h. The images were then captured at an excitation wavelength of TRITC (red, 480 nm), DAPI (blue, 340 nm), and GREEN (520 nm, green).

The codelivery of DOX and GFP-DNA into A549 cells was investigated by fluorescence microscopy. The hybrid micelles were mixed with GFP-DNA at different N/P ratios to form various complexes. As shown in Fig. 1, the red (DOX) and green (GFP-DNA) fluorescence in the fluorescence microscopy images represent the direct accumulation of DOX and genes in the cells. Moreover, the appearance of green fluorescence demonstrates that the gene was successfully transfected after reaching the tumor cells.

The combination therapy of DOX and p53 gene could be used for the treatment of cancer. The key point of codelivery of gene and drug is to achieve combination therapeutic effect. In order to verify that the hybrid micelles/p53 gene nanoparticles were better than that of the individual prodrug mPEG-*b*-PBYP-*hyd*-DOX micelles or gene vector mPEG-*b*-PBYP-*g*-DAE/p53 gene complexes, the cell viability against A549 and H1299 cells was investigated using MTT assay. One can see from Fig. 2 that at the selected N/P ratio of 30, the mixed micelles/p53 complexes showed a stronger anticancer effect than those of mPEG-*b*-PBYP-*hyd*-DOX and mPEG-*b*-PBYP-*g*-DAE/p53 complexes for two different cells, which was attributed to the combination therapy of DOX and p53 gene. To summarize, the above experimental results showed that p53 gene and DOX-coloaded nanoparticles have a synergistic inhibitory effect of drug and gene on lung cancer cells.

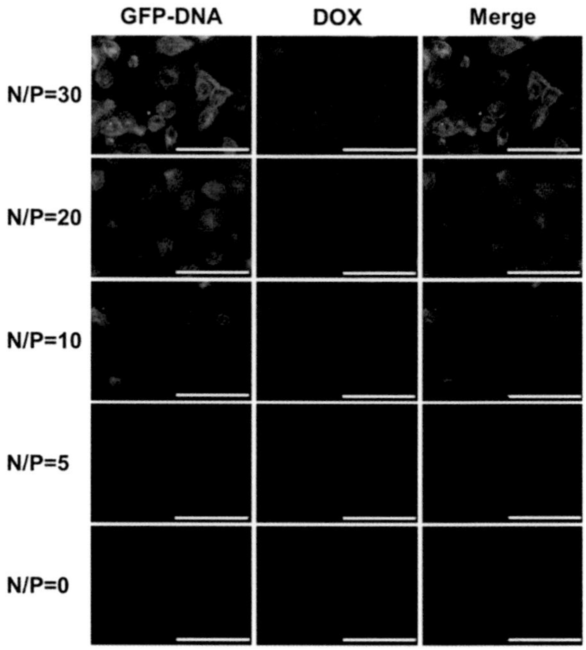


**Fig. 1** Fluorescence images of A549 cells incubated with the hybrid micelles/GFP-DNA complexes with different N/P ratios. For each panel, the images from left to right showed fluorescence of GFP (green), DOX (red), and the overlays of two images. The dosage of GFP-DNA was 3.0 mg $L^{-1}$. The scale bars corresponded to 50 μm in all images

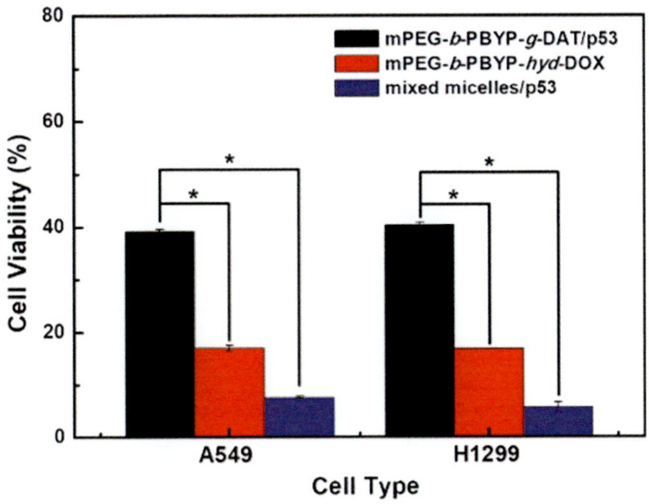


**Fig. 2** Cell viability of A549 cells and H1299 cells treated with different micelles at N/P ratios=30 for 48 h incubation (*$p < 0.05$)

## 3.14 Intracellular Release of DOX and p53 Genes

To demonstrate whether the nanoparticles could be efficiently internalized into tumor cells and increased intracellular drug accumulation and gene transfection, the cellular uptake and intracellular drug and gene release behaviors of hybrid micelles/p53-GFP genes nanoparticles were monitored using a live cell imaging system, which could simultaneously record the dynamic uptake process and the variation of fluorescence intensity inside A549 cells. Before the measurement, the cell nuclei were stained with H 33342 (blue), and the DOX is a fluorescent molecule, and p53-GFP gene could translate into fluorescence protein whose emission can be directly used to visualize cellular uptake without additional fluorescent probes.

As shown in Fig. 3A, when A549 cells were treated with mixed micelles/p53-GFP gene nanoparticles for 1 h, the red and blue fluorescence in cytoplasm could be observed. As time goes on, the intensity of fluorescence increased gradually, and the stronger fluorescence appeared in the nucleus. After 5 h incubation, the results demonstrated that the most nanoparticles were internalized by A549 cells via endocytosis. In contrast, the fluorescence intensity of A549 cells that were separately incubated with free DOX and free p53-GFP was weak, as shown in Fig. 3B. This is because the DOX enters into tumor cells by a diffusion process and passes through the cell membrane through a concentration gradient. Therefore, free drugs are easy to enter and escape from the tumor cells (Dai et al. 2011). Moreover, free p53 gene would be generally decomposed directly, and unable to replicate, survive stably, and express itself when entering cells. So it has stronger fluorescence intensity when incubated with hybrid nanoparticles than free DOX and free p53-GFP gene. All of

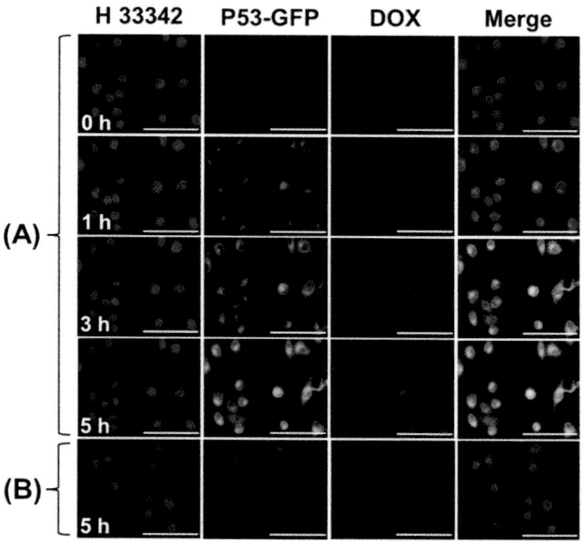


**Fig. 3** Live cell imaging system images of A549 cells incubated with: (**A**) the hybrid micelles/p53-GFP complex; and (**B**) free p53-GFP (DOX dosage was 13.5 mg $L^{-1}$, p53-GFP gene dosage was 3.0 mg $L^{-1}$, and weight ratio was 30) for different times. For each panel, images from left to right showed the cell nuclei stained with H 33342 (blue), the DOX fluorescence in cells (red), the GFP fluorescence in cell (green), and overlays of the blue, green, and red images. The scale bars were 100 μm in all images

these results illustrated that the hybrid micelles/p53-GFP gene could keep longer period to accumulate more drugs and genes in the lung tumor cells.

## 4 Notes

(1) Sodium azide ($NaN_3$) should be used carefully during the experiment (Preparation of pH-Responsive Doxorubicin Derivative DOX-*hyd*-$N_3$) to prevent explosion.
(2) Since phosphorous trichloride ($PCl_3$) is highly hygroscopic and reactive, it should be used in the experiment (Preparation of Cyclic Phosphoester Monomer BYP) right after it is distilled.
(3) The cyclic phosphoester molecules, such as 2-chloro-1,3,2-dioxaphospholane (CP), 2-chloro-2-oxo- 1,3,2-dioxaphospholane (COP), and 2-(but-3-yn-1-yloxy)-2-oxo-1,3,2-dioxaphospholane (BYP), should be sealed and stored in an inert atmosphere at −20 °C.
(4) When using hydrazine hydrate ($N_2H_4$ $H_2O$), prevent the vapor from leaking and being inhaled.
(5) Doxorubicin is a fluorescence molecule and should be handled in the dark.

## 5 Conclusion

This protocol introduces the preparations of pH-responsive prodrugs and p53 gene vectors for assembling into hybrid micelles and for coloading antitumor drug DOX and p53 gene. The methods mainly consist of the preparations of biodegradable polyphophoester-based copolymer, click reaction, and postmodification of copolymer, involving in various synthesis methods and self-assembly. In order to achieve the purpose of coordinated release of drugs and genes, the preparation of pH-sensitive prodrugs and the process of gene transfection are key steps. During selection of the preparation methods, the following factors should be considered: (i) the yield rate of the linking reaction between the alkynyl and azide groups, (ii) difficulty in purifying prodrug and polycation, (iii) repeatability and reproducibility of reaction, and (iv) whether the polymers can be biodegraded or not. The ideal synthesis method should have a higher yield and be conducive to self-assembly to load gene. Preferably, the operation is simple and easy to achieve. It is important to select an appropriate synthesis method based on the expected use and intended effect in the actual operation.

## References


Bildstein L, Dubernet C, Couvreur P (2011) Prodrug-based intracellular delivery of anticancer agents. Adv Drug Deliver Rev 63:3–23.

Cao DL, He JL, Xu JY, Zhang MZ, Zhao L, Duan GX, Cao YW, Zhou RH, Ni PH (2016) Polymeric prodrugs conjugated with reduction-sensitive dextran–camptothecin and pH-responsive dextran–doxorubicin: an effective combinatorial drug delivery platform for cancer therapy. Polym Chem 7:4198–4212

Chan JMW, Tan JPK, Engler AC, Ke XY, Gao SJ, Yang CA, Sardon H, Yang YY, Hedrick JL (2016) Organocatalytic anticancer drug loading of degradable polymeric mixed micelles via a biomimetic mechanism. Macromolecules 49:2013–2021

Chen XJ, Parelkar SS, Henchey E, Schneider S, Emrick T (2012) PolyMPC−Doxorubicin prodrugs. Bioconjug Chem *23*:1753–1763

Chenau J, Michelland S, de Fraipont F, Josserand V, Coll JL, Favrot MC, Seve M (2009) The cell line secretome, a suitable tool for investigating proteins released in vivo by tumors. Application to the study of p53-modulated proteins secreted in lung cancer Cells. J Proteome Res 8:4579–4591

Dai J, Lin SD, Cheng D, Zou SY, Shuai XT (2011) Interlayer-crosslinked micelle with partially hydrated core showing reduction and pH dual sensitivity for pinpointed intracellular drug release. Angew Chem Int Ed 50:9404–9408

Delplace V, Couvreur P, Nicolas J (2014) Recent trends in the design of anticancer polymer prodrug nanocarriers. Polym Chem 5:1529–1544

Ding XW, Liu Y, Li JH, Luo Z, Hu Y, Zhang BL, Liu JJ, Zhou J, Cai KY (2014) Hydrazone-bearing PMMA-functionalized magnetic nanocubes as pH-responsive drug carriers for remotely targeted cancer therapy in vitro and in vivo. ACS Appl Mater Interfaces 6:7395–7407

Fisher MD, Swisher SG, Nemunaitis J, Cunningham C (2001) Strategies to restore p53 function in patients with lung cancer. Clin Lung Cancer 3:99–101

Huang FS, Cheng R, Meng FH, Deng C, Zhong ZY (2015) Micelles based on acid degradable poly (acetal urethane): preparation, pH-sensitivity, and triggered intracellular drug release. Biomacromolecules 16:2228–2236

Jemal A, Bray F, Center MM, Ferlay J, Ward E, Forman D (2011) Global cancer statistics. CA Cancer J Clin 61:69–90

Jin Y, Song L, Su Y, Zhu LJ, Pang Y, Qiu F, Tong GS, Yan DY, Zhu BS, Zhu XY (2011) Oxime linkage: a robust tool for the design of pH-sensitive polymeric drug carriers. Biomacromolecules 12:3460–3468

Kim SS, Rait A, Kim E, Pirollo KF, Nishida M, Farkas N, Dagata JA, Chang EH (2014) A nanoparticle carrying the p53 gene targets tumors including cancer stem cells, sensitizes glioblastoma to chemotherapy and improves survival. ACS Nano 8:5494–5514

Lane DP, Cheok CF, Lain S (2010) p53-based cancer therapy. Cold Spring Harbor Perspect Boil 2: a001222

Li ZY, Zhang L, Li QS (2015a) Induction of apoptosis in cancer cells through N-acetyl-l-leucine-modified polyethylenimine-mediated p53 genedelivery. Colloids Surf B 135:630–638

Li YM, Xu B, Bai T, Liu WG (2015b) Co-delivery of doxorubicin and tumor-suppressing p53 gene using a POSS-based star-shaped polymer for cancer therapy. Biomaterials 55:12–23

Libiszowski J., Kaluzynski K., Penczek S (1978) Polymerization of cyclic esters of phosphoric acid. VI. Poly(alkly ethylene phosphates). Polymerization of 2-alkoxy-2-oxo-1,3,2-dioxaphospholans and structure of polymers. J Polym Sci Part A-Polym Chem 16:1275–1283

Lim YH, Heo GS, Cho S, Wooley KL (2013) Construction of a reactive diblock copolymer, polyphosphoester-*block*-poly(l-lactide), as a versatile framework for functional materials that are capable of full degradation. ACS Macro Lett 2:785–789

Lim YH, Tiemann KM, Heo GS, Wagers PO, Rezenom YH, Zhang SY, Zhang FW, Youngs WJ, Hunstad DA, Wooley KL (2015) Preparation and in vitro antimicrobial activity of silver-bearing degradable polymeric nanoparticles of polyphosphoester-*block*-poly(L-lactide). ACS Nano 9: 1995–2008

Liu J, He JL, Zhang MZ, Xu GQ, Ni PH (2018) A synergistic polyphosphoester-based co-delivery system of the anticancer drug doxorubicin and the tumor suppressor gene p53 for lung cancer therapy. J Mater Chem B 6:3262–3273

Li F, He JL, Zhang MZ, Ni PH (2015c) A pH-sensitive and biodegradable supramolecular hydrogel constructed from a PEGylated polyphosphoester-doxorubicin prodrug and α-cyclodextrin. Polym Chem 6:5009–5014

Pang X, Jiang Y, Xiao QC, Leung AW, Hua HY, Xu CS (2016) pH-responsive polymer–drug conjugates: design and progress. J Control Release 222:116–129

Steinbach T, Wurm FR (2015) Poly(phosphoester)s: a new platform for degradable polymers. Angew Chem Int Ed 54:6098–6108

Steinbach T, Schröder R, Ritz S, Wurm FR (2013) Microstructure analysis of biocompatible phosphoester copolymers. Polym Chem 4:4469–4479

Szymañska K, Hainaut P (2003) TP53 and mutations in human cancer. Acta Biochim Pol 50:231–238

Tseng SJ, Liao ZX, Kao SH, Zeng YF, Huang KY, Li HJ, Yang CL, Deng YF, Huang CF, Yang SC, Yang PC, Kempson IM (2015) Highly specific in vivo gene delivery for p53-mediated apoptosis and genetic photodynamic therapies of tumour. Nat Commun 6:6456

Torre LA, Bray F, Siegel RL, Ferlay J, Lortet-Tieulent J, Jemal A (2015) Global cancer statistics, 2012. CA Cancer J Clin 65:87–108

Wang HY, Wang HX, Liang JM, Jiang YF, Guo QQ, Peng HG, Xu Q, Huang YZ (2014) Cell-penetrating apoptotic peptide/p53 DNA nanocomplex as adjuvant therapy for drug-resistant breast cancer. Mol Pharm 11:3352–3360

Xu QX, Leong JY, Chua QY, Chi YT, Chow PKH, Pack DW, Wang CH (2013) Combined modality doxorubicin-based chemotherapy and chitosan-mediated p53 gene therapy using double-walled microspheres for treatment of human hepatocellular carcinoma. Biomaterials 34:5149–5162

Yang QQ, Yang Y, Li L, Sun W, Zhu X, Huang Y (2015) Polymeric nanomedicine for tumor-targeted combination therapy to elicit synergistic genotoxicity against prostate cancer. ACS Appl Mater Interfaces 7:6661–6673

Zan MH, Li JJ, Luo SZ, Ge ZS (2014) Dual pH-triggered multistage drug delivery systems based on host–guest interaction-associated polymeric nanogels. Chem Commun 50:7824–7827

Zeng X, Sun YX, Qu W, Zhang XZ, Zhuo RX (2010) Biotinylated transferrin/avidin/biotinylated disulfide containing PEI bioconjugates mediated p53 gene delivery system for tumor targeted transfection. Biomaterials 31:4771–4780

Zhang W, Shen JL, Su H, Mu G, Sun JH, Tan CP, Liang XJ, Ji LN, Mao ZW (2016) Co-Delivery of cisplatin prodrug and chlorin e6 by mesoporous silica nanoparticles for chemo-photodynamic combination therapy to combat drug resistance. ACS Appl Mater Interfaces 8:13332–13340

Zhang SY, Zou J, Zhang FW, Elsabahy M, Felder SE, Zhu JH, Pochan DJ, Wooley KL (2012a) Rapid and versatile construction of diverse and functional nanostructures derived from a polyphosphoester-based biomimetic block copolymer system. J Am Chem Soc 134: 18467–18474

Zhang SY, Li A, Zou J, Lin LY, Wooley KL (2012b) Facile synthesis of clickable, water-soluble, and degradable polyphosphoesters. ACS Macro Lett 1:328–333

Zhang QQ, He JL, Zhang MZ, Ni PH (2015) A polyphosphoester-conjugated camptothecin prodrug with disulfide linkage for potent reduction-triggered drug delivery. J Mater Chem B 3:4922–4932

Zhao D, Liu CJ, Zhuo RX, Cheng SX (2012) Alginate/$CaCO_3$ hybrid nanoparticles for efficient codelivery of antitumor gene and drug. Mol Pharmaceutics 9:2887–2893

# Preparation and Evaluation of siRNAsome as siRNA and Drug Delivery System 27

T. Jiang, M. Zheng, and Bingyang Shi

## Contents




T. Jiang · M. Zheng
Henan-Macquarie University Joint Centre for Biomedical Innovation, School of Life Sciences, Henan University, Kaifeng, China

Henan Key Laboratory of Brain Targeted Bio-nanomedicine, School of Life Sciences & School of Pharmacy, Henan University, Kaifeng, China
e-mail: mzheng@henu.edu.cn

B. Shi (✉)
Henan-Macquarie University Joint Centre for Biomedical Innovation, School of Life Sciences, Henan University, Kaifeng, China

Henan Key Laboratory of Brain Targeted Bio-nanomedicine, School of Life Sciences & School of Pharmacy, Henan University, Kaifeng, China

Department of Biomedical Sciences, Faculty of Medicine & Health Sciences, Macquarie University, Sydney, NSW, Australia
e-mail: bs@henu.edu.cn





H. Tian and X. Chen (eds.), *Gene Delivery*, Biomaterial Engineering,
https://doi.org/10.1007/978-981-16-5419-0_28

**Abstract**

Spherical nucleic acids (SNA) show great potential for gene regulation. However, lack of suitable SNA nanostructure to codeliver small interfering RNA (siRNA) and chemotherapeutic drug to treat cancer is still challenged. Here, we described the preparation of a novel SNA, siRNAsome, which can be prepared by the self-assembly of siRNA-disulfide-poly(N-isopropylacrylamide) (siRNA-SS-PNIPAM) diblock copolymers. This siRNAsome is capable of loading both hydrophilic and hydrophobic drugs while attaching the functional siRNA as both stabilizing shell and gene regulator. In addition, we also applied the reduction-responsive property onto this SNA, to enable its accumulative release of the attached siRNA and loaded drugs intracellularly. In this chapter, methods for siRNA-SS-PNIPAM diblock polymer synthesis, siRNAsome nanoparticle formation, biophysical characterization, and in vitro and in vivo evaluation of these siRNAsomes are described. Our results showed that, when such siRNAsomes are loaded with doxorubicin hydrochloride (DOX·HCl) and P-glycoprotein (Pgp) siRNA, which targets the Pgp drug exporter, synergistic therapy on multidrug-resistant (MDR) cancer cells is achieved.

**Keywords**

siRNAsome · Vesicle · siRNA · Drug delivery · Spherical nucleic acids

## 1 Introduction

Spherical nucleic acids (SNA) are a three-dimensional nanostructure commonly composed of a nanoparticle core and a highly oriented nucleic acid shell (Cutler et al. 2011, 2012). Compared with linear nucleic acids, which cannot readily enter cells without the assistance of transfection agents, the SNA structure is recognized by Class A scavenger receptors and has been demonstrated to be taken up rapidly by almost all cell types with no requirement of ancillary transfection agents (Patel et al. 2010; Choi et al. 2013; Mokhtarzadeh et al. 2019). Moreover, SNA protects immobilized nucleic acids from potent enzymatic digestion (Seferos et al. 2009), in sharp contrast to linear nucleic acids that suffer from rapid nuclease degradation in the blood (Zheng et al. 2018). Thus, these superior properties endow SNAs with high potential for gene manipulation via RNA interference (RNAi) pathways to disease treatment with no cocarrier-induced cytotoxicity and immunogenicity.

It is hypothesized that the codelivery of siRNA and small molecular drugs can allow one to independently access gene and protein targets, thereby circumventing drug resistance (Yu et al. 2012; Lu et al. 2016; Zheng et al. 2019), which is incompetent by one-dimensional therapeutic strategies. Yet, not enough SNA nanoparticles have been employed to codeliver siRNAs and small molecular drugs, due to the lack of suitable SNA nanostructures. To date, most frequently reported SNAs nanostructures are built with an inorganic core, such as gold (Rosi et al. 2006), silver (Lee et al. 2007), and quantum dots (Mitchell et al. 1999). These SNAs cores do not play a significant role but contribute to a nonbioresorbable metallic mass and are unable to be utilized as a reservoir for payload molecules, extremely limiting the full use of the entire nanostructure to realize the codelivery of siRNA and other drugs. Recently, drug-cored (Tan et al. 2015; Tan et al. 2016; Guo et al. 2019) or drug-loaded micellar SNAs (Zhu et al. 2018), in which drugs are anchored or encapsulated inside a polymer core together with a nucleic acid-immobilizing shell, represents a promising approach for nucleic acid and drug codelivery with no cationic materials. Nevertheless, the hydrophobic micellar core of these micellar SNA only allows loading of hydrophobic small molecules, excluding a myriad of hydrophilic molecules. Consequently, developing a kind of SNA that is capable of loading both hydrophobic and hydrophilic drugs is highly desired.

In this protocol, we described the preparation of a novel SNA nanostructure, siRNAsome (Zheng et al. 2019), which originated from the self-assembly of siRNA-disulfide-poly(N-isopropylacrylamide) (siRNA-SS-PNIPAM) diblock copolymers (Fig. 1). The siRNAsome consists of a hydrophilic siRNA stabilization shell, a temperature and intracellular reduction-sensitive hydrophobic median layer, and an empty aqueous interior. Notably, like polymersome performed (Meng and Zhong 2011; Lee and Feijen 2012), these siRNAsomes are capable of encapsulating biomacromolecules and hydrophilic drugs in its watery interior, and hydrophobic drugs in its hydrophobic membranes. Moreover, these siRNAsomes can also effectively release the attached siRNA and encapsulated drugs results from the cleavage of disulfide linker in the intracellular reduction milieu. In this chapter, not only the methods for siRNA-SS-PNIPAM copolymer synthesis, siRNAsome nanoparticle formation and characterization, are described in detail, but the evaluations of its reduction responsiveness, cellular uptake, gene silencing ability, biocompatibility, and therapeutic efficacy were also performed. Results showed these siRNAsomes are capable of overcoming DOX resistance in multidrug-resistant (MDR) cancer cells by codelivering doxorubicin hydrochloride (DOX·HCl) and siRNA that targets the P-glycoprotein (Pgp) drug exporter, inducing effective synergistic effect for cancer therapy.

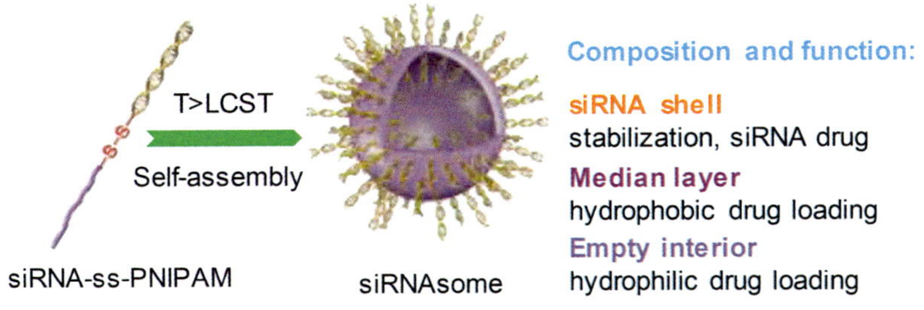


**Fig. 1** Illustration of siRNAsome formation, composition, and function. (Adapted from Zheng et al. 2019, with permission)

# 2 Materials

## 2.1 Synthesis and Characterization of siRNA-SS-PNIPAM

### 2.1.1 Synthesis of 2-(2-Pyridyldithio)Ethylamine Hydrochloride

1. 2-Mercaptoethylamine hydrochloride (Sigma-Aldrich)
2. Pyridine disulfide (Sigma-Aldrich)
3. Methanol (analytical grade)
4. Separatory funnel
5. Round-bottom flask
6. Magnetic stirrer
7. Rotary vacuum evaporator
8. Ethyl ether (analytical grade)
9. Isopropanol (analytical grade)
10. Deionized water (Milli-Q water)
11. Micropore filter membrane (0.2 μm)
12. Vacuum pump
13. Vacuum drying oven
14. Varian Inova Unity 400 NMR Spectrometer

### 2.1.2 Synthesis of Poly(N-Isopropylacrylamide) (PNIPAM)

1. N-isopropylacrylamide (NIPAM, Sigma-Aldrich)
2. 4-Cyano-4-(dodecylsulfanylthiocarbonyl)sulfanylpentanoic acid (DCT, a kind of reversible addition-fragmentation chain transfer (RAFT) polymerization agent, J&K Scientific)
3. 2,2′-Azobis(2-methylpropionitrile) (AIBN)
4. 1,4-dioxane (analytical grade)
5. Reaction tube
6. Oil bath
7. Magnetic stirrer
8. Hexanes (analytical grade)
9. Micropore filter membrane (0.2 μm)
10. Vacuum drying oven
11. Vacuum pump
12. Varian Inova Unity 400 NMR Spectrometer

### 2.1.3 Synthesis of PNIPAM-SS-Py

1. PNIPAM (from Sect. 2.1.2)
2. N-hydroxysuccinimide (NHS, Alfa Aesar)
3. N, N′-dicyclohexylcarbodiimide (DCC, Alfa Aesar)
4. Anhydrous dichloromethane (DCM, analytical grade)
5. Round-bottom flask

6. 2-(2-pyridyldithio)ethylamine hydrochloride (from Sect. 2.1.2)
7. Triethylamine (TEA, analytical grade)
8. Magnetic stirrer
9. Rotary vacuum evaporator
10. Ethyl ether
11. Micropore filter membrane (0.2 μm)
12. Vacuum drying oven
13. Dimethyl sulfoxide (DMSO, analytical grade)
14. Deionized water (Milli-Q water)
15. Vacuum freeze drier
16. Vacuum pump
17. Varian Inova Unity 400 NMR Spectrometer

### 2.1.4 Synthesis of siRNA-SS-PNIPAM

1. Thiol-terminated siRNA (GenePharma Co., Ltd. China)
2. Diethyl pyrocarbonate (DEPC) water
3. Acetic acid glacial (analytical grade)
4. DMSO (analytical grade)
5. RNase-free microcentrifuge tube
6. PNIPAM-SS-Py (from Sect. 2.1.3)
7. Deionized water (Milli-Q water)
8. Isopropanol (analytical grade)
9. Centrifuge

### 2.1.5 Characterization of siRNA-SS-PNIPAM

#### Ultraperformance Liquid Chromatography (UPLC) Analysis

1. Fluorescein isothiocyanate isomer I (FITC)-modified PNIPAM (FITC-PNIPAM)
2. siRNA (GenePharma Co., Ltd. China)
3. FITC-modified siRNA-SS-PNIPAM
4. Waters ACQUITY UPLC XEVO TQD system with ultraviolet/ visible (UV/ vis) detector
5. ACQUITY UPLC Peptide BEH 300 C18 column (1.7 μm, 2.1 mm × 50 mm)
6. 0.1 M triethylammonium acetate (TEAA, pH 7.0)
7. Acetonitrile (chromatographic grade)

#### Lower Critical Solution Temperature (LCST) of siRNA-SS-PNIPAM

1. siRNA-SS-PNIPAM (from Sect. 2.1.4)
2. 4-(2-hydroxyerhyl)piperazine-1-erhanesulfonic acid (HEPES) buffer (10 mM, pH 7.4)
3. Zetasizer Nano ZS instrument (Malvern Instruments, Worcestershire, UK), equipped with He-Ne laser (10 mW, 633 nm wavelength)
4. Low-volume quartz cuvette (ZEN3600, Malvern Instruments)

## 2.2 Formation and Characterization of siRNAsome

1. siRNA-SS-PNIPAM
2. HEPES buffer (10 mM, pH 7.4)
3. Incubator
4. Zetasizer Nano ZS instrument (Malvern Instruments, Worcestershire, UK), equipped with He-Ne laser (10 mW, 633 nm wavelength)
5. Low-volume quartz cuvette (ZEN3600, Malvern Instruments)
6. Transmission electron microscope (TEM, JEM-2100, JEOL, Tokyo, Japan)
7. 3 mm-mesh copper grids coated with carbon films
8. Uranyl acetate solution (1% w/v)
9. 2% agarose
10. Preheated 1 × TAE buffer
11. Gel electrophoresis equipment

## 2.3 Drug Encapsulation by siRNAsome

1. Doxorubicin hydrochloride (DOX·HCl)
2. Docetaxel (DTX)
3. DMSO
4. FITC-modified bovine serum albumin (FITC-BSA)
5. HEPES buffer
6. siRNA-SS-PNIPAM
7. DEPC water
8. 3.5 kDa and 250 kDa dialysis bag
9. SpectraMax i3x multimode microplate reader
10. Agilent 1260 Infinity HPLC system (Agilent Technologies, USA)
11. Sepax GP-C18 column (5 μm, 150 mm × 4.6 mm)
12. Acetonitrile (chromatographic grade)
13. Deionized water (Milli-Q water)
14. Micropore filter membrane (0.2 μm)
15. Bicinchoninic acid (BCA) protein assay kit

## 2.4 Reduction Responsiveness of siRNAsome

### 2.4.1 Size, Morphology Change, and siRNA Release

1. siRNAsome
2. DL-1,4-Dithiothreitol (DTT)
3. HEPES buffer (pH 7.4)
4. Zetasizer Nano ZS instrument (Malvern Instruments, Worcestershire, UK), equipped with He-Ne laser (10 mW, 633 nm wavelength)
5. Low-volume quartz cuvette (ZEN3600, Malvern Instruments)
6. TEM (JEM-2100, JEOL, Tokyo, Japan)

7. 2% agarose
8. Preheated 1 × TAE buffer
9. Gel electrophoresis equipment

#### 2.4.2 In Vitro DOX·HCl Release

1. DOX·HCl
2. siRNAsome
3. DTT
4. Phosphate-buffered saline (PBS) (137 mM NaCl, 2.7 mM KCl, 8 mM $Na_2HPO_4$, and 2 mM $KH_2PO_4$, pH 7.4)
5. Dialysis bag (MWCO 12,000)
6. Microcentrifuge tube
7. Fluorescence meter (FLS920) measurement (excitation at 480 nm)

### 2.5 In Vitro Evaluation of siRNAsome

#### 2.5.1 Flow Cytometry Assay

1. Multiple drug resistance (MDR) MCF-7 cell lines
2. 6-well culture plates
3. Dulbecco's modification of Eagle's medium (DMEM)
4. Penicillin-streptomycin solution
5. Heat-inactivated fetal bovine serum (FBS)
6. PBS (pH 7.4)
7. Free 5-carboxyfluorescein (FAM)-labeled siRNA
8. FAM-labeled siRNAsome
9. $CO_2$ cell incubator
10. 0.25% trypsin-EDTA
11. Vertical flow clean bench
12. Optical microscope
13. Flow cytometry (FACS Calibur, BD Bioscience, USA)

#### 2.5.2 Confocal Laser-Scanning Microscopy Assay

1. MDR MCF-7 cell lines
2. 24-well glass bottom plates
3. DMEM
4. Penicillin-streptomycin solution
5. FBS
6. PBS (pH 7.4)
7. Free FAM-siRNA
8. FAM-siRNAsome
9. 4% paraformaldehyde solution
10. 4′,6-diamidino-2-phenylindole (DAPI)
11. $CO_2$ cell incubator

12. Vertical flow clean bench
13. Confocal laser-scanning microscope (Leica SP8)

#### 2.5.3 In Vitro Cytotoxicity Assay of siRNAsome

1. MDR MCF-7 cell lines
2. 96-well culture plates
3. DMEM
4. Penicillin-streptomycin solution
5. FBS
6. PBS (pH 7.4)
7. siNRAsome
8. 3-[4,5-dimethylthiazol-2-yl]-3,5-diphenyltetrazolium bromide (MTT) solution
9. DMSO
10. $CO_2$ cell incubator
11. Vertical flow clean bench
12. SpectraMax i3x multimode microplate reader

#### 2.5.4 Real-Time Quantitative PCR Analysis

1. MDR MCF-7 cell lines
2. 6-well culture plates
3. DMEM
4. Penicillin-streptomycin solution
5. FBS
6. PBS (pH 7.4)
7. Free siRNA
8. Scramble (nonspecific) siRNA-based siRNAsome (Scr-siRNAsome)
9. P-glycoprotein (Pgp)-specific siRNA-based siRNAsome (Pgp-siRNAsome)
10. 0.25% trypsin-EDTA
11. RNAprep pure Cell/Bacteria Kit (Tiangen Biotech., Beijing, China)
12. PrimeScript RT Reagent Kit (Takara, Kyoto, Japan)
13. TB Green™ Premix Ex Taq™ (Takara, Kyoto, Japan)
14. $CO_2$ cell incubator
15. Vertical flow clean bench
16. Roche Light Cycle 480 Real-Time PCR instrument

### 2.6 In Vitro and In Vivo Evaluation of DOX·HCl-Loaded siRNAsome

#### 2.6.1 MTT Assay

1. MDR MCF-7 cell lines
2. 96-well culture plates
3. DMEM
4. Penicillin-streptomycin solution
5. FBS

6. PBS (pH 7.4)
7. Free DOX·HCl
8. Scr-siRNAsome loaded with DOX·HCl
9. Pgp-siNRAsome loaded with DOX·HCl
10. MTT solution
11. DMSO
12. $CO_2$ cell incubator
13. Vertical flow clean bench
14. SpectraMax i3x multimode microplate reader

#### 2.6.2 In Vivo Antitumor Assay in Subcutaneous MDR MCF-7 Tumor Model

1. Female BALB/c nude mice aged 6–8 weeks (18 ~ 21 g)
2. MDR MCF-7 cells
3. PBS (pH 7.4)
4. Free DOX·HCl
5. Scr-siRNAsome loaded with DOX·HCl.
6. Pgp-siNRAsome loaded with DOX·HCl
7. Vernier caliper
8. Mice-weighing scale
9. Syringe

## 3 Methods

### 3.1 Synthesis and Characterization of siRNA-SS-PNIPAM

#### 3.1.1 Synthesis of 2-(2-Pyridyldithio)Ethylamine Hydrochloride (Wang et al. 2016)

1. Dissolve 2-mercaptoethylamine hydrochloride (1.05 g, 10.0 mmol) and pyridine disulfide (6.6 g, 30.0 mmol) in 20 mL and 50 mL methanol at 0 °C, respectively (see Note 1).
2. Add the 2-mercaptoethylamine hydrochloride solution dropwise into the pyridine disulfide solution in a 150 mL round-bottom flask.
3. Stir the reaction mixture at ambient temperature with nitrogen atmosphere for 12 h.
4. Concentrate the reaction mixture to around 10 mL by rotary evaporator.
5. Precipitate the reaction mixture in cold ethyl ether (150 mL) three times (see Note 2).
6. Dissolve the precipitation in isopropanol/$H_2O$ (8/1, v/v) mixture and then maintain at −20 °C. The product was obtained as a white crystalline solid after recrystallization (see Note 3).
7. Filter the crystal through a micropore filter membrane (0.2 μm) via a vacuum pump and dry in a vacuum drying oven at 30 °C.
8. Confirm the structure of the product with $^1H$ NMR.

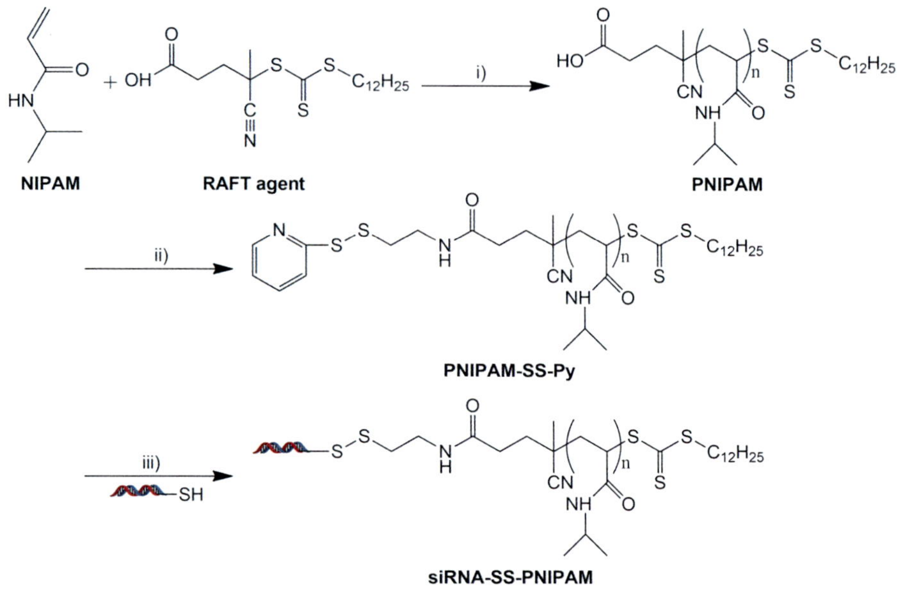


**Fig. 2** Synthetic pathway for siRNA-SS-PNIPAM. Conditions: (i) AIBN initiator, 1, 4-dioxane, 70 °C, 24 h; (ii) 2-(2-pyridyldithio)ethylamine, DCC/ NHS, DCM, room temperature, 24 h; and (iii) DMSO, 37 °C, 48 h. (Adapted from Zheng et al. 2019, with permission)

### 3.1.2 Synthesis of Poly(N-isopropylacrylamide) (PNIPAM, 19 kDa, Fig. 2(i)) (Li et al. 2010)

1. Purge with nitrogen for 30 min in a 50 mL reaction tube.
2. Add NIPAM monomer (1.00 g, 8.84 mmol), DCT (RAFT reagent, 17.8 mg, 0.044 mmol), and AIBN initiator (1.45 mg, 8.84 μmol) into 15 mL 1,4-dioxane solution in a reaction tube (see Note 4).
3. Seal and place the reaction tube in a preheated oil bath at 70 °C.
4. Stir the reaction tube for 24 h under nitrogen atmosphere.
5. Cease the polymerization reaction by rapid cooling and expose the polymerization solution to air.
6. Precipitate the polymerization solution in cold hexanes (225 mL) three times (see Note 5).
7. Collect the product by filter through a micropore membrane filter (0.2 μm) via a vacuum pump and dry in a vacuum drying oven at 30 °C.
8. Confirm the structure of the product with $^1$H NMR.

### 3.1.3 Synthesis of PNIPAM-SS-Py (Fig. 2(ii)) (Xu et al. 2009)

1. Purge with nitrogen for 30 mins in a 250 mL round-bottom flask.
2. Dissolve PNIPAM (0.5 g, 0.026 mmol), NHS (12.11 mg, 0.105 mmol), and DCC (21.72 mg, 0.105 mmol) in 100 mL of anhydrous dichloromethane solution in a round-bottom flask at 4 °C.

3. Let the solution react at room temperature for 20 h; then add 2-(2-pyridyldithio) ethylamine hydrochloride (17.56 mg, 0.079 mmol) and triethylamine (TEA, 21.30 mg, 0.211 mmol), and react at ambient temperature for another 24 h (see Note 6).
4. Concentrate the solution by rotary evaporator to around 10 mL, and precipitate the reaction solution in cold diethyl ether (150 mL) three times (see Note 2).
5. Collect the precipitate by filter through a micropore membrane filter (0.2 μm) via a vacuum pump and dry in a vacuum drying oven at 30 °C.
6. Dissolve the precipitate in 5 mL of DMSO and dialyze against Milli-Q water for 48 h (see Note 7).
7. Obtain the final product by lyophilization for 24 h.
8. Confirm the structure of the product with $^1$H NMR.

### 3.1.4 Synthesis of siRNA-SS-PNIPAM (Fig. 2(iii))

1. Dissolve thiol-terminated siRNA (100 μg, 7.58 nmol) in 20 μL DEPC aqueous solution (see Note 8).
2. Add thiol-terminated siRNA aqueous solution and 2 μL acetic acid glacial into 200 μL DMSO in a 1.5 mL RNase-free microcentrifuge tube.
3. Dissolve PNIPAM-SS-Py (19 kDa) (7.20 mg, 0.38 μmol) into the mixed solution.
4. Purge with nitrogen for 15 mins, and shake the reaction mixture at 37 °C for 48 h.
5. Dialyze the reaction solution against preheated Milli-Q water at 37 °C for 0.5 h to remove DMSO.
6. Add DEPC water to 1 mL and incubate at 37 °C for 0.5 h, then centrifuge 3 times (15,000 rpm, 20 min) to remove unreacted free siRNA.
7. Add 500 μL DEPC water and 350 μl isopropanol into the centrifuge tube, incubate at room temperature for 20 min, and centrifuge for 15 min at 10000 rpm.
8. Remove the supernatant-containing unreacted PNIPAM carefully and dialyze against Milli-Q water for 48 h to get the final product of siRNA-SS-PNIPAM (see Note 7).

### 3.1.5 Characterization of siRNA-SS-PNIPAM

#### Ultraperformance Liquid Chromatography (UPLC) Analysis

Analyze fluorescein isothiocyanate isomer I (FITC)-modified PNIPAM (FITC-PNIPAM), free siRNA, and FITC-labeled siRNA-SS-PNIPAM using a Waters ACQUITY UPLC XEVO TQD system, which is equipped with ACQUITY UPLC Peptide BEH 300 C18 column (1.7 μm, 2.1 mm × 50 mm) and ultraviolet/ visible (UV/vis) detector (see Note 9).

#### Lower Critical Solution Temperature (LCST) of siRNA-SS-PNIPAM

1. Determine the LCST of siRNA-SS-PNIPAM in terms of particle size using a Zetasizer Nano ZS instrument (Malvern Instruments, Worcestershire, UK) equipped with He-Ne laser (10 mW, 633 nm wavelength) (see Note 10).

2. Add 200 μL of siRNA-SS-PNIPAM solution (siRNA concentration at 200 nM) into a low-volume quartz cuvette (ZEN3600, Malvern Instruments), heat at determined temperature for 10 min, then measure the particle size of the samples.

### 3.2 Formation and Characterization of siRNAsome

1. Dissolve siRNA-SS-PNIPAM in HEPES buffer (10 mM, pH 7.4), incubate the solution at 37 °C for 30 min, and self-assemble into siRNAsome directly (see Note 8).
2. Determine the hydrodynamic size, polydispersity index (PDI) of siRNAsome at 37 °C by Zetasizer Nano ZS instrument (Fig. 3a).
3. Examine the morphology of siRNAsome using a transmission electron microscope (TEM, JEM-2100, JEOL, Tokyo, Japan) at an acceleration voltage of 200 kV and a beam current of 40 μA. Place each sample on 3 mm-mesh copper grids and stain with uranyl acetate solution (1% w/v) for 15 min (Fig. 3b, see Note 11).
4. Perform the gel retardation assay of siRNAsome by gel electrophoresis (2% agarose, preheated 1 × TAE buffer, 100 V, 30 min) (see Note 12).

### 3.3 Drug Encapsulation by siRNAsome (Table 1)

1. Dissolve different amount of free DOX·HCl, DTX, and BSA in HEPES buffer (10 mM, pH 7.4), DMSO, and HEPES buffer (10 mM, pH 7.4), respectively (see Note 13).
2. Dissolve siRNA-SS-PNIPAM with DEPC water. Then add free DOX·HCl, DTX, and BSA solution into siRNA-SS-PNIPAM solution, followed by shaking the mixture at room temperature for 3 h.

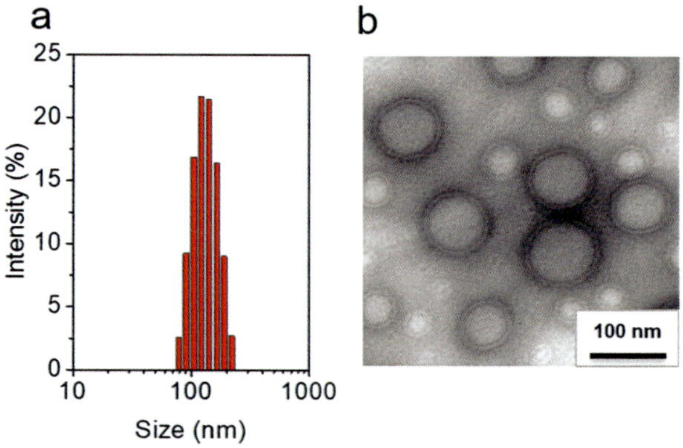


**Fig. 3** Characterization of the siRNAsome. (**a**) Size and (**b**) TEM image of siRNAsomes derived from PNIPAMs of 19 kDa in molecular weight. These results demonstrated this siRNAsome displayed a clear vesicular morphology with a diameter around 120 nm. (Adapted from Zheng et al. 2019, with permission)

**Table 1** Drug-loading content (DLC) and drug-loading efficiency (DLE) for DOX·HCl, DTX, and BSA with 19 kDa PNIPAM-derived siRNAsome and characterization of drug-loaded siRNAsome. (Adapted from Zheng et al. 2019, with permission)

| | DLC (*wt.* %) | | | Size | |
|---|---|---|---|---|---|
| Loaded drug | Theory | Determined | DLE (%) | (nm) | PDI |
| DOX·HCl | 10 | 4.42 | 41.4 | 131.5 | 0.088 |
| | 20 | 8.41 | 36.6 | 137.7 | 0.087 |
| DTX | 10 | 5.48 | 52.3 | 136.2 | 0.169 |
| | 20 | 9.74 | 43.2 | 138.6 | 0.165 |
| BSA | 10 | 4.69 | 44.3 | 164.2 | 0.569 |
| | 20 | 7.58 | 32.8 | 178.3 | 0.344 |

3. Adjust the temperature to 37 °C and shake for another 2 h to encapsulate the drugs (see Note 14).
4. Remove unloaded free DOX·HCl, DTX, and BSA by dialysis against preheated HEPES buffer (10 mM, pH 7.4) at 37 °C with 3.5 kDa, 3.5 kDa, and 250 kDa dialysis bag (see Note 15).
5. Determine the loading content of DOX·HCl, DTX, and BSA by multimode microplate reader (see Note 16), high-performance liquid chromatography (HPLC) (see Note 17), and BCA kit, respectively.

## 3.4 Reduction Responsiveness of siRNAsome

### 3.4.1 Size, Morphology Change, and siRNA Release

1. Incubate siRNAsome with 10 mM DTT (see Note 18) at 37 °C in 10 mM HEPES buffer (pH 7.4).
2. Visualize free siRNA release by gel electrophoresis (see Note 12; 2% agarose, preheated 1 × TAE buffer, 100 V, 30 min; Fig. 4a).
3. Determine the particle size changes by DLS at 6 and 24 h post-DTT treatment (Fig. 4b).
4. Examine the morphology disruption of siRNAsome by TEM (see Note 11) at 6 h post-DTT treatment (Fig. 4c).

### 3.4.2 In Vitro DOX·HCl Release

1. Add 500 μL DOX·HCl-loaded siRNAsome solution (containing 10 mM DTT) in a dialysis bag (MWCO 12,000), and then immerse the dialysis bag into 20 mL of the PBS-releasing medium (containing 10 mM DTT) in a 50 mL centrifuge tube (see Note 18).
2. Oscillate the tube at 200 rpm at 37 °C.
3. Pipette the solution outside the dialysis membrane (4 mL) and replace with the same volume of fresh PBS medium (containing 10 mM DTT) at the time point of 0.5, 1, 2, 4, 6, 8, 10, 12, 24, and 48 h.

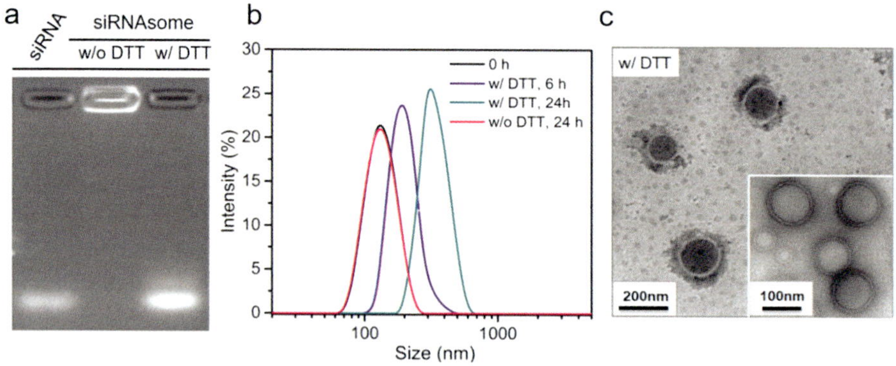


**Fig. 4** Responsiveness of siRNAsomes in a reducing environment. (**a**) siRNA release determined by gel electrophoresis; (**b**) modulation of nanoparticle size determined by DLS; and (**c**) siRNAsome structure disruption assessed by TEM (inset is unreduced siRNAsome structure). These results showed this kind of siRNA nanostructure is sensitive under the reduction of DTT. (Adapted from Zheng et al. 2019, with permission)

4. Determine the released DOX·HCl concentration using fluorescence meter (FLS920; excitation at 480 nm) based on the standard curve of DOX·HCl.
5. Conduct the release experiments in triplicates and present the averaged data with standard deviations.

## 3.5 In Vitro Evaluation of siRNAsome

### 3.5.1 Flow Cytometry Assay (Fig. 5a)

1. Seed MDR MCF-7 cells at a density of $3.0 \times 10^5$ cells/well in 6-well plates and culture in DMEM media (containing 10% FBS and 1% penicillin-streptomycin) (see Note 19). Culture overnight at 37 °C with 5% $CO_2$.
2. Remove the culture medium and replenish with 1.8 mL of fresh medium.
3. Add 200 μL of PBS, free FAM-siRNA, and FAM-siRNAsome in culture medium (see Note 20) with final siRNA concentrations at 200 nM.
4. Incubate the cells at 37 °C with 5% $CO_2$ for 12 h.
5. Remove all the medium, rinse the cells with PBS buffer three times, trypsinization for 3 min (see Note 21), centrifuge (1000 rpm, 3 min), and resuspend the cells in fresh PBS buffer (see Note 22).
6. Analyze all samples by flow cytometry (FACS Calibur, BD Bioscience, USA).

### 3.5.2 Confocal Laser-Scanning Microscopy Assay (Fig. 5b)

1. Seed MDR MCF-7 cells at a density of $1.0 \times 10^5$ cells/well in 24-well glass bottom plates and culture in DMEM media (containing 10% FBS and 1% penicillin-streptomycin). Culture overnight at 37 °C in the presence of 5% $CO_2$.
2. Remove the culture medium and replenish with 450 μL fresh medium.

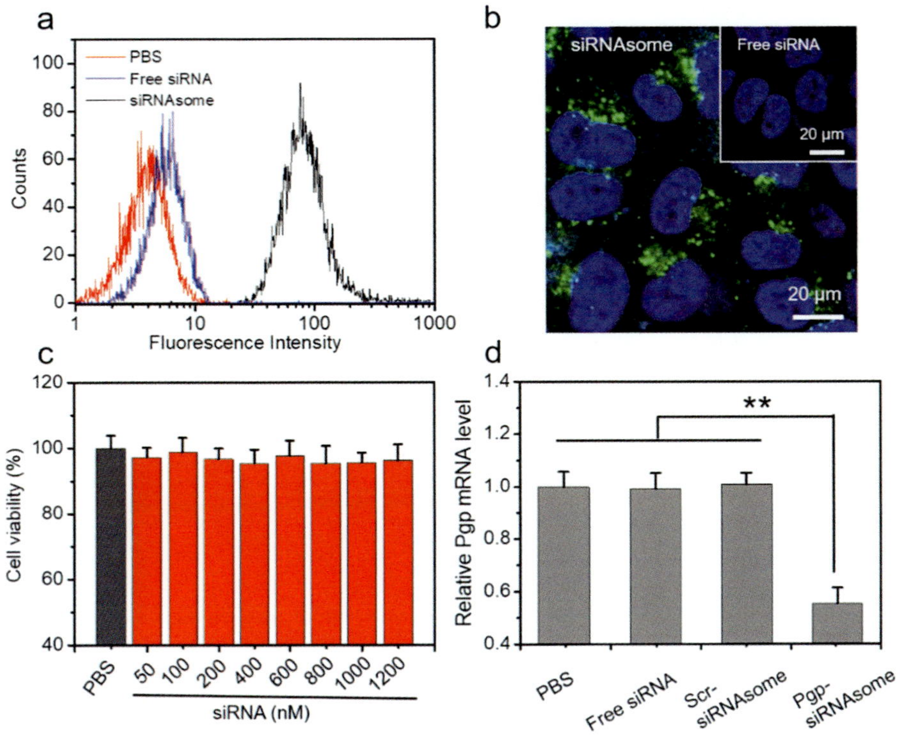


**Fig. 5** In vitro evaluation of siRNAsome. (**a**) Flow cytometry assays and (**b**) confocal microscopy assays show cellular uptake of siRNAsome; (**c**) cell viability assay of MDR MCF-7 cells incubated with siRNAsomes (siRNA concentration ranging from 50 to 1200 nm) shows ideal biocompatibility and safety; and (**d**) gene silencing of Pgp mRNA level as determined by RT-PCR assay. These results showed the siRNAsome displayed effective cellular uptake, excellent biocompatibility, and potent gene silencing capacity. (Adapted from Zheng et al. 2019, with permission)In Vitro and In Vivo Evaluation of DOX·HCl-Loaded siRNAsome

3. Add 50 μL of PBS, free FAM-siRNA, and FAM-siRNAsome in culture medium (see Note 20) with final siRNA concentrations at 200 nM.
4. Incubate the cells at 37 °C in the presence of 5% $CO_2$ for 12 h.
5. Remove all the medium, rinse the cells with PBS buffer three times, fix cells with 4% formaldehyde solution for 15 min, and stain with 10 μM DAPI for 10 min.
6. Image the fixed cells by confocal laser-scanning microscopy (Leica SP8).

### 3.5.3 In Vitro Cytotoxicity Assay of siRNAsome (Fig. 5c)

1. Seed MDR MCF-7 cells at a density of $5.0 \times 10^3$ cells/well in 96-well plates and culture in DMEM media (containing 10% FBS and 1% penicillin-streptomycin). Culture overnight at 37 °C in the presence of 5% $CO_2$.
2. Remove the culture medium and replenish with 90 μL fresh medium.
3. Add 10 μL of empty siRNAsome (in 37 °C solution) in culture medium, with a final siRNA concentration ranging from 50 to 1200 nM (see Note 23).

4. Incubate the cells at 37 °C in the presence of 5% $CO_2$ for 48 h.
5. Add 10 μL of MTT (5 mg/mL in PBS) into each well (see Note 24).
6. Incubate the cells for another 4 h, and remove all the medium carefully to avoid the purple crystal removal.
7. Add 150 μL DMSO into each well.
8. Determine the cell viability by measuring the absorbance of formazan at 492 nm or 570 nm using a microplate reader (see Note 25). Conduct the assay in quadruplicates and present the averaged data with standard deviations.

### 3.5.4 Real-Time Quantitative PCR Analysis (Fig. 5d)

1. Seed MDR MCF-7 cells at a density of $2.0 \times 10^5$ cells/well in 6-well plates and culture in DMEM media (containing 10% FBS and 1% penicillin-streptomycin). Culture overnight at 37 °C in the presence of 5% $CO_2$.
2. Remove the culture medium and replenish with 1800 μL fresh medium.
3. Add 200 μL of PBS, free siRNA, Scr-siRNAsome, and Pgp-siRNAsome into culture medium for final siRNA concentrations at 200 nM (see Note 26).
4. Incubate the cells at 37 °C in the presence of 5% $CO_2$ for 48 h.
5. Remove all the medium, and rinse the cells with PBS buffer three times, followed by trypsinization for 3 min and centrifuge (1000 rpm, 3 min).
6. Resuspend the cells with PBS and centrifuge (1000 rpm, 3 min).
7. Total RNA of centrifuged cells was obtained with an RNAprep pure Cell/Bacteria Kit (Tiangen Biotech., Beijing, China; see Note 27).
8. Total RNA was quantified and reversely transcribed into cDNA using a PrimeScript RT Reagent Kit (Takara, Kyoto, Japan). The amounts of Pgp and GAPDH mRNAs were then quantified by real-time PCR using TB Green™ Premix Ex Taq™ (Takara, Kyoto, Japan; see Note 28, Note 29).
9. The amount of Pgp mRNA was normalized to that of GAPDH mRNA. The Pgp mRNA level was analyzed by real-time qPCR.

### 3.5.5 MTT Assay (Fig. 6a)

1. Seed MDR MCF-7 cells at a density of $5.0 \times 10^3$ cells/well in 96-well plates and culture in DMEM media (containing 10% FBS and 1% penicillin-streptomycin) (see Note 23). Culture overnight at 37 °C in a cell incubator with 5% $CO_2$.
2. Remove the culture medium and replenish with 90 μL fresh medium.
3. Add 10 μL of PBS, free DOX·HCl, Scr-siRNAsome@DOX·HCl, and Pgp-siNRAsome@DOX·HCl in culture medium resulting a final siRNA concentration of 200 nM (corresponding DOX·HCl concentration is 0.59 μg/mL).
4. Incubate the cells at 37 °C with of 5% $CO_2$ for 72 h.
5. Add 10 μL of MTT (5 mg/mL in PBS) into each well (see Note 24).
6. Incubate the cells for another 4 h, and remove all the medium carefully to avoid the purple crystal removal.
7. Add 150 μL DMSO into each well.
8. Determine cell viability by measuring the absorbance of formazan at 492 nm or 570 nm using a microplate reader. Conduct the assay in quadruplicates and present the averaged data with standard deviations.

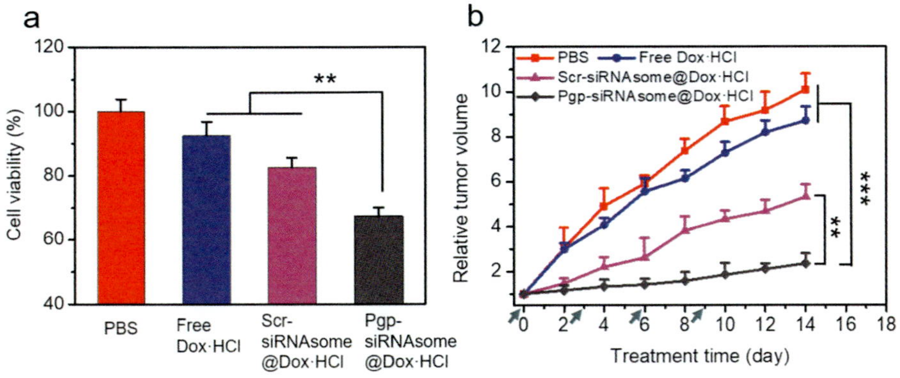


**Fig. 6** Synergistic therapy against MDR MCF-7 cancer cells and tumor model by using siRNAsomes to codeliver DOX·HCl and Pgp-siRNA. (**a**) Cell viability of MDR MCF-7 cells treated with DOX·HCl-loaded siRNAsomes and controls; and (**b**) tumor growth profiles of MDR MCF-7 tumor-bearing mice treated with DOX·HCl-loaded siRNAsomes and its controls. Both the in vitro and in vivo antitumor results showed the DOX·HCl-loaded siRNAsomes demonstrated effective synergistic therapy. (Adapted from Zheng et al. 2019, with permission)

### 3.5.6 In Vivo Antitumor Assay in Subcutaneous MDR MCF-7 Tumor Model (Fig. 6b)

1. House BALB/c nude mice under standard conditions of room temperature and dark-light cycles with plenty of food and water (see Note 30).
2. Resuspend MDR MCF-7 cells at a density of $5 \times 10^5$ cells in a volume of 0.1 mL PBS (see Note 31), then inject into subcutaneous tissue to build a subcutaneous tumor model.
3. Weigh the mice and randomly divide them into four groups ($n = 5$) after 10–15 days of tumor planting.
4. Intravenously inject PBS, free DOX·HCl, Scr-siRNAsome@DOX·HCl, and Pgp-siNRAsome@DOX·HCl (at a dose equivalent of 0.45 mg DOX equiv./kg and 2 mg siRNA equiv./kg) to MDR MCF-7 subcutaneous tumor mice through tail vein every 3 days for 10–15 days postimplantation (see Note 32), total four injections.
5. Measure the tumor volume every 2 days via vernier caliper.
6. Normalize the relative tumor size to initial volume size. Results are expressed as mean and standard deviation ($n = 5$).

## 4 Notes

1. The reagent requires anhydrous and oxygen-free environment. Long-term storage should also be avoided.
2. Better to precool ethyl ether at 4 °C for more than 30 min before using for precipitation.

3. The temperature of recrystallization needs to be carefully monitored: First dissolve the precipitate at room temperature, store at 4 °C for 2 h, and then overnight at −20 °C. Finally, white needle-like crystals with expected structure can be collected. If cooling too fast, the product might result with contaminations.
4. The RAFT reagent and AIBN initiator is sensitive; thus, the synthesis of PNIPAM requires strictly anhydrous and oxygen-free environment. Long-term storage should also be avoided.
5. Hexanes is suggested to be precooled at 4 °C for more than 30 min. before using for precipitation.
6. TEA possesses high toxicity and tends to be oxidized when exposed to light and heat. It also has strong corrosion and irritation ability, so protection measurement and good ventilation are essential across entire experimental procedure.
7. To completely remove excess by-product or impurity, the deionized water should be changed every 2–3 h.
8. Throughout all of the experiments, strict RNase-free conditions must be applied. Use RNase-free tubes and pipetting tips. Before the experiment, spray the bench, pipette, and gloves with a solution of DNase/ RNase inhibitor.
9. Maintain the analytical column at 25 °C. Perform the analysis at a flow rate of 0.3 mL/min using the eluent with the gradient of 0.1 M triethylammonium acetate (TEAA, pH 7.0) and acetonitrile.
10. Observe the critical point of stable particle size formation by increasing the temperature of siRNA solution from 25 °C to 37 °C.
11. Keep the temperature of the siRNAsome samples and copper mesh above at 37 °C during the experiment.
12. Preheat the 1 × TAE buffer to 37 °C and maintain at 37 °C during gel electrophoresis.
13. DOX·HCl is a kind of hydrophilic drug that is sensitive to light. Thus, exposure to light should be avoided during the entire conduct. DTX is a kind of hydrophobic drug.
14. The hydrophobic DTX can be loaded into the hydrophobic median layer of siRNAsome, while the hydrophilic DOX•HCl and BSA can be encapsulated into the watery interior of siRNAsome. The weak electrostatic interaction between siRNA and DOX•HCl also contributes to the loading efficiency improvement of DOX•HCl into the siRNAsome.
15. During the 12 h dialysis, deionized water should be changed every 1 h to sufficiently remove the impurities sufficiently.
16. The excitation wavelength of DOX·HCl is 492 nm, and the fluorescence intensity was measured using a microplate reader.
17. To ensure the accuracy of DTX-loading efficiency, a standard curve of DTX should be determined by HPLC first.
18. GSH maintains a millimolar concentration (3–10 mM) in the cytosol and subcellular compartments in cancer cells, but lower concentration (~2.8 μM) in cellular exterior such as plasma (Son et al. 2012). Therefore, simulated intracellular environment is set at a concentration of 10 mM DTT.

19. The cells should be passaged frequently and at regular intervals to maintain cells in midlog growth stage. Generation is suggested to subculture within 40 since primary culture. A subcultivation ratio of 1:3 is recommended.
20. Keep the siRNAsome solution at 37 °C before use.
21. Warm up the trypsin to 37 °C before use.
22. Try to ensure the viability and activity of cells by careful exercise during the washing process.
23. Edge wells in plates must be not used in experiment since the cells in those wells usually grow slower than inner-plate wells.
24. Once MTT is added, the plate should be protected from light.
25. Relative cell viability was calculated by the following equation: The viability (%) = $(OD_{sample}/OD_{control}) \times 100$. $OD_{control}$ is obtained in PBS while $OD_{sample}$ is obtained in the presence of siRNAsomes.
26. The siRNA sequences are as follows: Pgp-siRNA (sense: 5′-GAAACCAACUGUUAGUGUAdTdT-3′; antisense: 5′-UACACUGACA GUUGGUUUCdTdT-3′), scramble siRNA (sense: 5′-UUCUCCGAACGU GUCACGUdTdT-3′, antisense: 5′-ACGUGACAC GUUCGGAGAAdTdT-3′).
27. Allow all required reagents in the kit to reach 4 °C/R.T. before use.
28. The TB Green *Premix Ex Taq* solution should be performed away from light while using. The reaction time should be strictly controlled according to the assay kit instruction.
29. qRT-PCR primer sequences are as follows: forward primer 5′-CCATAGCTCGTGCCCTTGTTAGA-3′ and reverse primer 5′-CGGTGAGC AATCACAATGCAG-3′.
30. Laboratory mice should be selected as single gender for in vivo experiment.
31. Place MDR MCF-7 cells on ice or at 4 °C to maintain cell viability.
32. Prepare for injections of samples when tumor size exceeds 6 ~ 7 mm in diameter.

## 5 Conclusion

This protocol introduces the preparation of a novel reduction-sensitive polymersomal SNA, termed siRNAsome. This siRNAsome is able to encapsulate biomacromolecules and hydrophilic drugs in its hydrophilic interior, and hydrophobic drugs in its hydrophobic membranes. In addition, the intrinsic properties of SNA enable its siRNA shell not only capable of stabilizing the nanoparticle structure, but also be utilized as RNAi drug. Moreover, by taking advantage of intracellular reducing environment, attached siRNAs and loaded drugs can be accumulatively released once inside the cell. The siRNAsomes can be efficiently taken up by cells while displaying no cytotoxicity. When such novel SNA nanostructures loaded with Pgp-siRNA and DOX·HCl are applied in MDR MCF-7 cells, the two payloads together improved the cell-killing ability to MDR cancer cells, showing synergistic therapeutic effect.

## References


Choi CH, Hao L, Narayan SP et al (2013) Mechanism for the endocytosis of spherical nucleic acid nanoparticle conjugates. Proc Natl Acad Sci U S A 110(19):7625–7630

Cutler JI, Zhang K, Zheng D et al (2011) Polyvalent nucleic acid nanostructures. J Am Chem Soc 133(24):9254–9257

Cutler JI, Auyeung E, Mirkin CA (2012) Spherical nucleic acids. J Am Chem Soc 134(3): 1376–1391

Guo Y, Zhang J, Ding F et al (2019) Stressing the role of DNA as a drug carrier: synthesis of DNA-drug conjugates through grafting chemotherapeutics onto phosphorothioate oligonucleotides. Adv Mater 31(16):1807533

Lee JS, Feijen J (2012) Polymersomes for drug delivery: design, formation and characterization. J Control Release 161(2):473–483

Lee JS, Lytton-Jean AK, Hurst SJ et al (2007) Silver nanoparticle-oligonucleotide conjugates based on DNA with triple cyclic disulfide moieties. Nano Lett 7(7):2112–2115

Li M, De P, Li HM et al (2010) Conjugation of RAFT-generated polymers to proteins by two consecutive thiol-ene reactions. Polym Chem 1(6):854–859

Lu Y, Liu L, Wang Y et al (2016) siRNA delivered by EGFR-specific scFv sensitizes EGFR-TKI-resistant human lung cancer cells. Biomaterials 76:196–207

Meng FH, Zhong ZY (2011) Polymersomes spanning from nano- to microscales: advanced vehicles for controlled drug delivery and robust vesicles for virus and cell mimicking. J Phys Chem Lett 2(13):1533–1539

Mitchell GP, Mirkin CA, Letsinger RL (1999) Programmed assembly of DNA functionalized quantum dots. J Am Chem Soc 121:8122–8123

Mokhtarzadeh A, Vahidnezhad H, Youssefian L et al (2019) Applications of spherical nucleic acid nanoparticles as delivery systems. Trends Mol Med 25(12):1066–1079

Patel PC, Giljohann DA, Daniel WL et al (2010) Scavenger receptors mediate cellular uptake of polyvalent oligonucleotide-functionalized gold nanoparticles. Bioconjug Chem 21(12): 2250–2256

Rosi NL, Giljohann DA, Thaxton CS et al (2006) Oligonucleotide-modified gold nanoparticles for intracellular gene regulation. Science 312(5776):1027–1030

Seferos DS, Prigodich AE, Giljohann DA et al (2009) Polyvalent DNA nanoparticle conjugates stabilize nucleic acids. Nano Lett 9(1):308–311

Son S, Namgung R, Kim J et al (2012) Bioreducible polymers for gene silencing and delivery. Acc Chem Res 45(7):1100–1112

Tan X, Li BB, Lu X et al (2015) Light-triggered, self-immolative nucleic acid-drug nanostructures. J Am Chem Soc 137(19):6112–6115

Tan X, Lu X, Jia F et al (2016) Blurring the role of oligonucleotides: spherical nucleic acids as a drug delivery vehicle. J Am Chem Soc 138(34):10834–10837

Wang LH, Wu DC, Xu HX et al (2016) High DNA-binding affinity and gene-transfection efficacy of bioreducible cationic nanomicelles with a fluorinated core. Angew Chem Int Ed Engl 55(2): 755–759

Xu HF, Meng FH, Zhong ZY (2009) Reversibly crosslinked temperature-responsive nano-sized polymersomes: synthesis and triggered drug release. J Mater Chem 19(24):4183–4190

Yu YH, Kim E, Park DE et al (2012) Cationic solid lipid nanoparticles for co-delivery of paclitaxel and siRNA. Eur J Pharm Biopharm 80(2):268–273

Zheng M, Tao W, Zou Y et al (2018) Nanotechnology-based strategies for siRNA brain delivery for disease therapy. Trends Biotechnol 36(5):562–575

Zheng M, Jiang T, Yang W et al (2019) The siRNAsome: a cation-free and versatile nanostructure for siRNA and drug co-delivery. Angew Chem Int Ed Engl 58(15):4938–4942

Zhu S, Xing H, Gordiichuk P et al (2018) PLGA spherical nucleic acids. Adv Mater 30(22): 1707113

# Development of Cationic Lipid-Assisted PEG-*b*-PLA Nanoparticle for Nucleic Acid Therapeutics

# 28

Liang Zhao and Xianzhu Yang

## Contents



**Abstract**

Nucleic acid-based macromolecules, including protein-expressing plasmid DNA (pDNA) and messenger RNA (mRNA), antisense oligonucleotides (ASOs), small interfering RNA (siRNA), genome editing systems, and so on, have paved new avenues for the development of therapeutic interventions against various types of diseases. Several nucleic acid-based drug have been approved for clinical application, and many more are under clinical evaluation. However, it should be noted that their clinical translation is dependent on the successful delivery to the target site and cells. Among these formulations, the clinically validated polylactide (PLA)-based nanocarriers have attracted wide attention. Unfortunately, PLA nanocarriers inefficiently encapsulated nucleic acid. In this regard, a cationic lipid-assisted PEG-*b*-PLA nanoparticle (CLAN) is explored to high efficiently encapsulate nucleic acid drug inside its aqueous core through double emulsion method. In this protocol, siRNA is used as a model nucleic acid drug, and the preparation and characterization of siRNA-loaded CLAN are described. And, all nucleic acid drugs could be loaded into the CLAN formulation with the same

L. Zhao · X. Yang (✉)
School of Biomedical Sciences and Engineering, South China University of Technology, Guangzhou, China
e-mail: yangxz@scut.edu.cn



H. Tian and X. Chen (eds.), *Gene Delivery*, Biomaterial Engineering,
https://doi.org/10.1007/978-981-16-5419-0_29

procedures. The present results demonstrate that the CLAN formulation displayed an extreme high encapsulation efficiency (>95%), an efficient cellular uptake of siRNA-loaded CLAN by tumor cells, and thereby improving the downregulation of targeted gene in vitro and in tumor models.

**Keywords**

Cationic lipid-assisted nanoparticles · siRNA delivery · Gene silence · Nanomedicine · Nucleic acid therapeutics · Double emulsion

## 1 Overview

With robust potencies to regulate disease-related gene expression, nucleic acid drugs have been regarded as promising therapies for numerous diseases (Opalinska and Gewirtz 2002), such as genetic disorders, cancer, infectious diseases, and viral infections. The development of nucleic acid drug originated the concept of gene therapy during the 1960s and early 1970s, which was performed via the recombinant viruses carrying DNA to express the desired protein (Kong 1963; Friedmann and Roblin 1972; Rogers et al. 1973). So far, nucleic acid-based therapy has extended from the early concept of introducing a gene to express the desired protein to downregulating gene expression and editing genes (Setten et al. 2019; Anzalone et al. 2020). After years of hard work, a number of these therapeutics have already completed their clinical evaluation and are approved. Meanwhile, these delivery systems of nucleic acid drug have evolved from early viral vectors to nonviral vectors due to the safety concerns. For instance, the early gene therapy mainly relied on adenovirus or adeno-associated virus vector-mediated gene therapy (Glybera, Luxturna, and Zolgensma). And, with the rapid development of nanotechnology in recent decades, the success clinical translation of first siRNA drug, Onpattro, relies on lipid nanoparticle (LNP) technology (nonviral vector) for siRNA delivery to hepatocytes for inhibition of the disease-causing mutant transthyretin protein (Hoy 2018; Akinc et al. 2019). In addition, two mRNA-based vaccines have been given emergency use authorization for clinical therapeutics against the COVID-19 in the last year, and both of which are developed using lipid nanoparticles by Moderna and Pfizer/BioNTech, respectively (Khurana et al. 2021). Despite great progress in the nonviral vector, safe and efficient in vivo delivery systems of nucleic acids remain desired and still a major challenge (Van Den Berg et al. 2021).

During the latest decades, a remarkable progress has been made in the development of nonviral vectors (Yin et al. 2014). Despite the tremendous amount of effort, the cationic lipids or polymers remain the main materials to construct these vectors. Nevertheless, the potential cytotoxicity of cationic materials limited their clinical application (Lv et al. 2006). For instance, the trial of CALAA-01, a cationic cyclodextrin-based delivery system of siRNA, has been terminated due to 21% of the patients having an adverse event (Zuckerman et al. 2014). Furthermore, cationic delivery systems usually elicited rapid clearance by the reticuloendothelial system due to the enhanced adsorption of serum proteins (Moghimi and Patel 1998), which would decrease the delivery efficacy into targeted cells. Compared to these cationic delivery systems, clinically validated PLA and its analogues-based nanocarriers have attracted wide attention to be explored as the nonviral vector (Singh et al. 2000; Luu et al. 2003; Jilek et al. 2005). The several groups have used the PLA-based nanocarrier to encapsulate nucleic through double emulsion method (Murata et al. 2008; Patil and Panyam 2009; Cun et al. 2010), but the encapsulation efficacy was rather low (<60%) for pDNA and only ~20% for siRNA. As a result, the low encapsulation efficacies restricted its wide usage.

In order to improve the encapsulation efficacy of nucleic acid drugs, the cationic lipid assisted PEG-b-PLA nanoparticle (CLAN) has been explored for reaching this purpose. In this section, siRNA is used as a model nucleic acid drugs, and instructions to prepare the siRNA-encapsulated CLAN formulation are introduced. The characterization, cellular uptake, the silencing efficacy were comparatively evaluated. Due to the versatile design of the system, the CLAN system can be used to load different types of nucleic acid drugs.

## 2 Protocol

### 2.1 Materials

#### 2.1.1 Preparation of siRNA-Loaded CLAN Systems

1. The diblock copolymer $mPEG_{5K}$-$PLA_{25K}$ (the subscript number represents molecule weight of each block).
2. Cationic lipid N,N-bis(2-hydroxyethyl)-N-methyl-N-(2-cholesteryloxycarbonyl aminoethyl) ammonium bromide (BHEM-Chol)
3. RNase-free water.
4. Chloroform (reagent grade).
5. PVA solution (1.0%, w/v)
6. siRNA

#### 2.1.2 Determination of Encapsulation Efficiency, Drug Release, Particle Size, and Morphology

1. FAM-siRNA
2. HPLC system with fluorescence detector
3. Triethylammonium acetate buffer (0.1 M, pH 7.4)
4. Acetonitrile (chromatographic grade)
5. Phosphate buffer (0.01 M, pH 7.4)
6. Malvern Zetasizer Nano ZS90
7. Transmission electron microscopy (TEM)
8. Copper grids coated with carbon films

### 2.1.3 Cellular Uptake

1. Human hepatocellular liver carcinoma cell line HepG2
2. Dulbecco's modification of Eagle's medium (DMEM)
3. Heat-inactivated fetal bovine serum (FBS)
4. Phosphate-buffered saline (PBS, 0.01 M, pH 7.4)
5. 24-well tissue culture plates
6. Trypsin EDTA
7. $CO_2$ incubator
8. FAM-siRNA

### 2.1.4 Cell Transfection

1. Human hepatocellular liver carcinoma cell line HepG2
2. Dulbecco's modification of Eagle's medium (DMEM)
3. Heat-inactivated fetal bovine serum (FBS)
4. Phosphate-buffered saline (PBS, 0.01 M, pH 7.4)
5. 6-well tissue culture plates
6. Trypsin EDTA
7. $CO_2$ incubator

### 2.1.5 Cell Apoptosis

1. Human hepatocellular liver carcinoma cell line HepG2
2. Dulbecco's modification of Eagle's medium (DMEM)
3. Heat-inactivated fetal bovine serum (FBS)
4. Phosphate-buffered saline (PBS, 0.01 M, pH 7.4)
5. 24-well tissue culture plates
6. Trypsin EDTA
7. $CO_2$ incubator

### 2.1.6 Effects on the Anticancer Activity of Breast Tumor-Bearing Mice

1. BALB/c nude mice (4–6 weeks old)
2. Human breast cancer cell line MDA-MB-435 s
3. Phosphate-buffered saline (PBS, 0.01 M, pH 7.4)
4. Insulin needle

## 2.2 Methods

### 2.2.1 Preparation of siRNA-Loaded CLAN Systems (Notes 1, 2, 3, 4, 5, 6)

1. Add an aqueous solution of siRNA (0.2 mg in 25 μL of RNase-free water) into 0.5 mL chloroform containing 1.0 mg of BHEM-Chol and 25 mg of $mPEG_{5K}$-$PLA_{25K}$ over an ice bath.

2. The mixture solution was emulsified by sonication (80 W, for 30s) over an ice bath.
3. Add PVA solution (1.5 mL, 1.0%, w/v) into the resultant primary emulsion.
4. Emulsify by sonication (80 W for 2 min) over an ice bath to form a water-in-oil-in-water emulsion.
5. The mixture was then transferred into 25 mL of aqueous solution and further stirred for 3 h to evaporate most of chloroform.
6. Residual chloroform was removed using a rotary evaporator for 30 min under reduced pressure.
7. The resultant CLAN particles were collected by centrifugation (30,000 × g, 1 h) and washed twice with sterile water to remove PVA and possible unencapsulated siRNA. The obtained nanoparticles were stored at 4 °C for subsequent use.

### 2.2.2 Encapsulation Efficiency (Note 7)

1. The fluorescently labeled FAM-siRNA was used to prepare the siRNA-encapsulated CLAN systems. And, the unencapsulated siRNA in the supernatant was collected after centrifugation (30,000 × g, 1 h).
2. Measure FAM-siRNA by high-performance liquid chromatography (HPLC) analyses, using a Waters HPLC system consisting of a Waters 1525 binary pump, a Waters 2475 fluorescence detector, a 1500 column heater, and a Symmetry C18 column. HPLC grade triethylammonium acetate buffer (0.1 M, pH 7.4) with acetonitrile at a ratio of 72:28 (v/v) was used as the mobile phase at 30 °C with a flow rate of 0.5 mL $min^{-1}$. The fluorescence detector was set at 485 nm for excitation and 535 nm for emission and linked to Breeze software for data analysis.
3. Calculate the encapsulation efficiency of siRNA with the following formula: $EE = (1\text{-}W_{supernatant}/W_{total}) \times 100\%$, where EE is the encapsulation efficiency of siRNA, $W_{supernatant}$ is the measured amount of siRNA in the supernatant, and $W_{total}$ is the total amount of siRNA used for loading.

### 2.2.3 Drug Release

1. Suspend the CLAN formulation encapsulating FAM-siRNA in 5.0 mL of phosphate buffer (0.01 M, pH 7.4) and incubate at 37 °C with gentle shaking (70 rpm).
2. Take the samples at predetermined intervals and centrifuge (30,000 × g, 1 h) to collect supernatant and precipitate, respectively. The precipitate was resuspended in 5.0 mL of phosphate buffer (0.01 M, pH 7.4) to further perform the in vitro release experiment.
3. Measure FAM-siRNA in supernatant by HPLC system with fluorescence detector.
4. Calculate the release rate in Fig. 1.

### 2.2.4 Particle Size (Note 8)

1. Detect the particle sizes and zeta potential values of CLAN formulations using a zeta potential analyzer with dynamic light scattering (DLS, Malvern Zetasizer Nano ZS90)..

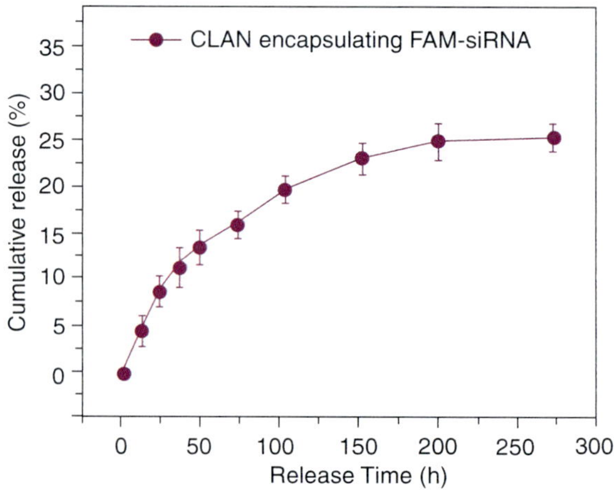


**Fig. 1** In vitro cumulative release of FAM-siRNA from CLAN system nanoparticles. (Adapted from Yang et al. (2011), with permission).

### 2.2.5 Determination of the Particle Morphology under TEM

1. Resuspend the CLAN formulation encapsulating siRNA in RNase-free water.
2. Add the suspension onto copper grids coated with carbon films.
3. Take out copper grids, and then dried in air.
4. Observe the samples by TEM at 120 kV.

### 2.2.6 Cellular Uptake (Notes 9, 10)

1. Seed HepG2 cells into 24-well plates at a density of $5 \times 10^4$ per well overnight.
2. Add CLAN formulation encapsulating FAM-siRNA into the 24-well plates. The final FAM-siRNA-concentration was 200 nM.
3. Aspirate the medium at different time points. Then, the treated HepG2 cells were rinsed twice with cold PBS.
4. Trypsinize the HepG2 cells, and washed by cold PBS twice.
5. Filter the cell suspension through 35 μm nylon mesh, and then subjected to flow cytometric analysis in Fig. 2.

### 2.2.7 Cell Transfection (Notes 11, 12, 13)

1. HepG2 cells in DMEM medium supplemented by 10% heat-inactivated FBS were seeded on 6-well plates ($1.0 \times 10^5$ per well) and allowed to grow until 50% confluence.
2. Aspirate the culture medium and rinse cells twice with cold PBS.
3. Add DMEM medium containing CLAN formulations. CLAN formulation encapsulating siRNA (siRNA targeting Plk1 mRNA (si*Plk1*, antisense strand, 5-′-UAAGGAGGGUGAUCUUCUUCAdTdT-3′) or scrambled sequence (si*N.C.*, antisense strand, 5′-ACGUGACACGUUCGGAGAAdTdT-3′).
4. Lipofectamine 2000 carrying 50 nM of si*Plk1* was used as the positive control and performed according the supplier's protocol.

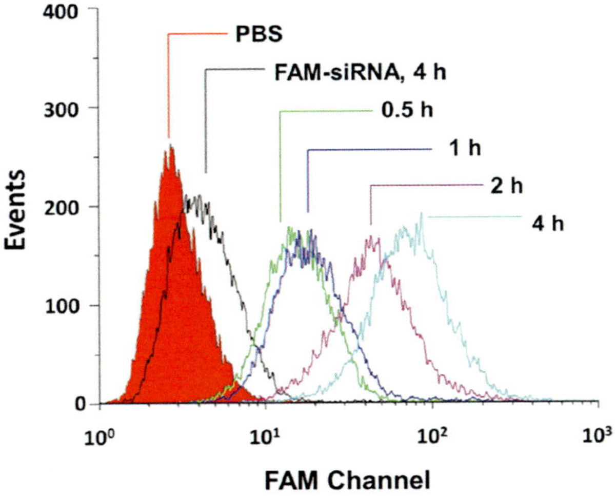


**Fig. 2** Flow cytometric analyses of HepG2 cells treated with CLAN formulation encapsulating FAM-siRNA for different periods of time. (Adapted from reference Yang et al. (2011), with permission)

5. After treatment for 24 h, total RNA from transfected cells was isolated using RNeasy mini-kit (Qiagen, Valencia, CA) according to the protocol of the manufacturer.
6. Two micrograms of total RNA were transcribed into cDNA using the PrimeScript™ first Strand cDNA Synthesis Kit (Takara, Dalian, China).
7. Two microliter of cDNA was subjected to quantitative real-time PCR analysis targeting Plk1 and glyceraldehyde 3-phosphate dehydrogenase (GAPDH) using the SYBR® Premix Ex Taq™ (Perfect Real Time) (Takara). Analysis was performed using the Applied Biosystems StepOne™ Real-Time PCR Systems. Relative gene expression values were determined by the ΔΔCT method using StepOne™ Software v2.1 (Applied Biosystems). Data are presented as the fold difference in Plk1 expression normalized to the housekeeping gene GAPDH as the endogenous reference and relative to the untreated control cells in Fig. 3.

### 2.2.8 Effects on the Apoptosis of HepG2 Cells (Note 14)

1. Seed HepG2 cells in DMEM medium supplemented by 10% heat-inactivated FBS on 24-well plates ($5.0 \times 10^4$ per well) overnight.
2. Aspirate the culture medium and rinse cells twice with cold PBS.
3. Add DMEM medium containing CLAN formulations. CLAN formulation encapsulating siPlk1 or si*N.C.*
4. Lipofectamine 2000 carrying 50 nM of si*Plk1* was used as the positive control and performed according to the supplier's protocol.
5. Trypsinize the HepG2 cells at 48 h posttreatment, washed by cold PBS twice.
6. Stain the treated cells using the Annexin V-FITC apoptosis detection kit I (BD Biosciences) according to the protocol of the manufacturer.

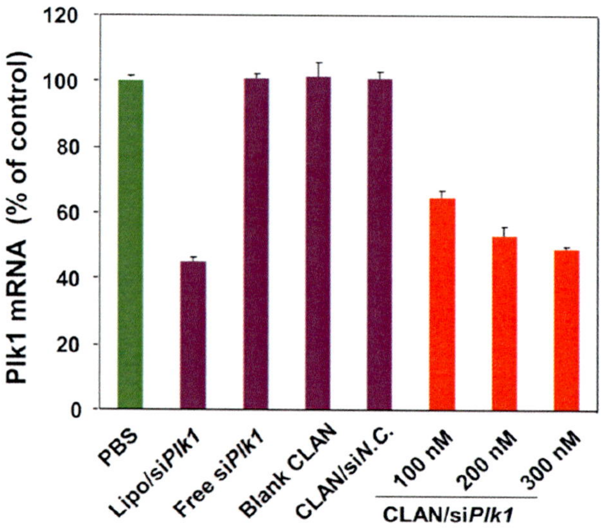


**Fig. 3** Plk1 mRNA expression in HepG2 cells determined by quantitative RT-PCR analysis following treatment with different formulations. Lipo/si*Plk1* represent the complexes of Lipofectamine 2000 with si*Plk1* (50 nM). Free si*Plk1* represent that cells were incubated with si*Plk1* at a dose of 300 nM. Blank CLAN and CLAN/si*N.C.* represent that cells were administered empty nanoparticles and nanoparticles encapsulating si*N.C.* (CLAN/si*N.C.*, 300 nM siRNA), respectively. (Adapted from Yang et al. (2011) with permission)

7. Filter the cell suspension through 35 μm nylon mesh and then subjected to flow cytometric analysis.
8. Analyzes the result using WinMDI 2.9 software in Fig. 4.

### 2.2.9 Effects on the Anticancer Activity of Breast Tumor-Bearing Mice (Note 15)

1. Implant approximate $5 \times 10^6$ MDA-MB-435 s cells/50 μL in PBS into the mammary fat pads of female mice (~20 g).
2. Measure tumor volume with a vernier caliper. Estimate the tumor volume according to the formula: tumor volume ($mm^3$) = $0.5 \times$ length $\times$ width$^2$.
3. Randomly divide the mice into five groups (five mice per group) at day 14 after tumor inoculation. The tumor volume reached around 50 $mm^3$.
4. Treat animals with PBS, and Blank CLAN formulation in control group.
5. Treat animals in other three groups with free siPlk1, CLAN/*siN.C.*, and CLAN/ si*Plk1* via tail vein at a dose of 20 μg per mouse per injection.
6. Administrate these formulations every 2 days with total six doses per mouse.
7. Measure tumor volume with a vernier caliper every 2 days.
8. Tumor growth curves for each group in Fig. 5.

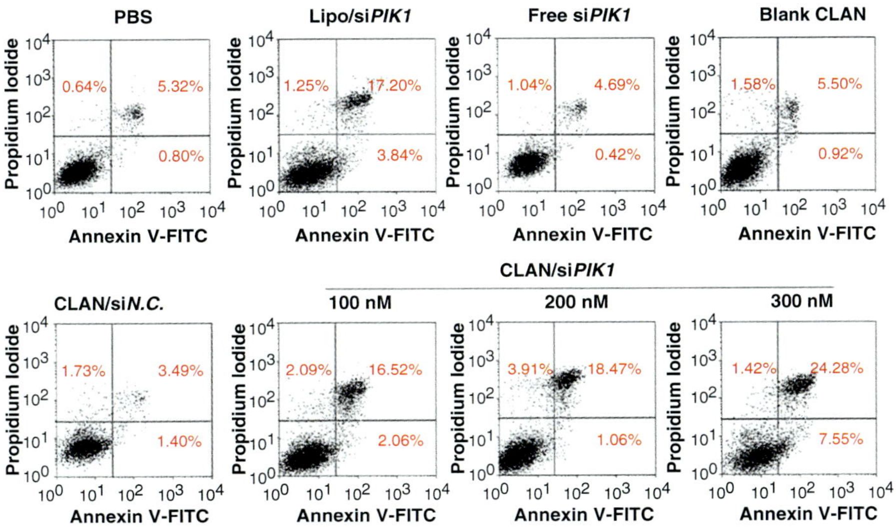


**Fig. 4** The influence of si*Plk1* delivery by CLAN formulation on apoptosis in HepG2 cells. Early apoptotic cells are presented in the lower right quadrant and apoptotic are presented in the upper right quadrant. Lipo/si*Plk1* represents the complexes of Lipofectamine 2000 with si*Plk1* (50 nM). Free si*Plk1* represent that cells were incubated with si*Plk1* at a dose of 300 nM. Blank CLAN and CLAN/si*N.C.* represent that cells were administered empty nanoparticles and CLAN nanoparticles encapsulating si*N.C.* (CLAN/si*N.C.*, 300 nM siRNA), respectively. (Adapted from Yang et al. (2011), with permission)

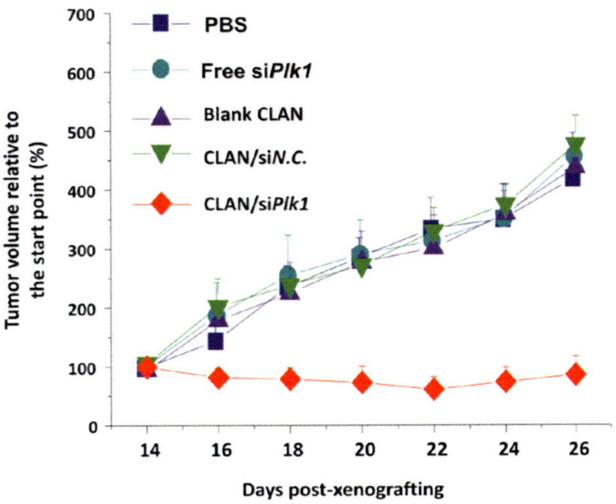


**Fig. 5** Inhibition of tumor growth in a MDA-MB-435 s xenograft murine model following i.v. injection of si*Plk1*-encapsulated nanoparticles. (Adapted from Yang et al. (2011), with permission)

## 3 Discussion

There are common mistakes when following the above procedure. Here are some notes which can be used to solve possible problems.

## 4 Notes

1. In the process of preparing a systemic delivery carrier for siRNA by double emulsification, the oil phase containing material and the inner water phase containing siRNA will form a water-in-oil primary emulsion under ultrasonic conditions, and then the outer water phase will be added to form water-in-oil-in-water multiple emulsion (Ding et al. 2019). Regarding the formulation structure, cationic lipids are assembled at the oil-water interface due to the amphiphilic property. On the one hand, it can reduce the surface tension, stabilize the emulsion, and prevent drug leakage caused by demulsification, and on the other hand, it can improve the encapsulation efficiency of siRNA through charge interaction.
2. The chloroform solution containing BHEM-Chol and $mPEG_{5K}$-$PLA_{25K}$ should be stored in a closed glass bottle at −20 °C to prevent volatilization.
3. When configuring the siRNA solution, centrifuge the siRNA powder at 12000 g for 1 min before dissolving it and ensure no enzyme operation to prevent degradation. The dissolved siRNA solution should be aliquoted and stored at −20 °C to avoid repeated freezing and thawing.
4. The mechanical vibration of the medium caused by ultrasound will release heat (Dominici et al. 2005). Excessive heat may cause the degradation of nucleic acid, so all reagents should be precooled over ice before use, and the pause time should be set in the ultrasonic conditions (primary emulsion on for 5 s and off for 2 s, multiple emulsion on for 10 s and off for 2 s).
5. During the rotary steaming process, the vacuum degree should be lowered slowly to prevent the precipitation of nanoparticles caused by the liquid evaporation too fast.
6. Due to the toxicity sensitivity at the cellular level, the chloroform in the particles must be fully removed by extra rotary steaming at 50 mbar for 30 min. And excessive PVA has obvious cytotoxicity, so it is necessary to wash the particles with RNase-free water several times.
7. In order to ensure the accuracy of the detection of the encapsulation rate, the standard product needs to be diluted with the supernatant of the blank particles under the same processing conditions to deduct the influence of the background on the detection results, and then use the HPLC to determine the encapsulation efficiency of siRNA.
8. The prepared nanoparticles were diluted with water to 1 mg/mL, and the particle size and potential were measured by dynamic light scattering (DLS). The instrument used is Zetasizer Nano ZS90 from Malvern Company, the light source is He-Ne, the wavelength of the light source is 633 nm, and the measurement is performed at a scattering angle of 90°.

9. FAM-siRNA should be performed away from light while using.
10. After diluting the nanoparticle solution with culture medium, make sure that the volume of the particle solution is less than 10% of the total volume, and set a blank control to ensure that the change of osmotic pressure has no effect on the experimental results.
11. Cell transfection has high requirements on the cell state, and it must ensure that the cell has a good shape, a clear outline, and an excellent proliferation condition. Select cells in the logarithmic growth phase for digestion and seeding.
12. The extraction of total RNA from cells needs to be carried out in an ultraclean bench, and strictly use enzyme-free reagents and consumables to prevent RNA degradation during the operation. Until A260/A280 is between 1.7 and 2.1, total RNA can be used in subsequent experiments.
13. The primers used in the quantitative real-time PCR for Plk1 and GAPDH were: Plk1-forward 5′-AGCCTGAGGCCCGATACTACCTAC-3′, Plk1-reverse 5′-ATTAGGAGTCCCACACAGGGTCTTC-3′, and GAPDH-forward 5′-TTCACCACCATGGAGAAGGC-3′, GAPDH-reverse 5′-GG-CATGGACTGTGGTCATGA-3′. PCR parameters consisted of 30 s of Taq activation at 95 °C, followed by 40 cycles of PCR at 95 °C × 5 s, 60 °C × 30 s, and 1 cycle of 95 °C × 15 s, 60 °C × 60 s and 95 °C × 15 s.
14. In the cell processing of apoptosis, attention should be paid to the time of trypsin digestion to prevent false positives caused by excessive trypsin digestion, or the increase of PI single-positive cell populations caused by insufficient digestion.
15. The nanoparticle solution is preprepared to be an isotonic solution with 10 × PBS before administration, and make sure to use it as soon as possible.

## 5 Conclusion

This protocol presents a kind of a cationic lipid-assisted PEG-*b*-PLA nanoparticle system for efficient siRNA encapsulation. The nanoparticle was prepared by a double emulsion-solvent evaporation technique with assistance of cationic lipid. Encapsulation efficiency, drug release, particle size, and morphology of the obtained nanoparticles are characterized. Results demonstrate that the CLAN systems exhibited a vesicle-like structure and efficient delivery siRNA into tumor cells, thereby improving the downregulation of Plk1 gene expression in human hepatocellular liver carcinoma cell line HepG2.

## References

Akinc A, Maier MA, Manoharan M, Fitzgerald K, Jayaraman M, Barros S, Ansell S, Du XY, Hope MJ, Madden TD, Mui BL, Semple SC, Tam YK, Ciufolini M, Witzigmann D, Kulkarni JA, Van Der Meel R, Cullis PR (2019) The Onpattro story and the clinical translation of nanomedicines containing nucleic acid-based drugs. Nat Nanotechnol 14(12):1084–1087

Anzalone AV, Koblan LW, Liu DR (2020) Genome editing with CRISPR–Cas nucleases, base editors, transposases and prime editors. Nat Biotechnol 38(7):824–844

Cun DM, Foged C, Yang MS, Frokjaer S, Nielsen HM (2010) Preparation and characterization of poly(DL-lactide-co-glycolide) nanoparticles for siRNA delivery. Int J Pharm 390(1):70–75

Ding SK, Serra CA, Vandamme TF, Yu W, Anton N (2019) Double emulsions prepared by two-step emulsification: history, state-of-the-art and perspective. J Control Release 295:31–49

Dominici JT, Clark S, Scheetz J, Eleazer PD (2005) Analysis of heat generation using ultrasonic vibration for post removal. J Endod 31(4):301–303

Friedmann T, Roblin R (1972) Gene therapy for human genetic disease? Science 175(4025):949–955

Hoy SM (2018) Patisiran: first global approval. Drugs 78(15):1625–1631

Jilek S, Merkle HP, Walter E (2005) DNA-loaded biodegradable microparticles as vaccine delivery systems and their interaction with dendritic cells. Adv Drug Deliver Rev 57(3):377–390

Khurana A, Allawadhi P, Khurana I, Allwadhi S, Weiskirchen R, Banothu AK, Chhabra D, Joshi K, Bharani KK (2021) Role of nanotechnology behind the success of mRNA vaccines for COVID-19. Nano Today 38:101142

Kong A (1963) Possible integration of viral nucleic acid into the genome of animal cells. Prog Med Virol 5:169–218

Luu YK, Kim K, Hsiao BS, Chu B, Hadjiargyrou M (2003) Development of a nanostructured DNA delivery scaffold via electrospinning of PLGA and PLA-PEG block copolymers. J Control Release 89(2):341–353

Lv HT, Zhang SB, Wang B, Cui SH, Yan J (2006) Toxicity of cationic lipids and cationic polymers in gene delivery. J Control Release 144(1):100–109

Moghimi SM, Patel HM (1998) Serum-mediated recognition of liposomes by phagocytic cells of the reticuloendothelial system – the concept of tissue specificity. Adv Drug Deliver Rev 32(1–2):45–60

Murata N, Takashima Y, Toyoshima K, Yamamoto M, Okada H (2008) Anti-tumor effects of anti-VEGF siRNA encapsulated with PLGA microspheres in mice. J Control Release 126(3):246–254

Opalinska JB, Gewirtz AM (2002) Nucleic-acid therapeutics: basic principles and recent applications. Nat Rev Drug Discov 1(7):503–514

Patil Y, Panyam J (2009) Polymeric nanoparticles for siRNA delivery and gene silencing. Int J Pharm 367(1–2):195–203

Rogers S, Lowenthal A, Terheggen HG, Columbo JP (1973) Induction of arginase activity with the Shope papilloma virus in tissue culture cells from an argininemic patient. J Exp Med 137(4):1091–1096

Setten RL, Rossi JJ, Han SP (2019) The current state and future directions of RNAi-based therapeutics. Nat Rev Drug Discov 18(6):421–446

Singh M, Briones M, Ott G, O'Hagan D (2000) Cationic microparticles: a potent delivery system for DNA vaccines. Proc Natl Acad Sci U S A 97(2):811–816

Van Den Berg AIS, Yun CO, Schiffelers RM, Hennink WE (2021) Polymeric delivery systems for nucleic acid therapeutics: approaching the clinic. J Control Release 331:121–141

Yang XZ, Dou S, Sun TM, Mao CQ, Wang HX, Wang J (2011) Systemic delivery of siRNA with cationic lipid assisted PEG-PLA nanoparticles for cancer therapy. J Control Release 156(2):203–211

Yin H, Kanasty RL, Eltoukhy AA, Vegas AJ, Dorkin JR, Anderson DG (2014) Non-viral vectors for gene-based therapy. Nat Rev Genet 15(8):541–555

Zuckerman JE, Gritli I, Tolcher A, Heidel JD, Lim D, Morgan R, Chmielowski B, Ribas A, Davis ME, Yen Y (2014) Correlating animal and human phase Ia/Ib clinical data with CALAA-01, a targeted, polymer-based nanoparticle containing siRNA. Proc Natl Acad Sci U S A 111(31):11449–11454

# Index




H. Tian and X. Chen (eds.), *Gene Delivery*, Biomaterial Engineering,
https://doi.org/10.1007/978-981-16-5419-0